Ferrets, Rabbits, and Rodents

CLINICAL MEDICINE AND SURGERY

Ferrets, Rabbits, and Rodents

CLINICAL MEDICINE AND SURGERY

Elizabeth V. Hillyer, DVM
■ Oldwick, New Jersey

Katherine E. Quesenberry, DVM
■ The Animal Medical Center, New York, New York

W.B. SAUNDERS COMPANY
A Division of Harcourt Brace & Company
Philadelphia London Toronto Montreal Sydney Tokyo

W.B. Saunders Company
A Division of Harcourt Brace & Company

The Curtis Center
Independence Square West
Philadelphia, Pennsylvania 19106

Library of Congress Cataloging-in-Publication Data

Hillyer, Elizabeth V.
Ferrets, rabbits and rodents : clinical medicine and surgery / Elizabeth V. Hillyer, Katherine E. Quesenberry.—1st ed.

p. cm.
ISBN 0–7216–4023–0

1. Ferrets—Diseases. 2. Rabbits—Diseases. 3. Rodents—Diseases. 4. Ferrets—Surgery. 5. Rabbits—Surgery. 6. Rodents—Surgery. I. Quesenberry, Katherine E. II. Title.

SB997.5.F7H54 1997 636'.932—dc20

DNLM/DLC 95-37114

FERRETS, RABBITS, AND RODENTS: Clinical Medicine and Surgery

ISBN 0–7216–4023–0

Printed in the United States of America

Last digit is the print number: 9 8 7 6 5 4 3 2 1

I dedicate this book, with love, to my husband Steve and my daughters Charlotte and Ellie.

EVH

This book is dedicated with gratitude to my family, my husband Robert, and my children Zachary and Chelsea.

KEQ

We give a special thanks to the late Emil Dolensek, who guided us in the early years of our veterinary careers.

NOTICE

Companion animal practice is an ever-changing field. Standard safety precautions must be followed, but as new research and clinical experience grow, changes in treatment and drug therapy become necessary or appropriate. The authors and editors of this work have carefully checked the generic and trade drug names and verified drug dosages to assure that dosage information is precise and in accord with standards accepted at the time of publication. Readers are advised, however, to check the product information currently provided by the manufacturer of each drug to be administered to be certain that changes have not been made in the recommended dose or in the contraindications for administration. This is of particular importance in regard to new or infrequently used drugs. Recommended dosages for animals are sometimes based on adjustments in the dosage that would be suitable for humans. Some of the drugs mentioned here have been given experimentally by the authors. Others have been used in dosages greater than those recommended by the manufacturer. In these kinds of cases, the authors have reported on their own considerable experience. It is the responsibility of those administering a drug, relying on their professional skill and experience, to determine the dosages, the best treatment for the patient, and whether the benefits of giving a drug justify the attendant risk. The editors cannot be responsible for misuse or misapplication of the material in this work.

THE PUBLISHER

CONTRIBUTORS

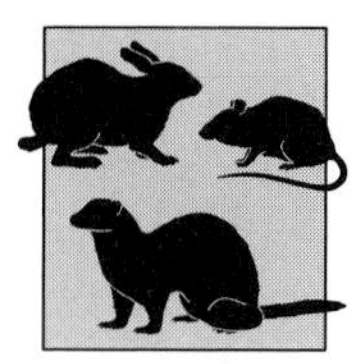

NATALIE ANTINOFF, DVM
Resident, Avian and Exotic Pet Medicine, The Animal Medical Center, New York, New York
Ferrets—Musculoskeletal and Neurologic Diseases

LOUISE BAUCK, MVSc, DVM
Director of Veterinary Services, Hagen Agricultural Research Institute, Rolf C. Hagen, Inc., Montréal, Québec, Canada
Small Rodents—Basic Anatomy, Physiology, Husbandry, and Clinical Techniques

JUDITH A. BELL, DVM, MSc, PhD
Clyde, New York
*Ferrets—*Helicobacter mustelae *Gastritis, Proliferative Bowel Disease, and Eosinophilic Gastroenteritis; Ferrets—Periparturient and Neonatal Diseases*

CRAIG BIHUN, DVM, DVSc
Head, Veterinary Diagnostic Section, Health Canada, Ottawa, Ontario, Canada
Small Rodents—Basic Anatomy, Physiology, Husbandry, and Clinical Techniques

DALE L. BROOKS, DVM, PhD
Department of Medicine and Epidemiology, and Director, Animal Resources Service, School of Veterinary Medicine, University of California—Davis, Davis, California
Rabbits—Nutrition and Gastrointestinal Physiology

SUSAN A. BROWN, DVM
Partner/Staff Veterinarian, Midwest Bird and Exotic Animal Hospital, Westchester, Illinois
Ferrets—Basic Anatomy, Physiology, and Husbandry; Ferrets—Neoplasia

PETRA M. BURGMANN, BSc, DVM, Diplomate, ABVP (Avian Practice)
Staff Veterinarian, High Park Animal Clinic, Toronto, Ontario, Canada
Other Topics—Formulary

JAMES W. CARPENTER, MS, DVM, Diplomate, ACZM
Associate Professor, Exotic Animal, Wildlife, and Zoo Animal Medicine Service, College of Veterinary Medicine, Kansas State University, Manhattan, Kansas
Rabbits—Neurologic and Musculoskeletal Disease

BARBARA J. DEEB, DVM, MS
Clinical Assistant Professor, Department of Comparative Medicine, University of Washington; Veterinarian—Small Mammals, Pet Corner Veterinary Clinic, Seattle, Washington
Rabbits—Respiratory Disease and the Pasteurella Complex

THOMAS M. DONNELLY, BVSc, Diplomate, ACLAM
Senior Scientist, The Picower Institute for Medical Research, Manhasset, New York
Rabbits—Basic Anatomy, Physiology, and Husbandry; Guinea Pigs and Chinchillas—Biology, Husbandry, and Clinical Techniques; Guinea Pigs and Chinchillas—Disease Problems of Guinea Pigs and Chinchillas; Small Rodents—Disease Problems of Small Rodents

EDWARD J. GENTZ, MS, DVM
Clinical Instructor, Exotic Animal Medicine and Wildlife Health, College of Veterinary Medicine, Cornell University, Ithaca, New York
Rabbits—Neurologic and Musculoskeletal Disease

ELIZABETH V. HILLYER, DVM
Medical writer and editor, Oldwick, New Jersey
Ferrets—Urogenital Diseases; Ferrets—Cardiovascular Diseases; Rabbits—Dermatologic Diseases; Guinea Pigs and Chinchillas—Biology, Husbandry, and Clinical Techniques; Appendices

HEIDI L. HOEFER, DVM, Diplomate, ABVP (Avian Practice)
Staff Veterinarian, Avian and Exotic Pet Medicine, The Animal Medical Center, New York, New York
Ferrets—Gastrointestinal Diseases; Other Topics—Small Mammal Radiology

JEFFREY R. JENKINS, DVM, Diplomate, ABVP (Avian Practice)
Avian and Exotic Animal Hospital of San Diego, San Diego, California
Rabbits—Gastrointestinal Diseases; Rabbits—Soft Tissue Surgery and Dental Procedures

AMY KAPATKIN, DVM
Lecturer in Surgery, University of Pennsylvania School of Veterinary Medicine, Department of Clinical Studies, Philadelphia, Pennsylvania
Other Topics—Orthopedics in Small Mammals

SUSAN E. KIRSCHNER, DVM, Diplomate, ACVO
Staff Ophthalmologist, The Oregon Veterinary Referral Center, Portland, Oregon
Other Topics—Ophthalmologic Diseases in Small Mammals

DOUGLAS R. MADER, MS, DVM, Diplomate, ABVP (Canine and Feline Practice)
Associate Clinical Professor, Department of Medicine and Epidemiology, School of Veterinary Medicine, University of California—Davis, Davis; Veterinarian, Long Beach Animal Hospital, Long Beach; Staff Veterinarian, Santa Ana Zoo, Prentice Park, Santa Ana; Attending Veterinarian, Allergan Pharmaceuticals, Irvine, California
Rabbits—Basic Approach to Veterinary Care

DIANE E. MASON, DVM, MS, Diplomate, ACVA
Instructor, Department of Anatomy and Physiology, College of Veterinary Medicine, Kansas State University, Manhattan, Kansas
Other Topics—Anesthesia, Analgesia, and Sedation for Small Mammals

MICHAEL S. MILLER, MS, VMD
Director, Cardiology—Ultrasound Referral Service, Thornton, Pennsylvania
Ferrets—Cardiovascular Diseases

JAMES K. MORRISEY, DVM
Resident, Avian and Exotic Pet Medicine, The Animal Medical Center, New York, New York
Appendices

HOLLY MULLEN, DVM, Diplomate, ACVS
Chief of Surgery, California Veterinary Surgical Practice, Emergency Animal Hospital and Referral Center of San Diego, San Diego, California
Ferrets—Soft Tissue Surgery; Guinea Pigs and Chinchillas—Soft Tissue Surgery; Small Rodents—Soft Tissue Surgery

CONNIE ORCUTT, DVM, Diplomate, ABVP (Avian Practice)
Avian and Exotic Pet Medicine, Angell Memorial Animal Hospital, Boston, Massachusetts
Ferrets—Dermatologic Diseases

JOANNE PAUL-MURPHY, DVM, Diplomate, ACZM
Assistant Professor, Department of Surgical Sciences, University of Wisconsin School of Veterinary Medicine, Madison, Wisconsin
Rabbits—Reproductive and Urogenital Disorders

KATHERINE E. QUESENBERRY, DVM, Diplomate, ABVP (Avian Practice)
Service Head, Avian and Exotic Pet Medicine, The Animal Medical Center, New York, New York
Ferrets—Basic Approach to Veterinary Care; Ferrets—Endocrine Diseases; Guinea Pigs and Chinchillas—Biology, Husbandry, and Clinical Techniques; Apendices

KAREN L. ROSENTHAL, DVM, MS, Diplomate, ABVP (Avian Practice)
Staff Veterinarian, Exotic and Avian Pet Medicine, The Animal Medical Center, New York, New York
Ferrets—Respiratory Diseases; Ferrets—Endocrine Diseases

DORCAS O. SCHAEFFER, DVM, MS, Diplomate, ACLAM
Assistant Professor and Director, Laboratory Animal Facilities, Department of Comparative Medicine, College of Veterinary Medicine, Knoxville, Tennessee
Guinea Pigs and Chinchillas—Disease Problems of Guinea Pigs and Chinchillas

DALE A. SMITH, DVM, DVSc
Associate Professor, Department of Pathobiology, Ontario Veterinary College, University of Guelph, Guelph, Ontario, Canada
Other Topics—Formulary

MARK E. STAMOULIS, DVM, Diplomate, ACVIM (Cardiology)
Clinical Assistant Professor, Department of Medicine, Tufts University School of Veterinary Medicine, Vice President, New England Veterinary Specialists, Framingham, Massachusetts
Ferrets—Cardiovascular Diseases

JOSEPH D. STEFANACCI, VMD, Diplomate, ACVR
Staff Radiologist, and Supervisor, Department of Radiology, The Animal Medical Center, New York, New York
Other Topics—Small Mammal Radiology

PREFACE

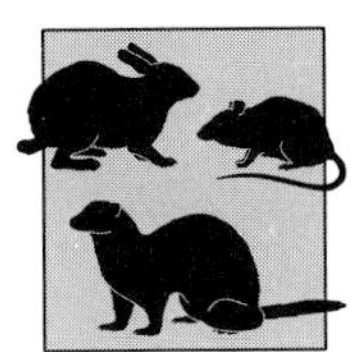

Only 10 years ago, we were faced with the diagnostic dilemma of a 2-year-old spayed female ferret with a swollen vulva, hair loss, and yet no evidence of a remnant ovary on two abdominal exploratory surgeries. Today, most veterinarians who treat ferrets would suspect that the ferret had an adrenocortical tumor, which, indeed, she did.

Our knowledge of the clinical medicine of small mammals, such as ferrets, rabbits, and rodents, has expanded greatly over the past 10 years, thanks largely to the pioneering work of practicing veterinarians who work daily with these species. We are pleased to have many of these veterinarians represented in this book as contributing authors. Our contributors work in different arenas of small mammal medicine, including private practice, academia, research laboratories, and breeding facilities. They bring their varied perspectives based on many combined years of experience working with small mammals. Their differences in approach are sometimes evident; however, we think that these differences are seldom contradictory and, in fact, are instructive. We feel very fortunate to have been able to compile the work of these authors, and we thank them for their participation and concerted efforts.

This book is intended to address the common questions and concerns of the practicing veterinarian who works with small mammals. In addition, we believe that it will be a useful reference for veterinary students, veterinary technicians, research scientists, pet shop owners, and dedicated pet owners and breeders. The publication of a user-friendly veterinary reference, especially for the management of ferrets and rabbits, is long overdue.

A large component of small mammal medicine is preventive medicine. For this reason, we have included chapters on basic biology, husbandry, and routine care of the healthy animal, in addition to chapters on disease management, surgery, and radiology. We hope that this book will be valuable as a user-friendly source of quick answers (see the tables of differential diagnoses in the Appendices, as well as the Formulary), as a guide to approaching both straightforward and complex medical and surgical problems, and, finally, as a source of in-depth reference material.

We encourage readers to write to us with comments and suggestions for improving subsequent editions of this book. Moreover, we encourage veterinarians to investigate common and uncommon problems and to publish their findings. Much basic work remains to be done, such as determining normal urinalyses and coagulation profiles in ferrets, determining the cause of the high incidence of neoplasia in ferrets in the United States, and improving treatment regimens for abscesses in rabbits, anorexia in guinea pigs, and fractures in small rodents.

Ferrets, rabbits, guinea pigs, rats, and mice have been domesticated for centuries, whereas gerbils, hamsters, and chinchillas were domesticated more recently. Ideas and help toward solving unusual medical problems in small mammals can often be found in the existing literature, be it in laboratory animal medicine, human medicine, or other fields of clinical veterinary medicine—particularly canine, feline, and equine medicine and surgery. Ten years ago, as clinical veterinarians we narrowly avoided embarking on a search for cancer in a seemingly healthy rabbit with a high serum calcium level. We found an reference in the laboratory animal literature that stated that serum calcium concentrations in rabbits can fluctuate with dietary calcium intake, a fact that is now common knowledge among small mammal practitioners. Hopefully, the next 10 years will witness greater cohesiveness and sharing of knowledge between laboratory animal medicine and clinical medicine and surgery.

This book was made possible through the support of many people. Our special thanks go to Ray Kersey at W.B. Saunders Company for believing in this project and giving us the support to make it a reality. We are indebted to the ever-patient and understanding staff at W.B. Saunders Company, especially Sandra Valkhoff, Frank Messina, and Denise LeMelledo. We extend our thanks also to Dr. Les Sealing, who labored through many revisions to produce the line drawings that grace this book. Finally, we thank our families for their forbearance and good humor during the innumerable late nights and working weekends of this project.

ELIZABETH V. HILLYER
KATHERINE E. QUESENBERRY

CONTENTS

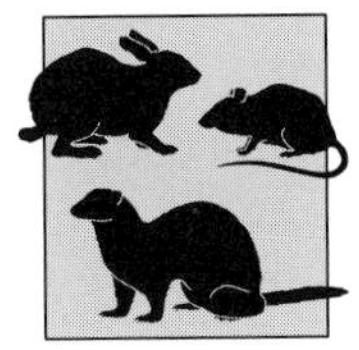

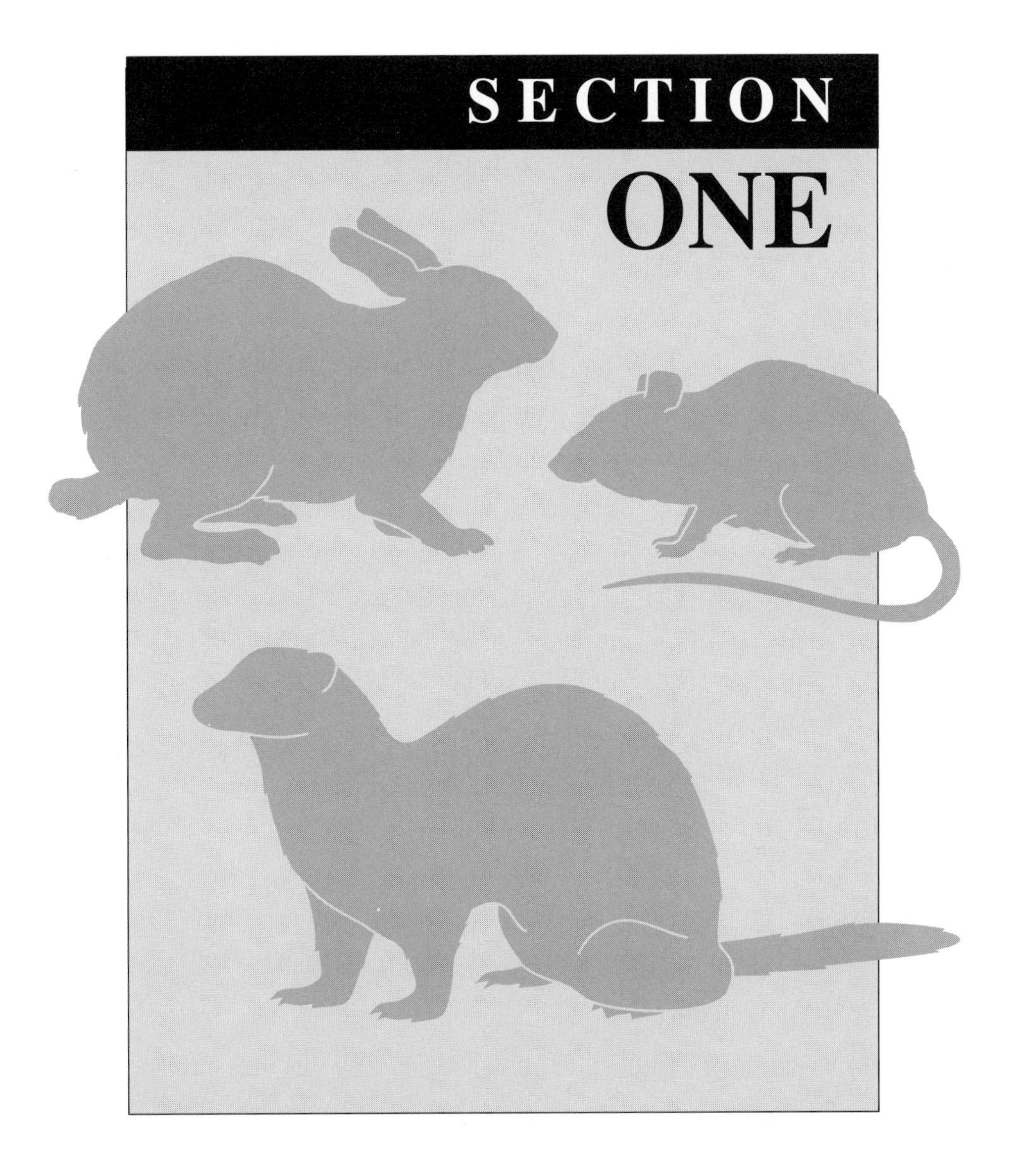

Ferrets

CHAPTER 1

Basic Anatomy, Physiology, and Husbandry

Susan A. Brown, DVM

HISTORY AND USE

Domestic ferrets *(Mustela putorius furo)* belong to the order Carnivora and to the family Mustelidae. Other members of this family include stoats (ermines), weasels, mink, martens, sables, badgers, otters, and skunks. According to writings by ancient Greek authors, domestic ferrets were used as working pets as long ago as 4 BC.[4] Domestic ferrets are probably most closely related to the European polecat *(Mustela putorius),* which still inhabits Northern Europe and the United Kingdom. However, some speculate that they may also be related to the steppe polecat *(Mustela eversmanni),* which has its origin in the area of the Russian Steppes.

The only other member of the ferret group is the black-footed ferret *(Mustela nigripes)* of North America. The black-footed ferret preys primarily on prairie dogs. During the settlement of what is now the western United States, prairie dogs were poisoned so that cattle and sheep could be raised. Consequently, the black-footed ferret nearly became extinct. Currently, captive breeding programs are attempting to re-establish this interesting creature back in the wild. Keeping a black-footed ferret as a pet is illegal. Despite such efforts, however, the fate of the species is still uncertain.

Initially, domestic ferrets were used as hunting animals for the control of wild or native rabbits and rodents. In Europe, Australia, and New Zealand, ferrets are still used in this capacity. Also, ferret pelts (known as "fitch") have been used in the fur industry, and ferrets are still being bred for this purpose in some areas of Northern Europe. In North

America, where they were introduced approximately 300 years ago, domestic ferrets have primarily been maintained as pets. In more recent years, they have also been used in research—in particular, in physiology, toxicology, and the study of infectious diseases.

Since the mid-1970s, the ferret's popularity as a pet in the United States has increased at an astounding rate. It is estimated that more than 7 million ferrets are kept as pets in this country.[10] Hunting that involves the use of ferrets is forbidden in most states. Their popularity is related to their small size, ease of care, comical personalities, and suitability for keeping in small living spaces.

It should be noted that keeping domestic ferrets as pets is not legal in all states. In addition, the laws of some cities located within ferret-legal states forbid the keeping of ferrets. Currently, no state recognizes the ferret as a domestic animal; therefore, regulations regarding this species usually are enforced by state fish and wildlife or conservation departments. Some areas require that those who wish to own or breed ferrets obtain a permit, and various laws exist regarding the management of ferret bites. (In some areas, ferrets can be destroyed legally in order to test for rabies, even in the presence of a current rabies vaccination.) It is, therefore, important for veterinarians to be familiar with legislation in their localities regarding the keeping of ferrets before they engage in their veterinary care.

ANATOMY AND PHYSIOLOGY

The following is a brief overview of the anatomic and physiologic features of domestic ferrets that are important to the practitioner. Refer to the extensive literature on the anatomy and physiology of the ferret for a more detailed discussion (see references 1 and 2). The skeletal anatomy is depicted in Figure 1–1, and the visceral anatomy is presented in Figure 1–2.

Body Shape

Ferrets have a long tubular body with short legs; this body shape allows them to get into and out of small holes in the ground in their hunting efforts. Consequently, the owner must block off all openings in a ferret's environment through which it might escape. The ferret's spine is very flexible, enabling the animal to easily turn 180° in a narrow passageway. The ferret's neck is long and thick and of approximately the same diameter as the mandibular area; this anatomy makes it difficult for owners to use collars on this animal. Even though their legs are short and their claws are primarily used for traction and digging, ferrets can climb along surfaces such as screen or wire mesh and may reach dangerous heights.

If male ferrets are allowed to reach sexual maturity before they are neutered, their body size is normally twice that of unneutered female ferrets. The body weight of intact male ferrets ranges from 1 to 2 kg, and that of intact females from 0.5 to 1 kg. When neutered before weaning, female ferrets become larger and male ferrets stay smaller than intact individuals of the same sex. Most ferrets that have been neutered early weigh between 0.8 and 1.2 kg. Also, males that have been neutered early do not develop the heavy muscular neck and shoulder area or the overall body weight that is characteristic of intact animals.

Ferrets experience a normal seasonal change in body fat—that is, they lose weight in the summer and gain it back in the winter. In intact animals, the weight change is most dramatic: the weight difference that occurs from season to season may be as great as 40%. In addition, I have observed that neutered ferrets younger than 1 year of age are at their greatest weight; as they age, these animals' fluctuations in weight become less and less dramatic, with their "summer weight" eventually becoming the year-round body condition.

Hair Coat and Skin

The "wild," or natural, coloring of domestic ferrets is probably *sable* (known as "fitch" in other countries). Sable ferrets have black guard hair with a cream colored undercoat, black feet and tail, and a black mask on the face. This is the approximate coloring of the European polecat *(M. putorius)*. The other two naturally occurring colors are *albino* and *cinnamon* (also known as "sandy") (Fig. 1–3*A through C*). Interestingly, the cinnamon coloring that is seen commonly in domestic ferrets in Europe (beige guard hair with a cream-colored undercoat and a lack of mask) is the natural coloring of the steppe polecat (*M. eversmanni)*. In the United States, more than 30 color variations are recog-

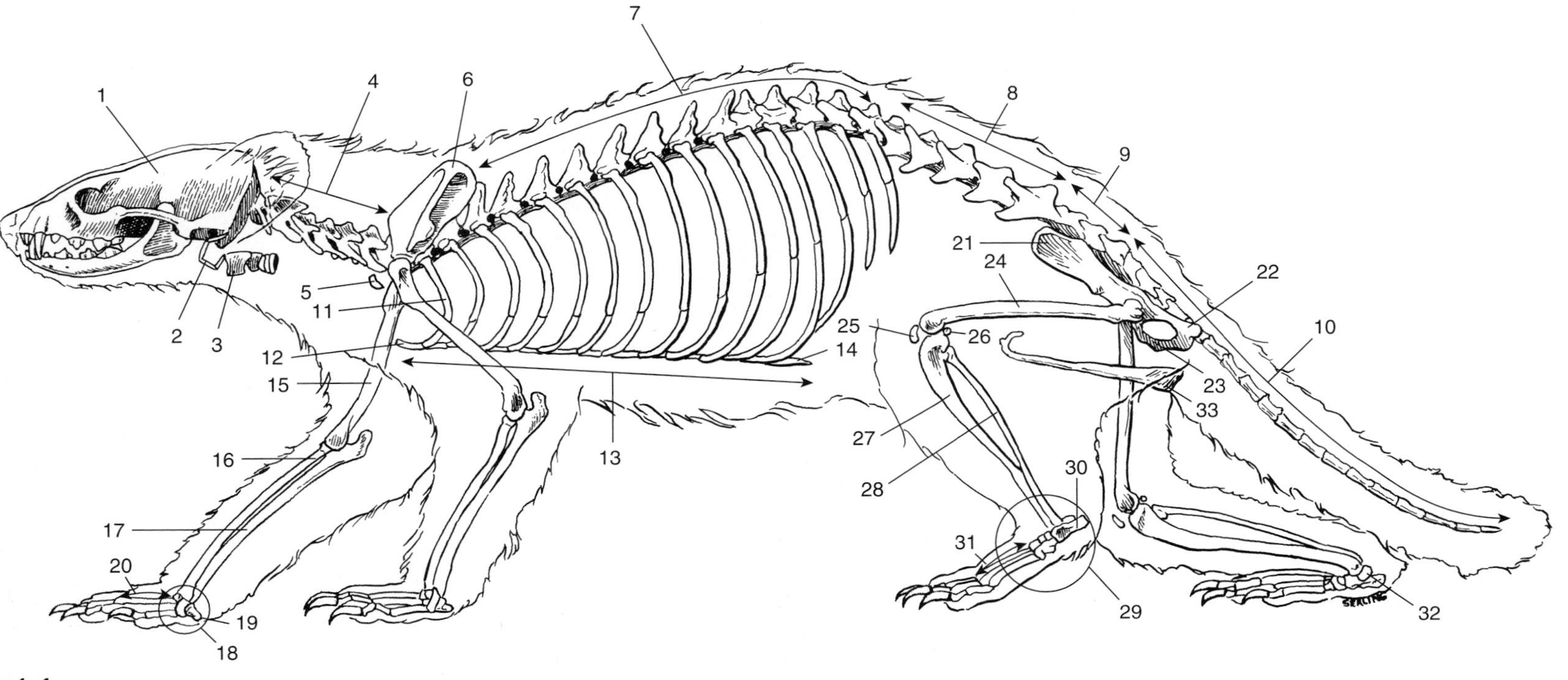

Figure 1–1
Skeletal anatomy of a ferret. (Adapted from An NQ, Evans HE: Anatomy of the ferret. *In* Fox JG, ed: Biology and Diseases of the Ferret. Philadelphia, Lea & Febiger, 1988, pp 14–65.)

1, calvaria; 2, hyoid apparatus; 3, larynx; 4, seven cervical vertebrae; 5, clavicle; 6, scapula; 7, 15 thoracic vertebrae; 8, five lumbar vertebrae; 9, three sacral vertebrae; 10, 18 caudal vertebrae; 11, first rib; 12, manubrium; 13, sternum; 14, xiphoid process; 15, humerus; 16, radius; 17, ulna; 18, carpal bones; 19, accessory carpal bone; 20, metacarpal bones; 21, ilium; 22, ischium; 23, pubis; 24, femur; 25, patella; 26, fabella; 27, tibia; 28, fibula; 29, tarsal bones; 30, calcaneus; 31, metatarsal bones; 32, talus; 33, os penis.

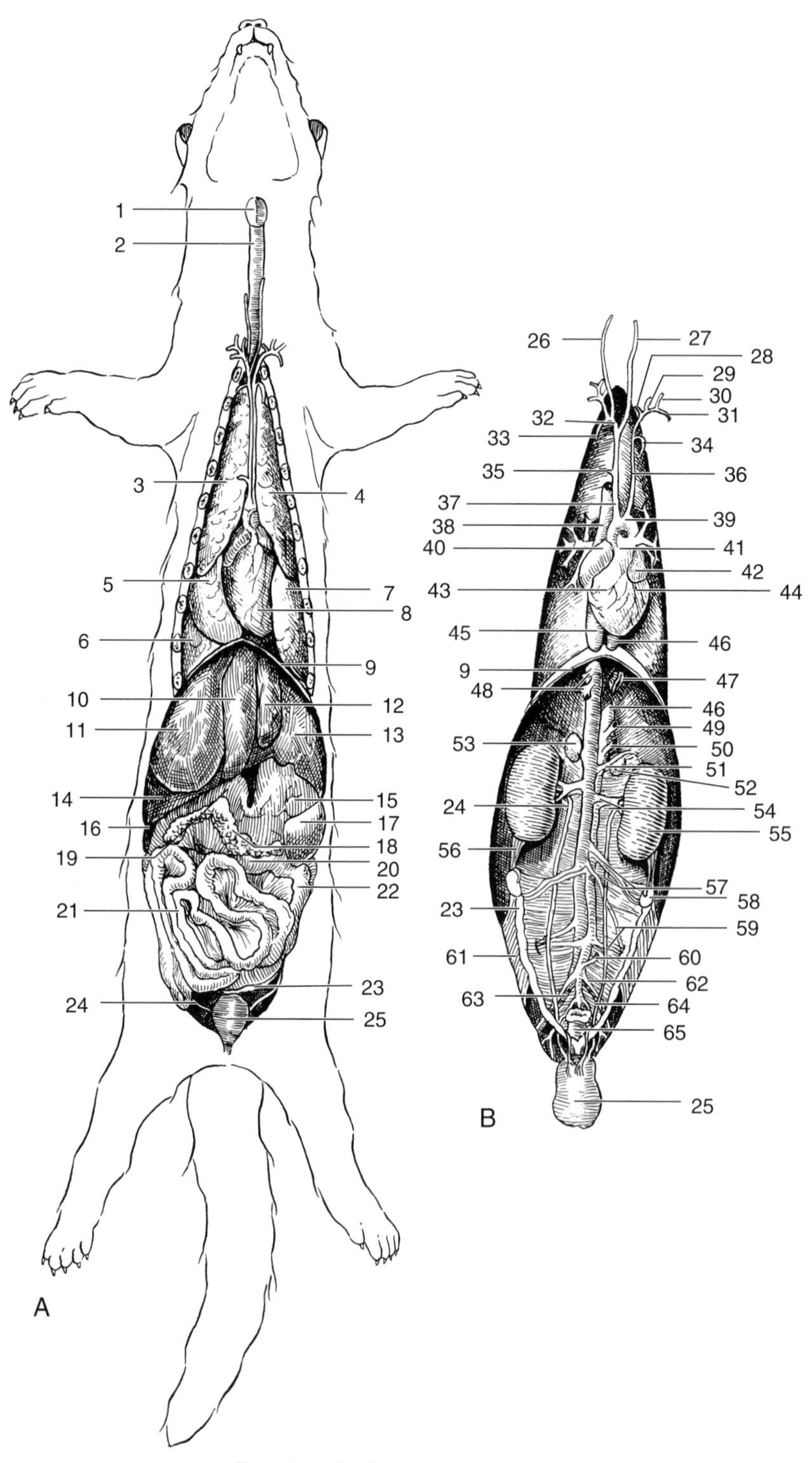

Figure 1–2 *See legend on opposite page*

nized. Color variations include silver (dark gray guard hair with a cream-colored undercoat and little or no mask), black-eyed white (white body hair but pigmented irises), chocolate (similar to sable but with dark brown rather than black guard hair), Siamese (guard hairs that are a lighter brown than chocolate and a light-colored mask), panda (white hair on the head and shoulders, and body hair of various colors), and shetland sable (sable body coloring but with a white stripe running vertically on the face from the nose to the top of the head; see Figure 1–3*D*).

Ferrets molt in the spring and the fall, concomitantly with their change in weight. The molting can be subtle or dramatic. The hair itself may vary in length from season to season, typically being shorter in the summer and longer in the fall. Hair color also may change, usually being lighter in the winter and darker in the fall. A large percentage of silver ferrets become black-eyed whites as they mature in years. Ferrets may lose or change their mask configuration from season to season and from year to year; for this reason, it is not a good idea to depend on photographs alone for pet identification. I recommend the use of a more permanent form of identification, such as microchipping or tattooing.

Ferrets have a pair of well-developed anal glands, as do all members of the Mustelidae family. These glands produce a serous yellow liquid that has a very powerful odor. Young ferrets or animals that are frightened or threatened may express this material suddenly. They are not able to project the fluid over a long distance as can skunks, and the fluid's odor lasts only a few minutes. As ferrets mature, they express the fluid from their anal glands infrequently, with only momentary foul-smelling results. In my opinion, routine removal of the anal glands (a procedure known as "descenting"; see Chapter 13) is not necessary because the anal gland secretion is not responsible for the musky body odor of ferrets. Rather, it is the sebaceous secretions of the skin that produce these animals' overall odor. Nevertheless, pet ferrets originating from large breeding farms are routinely descented when they are 5–6 weeks of age.

The skin of ferrets is amazingly thick, especially over the neck and shoulders. In health, it should have a smooth appearance and be without flakes or scales. Occasionally, small reddish brown patches might be seen on otherwise normal skin; these patches represent dried sebaceous secretions. They can be removed easily with bathing. Ferrets do not have sweat glands in their skin and thus quickly succumb to heat prostration.[9] Ferrets have very active sebaceous glands, which account for their body odor. During the breeding season, intact animals have increased sebaceous secretions; this increase results in a noticeable increase in body odor, yellow discoloration of the undercoat, and oily fur.

Skeletal System

The vertebral formula for the ferret is C7, T15, L5(6), S3, Cd18.[1] Ferrets have 14–15 pairs of ribs, and some ferrets have 14 on one side and 15 on the other. The first 10 ribs are attached to the sternum, and the remaining 4–5 become the costal arch. In ferrets, the thoracic inlet is bordered by the first pair of ribs and the sternum and is very small.[1] The presence of anterior thoracic masses or megaesophagus can result in dysphagia or dyspnea.

Each of the ferret's four feet has five clawed digits. The first digit on each foot has only two phalanges, whereas each of the other digits has three.[1] The claws are not retractable as in cats and thus must be trimmed periodically. I do not recommend the declawing of ferrets as a routine procedure, in part because declawed ferrets have difficulty with traction when on smooth surfaces.

Male ferrets have a J-shaped os penis, which can complicate urethral catheterization.

Figure 1–2

A, Ventral aspect of the viscera of a ferret in situ. *B,* Anatomy of the viscera and most important blood vessels as seen after removal of the lungs, liver, and gastrointestinal tract. (Adapted from An NQ, Evans HE: Anatomy of the ferret. *In* Fox JG, ed: Biology and Diseases of the Ferret. Philadelphia, Lea & Febiger, 1988, pp 14–65.)

1, larynx; 2, trachea; 3, right cranial lobe of lung; 4, left cranial lobe of lung; 5, right middle lobe of lung; 6, right caudal lobe of lung; 7, left caudal lobe of lung; 8, heart; 9, diaphragm; 10, quadrate lobe of liver; 11, right medial lobe of liver; 12, left medial lobe of liver; 13, left lateral lobe of liver; 14, right lateral lobe of liver; 15, stomach; 16, right kidney; 17, spleen; 18, pancreas; 19, duodenum; 20, transverse colon; 21, jejunoileum; 22, descending colon; 23, uterus; 24, ureter; 25, urinary bladder; 26, right common carotid artery; 27, left common carotid artery; 28, vertebral artery; 29, costocervical artery; 30, superficial cervical artery; 31, axillary artery; 32, right subclavian artery; 33, right internal thoracic artery; 34, left internal thoracic artery; 35, branch to thymus; 36, left subclavian artery; 37, brachiocephalic (innominate) artery; 38, cranial vena cava; 39, aortic arch; 40, right atrium; 41, pulmonary trunk; 42, left atrium; 43, right ventricle; 44, left ventricle; 45, caudal vena cava; 46, aorta; 47, esophagus; 48, hepatic veins; 49, celiac artery; 50, cranial mesenteric artery; 51, left adrenolumbar vein; 52, left adrenal gland; 53, right adrenal gland; 54, left renal artery and vein; 55, left kidney; 56, suspensory ligament of ovary; 57, left ovarian artery and vein; 58, left ovary; 59, left deep circumflex iliac artery and vein; 60, caudal mesenteric artery; 61, broad ligament of uterus; 62, left external iliac artery; 63, right common iliac vein; 64, left internal iliac artery; 65, rectum.

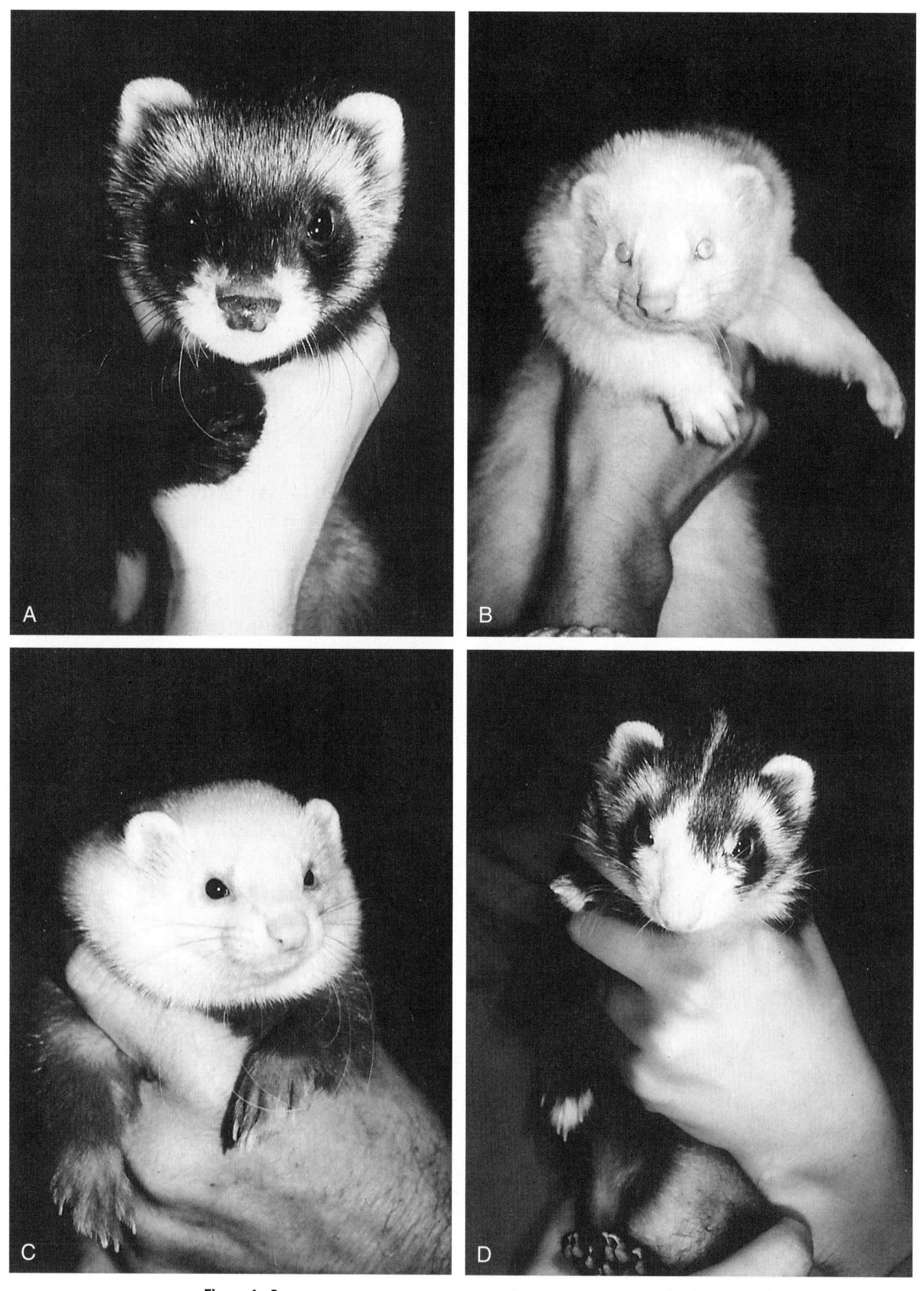

Figure 1–3
Four ferret color types. *A,* Sable. *B,* Albino. *C,* Cinnamon. *D,* Shetland sable.

Digestive Tract

The dental formula for the ferret is $2(I^3_3\ C^1_1\ P^3_3\ M^1_2) = 34$. The deciduous teeth erupt at 20–28 days of age, and the permanent teeth erupt at 50–74 days of age.[1] The upper incisors are slightly longer than the lower incisors and cover the lower ones when the mouth is closed. The canines are prominent as in other members of the order Carnivora.[1] In some ferrets, the tips of the upper canines extend beyond the most ventral portion of the chin. The canine roots are longer than the crown; this fact must be considered when extraction is necessary. Upper premolars 1 and 2 and all three of the lower premolars have two roots. The third upper premolar, or carnassial tooth, and the upper molar have three roots. The second lower molar is very tiny and has only one root.[1]

Ferrets have 5 pairs of salivary glands: the parotid, the zygomatic, the molar, the sublingual, and the mandibular.[1] Mucoceles are rare in ferrets (see Chapter 3). The mandibular lymph node lies cranial to the mandibular salivary gland and closer to the angle of the jaw. This lymph node can become enlarged, particularly in some cases of lymphoma, and thus may be confused with the salivary gland. Obtain a fine-needle aspirate of the mass and examine it cytologically in order to differentiate the two.

Ferrets have a simple stomach that can expand greatly to accommodate large amounts of food.[1] It fits into the curve of the liver in the cranial abdomen. The pylorus is well developed and is easily distinguished grossly. Ferrets have the ability to vomit but do not always do so in the presence of gastric foreign bodies. Before vomiting, ferrets usually "back up," hold the head low, squint the eyes, and, frequently, hypersalivate.

The small intestine is short, being approximately 182–198 cm in length. This length results in a short gastrointestinal transit time of about 3–4 hours in the adult animal.[1] The gut flora is simple, and therefore it is rare to see gastrointestinal upset with use of antibiotics.[3] The ileum and jejunum are indistinguishable on gross examination. Ferrets do not have a cecum or ileocolic valve.[9] The large intestine of the ferret is approximately 10 cm in length.[1]

The ferret's pancreas has two limbs that are connected at the midline near the pylorus.[1] The right limb is longer than the left and extends along the descending part of the duodenum. The left limb extends along an area between the stomach and the spleen. The liver has six lobes: the left lateral, the left medial, the quadrate, the right medial, the right lateral, and the caudate. The pear-shaped gallbladder is located between the quadrate and the right medial lobes.

Heart, Lungs, and Major Blood Vessels

The heart lies approximately between the 6th and 8th ribs.[1] It is cone-shaped, and, on a ventrodorsal view of the chest, its apex is directed to the left of midline. The ligament that connects the heart to the sternum can be surrounded by a varying amount of fat.[1] On lateral radiographic views, this gives the impression that the heart shadow is raised above the sternum. Loss of this raised effect (i.e., the heart shadow is in direct contact with the sternum) is one of the early signs of cardiac enlargement.*

The lungs of the ferret have six lobes. The left lung comprises two lobes—the left cranial and the left caudal lobes—whereas the right lung comprises four lobes—the right cranial, the right middle, the right caudal, and the accessory lobes.[1]

The anatomy of the major arteries exiting the aorta in the direction of the head is unusual. In place of bilateral carotid arteries, ferrets have a single central artery, *innominate artery 1* or the *brachiocephalic artery,* which exits the aortic arch just proximal to the left subclavian artery.[11] The brachiocephalic artery divides into the left carotid, the right carotid, and the right subclavian arteries at the level of the thoracic inlet. This central artery may be an anatomic adaptation that allows the ferret to maintain blood flow to the brain while it turns its head 180°.[11]

Spleen

The ferret spleen varies greatly in size, depending on the animal's age and state of health. The spleen is located along the greater curvature of the stomach and is attached to the stomach and liver by the gastrosplenic ligament.[1] The caudal splenic tip can be located anywhere from the cranial pole of the left kidney to the caudal pole of the right kidney, de-

---

*As described by Sam Silverman, DVM, PhD, in a lecture presented at the North American Veterinary Conference, Orlando, FL, January 1992.

pending on its size. When enlarged, the spleen extends in a diagonal fashion from the upper left to the lower right of the abdominal cavity.

Urogenital Tract and Adrenal Glands

The right kidney lies cranial to the left kidney in the retroperitoneal fat. The cranial end of the right kidney is covered by the caudate lobe of the liver. The bladder is small and easily holds 10 mL of urine at a low pressure.[2] Male ferrets have a small prostate gland that is located at the base of the bladder and surrounds the urethra.[1] When the prostate is grossly enlarged, as in the presence of paraurethral or prostatic cysts, it appears on lateral radiographic views as a round mass just dorsal to the neck of the bladder.

Ferrets are easily sexed. The preputial opening in male ferrets is located on the ventrum, as in male dogs, just caudal to the umbilical area. The os penis is readily palpable (see Fig. 1–1). In female ferrets, the urogenital opening is located in the perineal region ventral to the anus. The urogenital opening looks like a slit in nonestrous females; during estrus, the vulva becomes swollen and protuberant, appearing like a doughnut of tissue (see Chapters 5 and 9).

The natural breeding season for ferrets is from March to August in most climates. Fertility for both males and females depends on the photoperiod. Under artificial lighting conditions, they can be induced to breed year-round. Spermatogenic activity occurs in the seminiferous tubules from December to July; the testicles enlarge during this time.

Female ferrets are seasonally polyestrous and induced ovulators. Ovulation occurs 30–40 hours after copulation; normal gestation is 41–42 days. If fertilization does not occur, pseudopregnancy that lasts 41–43 days results. If not bred, roughly half of estrous females remain in estrus and develop bone marrow toxicity secondary to elevated estrogen levels (see Chapter 5).

The left adrenal gland lies in fatty tissue just medial to the cranial pole of the left kidney. It is approximately 6–8 mm in length and is usually crossed by the adrenolumbar vein on the ventral surface.[6] Two or more branches of the left adrenolumbar artery supply blood. The right adrenal gland lies more dorsal than the left one and is covered by the caudate lobe of the liver. It is intimately attached to the caudal vena cava. The caudal vena cava may lie over part or all of the gland. The right adrenal gland is slightly larger than the left one and is longer, being approximately 8–11 mm in length. The right adrenal is supplied by three to five separate vessels that come from a combination of the right renal artery, the right adrenolumbar artery, and the aorta.[6] An and Evans[1] do not address adrenal blood supply; however, the adrenolumbar artery and vein may be synonymous with their phrenicoabdominal artery and vein.

In one study, accessory nodules of adrenal cortical tissue were found in 11 of 135 ferrets.[6]

Physiologic values for domestic ferrets are presented in Table 1–1.

HUSBANDRY

The following discussion of husbandry focuses on the keeping of domestic ferrets as pets. The literature contains ample information about maintaining ferrets as laboratory animals; thus, this topic is not addressed here.

Overall, ferrets are easy to maintain in a household. They are small, have inexpensive feeding requirements, and are relatively quiet.

TABLE 1–1
PHYSIOLOGIC VALUES FOR DOMESTIC FERRETS

Life span	5–8 y average in the United States*
Sexual maturity	4–8 mo of age (usually reached in first spring after birth)
Gestation period	41–42 d
Litter size	1–18 kits (average, 8; primiparous jill average, 10)
Normal weight at birth	8–10 g
Eyes and ears open	21–37 d of age (usually, 30–35 d)
Weaning age	6–8 wk
Rectal temperature	37.8–40°C (100°–104°F)†
Average blood volume	mature male, 60 mL; mature female, 40 mL†
Heart rate	180–250 beats per min
Urine volume	26–28 mL/24 h†

*Some ferrets may reach 12 years of age.
†Data from Fox JG: Normal clinical and biologic parameters. *In* Fox JG, ed: Biology and Diseases of the Ferret. Philadelphia, Lea & Febiger, 1988, pp 159–173.

Housing

Up to two ferrets can easily be maintained in a wire cage (of the type used for rabbits) that measures 24 × 24 × 18 inches in height. The floor can be either solid or of wire. Glass tanks are not suitable for caging ferrets because they provide poor ventilation. Custom-built wooden cages can also be constructed, but care must be taken to protect corners, the lower third of walls, and the floor from urine absorption. Many ferret owners line their wooden cages with self-adhesive floor tiles or linoleum and plastic molding for ease of cleaning.

Ferrets can be maintained either indoors or outdoors. If they are kept outdoors, shade a portion of the cage for protection from extremes of heat and cold, and provide a well-insulated nest box. They do not tolerate temperatures over 90°F, especially in the presence of high humidity, and may need to be brought indoors. In climates where the temperatures drop below 20°F, a heated shelter is necessary. When caring for ferrets in veterinary hospitals, make sure that cages used to house ferrets are "escape proof." Because of their tubular shape and flexibility, ferrets can pass between the bars of the average clinic cage and escape.

Cage furniture should include some type of sleeping enclosure. Ferrets like to sleep in dark, enclosed spaces, and they become anxious if they do not have access to such areas. Towels, old shirts, and cloth hats can be used to the delight of the pet. Specific products designed for ferrets to sleep in, such as cloth tubes and tents, also are available. For the occasional ferret that insists on eating its cloth sleeping material, use a small cardboard, plastic, or wooden box with an access hole cut into it. To provide additional sleep and play areas, some owners use slings, hammocks, or shelves that are built into the cage.

Ferrets can be trained to use a litterbox relatively easily. However, because of their short digestive transit time, they may not always make it back to the cage to use the litterbox if it is not close by. Therefore, advise owners to have several litterboxes available in various rooms of the house for use by the pet when it is uncaged.

If ferrets are allowed out of their cages, the house must be "ferret proofed"—that is, all holes to the outside or to areas from which the ferrets cannot be retrieved must be blocked off. In addition, ferrets like to burrow into the soft foam rubber of furniture and mattresses. I recommend covering the bottom of all couches, chairs, and mattresses with either a piece of thin wood or hardware cloth. The burrowing is not only destructive but also potentially life threatening, as ferrets may swallow the foam rubber and develop gastrointestinal obstructive disease. Reclining chairs have been implicated in the deaths of many ferrets and should be removed from the environment. In addition, remove all access to any foam or latex rubber items such as athletic shoes, rubber bands, stereo speakers and headphones, and pipe insulation. Ferrets love to chew these substances, and ingestion of rubber foreign bodies is the most frequent cause of gastrointestinal obstruction, particularly in ferrets younger than 1 year of age.

Toys for ferrets should not include any latex rubber toys intended for dogs or cats. Instead, try paper bags, cloth toys for cats or babies, or hard plastic or metal toys. Ferrets love to run through cylindrical objects such as polyvinyl chloride pipe, large mailing tubes, and dryer vent tubing; these items make good toys and promote exercise.

Bathing

Ferrets, like cats, do not require routine bathing. Intact ferrets of both sexes develop a very strong body odor during the breeding season. Neutered animals have only a slight musky odor. Owners bathe their pets either to reduce this odor or to minimize allergic reactions they may have to ferret dander and fur. Frequent bathing may strip the skin of essential oils and produce a pruritic condition; therefore, I recommend bathing with a mild cat or ferret shampoo no more frequently than once a month, if the owner feels that it is absolutely necessary.

Behavior

Ferrets are lively, comical animals, and it is this behavior that endears them to people as pets. Ferrets are capable of making a variety of noises. They make a low-pitched, mumbling sound when they are roaming an area in search of an item. They chuckle and hiss happily when playing. There is loud squealing and screaming when they are fighting with or threatened by another ferret. They also scream when they are in pain or frightened, or during seizures.

When ferrets fight, they bite each other on the back of the neck. The skin in this area is very thick, and I have never seen an infected wound from fighting among even the most aggressive of ferrets. Also, the male ferret grasps the female ferret in this area during copulation. The grasping ferret can hang on tenaciously, causing the other ferret to scream. To minimize biting, I have found it helpful to apply a bitter-tasting product to the neck area of both ferrets. This type of product is also helpful when sprayed on an owner's hands, feet, or shoes to prevent nipping by a playful pet.

When a ferret is enticing a human or another ferret to play, it backs up rapidly across a room, usually chattering and hissing at the same time. Ferrets also like to leap and jump when they play. Ferret eyesight is good only at short distances, and they are most visually aware of rapid movements (e.g., those that would be noticed during the movement of prey).[2] They depend heavily on their sense of smell and on their hearing. Ferrets spend a lot of time with their noses to the floor investigating their environment. This behavior results in the inhalation of dust and debris and a subsequent loud sneeze. A ferret's sneeze, which is very loud and sounds like something between a cough and a sneeze, may be alarming to its owner. Unless sneezing is frequent or associated with other clinical signs, owners need not be alarmed.

Ferrets play intensely for short periods of time and then sleep soundly for several hours. I have observed that they are active about 25–30% of the day and asleep the remaining 70–75%. Ferrets can sleep so deeply that initially they may be difficult to wake. However, once awake, the normal ferret is bright and alert.

Nutrition

The complete dietary requirements of domestic ferrets are still a matter of some controversy, with no one particular diet being promoted as the best. Ferrets are strict carnivores that depend primarily on meat protein and fats for their dietary requirements.[8] The protein in the diet should be of high quality and easily digestible because of the ferret's very short gastrointestinal transit time of 3–4 hours.[3] They do not appear to need significant amounts of carbohydrates for energy.[8] Indeed, because of the absence in ferrets of significant intestinal flora that can break down these materials, it is recommended that these animals not be fed a diet rich in complex carbohydrates.[3] Ferrets love the taste of sweet foods, but they eat to their caloric requirements; thus, providing a diet rich in carbohydrates can lead to reduced intake of valuable protein and fat, which can result in disease.

Ferrets do not have the ability to digest large amounts of fiber. If they lived in the wild, they would encounter fiber primarily in the form of ingesta in the stomachs of their prey. Therefore, do not feed ferrets a diet that is high in fiber.

Most sources agree that domestic ferrets need a diet high in good-quality meat protein and fat and low in complex carbohydrates and fiber.[3, 8] High levels of protein from plant sources have been associated with urolithiasis in mustelids and are therefore undesirable.[3] The protein requirement is approximately 30–40% in adult, nonbreeding animals. In reproductively active animals and in young ferrets that have not reached sexual maturity, the protein requirement is a minimum of 35%.

The fat requirement for adult animals is approximately 18–30%.[3] In lactating females and in young preweaned kits, the fat requirement is a minimum of 25%. A fat level of 18–20% is adequate for nonbreeding adult animals. Add additional fat to the diet in the form of liquid fatty acid supplements, meat fat, or egg yolk. One of the most common signs of dietary fat deficiency is a dry, dull coat. Adding sufficient fat to the diet can improve the coat quality within 2 weeks. Obesity is rarely encountered in domestic ferrets.

Owing to the high metabolic rate of ferrets, a dry ration is preferred over a canned product. I recommend a high-quality dry kitten food or ferret food because of the higher concentration of calories and because of the decreased incidence of dental calculi associated with its use. For added fat, use a commercially available fatty acid supplement, such as Linatone (Lambert Kay, Cranbury, NJ), 1 mL/d for each ferret. Alternatively, use raw meat fat or egg yolk. Avoid giving sugary treats. Acceptable snack foods include fresh meat scraps, meat baby food, and liver or fish feline treats. Although ferrets cannot digest large amounts of fiber, many enjoy a small amount of vegetable or fruit, and up to 1 tsp/d of these items may be given.

If a ferret is to be fasted, as for blood testing or radiography, food can safely be withheld for a minimum of 4 hours but not longer than 6 hours. If fasted for too long, ferrets may become irritable and difficult to manage. In addition, if insulinoma is present, a ferret may show signs of severe hypoglycemia (including seizures and coma) if an extended fast is attempted.

Always make water available in either a sipper bottle or a heavy crock-type bowl. Ferrets love to play in the water, so the bowl should not be easy to overturn. Do not add any supplements to the ferrets' water supply.

Domestic ferrets are prone to the development of gastric trichobezoars. I recommend the use of a cat hairball laxative paste (1–2 mL q48–72h) as a preventive. Ferrets love the paste's sweet taste, and thus it also can be used to hide unpleasant or difficult-to-administer medications, such as pills.

REFERENCES AND FURTHER READING

1. An NQ, Evans HE: Anatomy of the ferret. *In* Fox JG, ed: Biology and Diseases of the Ferret. Philadelphia, Lea & Febiger, 1988, pp 14–65.
2. Andrews PLR: The physiology of the ferret. *In* Fox JG, ed: Biology and Diseases of the Ferret. Philadelphia, Lea & Febiger, 1988, pp 100–134.
3. Bell J: Ferret nutrition and diseases associated with inadequate nutrition. Proceedings of the North American Veterinary Conference, Orlando, FL, 1993, pp 719–720.
4. Fox JG: Taxonomy, history, and use. *In* Fox JG, ed: Biology and Diseases of the Ferret. Philadelphia, Lea & Febiger, 1988, pp 3–13.
5. Fox JG: Normal clinical and biologic parameters. *In* Fox JG, ed: Biology and Diseases of the Ferret. Philadelphia, Lea & Febiger, 1988, pp 159–173.
6. Holmes RL: The adrenal glands of the ferret, *Mustela putorius*. J Anat 1961; 95:325–339.
7. Kawasaki TA: Normal parameters and laboratory interpretation of disease states in the domestic ferret. Semin Avian Exotic Pet Med 1994; 3:40–47.
8. McLain DE, Thomas JA, Fox JG: Nutrition. *In* Fox JG, ed: Biology and Diseases of the Ferret. Philadelphia, Lea & Febiger, 1988, pp 135–152.
9. Moody KD, Bowman TA, Lang CM: Laboratory management of the ferret for biomedical research. Lab Anim Sci 1985; 35:272–279.
10. Rupprecht CE, Gilbert J, Pitts R, et al: Evaluation of an inactivated rabies virus vaccine in domestic ferrets. J Am Vet Med Assoc 1990; 193:1614–1616.
11. Willis LS, Barrow MV: The ferret *(Mustela putorius furo* L.*)* as a laboratory animal. Lab Anim Sci 1971; 21:712–716.

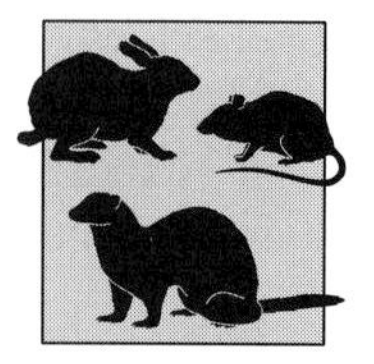

CHAPTER 2

Basic Approach to Veterinary Care

Katherine E. Quesenberry, DVM

Ferrets can easily be accommodated in an existing small animal veterinary practice. Special equipment needs are minimal, and the approach to handling ferrets in many ways is similar to that for dogs and cats. Ferret owners regularly seek veterinary care for a variety of reasons: ferrets need yearly preventive vaccinations; ferret owners generally are very attuned to their pets and are responsible pet owners; ferrets have a relatively short life span compared with cats and dogs; ferrets have a high incidence of disease beginning early in life; and many of the diseases common to ferrets are not easily ignored by the pet owner (e.g., alopecia resulting from adrenal disease and hypoglycemic episodes caused by insulinoma).

RESTRAINT AND PHYSICAL EXAMINATION

Restraint

Most ferrets are docile and can be examined easily without assistance for restraint. However, an assistant is usually needed when the rectal temperature is taken, when injections or oral medications are administered, or if an animal has a tendency to bite. Animals that may bite during an examination include nursing females and ferrets that are handled infrequently; young ferrets may nip. Like dogs and cats, even docile ferrets may attempt to bite during a procedure; take precautions accordingly.

Depending on the ferret's disposition, one of two basic restraint methods can be used for physical examination. For very active animals or those with a

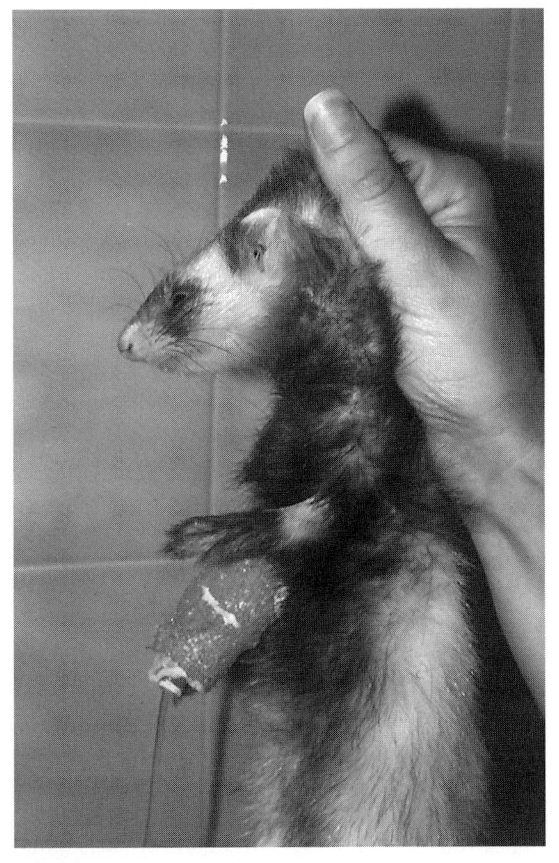

FIGURE 2–1
Restrain an active ferret by scruffing the loose skin on the back of the neck. A cephalic catheter is in place in this ferret.

tendency to bite, have the assistant scruff the animal at the back of the neck and suspend it with all four legs off the table (Fig. 2–1). With this hold, most ferrets become very relaxed, and the veterinarian is able to examine the oral cavity, head, and body, auscult the chest, and palpate the abdomen easily.

For more tractable animals, lightly restrain the ferret on the examination table. Examine the mucous membranes, oral cavity, head, and integument. Then, pick the ferret up with one hand for support under the body while ausculting the thorax or palpating the abdomen. At any time, the ferret can be scruffed for vaccination, ear cleaning, or any other procedure that may elicit an attempt to escape or bite.

To restrain a ferret for procedures such as venipuncture or ultrasound, hold it firmly by the scruff of the neck and around the hips without pulling the legs back. Most ferrets struggle if their legs are extended by pulling on the feet. Many animals can be distracted by feeding Nutri-Cal (EVSCO Pharmaceuticals, Buena, NJ) by syringe during a procedure. Leather gloves are not recommended because (1) they interfere with the handler's dexterity, (2) they cannot be disinfected between animals, and (3) a determined ferret could bite through them.

Physical Examination

Most ferrets strenuously object to having their temperature taken with a rectal thermometer. Always try to take the body temperature of ferrets at the beginning of the physical examination. If a ferret struggles during the examination and the temperature is then taken, it may be artificially elevated. You can use a glass rectal thermometer, but always hold the end of the thermometer to prevent it from breaking should the ferret struggle. A digital plastic thermometer may be preferable because it is unbreakable, and the temperature can be recorded in less time. The normal body temperature of a ferret is reported to be 100–104°F (37.8–40°C), with the average being 101.9°F (38.8°C).[19] However, in clinical practice, the normal temperature is usually not above 103°F unless the ferret is excited or the ambient temperature is high.

The physical examination of a ferret is basically the same as that of any small animal and can be quick and efficient if a few simple guidelines are followed. Note the attitude and alertness of the animal. Ferrets are nocturnal and may sleep in the carrier in the veterinary office; however, once awakened for the examination, ferrets should be alert and responsive. Assess hydration by noting the skin turgor of the eyelids, the tenting of the skin at the back of the neck, and the moistness of the oral mucous membranes. Skin turgor may be difficult to evaluate in cachectic animals. Estimate the capillary refill time by digitally pressing on the gingiva above the teeth.

Examine the eyes, nose, ears, and facial symmetry. Cataracts can occur in both juvenile and adult animals. Retinal degeneration is another ophthalmic disorder seen in ferrets and may be indicated by abnormal pupillary dilation. Inspect for nasal discharge and ask the owner about any history of sneezing or coughing. The ears may have a brown waxy discharge, but the presence of excessive brown exudate may indicate infestation with ear mites *(Otodectes cynotis)*.

The teeth of ferrets should be clean and their gums pink. Dental disease and dental tartar are commonly present and are exacerbated by the feeding of soft foods or treats such as raisins. Tartar most commonly accumulates on the first and second premolars of the upper dental arcade. Moderate dental tartar can be removed easily with a dental scraper without sedation in most ferrets. Alternatively, ferrets can be anesthetized and intubated, and the teeth cleaned with an ultrasonic scaler. Application of tartar control toothpaste to the teeth may decrease the formation of dental calculi.[10] Ferrets often break off the tip of one or both canine teeth; this is not usually a problem unless the tooth turns dark or the ferret exhibits sensitivity when eating. In these situations, recommend a root canal or extraction, depending on the degree of damage to the tooth. Gingival disease, which is manifest by erythematous gums that sometimes bleed, is a common sequela of the presence of excessive dental tartar. Clean the teeth of affected animals, and prescribe antibiotics if the gingival inflammation is severe.

Observe the symmetry of the face. Although uncommon, salivary mucoceles do occur in ferrets and are noticeable as asymmetric masses on either side of the face in the cheek area.

Palpate the regional lymph nodes of the neck, axillary, popliteal, and inguinal areas. Nodes should be soft and may sometimes feel enlarged in large or overweight animals because of surrounding fat. Any degree of firmness or asymmetry is suspicious and warrants close monitoring. If all nodes are consistently enlarged and firm, a full diagnostic workup is indicated.

Auscult the heart and the lungs in a quiet room. Ferrets have a rapid heart rate (180–250 beats per minute) and often a very pronounced sinus arrhythmia. If a ferret is excited and has a very rapid heart rate, subtle murmurs may be missed. Cardiomyopathies are seen frequently in ferrets, and any murmur or abnormal heart rhythm should be investigated further.

Palpate the abdomen while holding the ferret off the table, either with one hand supporting the ferret under the thorax or by scruffing the ferret. This allows the abdominal organs to displace downward, making palpation easier. If the history is consistent with the presence of a gastrointestinal foreign body or urinary blockage, palpate gently to avoid causing iatrogenic injury. Palpate the cranial abdomen while devoting particular attention to the presence of gas or any irregularly shaped mass in the stomach area, especially in ferrets with a history of vomiting or melena. The spleen is commonly enlarged in ferrets; this may or may not be significant, depending on other clinical findings. A very enlarged spleen may indicate systemic disease or, rarely, idiopathic hypersplenism, and further diagnostic workup is warranted. Always note any degree of splenic enlargement in the medical record so that this finding can be rechecked at future examinations.

Examine the genital area, noting particularly the size of the vulva in females. Vulvar enlargement in a spayed female is consistent with either adrenal disease or an ovarian remnant; the former is more common. If the vulva is of normal size, point this out to the owner so that any future enlargement of the vulva will be noticed. Examine the size of the testicles of male ferrets; testicular tumors are sometimes seen.

Check the furcoat for evidence of alopecia. Alopecia of the tail tip is common in ferrets and may be incidental and transient or an early sign of adrenal disease. Symmetric, bilateral alopecia or thinning of the hair coat that begins at the tail base and progresses cranially is a common clinical finding in ferrets with adrenal disease. Examine the skin on the back and neck for evidence of scratching or alopecia. Pruritus may be present with ectoparasites (fleas, *Sarcoptes scabiei*) or with adrenal disease. Check closely both visually and by searching through the haircoat with your hands for evidence of skin masses. Mast cell tumors are very common and can range in size from a small pimple to the size of a nickel. Often, the fur around a mast cell tumor is parted and matted with dark blood from the animal's scratching. Other types of skin tumors also commonly occur. Any bump or lump found on the skin should be excised and biopsied.

PREVENTIVE MEDICINE

Ferrets should be given a health examination on an annual basis until they are 4 to 5 years of age. Subsequently, twice yearly examinations are advised because of the high incidence of metabolic disease and neoplasia in older animals. Young, recently purchased ferrets need serial distemper vaccinations until they are 13 to 14 weeks of age. Recommend that routine blood tests (consisting of a complete blood count and serum biochemistry analysis) be done on an annual basis for older animals. Blood glucose concentrations should be measured twice yearly in healthy ferrets 4 years of age and older;

more frequent monitoring is needed in ferrets with insulinomas.

Vaccinations

Canine Distemper

Ferrets must be vaccinated against canine distemper virus. Currently, only one vaccine is USDA-approved for use in ferrets (Fervac-D, United Vaccines, Madison, WI). Although several other distemper vaccines are used and appear safe, efficacy trials have not been conducted with these products. Never use canine combination vaccines or vaccines of ferret cell or low-passage canine cell origin because of the possibility of vaccine-induced disease, especially in immunosuppressed or sick ferrets. The half-life of maternal antibody to canine distemper virus in ferrets is 9.4 days.[1] Give ferrets serial vaccines at 6–8 weeks of age, 10–12 weeks of age, and 13–14 weeks of age. Administer booster vaccinations yearly.

There are anecdotal reports of vaccine reactions following distemper vaccination of ferrets. Ferrets may vomit, have diarrhea, and develop erythematous skin and a high fever. Ferrets should be monitored in the waiting room or by the owner for 30 minutes after receiving a canine distemper vaccine. If a ferret has an adverse reaction, administer an antihistamine (e.g., diphenhydramine hydrochloride [Benadryl, Parke-Davis, Morris Plains, NJ], 0.5–2 mg/kg IV or IM) or, for severe reactions, epinephrine, 20 μg/kg IV, IM, SC, or intratracheally, and administer supportive care following standard protocols used in small animal medicine. It has been suggested that reactions are best prevented with the administration of distemper and rabies vaccinations separately at different visits and by carefully following the manufacturer's instructions for administration.

It is difficult to decide how to handle ferrets that have had an adverse reaction in the past. Possible options include no further canine distemper vaccinations or administration of diphenhydramine 15 minutes before vaccination. Alternatively, another canine distemper vaccine, Galaxy-D (Solvay Animal Health, Inc., Mendota Heights, MN), could be administered. However, Galaxy-D is not approved for use in ferrets nor has it been proved protective against canine distemper in this species. Discuss the options with the owner and obtain owner permission before using any nonapproved product.

Rabies

Vaccination against rabies is recommended, especially in rabies-endemic areas. An inactivated rabies vaccine is approved for use in ferrets (Imrab, Rhone Merieux Inc., Athens, GA) and is effective in producing immunity. Vaccinate healthy ferrets at 3 months of age at a dose of 1 mL administered SC; give booster vaccinations annually.[17]

Little is known about natural rabies infection in ferrets, including the virus' incubation period and shedding in the saliva as well as clinical signs. In ferrets with experimentally induced rabies, only mild clinical signs were noted before death.[4] Ferrets exhibited restlessness and apathy, and some showed paresis of the legs. Sick animals did not attempt to bite when threatened, and virus was not excreted in the submaxillary salivary glands of animals that died. In this study, it was concluded that ferrets are 50,000 times less susceptible to rabies than the fox, and 300 times less susceptible than the hare. In another study, ferrets that were fed up to 25 carcasses of mice infected with rabies did not develop the disease; in contrast, skunks became fatally infected after the consumption of only one carcass.[3]

Local state and city regulations regarding rabies vaccination in ferrets can vary, and veterinarians should contact their local governmental agencies regarding this issue. A person that has been bitten by a rabies-vaccinated ferret may be less likely to undergo rabies prophylaxis because of the decreased suspicion of rabies in that animal; however, the animal will not be legally protected by a vaccination history. Unlike dogs, which are held for an observation period after a bite exposure, ferrets are euthanized for laboratory rabies examination if there is any suspicion of disease.

Parasites

Gastrointestinal parasitism is uncommon in ferrets compared with dogs and cats. There are no reports of hookworms or roundworms naturally infecting ferrets or mink.[2] Rarely, ferrets may become infected with nematodes from other natural hosts through intermediate hosts or vectors. Nonetheless, do routine fecal flotation and direct fecal smears for all young ferrets at the initial examination, as protozoan parasites are seen occasionally.

Coccidiosis (*Isospora* species) can occur in young ferrets, with oocysts usually being shed between 6 and 16 weeks of age.[2] The infection is usually subclinical; occasionally, however, ferrets may have bloody diarrhea. Treatment of ferrets with coccidiosis is similar to that of small animals and should be continued for at least 2 weeks. Coccidiostats such as sulfadimethoxine and amprolium are effective and safe. The *Isospora* species that infect ferrets may cross infect dogs and cats, so check or treat other animals kept in households with multiple pets.

Giardiasis is occasionally seen in ferrets and probably occurs after exposure to infected dogs or cats in pet stores.[2] *Giardia* species can be detected on routine examination of a fresh fecal smear. Treat ferrets with giardiasis with metronidazole (10–20 mg/kg q12h perorally) for 10 days.

Cryptosporidiosis can occur in a high percentage of young ferrets.[16] Infection is usually subclinical in both immunocompetent and immunosuppressed animals and can persist for several weeks. Most immunocompetent animals recover from infection within 2–3 weeks, but infection can persist for months in immunosuppressed animals. Oocysts of *Cryptosporidium* are small (3–5 μm) and difficult to detect but can be found in samples of fresh feces examined immediately after acid-fast staining.[2,16] There is no treatment for *Cryptosporidium* infection, and because of the potential of zoonotic disease, ferrets may be a potential source of infection for humans, especially immunocompromised individuals with acquired immunodeficiency syndrome.[16]

Ear mites *(O. cynotis)* are very common in ferrets, but affected animals rarely show pruritus or irritation from infestation. This species also affects dogs and cats, and animals in households with multiple pets can pass the infection to other animals. The presence of a reddish-brown, thick, waxy discharge in the ear canal and pinna is characteristic of infestation. A direct smear of the exudate reveals adult mites or eggs. Ferrets normally have a brownish ear wax, and it is difficult to identify affected ferrets on the basis of the appearance of the exudate alone. Check all ferrets for ear mites at the initial examination, and do follow-up checks at the annual examination, especially in pets kept in multianimal households. (See Chapter 11 for a discussion of treatment options.)

Heartworms *(Dirofilaria immitis)* can cause disease in ferrets. Ferrets that are housed outdoors in heartworm-endemic areas are most susceptible to infection; however, all ferrets in endemic areas should be given preventive medicine throughout the year. Oral administration of ivermectin is currently the most practical preventive measure because it is administered once per month (see Chapter 7).

Flea infestation (*Ctenocephalides* species) is most common in ferrets kept in households with dogs or cats, and affected ferrets can become severely anemic from chronic infestations. Check all ferrets during the physical examination for signs of fleas or flea dirt. Treat infested animals with products safe for use in cats, and institute flea control measures. Lufenuron (Program, Ciba Animal Health, Ciba-Geigy Corp., Greensboro, NC) given at dosages used in cats may be effective for flea control in ferrets.

HOSPITALIZATION

Ferrets can be hospitalized in standard stainless steel small animal cages with some adaptations. Ferrets are agile escape artists and can squeeze through even very small openings. The bar spacing is too wide in many cages used for dogs and cats, allowing an easy avenue of escape. For housing ferrets, use only cages with very small spacing between vertical bars, or use cages with small crossbars. If this type of caging is not available, standard cages can be adapted for use by attaching a Plexiglass plate at least one-half the height of the cage door or higher to the front of the cage. The plate will prevent escape through the bars yet can be easily detached and cleaned.

Special hospital cages with Plexiglass fronts and circular access ports that are marketed for birds make excellent cages for ferrets (Fig. 2–2). There is no avenue of escape, and ferrets are visible at all times. Acrylic animal intensive care cages (Animal Care Products, Lyon Electric Company, Inc., Chula Vista, CA; Aquabrood, D & M Bird Farm, San Diego, CA) also can be used to house ferrets and are especially useful for animals that need supplemental heat or oxygen. Cages should be large enough to accommodate a sleeping area or box and an area for defecation and urination. Ferrets are very careful about not soiling their sleeping area, even when very sick.

Glass aquariums, although less than ideal be-

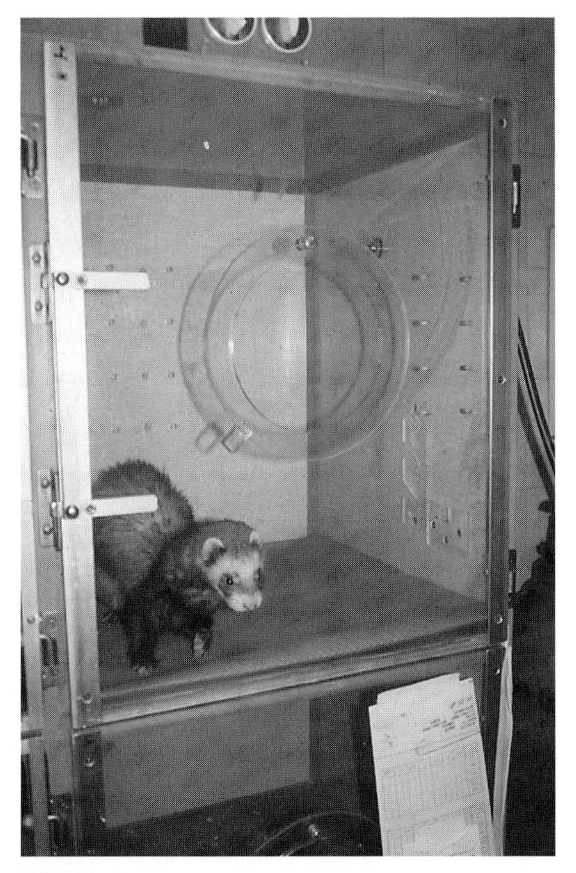

FIGURE 2–2
Special cages with Plexiglass fronts are good for hospitalized ferrets. Ferrets cannot escape from these cages and are visible to the observer.

cause of poor ventilation, can be used for hospitalized ferrets. Aquariums should have a wire lid that can be securely attached and should be used only in a well-ventilated area. Standard 10-gallon aquariums are too small for most male ferrets and many females; such aquariums also have the additional disadvantage that IV fluid administration sets cannot be used unless a hole is cut in the wire lid.

All ferrets like to burrow and should be given opportunity to do so while hospitalized. Clean towels make excellent burrowing material. Alternatively, a mound of shredded paper provides much satisfaction to hospitalized animals. If not provided with burrowing material, many ferrets will burrow underneath the cage paper.

An oxygen cage should be available for use at all times for dyspneic animals. Monitor the temperature in commercial oxygen cages closely, as ferrets can become hypothermic quickly at cool cage temperatures that are standard for dogs and cats. Conversely, ferrets overheat at temperatures used for avian patients.

Provide water for hospitalized ferrets in either water bottles or small weighted bowls (or both). Ask the owner which type of watering system the ferret is accustomed to before hospitalization.

Ferrets can be finicky eaters and should be fed their regular diet while hospitalized, if possible. Otherwise, feed a premium quality, high-protein cat or kitten chow or use a very palatable ferret food. If dietary changes are needed in the regular diet, recommend that changes be made gradually after the ferret has been released from the hospital.

CLINICAL AND TREATMENT TECHNIQUES

Venipuncture

Obtaining a blood sample from a ferret is relatively easy and usually does not require anesthesia. There are several readily accessible venipuncture sites; the technique and site chosen depend on how much blood is needed and on the availability of assistants for restraint. Anesthesia can be used if assistants are unavailable, but alterations in blood values may occur.[14] Ferrets can often be distracted during restraint for venipuncture by offering food or Nutri-Cal by syringe. However, draw blood for glucose determination or other fasting samples before offering any food.

Most veterinary laboratories can do complete hematologic and biochemical analysis with 1.5–2 mL of blood. The blood volume of healthy ferrets is approximately 40 mL in average-sized females weighing 750 g, and 60 mL in males weighing 1 kg.[7] Up to 10% of the blood volume can be safely withdrawn at one time in a normal ferret.

Two techniques are commonly used for obtaining a blood sample that is adequate for hematologic and biochemical analysis. For jugular venipuncture, the technique is similar to that used in cats, with the forelegs of the ferret extended over the edge of a table and the neck extended up (Fig. 2–3). Use a 22- or 25-gauge needle with a 3-mL syringe for venipuncture in most ferrets; a 20- or 22-gauge needle can be used in big males. Shave the neck at the venipuncture site to enhance visibility of the jugular vein. The vein is usually more lateral in the neck than it is in a dog or cat, and it is sometimes difficult to locate in big males. Once the needle is inserted, the blood should flow easily into the syringe. If the neck is overextended and the head is arched

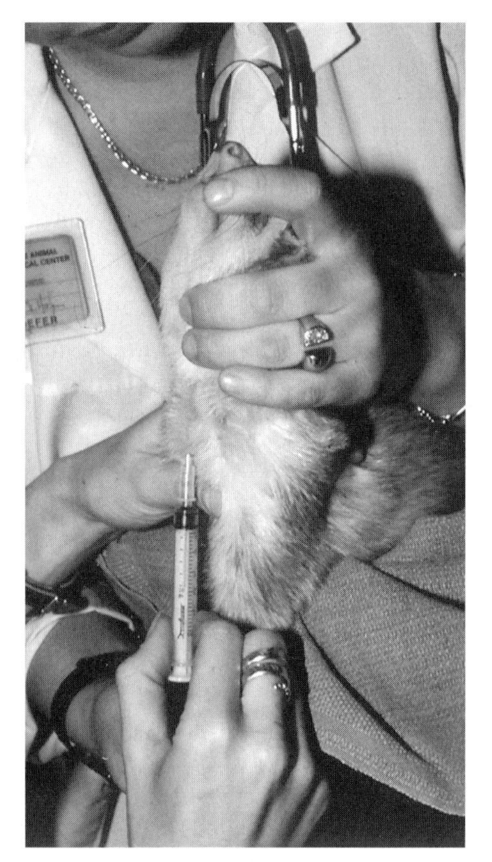

FIGURE 2–3
Jugular venipuncture in a ferret. The forelegs of the ferret are extended over the edge of the table, and the neck is extended upward.

back, the blood may not flow readily from the vein. Relax the hold on the head or gently "pump" the vein by moving the head slowly up and down to enhance blood flow into the syringe.

The second technique is venipuncture of the anterior vena cava. Restrain the ferret on its back with the forelegs held against its sides and the head and neck extended (Fig. 2–4). Usually two assistants are needed, one for restraint of the forelegs and head and the other for restraint of the rear legs. Insert a 25-gauge needle with an attached 3-mL syringe into the thoracic cavity between the first rib and the manubrium at a 45° angle to the body. Direct the needle toward the opposite rear leg and insert it almost to the hub. Pull back on the plunger as the needle is slowly withdrawn until blood fills the syringe. If the ferret struggles, quickly withdraw the needle and wait until the ferret is quiet before making a second attempt.

The lateral saphenous or the cephalic vein can be used if only a small amount of blood is needed for a packed cell volume (PCV) or blood glucose analysis, for example. To prevent collapse of the vein, use a tuberculin syringe with a 27-gauge needle or an insulin syringe with an attached 28-gauge needle for venipuncture. The saphenous vein lies just above the hock joint on the lateral surface of the leg (Fig. 2–5); the cephalic vein is in the same anatomic location as in a dog. Shave the fur from the area to enhance visibility of the vein before venipuncture.

Venipuncture of the tail artery can be used for obtaining blood samples in nonanesthetized ferrets.[5] For this technique, place the ferret in a heated environment for several minutes to facilitate blood flow. Then, remove the ferret from this environment and restrain it on its back. Insert a syringe with a 21- or 20-gauge needle directed toward the body into the ventral side of the tail, in the groove along the midline. The artery is located 2–3 mm deep to the skin. Once the artery is entered, slowly

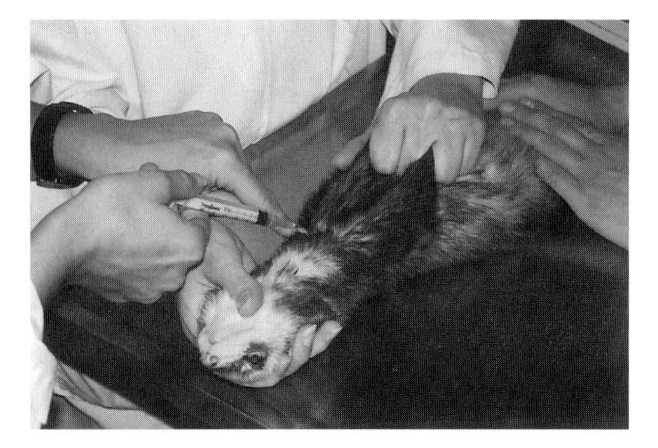

FIGURE 2–4
A ferret is restrained for venipuncture of the anterior vena cava. Both forelegs are pulled back, and the neck is extended.

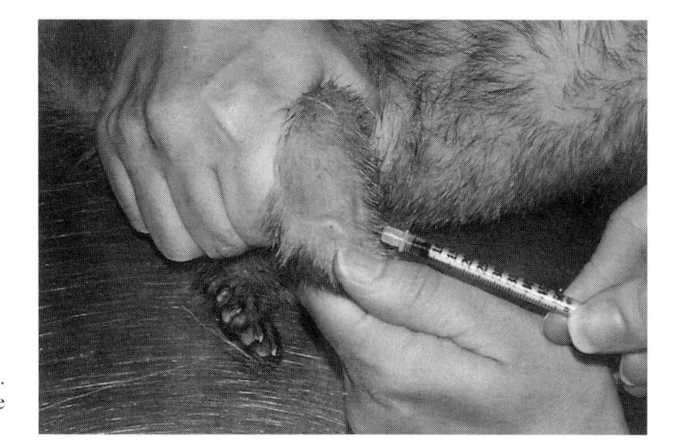

FIGURE 2–5
The lateral saphenous vein is visible just above the hock. Shaving the fur from the leg enhances visibility of the vein. (The head of the ferret is to the right.)

withdraw the plunger until blood fills the syringe. Approximately 3–5 mL of blood can be withdrawn with this technique. Apply pressure to the venipuncture site for 2–3 minutes after the needle has been withdrawn.

Reference Ranges

Published reference ranges for hematologic and serum biochemistry analyses in ferrets are listed in Tables 2–1 and 2–2. Most of these values were reported in early studies of laboratory ferrets. Ideally, each clinical laboratory should establish reference ranges for ferrets.

The hematocrit of ferrets is high relative to that of other species and may be as high as 63% in a normal animal. The white blood cell count tends to be lower than that of other species. Although published ranges for white blood cell counts are $2.5–19.1 \times 10^3/\mu L$,[7, 9, 18] at our laboratory the normal range is lower ($3–8 \times 10^3/\mu L$), with most normal white blood cell counts being $4–6 \times 10^3/\mu L$. Elevated white blood cell counts are not seen as commonly in ferrets as in dogs and cats, perhaps in part because infectious diseases are not common in ferrets. These findings have been corroborated in conversations with other clinicians who work with pet ferrets.

Little work has been published regarding reference ranges for blood coagulation times in ferrets. In male ferrets, the mean prothrombin time was 15.7 seconds, and the normal range was 14.4–16.5 seconds.[18]

Isoflurane anesthesia can cause decreases in all hematologic values, beginning at induction of anesthesia and becoming maximal at 15 minutes after induction.[14] Therefore, the values obtained from the analysis of blood samples collected while a ferret is anesthetized must be carefully interpreted.

Urine Collection, Urinalysis, and Urinary Catheterization

Urine samples can be collected by cystocentesis or free catch after natural voiding or gentle manual expression of the bladder. The techniques for manual bladder expression and cystocentesis are the same as those used in dogs and cats. Use a 25-gauge needle for cystocentesis.

Reference values for urinalysis are listed in Table 2–3.[6, 18, 19] The normal pH of urine in ferrets was reported in one study to be 6.5–7.5[19]; however urine pH can vary according to the diet, and the normal urine pH in ferrets on a high-quality, meat-based diet is approximately 6.0.*

Urinary catheterization is difficult in ferrets, but it can be done successfully with techniques that have been described for male and female ferrets.[13] After tranquilization or anesthesia with isoflurane, position females in ventral recumbency and elevate the rear quarters with a rolled towel. With a vaginal speculum, locate the urethral opening in the floor of the urethral vestibule, approximately 1 cm cranial to the clitoral fossa. Introduce a 3.5-French, red rubber urethral catheter fitted with a wire stylet into the ure-

*Bell J: Personal communication, 1995.

TABLE 2–1
REFERENCE RANGES FOR HEMATOLOGIC VALUES IN FERRETS

		Fitch Ferrets*[9]		Albino Ferrets†[18]	
Value	**Sex**	***Range***	***Mean***	***Range***	***Mean***
Hematocrit (%)	♂	46–57	49.1	44–61	55.4
	♀	47–51	48.4	42–55	49.2
Hemoglobin (g/dL)	♂	15.2–17.7	16.1	16.3–18.2	17.8
	♀	15.2–17.4	15.9	14.8–17.4	16.2
Red blood cells ($\times 10^6/\mu L$)	♂			7.30–12.18	10.23
	♀			6.77–9.76	8.11
Reticulocytes (%)	♂			1–12	4.0
	♀			2–14	5.3
White blood cells ($\times 10^3/\mu L$)	♂	5.6–10.8	7.3	4.4–19.1‡	9.7
	♀	2.5–8.6	5.9	4.0–18.2‡	10.5
Neutrophils	♂	616–7020/μL	2659/μL	11–82%	57.0%
	♀	725–2409/μL	1825/μL	43–84%	59.5%
Lymphocytes	♂	1728–4704/μL	3791/μL	12–54%	35.6%
	♀	1475–5590/μL	3426/μL	12–50%	33.4%
Monocytes	♂	0–432/μL	176/μL	0–9%	4.4%
	♀	100–372/μL	263/μL	2–8%	4.4%
Eosinophils	♂	112–768/μL	378/μL	0–7%	2.4%
	♀	50–516/μL	214/μL	0–5%	2.6%
Basophils	♂	0–112/μL	50/μL	0–2%	0.1%
	♀	0–172/μL	48/μL	0–1%	0.2%
Bands	♂	0–972/μL	233/μL		
	♀	0–248/μL	99/μL		
Platelets ($\times 10^3/\mu L$)	♂			297–730	453
	♀			310–910	545
Mean corpuscular volume (μm^3)	♂				54
	♀				61
Mean corpuscular hemoglobin (pg)	♂				17.6
	♀				19.9
Mean corpuscular hemoglobin concentration (%)	♂				32.2
	♀				32.8

*Males all castrated.
† Males all intact.
‡ These white blood cell counts are higher than those currently seen in clinical practice. At our laboratory, the normal white blood cell count is $3-8 \times 10^3/\mu L$, and most are $4-6 \times 10^3/\mu L$.
Adapted with permission from Lee EJ, Moore WE, Fryer HC, Minocha HC: Hematological and serum chemistry profiles of ferrets *(Mustela putorius furo)*. Lab Anim 1982; 16:133–137, and Thornton PC, Wright PA, Sacra PJ, Goodier TEW: The ferret, *Mustela putorius furo*, as a new species in toxicology. Lab Anim 1979; 13:119–124. Copyright 1979 and 1982, Macmillan Magazines Limited.

thral orifice. In male ferrets, exteriorize the penis from the prepuce and pass a catheter without a stylet into the urethral orifice. Once the catheter is in place, secure it with butterfly tape strips sutured to the skin.

Splenic Aspiration

Splenic aspiration is a common diagnostic technique that is used in ferrets with enlarged spleens (see Chapter 7). The technique is simple and can be done in unanesthetized ferrets. Restrain the ferret on its back or in lateral recumbency and shave and aseptically prepare the abdominal skin in an area over the spleen. Palpate and immobilize the spleen directly under the prepped area with one hand while directing a 3-mL syringe with an attached 25-gauge needle into the spleen with the other hand. Quickly aspirate the spleen and withdraw the needle; a positive aspirate appears bloody. Prepare several slides for cytologic staining. Obtain an aspirate from two sites. Results of cytologic examination of a splenic aspirate are usually reported as compatible with extramedullary hematopoiesis, lymphoid hyperplasia, or lymphoma.

TABLE 2-2
REFERENCE RANGES FOR SERUM BIOCHEMISTRY VALUES IN FERRETS

Value	Albino*	Fitch†
Total protein (g/dL)	5.1–7.4	5.3–7.2
Albumin (g/dL)	2.6–3.8	3.3–4.1
Glucose (mg/dL)	94–207	62.5–134
Fasting glucose (mg/dL)		90–125‡
Blood urea nitrogen (mg/dL)	10–45	12–43
Creatinine (mg/dL)	0.4–0.9	0.2–0.6
Sodium (mmol/L)	137–162	146–160
Potassium (mmol/L)	4.5–7.7	4.3–5.3
Chloride (mmol/L)	106–125	102–121
Calcium (mg/dL)	8.0–11.8	8.6–10.5
Phosphorus (mg/dL)	4.0–9.1	5.6–8.7
Alanine aminotransferase (U/L)		82–289 78–149§
Aspartate aminotransferase (U/L)	28–120	57–248§
Alkaline phosphatase (U/L)	9–84	30–120 31–66§
Bilirubin (mg/dL)	<1.0	0–0.1§
Cholesterol (mg/dL)	64–296	119–209§
Carbon dioxide (mmol/L)	16.5–28	16–28§

*Combined values of male (N = 40) and female (N = 24) ferrets from reference 18.
†Combined values of intact male, female, and castrated male ferrets (total N = 13, aged 4–8 mo) from reference 9, except where noted.
‡From Brown S: Personal communication, 1995.
§Combined values from cardiac and orbital venipuncture of male ferrets (N = 16) from reference 7.

Bone Marrow Aspiration

Evaluation of the bone marrow is a valuable diagnostic tool in many disease conditions, including anemia, thrombocytopenia, pancytopenia, proliferative abnormalities, and suspected hematopoietic malignancies. Anesthesia is required for bone marrow aspiration in ferrets, and isoflurane is preferred over injectable tranquilizers in clinically ill animals.

The iliac crest, proximal femur, and humerus are possible sites for bone marrow collection, although the proximal femur is usually the most readily accessible site. Place the ferret in lateral recumbency, then shave and aseptically prepare the area around the proximal femur. In accordance with one described technique,[15] make a small incision through the skin over the greater trochanter with a No. 15 scalpel blade. Hold and stabilize the femur with one hand while inserting a 20-gauge, 1.5-inch spinal needle into the bone medial to the greater trochanter. Use steady pressure and an alternating rotating motion to advance the needle into the marrow cavity. Withdraw the stylet, and attach a 6- to 12-mL syringe to the needle. Aspirate the marrow sample into the syringe, stopping suction as soon as the sample is visible (to prevent blood contamination).

Intravenous Catheters

Indwelling IV catheters are used routinely in ferrets. Catheters can be placed in the lateral saphenous or cephalic veins. Jugular vein catheters are more difficult to place and are used less frequently. Catheter placement is done with the ferret under isoflurane anesthesia administered by face mask. First puncture the skin over the vein with a 20- or 22-gauge needle, taking care to avoid the vein; then, introduce a short 24- or 25-gauge over-the-needle catheter into the vein. After placement, attach a T-connector to the catheter and wrap the leg securely

TABLE 2-3
REFERENCE RANGES FOR URINALYSIS IN FERRETS

Value	Mean ± SD*	Range
24-h urine volume (mL)	24.93 ± 14.31[6] 26 ♂[18] 28 ♀[18]	 8–48 ♂[18] 8–140 ♀[18]
pH		6.5–7.5[19]
Urine protein (mg/dL)		7–33 ♂[18] 0–32 ♀[18]
Exogenous creatinine clearance (mL/min per kg)	3.32 ± 2.16♀[6]	
Inulin clearance (mL/min per kg)	3.02 ± 1.78♀[6]	
Endogenous creatinine clearance (mL/min per kg)	2.50 ± 0.93[6]	

*Mean 24-h urine volume and endogenous creatinine clearance from reference 6 are based on values from 25 female and 2 male ferrets.

with a soft padded bandage. Maintain the catheter routinely, flushing with a small volume of 0.9% saline to maintain patency. Closely monitor ferrets with indwelling catheters to prevent entanglement in the fluid line or overhydration. Most ferrets do not chew a catheter once it is placed and do not require an Elizabethan collar.

Fluid Therapy

Hospitalized ferrets often require fluid therapy for maintenance of hydration and correction of dehydration. Daily fluid requirements for ferrets have not been determined; however, use of 75–100 mL/kg per day appears to be adequate for maintenance. Calculate fluid requirements at this rate, and provide additional fluids to compensate for excessive ongoing fluid loss and to correct dehydration calculated as a percentage of the body weight. Give fluids SC or IV; IV fluids are preferred in very ill animals.

Administer SC fluids in the loose skin along the back and dorsal cervical area, dividing the calculated daily fluid volume into doses given two or three times a day. Ferrets often react painfully to SC fluid administration, and good restraint is needed if ferrets are to be prevented from biting their handlers.

Administer IV fluids with a Buretrol device (Baxter Healthcare, Deerfield, IL), control flow regulator, or infusion pump to prevent overhydration. Divide the daily calculated fluid volume into two or three doses, or administer the fluids by continuous infusion. Depending on the clinical condition of the ferret, add dextrose (2.5–5%), B vitamins, or potassium to maintenance fluids, using the same criteria and calculations as those used for dogs and cats.

Blood Transfusion

Blood transfusions may be needed in ferrets that are anemic from chronic disease, estrogen toxicity, or blood loss. As for other species, evaluate the need for a transfusion based on the ferrets' PCV and clinical status. One rule of thumb is to consider a transfusion once the PCV falls below 15%. If anemia has developed gradually, a ferret may tolerate a PCV as low as 12% without the need for a transfusion.

Ferrets lack detectable blood groups, and there is little risk of transfusion reaction, even without crossmatching.[11] Large male ferrets are preferred as donors because they have a larger blood volume than females. Depending on the size of the donor ferret, 6–12 mL of blood can be safely collected for transfusion. Collect blood into an anticoagulant such as acid-citrate-dextrose at a ratio of 1 mL of anticoagulant to 6 mL of donor blood.[8] For blood collection, anesthetize the donor ferret with isoflurane, and collect blood from the jugular vein or the anterior vena cava with a small-gauge butterfly catheter or a 22- to 25-gauge needle attached to a 6- or 12-mL syringe (see section on Venipuncture for techniques). Immediately administer the donor blood by slow bolus or infusion with a syringe pump into a catheter placed in the jugular vein of the recipient ferret. Intraosseous blood transfusions can be given to ferrets if an IV catheter cannot be placed (Fig. 2–6).

Antibiotic and Drug Therapy

Ferrets are given antibiotics and other drugs at dosages (on a per weight basis) similar to those used in cats (see Chapter 33). IV antibiotics are preferred in very sick animals if an indwelling catheter is in place. IM antibiotics can be given, but SC administration is preferred if therapy continues over several

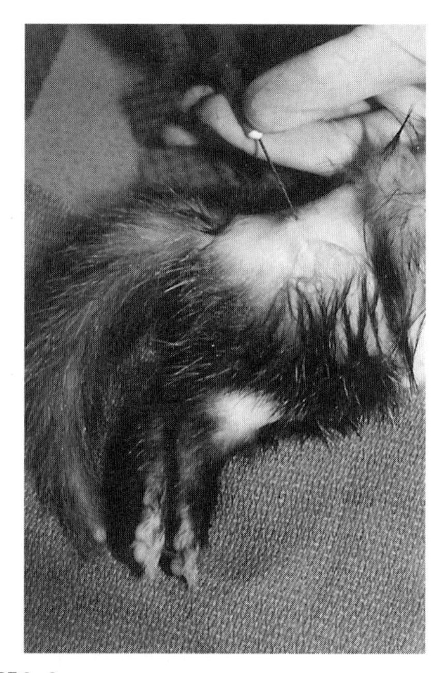

FIGURE 2–6
An intraosseous blood transfusion can be given if a vein is not easily accessible.

days because of the limited muscle mass in these animals. Oral medications are most easily given in a liquid form because ferrets are difficult to treat with pills.

Nutritional Support

Anorectic ferrets can be force-fed high-energy paste supplements (e.g., Nutri-Cal), liquid soy-based formulas (e.g., Isocal, Mead Johnson Nutritionals, Evansville, IN), meat-based baby foods, or meat-based soft foods marketed for hospitalized dogs and cats (Prescription Diet Canine/Feline a/d, Hills Pet Products, Topeka, KS), or mixtures of any of these. Use Nutri-Cal alone only on a short-term basis (1 day or less) or to supplement the diet of a ferret with a poor appetite. Use a more complete diet for force-feeding for a period longer than 1 day.

Force-feed anorectic ferrets as much as they will take comfortably (usually 2–5 mL) three to four times daily. Use a syringe to administer food. Once ferrets develop a taste for the supplement, they may take it directly from a bowl or tip of a tongue depressor. Force-feeding is very important for preventing hypoglycemia in the management of anorectic ferrets with insulinomas.

ZOONOTIC DISEASES

Influenza (orthomyxovirus) is the only documented zoonotic disease of ferrets.[12] Ferrets are very susceptible to influenza virus, and the potential for transmission from humans to ferrets is much greater than that for transmission from ferrets to humans. Potential bacterial zoonotic diseases include leptospirosis, listeriosis, salmonellosis, campylobacteriosis, and tuberculosis. These diseases occur in ferrets with varying frequencies, but transmission from ferrets to humans has not been documented. Ferrets are susceptible to rabies; however, little is known about natural rabies infection, and there are no reports of rabies transmission from ferrets to humans. Cryptosporidiosis is potentially transmissible, especially to humans that are immunosuppressed. Ferrets are susceptible to dermatophytosis from *Microsporum canis* and *Trichophyton gypseum*; therefore, take precautions when handling affected ferrets to prevent transmission. Potentially zoonotic parasitic diseases of ferrets include scabies *(S. scabiei)*, giardiasis (*Giardia* species), and helminthiasis.

REFERENCES

1. Appel MJ, Harris WV: Antibody titers in domestic ferret jills and their kits to canine distemper virus vaccine. J Am Vet Med Assoc 1988; 193:332–333.
2. Bell JA: Parasites of domesticated pet ferrets. Compend Contin Educ Pract Vet 1994; 16:617–620.
3. Bell JF, Moore GJ: Susceptibility of carnivora to rabies virus administered orally. Am J Epidemiol 1971; 93:176–182.
4. Blancou J, Aubert MFA, Artois M: Experimental rabies in the ferret *(Mustela [putorius] furo)*: susceptibility—symptoms—excretion of the virus. Rev Med Vet 1982; 133:553–557.
5. Bleakley SP: Simple technique for bleeding ferrets *(Mustela putorius furo)*. Lab Anim 1980; 14:59–60.
6. Esteves MI, Marini RP, Ryden EB, et al: Estimation of glomerular filtration rate and evaluation of renal function in ferrets *(Mustela putorius furo)*. Am J Vet Res 1994; 55:166–172.
7. Fox JG: Normal clinical and biologic parameters. *In* Fox JG, ed.: Biology and Diseases of the Ferret. Philadelphia, Lea & Febiger, 1988, pp 159–173.
8. Hoefer HL: Transfusions in exotic species. *In* Hohenhaus AE, ed.: Transfusion Medicine. Philadelphia, JB Lippincott, 1992, pp 625–635.
9. Lee EJ, Moore WE, Fryer HC, Minocha HC: Haematological and serum chemistry profiles of ferrets *(Mustela putorius furo)*. Lab Anim 1982; 16:133–137.
10. Mann PH, Harper DS, Regnier S: Reduction of calculus accumulation in domestic ferrets with two dentifrices containing pyrophosphate. J Dent Res 1990; 69:451–453.
11. Manning DD, Bell JA: Lack of detectable blood groups in domestic ferrets: implications for transfusion. J Am Vet Med Assoc 1990; 197:84–86.
12. Marini RP, Adkins JA, Fox JG: Proven or potential zoonotic diseases of ferrets. J Am Vet Med Assoc 1989; 195: 990–994.
13. Marini RP, Esteves MI, Fox JG: A technique for catheterization of the urinary bladder in the ferret. Lab Anim 1994; 28:155–157.
14. Marini RP, Jackson LR, Esteves MI, et al: Effect of isoflurane on hematologic variables in ferrets. Am J Vet Res 1994; 55:1479–1483.
15. Palley LS, Marini RP, Rosenbald WD, Fox JG: A technique for femoral bone marrow collection in the ferret. Lab Anim Sci 1990; 40:654–655.
16. Rehg JE, Gigliotti F, Stokes DC: Cryptosporidiosis in ferrets. Lab Anim Sci 1988; 38:155–158.
17. Ruprecht CE, Gilbert J, Pitts R, et al: Evaluation of an inactivated rabies vaccine in domestic ferrets. J Am Vet Med Assoc 1990; 196:1614–1619.
18. Thornton PC, Wright PA, Sacra PJ, Goodier TEW: The ferret, *Mustela putorius furo*, as a new species in toxicology. Lab Anim 1979; 13:119–124.
19. Williams CSF: Practical Guide to Laboratory Animals. St. Louis, CV Mosby, 1976, p 66.

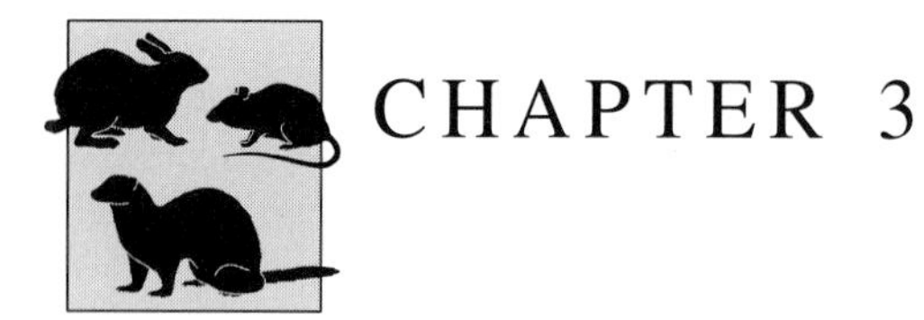

CHAPTER 3

Gastrointestinal Diseases

Heidi L. Hoefer, DVM

Disease of the gastrointestinal (GI) tract is common in ferrets. It is important for the clinician to be familiar with the more common GI disorders, to recognize clinical signs, and to differentiate among potential diagnoses.

DENTAL DISEASE

Dental tartar, gingivitis, and periodontal disease are common in middle-aged and older ferrets. Moist or semimoist diets may predispose these animals to dental calculus formation and periodontal disease.[19] Biting and gnawing habits often result in discoloration, wearing, and breaking of the tips of the canine teeth (Fig. 3–1). Broken canine teeth do not usually result in obvious discomfort or pain unless the dental pulp is exposed. Root canal restoration or surgical removal of the affected teeth may be necessary in some ferrets.[20] Tooth root abscesses are not common but can occur at any age.

Although dysphagia and drooling are sometimes seen, dental disease is often an incidental finding during physical examination. Dental extractions and scaling can be performed with the animal under anesthesia. Follow the basic principles for dental disease management that apply in the care of the dog or cat.

SALIVARY MUCOCELE

Ferrets have five major pairs of salivary glands: the parotid, submandibular, sublingual, molar, and zygomatic.[24] Trauma to a gland can result in extravasation of saliva and salivary mucocele formation. Although this lesion is uncommon in the ferret, mucocele diagnosis and treatment have been described.[1, 22]

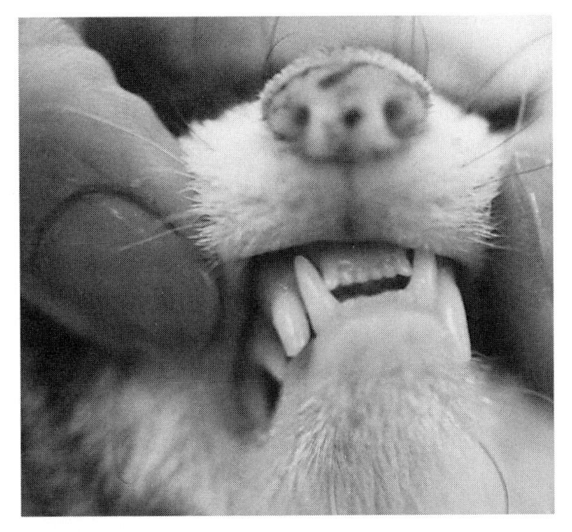

FIGURE 3–1
Broken canine teeth are a common finding in ferrets.

Diagnosis of a mucocele is relatively straightforward. Facial swellings are often seen in the commissures of the mouth, or in the orbital area in the case of a zygomatic mucocele. Other locations also are possible. Aspirate the mass to obtain samples for cytologic analysis. The fluid is viscous or mucinous and clear or blood-tinged. Cytologic examination reveals amorphous debris and occasional red blood cells.

Treatment for salivary mucoceles is usually surgery. In one reported case, scalpel blade lancing of the medial wall of the mucocele resulted in drainage and no recurrence.[1] Marsupialization into the mouth with the use of a wide circular incision in the medial wall of the mucocele may be effective for mucoceles that bulge into the oral cavity (Fig. 3–2). Surgical excision of the affected salivary gland is ideal for avoiding recurrence (see Chapter 13). It may be possible to inject contrast medium into the mucocele in an effort to trace the origin of the saliva. Review the superficial anatomy of the head and neck region of the ferret before attempting surgical excision of a salivary gland.[24] Recurrence is possible.

ESOPHAGEAL DISEASE

Diseases of the esophagus are rare in ferrets. Acquired megaesophagus has been reported in ferrets and I have seen the condition several times in my practice.[4, 18] *Megaesophagus* describes an esophagus that is enlarged (dilated) on radiographic examination and that lacks normal motility. It is important to recognize this disease because the prognosis in ferrets with megaesophagus is poor. Clinical signs include lethargy, inappetence or anorexia, dysphagia, and weight loss. Regurgitation is common. Coughing or choking motions are sometimes described, and some ferrets have labored breathing. Differential diagnosis includes the presence of an esophageal or GI foreign body, gastritis, influenza, and respiratory diseases.

Diagnosis is based on clinical signs and radiographic evidence. The esophagus is often dilated in both the cervical and thoracic segments (Fig. 3–3). Food may be visualized in the esophagus. Aspiration pneumonia and gastric gas are sometimes evident in addition to esophageal dilation. Use radiography of the abdomen to exclude lower GI disease. Administer barium (10 mL/kg PO) to delineate the esophagus and to evaluate mural lesions, strictures, or obstructions (Fig. 3–4). An endoscope can also be used for evaluation of the esophagus. Use fluoroscopy, if available, to determine the motility of the esophagus following a barium swallow.

The cause of megaesophagus in the ferret is unknown. Consider possibilities in the differential diagnosis as for dogs and tailor the diagnostic workup accordingly. The management of ferrets with megaesophagus is similar to that of canine patients, but is usually less successful. Supportive care and antibiotics are palliative at best. Administration of a gastrointestinal motility enhancer such as metoclopramide (Reglan, AH Robins Company, Inc., Richmond, VA) or cisapride (Propulsid, Janssen Pharmaceutica, Inc., Titusville, NJ) may be helpful. Administer metoclopramide at 0.2 to 1 mg/kg

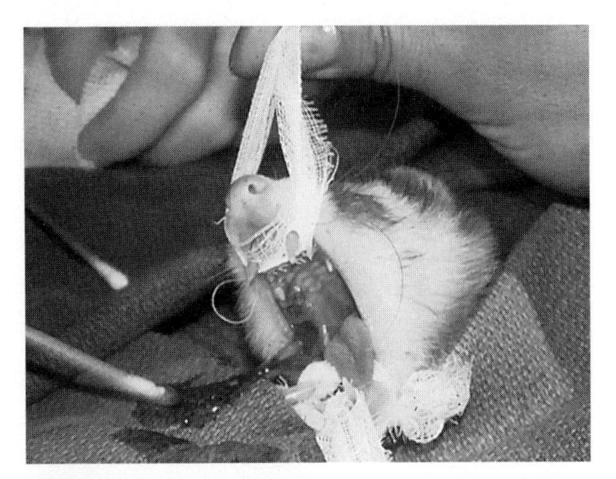

FIGURE 3–2
Surgical correction of a salivary mucocele. The medial aspect of the mucocele is marsupialized into the mouth.

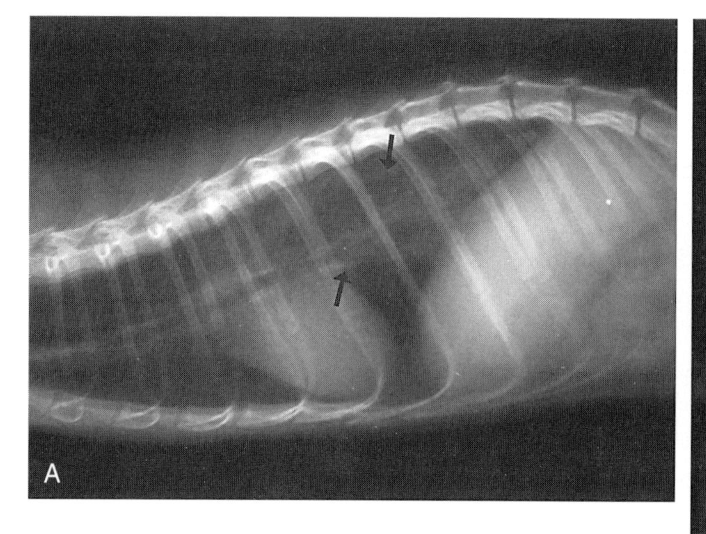

FIGURE 3–3
A, Lateral thoracic radiograph of a ferret with megaesophagus. Note the subtle dilation of the thoracic esophagus *(arrows)*. *B*, Ventrodorsal radiograph of the same ferret in *A*. The cranial thoracic esophagus is dilated *(arrow)* and is much easier to visualize in this view than in the lateral view.

q6–8h PO or SC. Cisapride, which is used for gastroesophageal reflux and gastroparesis in humans, has shown some promise in reducing the frequency of regurgitation in dogs with megaesophagus when it is given at 0.5 mg/kg q8–24h PO.[30] Its use in ferrets has not been evaluated. The 10-mg tablets can be made into a suspension by a compounding pharmacist (see Chapter 33). If esophagitis is suspected, add an H_2 receptor blocker, such as cimetidine or ranitidine (Zantac, Glaxo Pharmaceuticals, Research Triangle Park, NC).

The prognosis for ferrets with megaesophagus is poor; generally, they die or are euthanized within days of diagnosis. Affected ferrets are debilitated

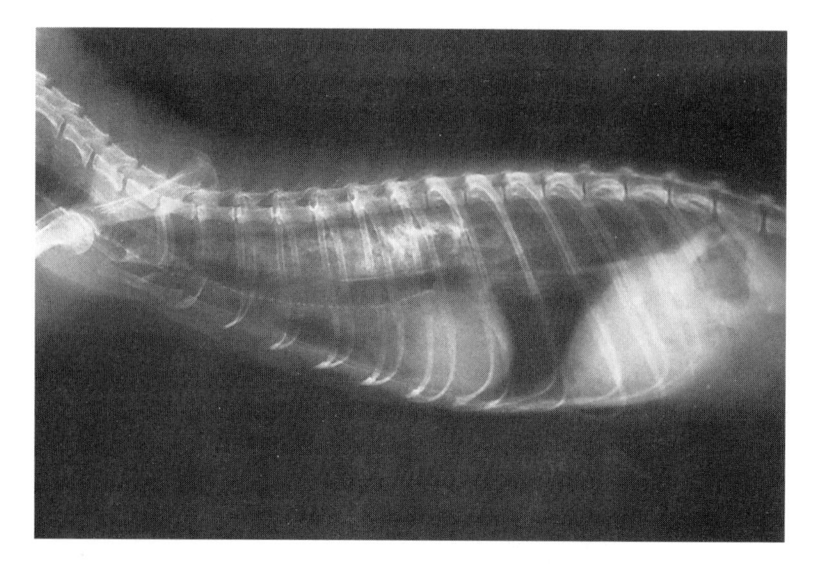

FIGURE 3–4
Lateral radiograph of a ferret with megaesophagus. Orally administered barium sulfate delineates the esophagus.

and suffer from malnutrition, hepatic lipidosis, and aspiration pneumonia.

Other causes of esophageal disease in the ferret are rare. Esophageal foreign body has been reported in a ferret and was successfully managed surgically.[7]

GASTRITIS AND ULCERATION

Gastric and duodenal ulceration has been reported in laboratory ferrets and is seen sporadically in pet ferrets. Causes of GI ulceration include foreign body or toxin ingestion, *Helicobacter mustelae* infection, treatment with ulcerogenic drugs, GI neoplasia, and azotemia secondary to renal disease. The presence of a GI foreign body is probably the most common cause in pet ferrets (see below).

The laboratory ferret is used as an animal model for the study of *H. pylori* infection in humans. *H. mustelae* isolated from the gastric mucosa of ferrets shares many molecular and biochemical features of *H. pylori*. *H. mustelae* infection in ferrets is associated with varying degrees of gastritis, with or without duodenitis, and it can result in ulcer formation.[13] See Chapter 4 for a discussion of *H. mustelae* infection.

Ulcerogenic drugs such as nonsteroidal and steroidal anti-inflammatory agents can be associated with ulcer formation. It is rare for ferrets to have GI bleeding when receiving corticosteroids at appropriate dosages; however, ulceration is possible with the prolonged use of other anti-inflammatory agents. For example, I have treated a ferret for melena, anorexia, and weight loss secondary to renal disease caused by ibuprofen overdose. Severe uremia and associated melena can occur in ferrets with primary renal disease, but this is uncommon.

Gastritis in ferrets may be acute or chronic. Clinical signs may include weight loss and vomiting. Affected ferrets may hypersalivate and display tooth-grinding, which are indicative of nausea and abdominal pain. Clinical signs of gastric or duodenal ulceration include melena, anorexia, lethargy, and weight loss.

Basic diagnostic testing includes whole-body radiography and screening blood tests. Fast the ferret for a short time (2–4 hours) in order to facilitate visualization of a gastric foreign body. The diagnosis of *H. mustelae* gastritis may be a diagnosis of exclusion of other more common disorders, such as the presence of a GI foreign body, and treatment for *H. mustelae* gastritis is often based on a presumptive diagnosis. Establish definitive diagnosis of *Helicobacter* infection by histopathologic study of gastric mucosa by endoscopy or at surgery (see Chapter 4). Specialized techniques are necessary for culturing the organism, which is not shed consistently in feces of infected ferrets.[15]

Treat gastritis and gastric ulceration with both specific therapy (according to the diagnosis) and supportive care. Hospitalize sick and anorectic ferrets for fluid therapy and parenteral treatment. A broad-spectrum antibiotic, administered parenterally, is indicated for sick ferrets. For ferrets that are not vomiting, offer multiple small feedings of a bland, moist, high-carbohydrate diet; avoid dry, high-fiber foods. For vomiting animals, withhold food for 6–12 hours, while closely monitoring for any sign of hypoglycemia (older ferrets often have subclinical insulinomas); then, if vomiting has resolved, introduce small frequent feedings.

Bismuth compounds have action against pepsin, a proteolytic enzyme believed to be an important factor in the development of peptic ulcers. Administer bismuth subsalicylate at a dose of 1 mL/kg q8h PO. Sucralfate (Carafate, Marion Merrell Dow, Inc., Kansas City, MO) is a cytoprotective agent that binds to the erosion site and helps to form a protective barrier. It is a safe and useful adjunct to ulcer treatment. One-eighth to 1/10th of a tablet is given to a ferret q6h PO.

Systemic H_2 receptor antagonists, such as cimetidine and ranitidine, are often used to treat gastric ulceration because they block the histamine receptor on the gastric parietal cell and reduce gastric acid secretion. The proton pump inhibitors, such as omeprazole (Prilosec, Astra Merck, Inc., Wayne, PA), are not useful for ferrets because they are not currently available in liquid form and cannot be made into a suspension.

Antacid therapy may not be helpful in the treatment of *Helicobacter* infection because affected ferrets usually develop hypochlorhydria.[15] The standard treatment for *Helicobacter* infection in humans is "triple therapy" with amoxicillin, metronidazole, and bismuth (see Chapter 4). Bismuth interferes with the colonization of *H. pylori* in humans and suppresses colonization of *H. mustelae* in ferrets.[29]

Surgical removal is the treatment of choice for GI foreign bodies.

GASTROINTESTINAL POLYPS

Two ferrets with GI polyps have been seen at the Animal Medical Center (New York, NY). Both ferrets showed lethargy, inappetence, melena, and weakness secondary to anemia. Abdominal radiographs suggested GI abnormalities. On surgical abdominal exploration, one ferret had a gastric polyp and the other had a small intestinal polyp. Both ferrets did well after surgical resection of the polyps, which were histologically benign.

GASTRIC BLOAT

Gastric bloat is rarely seen in pet ferrets, but it has been reported on domestic ferret farms and in black-footed ferrets (*Mustela nigripes*).[10, 27] Clinical signs are usually observed in weanling ferrets and include acute gastric distention, dyspnea, and cyanosis. Sudden death can occur.

The cause of gastric bloat is unknown but is thought to be related to overgrowth of *Clostridium perfringens (C. welchii)*. Certain conditions may predispose to clostridial overgrowth, including increased concentration of carbohydrates in the GI tract from overeating, diet changes, and intestinal hypomotility. *C. perfringens* multiplies rapidly, producing enterotoxins that attack the villous epithelial cells of the gut. Gas production by the bacteria results in abdominal distention.

Prevention and treatment of the disease are difficult because of the ubiquitous nature of the organism and the short course of disease. These animals are in shock and need immediate aggressive therapy. Relieve gastric pressure by trocharization or placement of an orogastric tube. Follow therapeutic protocols as for bloat in canine patients.

GASTROINTESTINAL FOREIGN BODIES

GI foreign bodies are very common in ferrets.[23] Ferrets are naturally very inquisitive and like to chew on miscellaneous environmental objects, particularly rubber or sponge products. Rubber foreign bodies are most commonly ingested by young ferrets (younger than 2 years of age); in contrast, trichobezoars (hair balls) are more common in older ferrets. Linear foreign bodies, commonly ingested by cats, are rare in ferrets.

The most common clinical signs of GI foreign body in ferrets include lethargy, inappetence or anorexia, and diarrhea. Vomiting is often *not* reported by the owner. However, if vomiting is noted by the owner, a GI foreign body is the most likely cause. Some ferrets display signs of nausea, including bruxism, ptyalism, and face rubbing. Weakness can be profound in acutely obstructed animals; some of these ferrets are recumbent and reluctant to ambulate. If a GI foreign body is suspected, palpate the abdomen carefully. Foreign bodies in the small intestine often are associated with very localized discomfort or pain. Gastric foreign bodies are more difficult to palpate. Take whole-body survey radiographs in these cases. Although uncommon, esophageal disease is an important differential diagnosis in the anorectic, "vomiting" ferret. Abnormal abdominal radiographic findings include segmental ileus, gaseous distention of the stomach, and occasionally, a visible foreign object or trichobezoar (Fig. 3–5). Contrast (barium) studies are rarely needed. Base the diagnosis on history, clinical signs, palpation, and the results of radiography. At a minimum, perform a complete blood count and serum chemistry for ferrets sick for longer than 2 or 3 days.

Ferrets rarely pass GI foreign bodies unassisted. Occasionally, a small, partially obstructing object may pass with the administration of intestinal lubricants (cat laxatives) q8h and replacement fluids. However, most GI foreign bodies must be removed surgically. Stabilize debilitated ferrets before surgery. Parenteral fluids are usually essential as these ferrets often present with varying degrees of dehydration. Perform an exploratory laparotomy as soon as possible in the sick ferret. Collect biopsy specimens from the liver, the spleen (if enlarged), and the stomach or intestines (if ulcerated or abnormal in appearance). Some of these ferrets may also have *H. mustelae* gastritis or GI lymphoma. Check the adrenal glands and the pancreas in older ferrets; it is not unusual to discover concurrent abdominal disease during surgery. (See Chapter 13 for a description of the surgical procedure.) In most instances, recovery is rapid after GI foreign body removal, and ferrets are able to eat soft foods 24 hours following surgery. Most ferrets can be discharged within 36–48 hours after surgery.

Prevention of foreign body obstructions includes recommendation of the regular use of a cat laxative preparation during active shedding seasons and

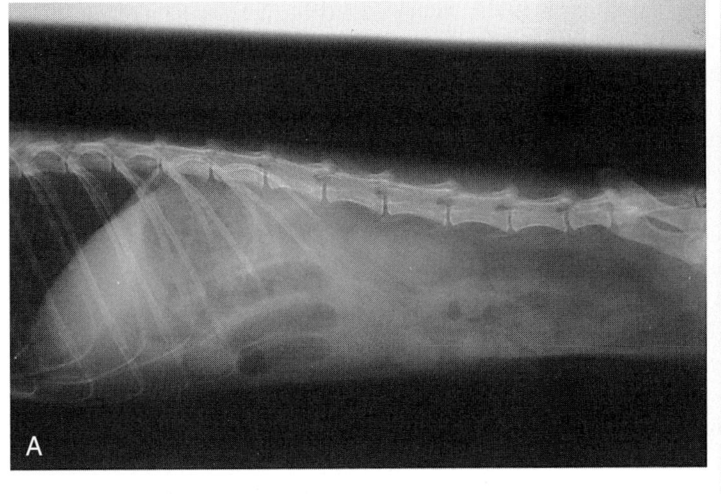

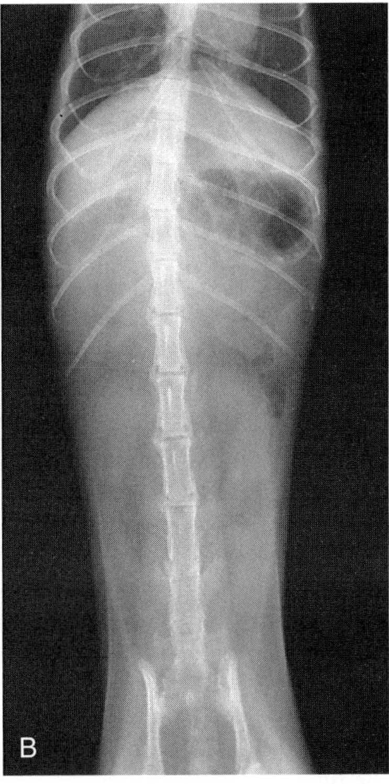

FIGURE 3–5
Lateral and ventrodorsal radiographic views of a ferret with gastrointestinal foreign body. There is a moderate amount of gastric gas present, and the proximal small intestine is markedly dilated. The foreign body is not visualized.

"ferret-proofing" the household. Ferrets should not be left uncaged or unsupervised. Advise owners to avoid giving small rubber "squeak" toys to pet ferrets.

GASTROINTESTINAL PARASITISM

GI parasites are uncommon in ferrets. However, any ferret with diarrhea should have a complete fecal parasite check, including a direct fresh wet mount and fecal flotation. Nematodiasis is rare in juvenile ferrets; however, coccidiosis and giardiasis are occasionally seen. Coccidiosis can be subclinical in ferrets or it may be associated with diarrhea, lethargy, and dehydration.[5] Rectal prolapse is possible. Base the diagnosis of coccidiosis on fecal testing, either by direct wet mount and microscopic examination or by fecal flotation. Follow the same treatment protocols as for canine and feline patients with coccidiosis.

Cryptosporidiosis is described in ferrets but may not result in clinical disease.[2, 25] Young ferrets can have a subclinical infection that can persist for several weeks. The oocysts can be shed in the feces of clinically normal ferrets. Histologically, the organism may be associated with an eosinophilic infiltrate in the lamina propria of the small intestine. It is not known whether zoonotic transmission of ferret cryptosporidia is possible; however, warn immunocompromised owners if the oocysts are detected in their ferrets.

ENTERITIS AND DIARRHEA

Salmonellosis

Salmonellosis is a contagious disease characterized by fever, bloody diarrhea, and lethargy. Conjunctivitis and anemia also may be present. *Salmonella newport*, *S. typhimurium*, and *S. choleraesuis* may be involved.[21] The incidence of salmonellosis in pet ferrets is very low and the infection may be associated with the feeding of uncooked meat, poultry, and meat byproducts. Isolation of *Salmonella* organisms usually requires the collection of multiple fecal samples and the use of selective media. Treatment consists of aggressive supportive care, use of antimicrobials, and shock therapy as needed.

Mycobacteriosis

Ferrets may be naturally or experimentally infected by the bovine, avian, and human tubercle bacilli.[6, 9, 28] *Mycobacterium bovis* and *M. avium* infections have been recognized in research and farm ferrets in England, Europe, and New Zealand. These infections may have been associated with the feeding of raw meat and poultry and unpasteurized dairy products. More recently, a pet ferret was reported to have a visceral infection caused by *M. avium*.[28] The ferret had a chronic history of weight loss, diarrhea, and vomiting that was unresponsive to treatment. Intestinal biopsy revealed granulomatous inflammation and acid-fast bacteria.

Base the diagnosis of mycobacteriosis on the findings of tissue biopsy, including histopathology with acid-fast staining and culture. *M. avium* can be detected in the small intestine, liver, spleen, and lymph nodes of affected ferrets. Because of the zoonotic potential, treatment is not recommended.

Campylobacteriosis

Campylobacter jejuni is a bacterial enteric pathogen that is associated with diarrhea and enterocolitis in humans and several animal species, including dogs, cats, calves, and sheep. *C. jejuni* can be isolated from the feces of normal ferrets. For several years during the 1980s, it was suspected to be the cause of proliferative colitis, which has since been renamed "proliferative bowel disease" in ferrets.[11, 12] However, inoculation of *C. jejuni* in 54 conventionally reared and two gnotobiotic ferrets caused diarrhea but not the full spectrum of clinical signs and histopathologic lesions seen in proliferative bowel disease (see Chapter 4).[2] The agent of porcine proliferative enteropathy, which is identical to that causing proliferative bowel disease in ferrets,[14] has recently been assigned the new genus and species name *Lawsonia intracellularis* (see Chapter 4). The importance of *C. jejuni* as a primary pathogen in pet ferrets is not known.

Viral Diarrhea

Rotavirus infection causes diarrhea in young ferrets. Farm outbreaks of diarrhea are associated with high morbidity and mortality rates in neonatal kits from 2 to 6 weeks of age.[3, 31] The morbidity is low in adult ferrets, but infection may result in a transient green mucoid diarrhea. No antemortem testing is available for the diagnosis of rotaviral infection in ferrets. Treatment is supportive; administer fluids and antibiotics to affected ferrets.

Canine distemper virus is a highly contagious paramyxovirus that causes fatal disease in unvaccinated ferrets. Clinical signs are variable but often include diarrhea in conjunction with nasal and ocular discharges and a generalized orange-tinged dermatitis (see Chapter 8). Diarrhea may be acute or intermittent. Fortunately, the widespread use of vaccinations against canine distemper virus has greatly limited the occurrence of distemper in ferrets, which now has become an uncommon disease. "Coldlike" symptoms and diarrhea in newly purchased, unvaccinated ferrets should arouse suspicion. There is no treatment for distemper.

Ferrets affected with the human influenza virus (an orthomyxovirus) are sometimes observed to have a transient diarrhea. The virus also produces upper respiratory disease associated with coughing, sneezing, inappetence, and lethargy. Affected ferrets are often febrile (see Chapter 8).

Reports of a new, highly transmissible diarrheal disease of ferrets have appeared sporadically in several rescue and breeder operations in the United States, especially in the Mid-Atlantic States. Although a causative agent has not yet been identified, histologic findings on intestinal biopsy are consistent with a viral infection, most likely with a rotavirus or a coronavirus.* Affected ferrets are lethargic and anorectic and develop a profuse, bright green diarrhea (hence, the term "green slime disease"). The morbidity is high. Treat affected ferrets aggressively; the use of shock fluids and antimicrobials as well as isolation is indicated.

LIVER DISEASE

Hepatic neoplasia is probably the most frequent condition seen in the liver of ferrets. Lymphoma is the most common hepatic neoplasm seen at the Animal Medical Center (New York, New York). Other reported hepatic neoplasms include hemangiosarcoma, adenocarcinoma, and hepatocellular adenoma.[17] Beta-cell carcinomas of the pancreas can eventually metastasize to the liver. Prognosis is guarded regardless of tumor type.

Other than neoplastic diseases, primary hep-

*Williams BH: Personal communication, 1995.

atopathies are uncommon in ferrets. Vascular shunts have not been reported. Hepatic lipidosis can be found in association with long-term anorexia. Chronic GI diseases (e.g., trichobezoar formation) can lead to hepatic lipidosis. Chronic-active lymphocytic hepatitis and cholangiohepatitis have been found on biopsy examination in several ferrets undergoing abdominal exploration at my hospital. The cause of these entities is unknown. Steroid hepatopathy is rare in ferrets, even with long-term steroid administration or hyperadrenocorticism.

Copper toxicosis was diagnosed in two sibling ferrets on the basis of high hepatic copper concentrations and histologic changes in hepatic tissue.[16] Clinical signs in these two ferrets were mostly nonspecific and included severe central nervous system depression with hypothermia and hyperthermia, respectively. One ferret was icteric. Both ferrets died within a few days of clinical evaluation despite supportive care. A genetic predisposition to copper toxicosis in these two ferrets was proposed because they were siblings with the same phenotypic coat color and because no environmental source of copper could be identified.

Persistent elevation of alanine aminotransferase level (>275 IU/L) is present on biochemical analysis in most cases of liver disease. Alkaline phosphatase concentration is sometimes elevated. Elevated total bilirubin levels are uncommon, and ferrets are rarely icteric. Base the diagnosis of liver disease on observation of persistent elevation of liver enzyme levels, radiographic and ultrasound findings, and for definitive diagnosis, liver biopsy analysis. Ultrasound-guided needle biopsy of the liver is possible, but full abdominal exploration is often recommended because of the likelihood of concomitant disease in ferrets.

NEOPLASIA

The GI tract is not a common site of primary neoplasia in ferrets. The oral cavity is a rare location for neoplastic lesions. A pyloric adenocarcinoma has been reported,[26] and I have found intestinal adenocarcinoma in one ferret. Lymphoma can also affect the GI tract of ferrets. Visceral and mesenteric lymph nodes and the liver are common sites for lymphoma; intestinal lymphoma is uncommon. Treatment involves surgical resection and debulking whenever possible. Chemotherapy for lymphoma is described in Chapter 10.

RECTAL DISEASE

Rectal prolapse can occur in ferrets. It is most often associated with diarrhea and is usually a disease of young ferrets. Possible causes include coccidiosis, proliferative bowel disease, colitis, campylobacteriosis, and neoplasia.

Diagnostic tests should include a fecal wet mount and flotation to check for parasites. GI parasitism other than coccidiosis is uncommon. Treat with antibiotics and antiparasitics, as indicated. Use rectal pursestring sutures if the prolapse is extensive; these sutures can be left in place for 2–3 days. However, small prolapses often resolve spontaneously or with treatment of the causative condition.

Include a careful rectal examination (visualization and palpation) in all ferret examinations. Undescented ferrets may develop anal gland disease, including impactions and abscessation. Palpation of the anal area may reveal either unilateral or 360° perianal swelling. Manage anal gland disease as in the dog. Be forewarned: anal gland odor is quite noxious and offensive. Anal gland removal is described in Chapter 13.

Neoplasia is rare in the rectal area, although I have seen one descented ferret with leiomyosarcoma that surrounded the rectal opening (Fig. 3–6).

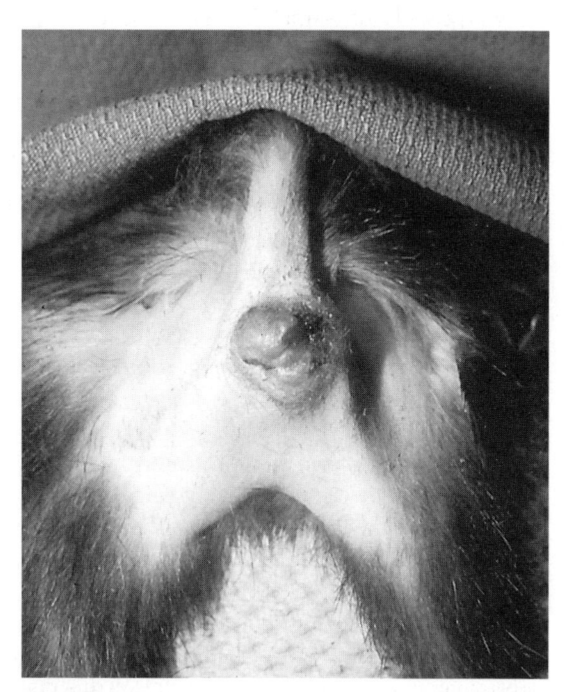

FIGURE 3–6
Rectal leiomyosarcoma in a ferret that presented for a recurrent rectal prolapse.

The ferret presented for a rectal prolapse, and a tumor was found on palpation. Treatment involves surgical debulking and, possibly, a rectoplasty. Prognosis is poor.

APPROACH TO VOMITING

Owners may describe "vomiting" in their ferrets, but some of these animals may actually be regurgitating. In light of this, the differential diagnoses for emesis in ferrets include both esophageal diseases and gastroenteric disorders. It is interesting to note that vomiting is not as frequently described in ferrets as it is in canine or feline patients. For example, ferrets rarely vomit hairballs, and often vomiting is not part of the clinical history characteristic for foreign body ingestion. The reason for this is unclear. No anatomic feature prevents emesis in ferrets; in fact, ferrets have long been laboratory animal models for human emesis studies because vomition can readily be induced in them in a laboratory setting.[8]

The major differential diagnoses for vomiting or regurgitation in ferrets include the presence of a GI foreign body, *H. mustelae* gastritis, gastroenteritis, and megaesophagus. It is uncommon for ferrets with metabolic problems such as azotemia or hepatic disease to vomit. Although definitive diagnosis is not always possible, it is important to recognize whether medical or surgical treatment is required. For example, most foreign body–related obstructions require surgery; gastroenteritis is a medical disease; and megaesophagus is essentially untreatable.

Diagnosis begins with taking of the history. Pointedly question an owner as to the chewing habits of his or her ferret: Does the ferret have a squeak toy? Is it unsupervised in the household or usually caged? Has vomiting been observed? The description of any vomiting behavior is significant. Also, question the owner regarding the animal's appetite, and obtain a description of the feces.

On physical examination, some foreign bodies in the small intestine can be distinctly palpated. However, enlarged mesenteric lymph nodes can sometimes feel like foreign objects. Also, remember that foreign bodies in the stomach are difficult to detect on palpation. Proliferative bowel disease may result in palpably thickened intestines in the ferret; however, vomiting is not usually a feature of this disease.

Radiography is the most important diagnostic test in the workup of the vomiting ferret. Perform whole-body radiography that includes all of the esophagus. Radiographic signs of megaesophagus can be subtle. The heart may appear small secondary to hypovolemia from dehydration. Varying amounts of gas can be seen with foreign body–related obstruction, and sometimes the incriminating object is visible. Segmental ileus or a dilated and gas- or fluid-filled stomach is a typical radiographic sign of obstruction (see Fig. 3–5; see also Chapter 31). Not all cases of GI foreign body are radiographically obvious. If evidence of foreign body obstruction is not well defined, consider medical therapy and perform repeat radiography in 24 hours. Alternatively, give barium contrast for a series of contrast-enhanced films.

If there is a strong indication of the presence of a foreign body, perform abdominal exploration the same day, preferably after parenteral fluid therapy has been started. Biopsy tissues as needed (e.g., from the liver or spleen), and save the incriminating object to show to the owner. Always check the entire gut for lesions and examine the pancreas and adrenal glands, especially in older ferrets. If a foreign body is not found, collect gastric and duodenal biopsies and request silver staining. *Helicobacter* infection is associated with gastritis, especially in the antral region and the proximal duodenum. Although it is rare to have negative findings on exploratory surgery in a ferret, the owner should realize that this is possible.

If surgery is not an option or is not recommended, consider treatment for *H. mustelae* gastritis (see Chapter 4). If obstruction is still a possibility, administer a cat hairball preparation (Laxatone [EVSCO Pharmaceuticals, Buena, NJ]) or Petromalt [VRx Products, Harbor City, CA]) at 1 mL q8–12h. Carefully examine all feces passed in the hospital; sometimes, foreign objects or matter may be found in the stool.

APPROACH TO DIARRHEA

Normal ferrets nibble on food all day. Their GI transit time is short (3 hours), so defecation is frequent in the healthy state. The normal stool is slightly soft and formed. Diarrhea can range from mucoid and green to hemorrhagic. Diarrhea in ferrets is difficult to classify as originating in the small intestine or the large intestine, as is the case in canine patients.

More important are the onset, duration, and severity of the diarrhea as well as concurrent clinical signs.

Several causes of diarrhea in ferrets are recognized. These can be separated into diseases of young ferrets and those of older ferrets as well as into infectious and noninfectious causes. The most common noninfectious causes of diarrhea include dietary indiscretion, foreign body ingestion, and trichobezoar. Occasionally, severe metabolic disease can result in a green (bile-tinged) mucoid diarrhea. Eosinophilic gastroenteritis typically affects mature ferrets but is uncommon.

Infectious agents are rare causes of diarrhea in closed groups or isolated ferrets, such as those kept as individual household pets. Ferrets do not usually have GI parasites, but coccidia can be present in young, newly purchased ferrets. Proliferative bowel disease is a disease of young ferrets. Rotavirus can cause outbreaks of severe diarrhea, but most reports of this are in very young, unweaned ferrets. Show ferrets may be susceptible to the newly recognized contagious viral diarrheal disease dubbed "green slime disease." Canine distemper virus in the epitheliotropic form causes diarrhea in conjunction with respiratory and integumentary disease in unvaccinated ferrets.

The clinical approach to the diagnosis of diarrhea depends on the severity and duration of clinical signs. Obtain a vaccination and diet history and perform a direct fecal wet mount and flotation for the detection of parasitism. Treat mild diarrhea without anorexia or vomiting on an outpatient basis with an antibiotic such as chloramphenicol or sulfadimethoxine or with a cat hairball preparation if a trichobezoar is a possibility. Sick ferrets need a more comprehensive workup that includes radiography to check for obstructive lesions and a complete blood count and a biochemistry analysis to assess metabolic conditions. If simple diagnostic tests are unrevealing and therapy is unsuccessful, consider exploratory surgery for gastrointestinal evaluation and biopsies. Endoscopy can be difficult in smaller ferrets but may be an alternative to surgery. Perform colonoscopy in ferrets with chronic colitis. Culture the feces for *C. jejuni* or *Salmonella* species, especially if the ferret is febrile or the feces are hemorrhagic.

Hospitalize sick or dehydrated ferrets for supportive care and a diagnostic workup. Give fluids subcutaneously if a ferret is stable, or intravenously if it is weak and dehydrated. Administer antibiotics parenterally. Metronidazole, chloramphenicol, and amoxicillin are good choices for GI disease in the ferret. Oral chloramphenicol does not usually cause the nausea and anorexia that it produces in some cats. Drugs that affect the motility of the gastrointestinal tract should never be administered without an initial diagnosis. Motility-enhancing drugs such as metaclopramide and cisapride are contraindicated if a GI obstruction is present, and anticholinergic drugs can produce an ileus that may be difficult to interpret radiographically.

REFERENCES

1. Bauck LS: Salivary mucocele in 2 ferrets. Mod Vet Pract 1985; 66:337–339.
2. Bell JA, Manning DD: Evaluation of *Campylobacter jejuni* colonization of the domestic ferret intestine as a model of proliferative colitis. Am J Vet Res 1991; 52:826–832.
3. Bernard SL, Gorham JR, Ryland LM: Biology and diseases of ferrets. *In* Fox JG, Cohen BJ, Loew FM, eds: Laboratory Animal Medicine. New York, Academic Press, 1984, pp 385–397.
4. Blanco MC, Fox JG, Rosenthal K, et al: Megaesophagus in nine ferrets. J Am Vet Med Assoc 1994; 205:444–447.
5. Blankenship-Paris TL, Chang J, Bagnell CR: Enteric coccidiosis in a ferret. Lab Anim Sci 1993; 43:361–363.
6. Bryant JL, Hanner TL, Fultz DG, et al: A chronic granulomatous intestinal disease in ferrets caused by an acid-fast organism morphologically similar to *Mycobacterium paratuberculosis*. Lab Anim Sci 1988; 38:498–499.
7. Caliguiri R, Bellah JR, Collins BR, Ackerman N: Medical and surgical management of esophageal foreign body in a ferret. J Am Med Vet Assoc 1989; 195:969–971.
8. Florczyk AP, Schurig JE, Bradner WT: Cisplatin-induced emesis in the ferret: a new animal model. Cancer Treat Rep 1982; 66:187–189.
9. Fox JG: Bacterial and mycoplasmal diseases. *In* Fox JG, ed: Biology and Diseases of the Ferret. Philadelphia, Lea & Febiger, 1988, 210–211.
10. Fox JG: Systemic diseases. *In* Fox JG, ed: Biology and Diseases of the Ferret. Philadelphia, Lea & Febiger, 1988, pp 258–259.
11. Fox JG, Ackerman JI, Newcomer CE: Ferret as a potential reservoir for human campylobacteriosis. Am J Vet Res 1983; 44:1049–1052.
12. Fox JG, Ackerman JI, Taylor N, et al: *Campylobacter jejuni* infection in the ferret: an animal model of human campylobacteriosis. Am J Vet Res 1987; 48:85–90.
13. Fox JG, Correa P, Taylor NS, et al: *Helicobacter mustelae*–associated gastritis in ferrets: an animal model of *Helicobacter pylori* gastritis in humans. Gastroenterology 1990; 99:352–361.
14. Fox JG, Dewhirst FE, Fraser GJ, et al: Intracellular *Campylobacter*-like organism from ferrets and hamsters with proliferative bowel disease is a *Desulfovibrio* sp. J Clin Microbiol 1994; 32:1229–1237.
15. Fox JG, Paster BJ, Dewhirst FE, et al: *Helicobacter mustelae* isolation from feces of ferrets: evidence to support fecal-oral transmission of a gastric *Helicobacter*. Infect Immun 1992; 60:606–611. (Published erratum appears in Infect Immun 1992; 60:4443.)
16. Fox JG, Zeman DH, Mortimer JD: Copper toxicosis in sibling ferrets. J Am Vet Med Assoc 1994; 205:1154–1156.
17. Goad ME, Fox JG: Neoplasia in ferrets. *In* Fox JG, ed: Bi-

ology and Diseases of the Ferret. Philadelphia, Lea & Febiger, 1988, 281–282.
18. Harms CA, Andrews GA: Megaesophagus in a domestic ferret. Lab Anim Sci 1993; 43:506–508.
19. Harper DS, Mann PH, Regner S: Measurement of dietary and dentrifice effects upon calculus accumulation rates in the domestic ferret. J Dent Res 1990; 69:447–450.
20. Johnson-Delaney CA, Nelson WB: A rapid procedure for filling fractured canine teeth of ferrets. J Sm Exotic Anim Med 1992; 1:100–102.
21. Marini RP, Adkins JA, Fox JG: Proven or potential zoonotic diseases of ferrets. J Am Vet Med Assoc 1989; 195:990–993.
22. Miller PE, Pickett JP: Zygomatic salivary gland mucocele in a ferret. J Am Vet Med Assoc 1989; 194:1437–1438.
23. Mullen HS, Scavelli TD, Quesenberry KE, Hillyer E: Gastrointestinal foreign body in ferrets: 25 cases (1986–1990). J Am Anim Hosp Assoc 1989; 28:13–19.
24. Poddar S, Jacob S: Gross and microscopic anatomy of the major salivary glands of the ferret. Acta Anat (Basel) 1977; 98:434–443.
25. Rehg JE, Gigliotti F, Stokes DC: Cryptosporidiosis in ferrets. Lab Anim Sci 1988; 38:155–158.
26. Rice LE, Stahl SJ, McLeod C Jr: Pyloric adenocarcinoma in a ferret. J Am Vet Med Assoc 1992; 200:1117–1118.
27. Schulman FY, Montali RJ, Hauer PJ: Gastroenteritis associated with *Clostridium perfringens* Type A in black-footed ferrets (*Mustela nigripes*). Vet Pathol 1993; 30:308–310.
28. Schultheiss PC, Dolginow SZ: Granulomatous enteritis caused by *Mycobacterium avium* in a ferret. J Am Vet Med Assoc 1994; 204:1217–1218.
29. Stables R, Campbell C, Clayton N, et al: Gastric anti-secretory, mucosal protective, anti-pepsin and anti-*Helicobacter* properties of ranitidine bismuth citrate. Aliment Pharmacol Ther 1993; 7:237–246.
30. Tams TR: Cisapride: clinical experience with the newest GI prokinetic drug. Proceedings of the Twelfth American College of Veterinary Internal Medicine Forum, San Francisco, 1994, pp 100–101.
31. Torres-Medina A: Isolation of an atypical rotavirus causing diarrhea in neonatal ferrets. Lab Anim Sci 1987; 37:167–171.

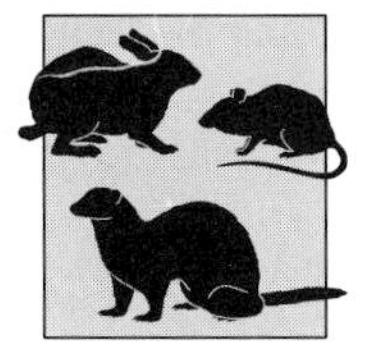

CHAPTER 4

Helicobacter mustelae Gastritis, Proliferative Bowel Disease, and Eosinophilic Gastroenteritis

Judith A. Bell, DVM, PhD

Helicobacter mustelae gastritis, proliferative bowel disease (PBD), which is also known as proliferative colitis or ileitis, and eosinophilic gastroenteritis all cause diarrhea and wasting in ferrets. Eosinophilic gastroenteritis has been infrequently diagnosed, and no specific causative agent for it has been found. *H. mustelae* gastritis and PBD are associated with bacterial agents and are relatively common in pet ferrets. Diagnosis becomes more complex when gastritis occurs concurrently with colitis/ileitis or with another systemic disease. Other entities to be ruled out include the presence of gastrointestinal foreign body, lymphoma, Aleutian disease, and diarrhea associated with corona virus.

HELICOBACTER MUSTELAE GASTRITIS

H. mustelae is a gram-negative rod morphologically similar to *Campylobacter* and requiring a microaerophilic environment for growth on artificial media. It is antigenically related and biochemically similar to *H. pylori,* a human pathogen associated with gastritis and ulcers.[3] Colonization of the stomach and pyloric area of the duodenum with *H. mustelae* is very common in domestic ferrets[10] and is accompanied by a specific immune response.[3] Although colonized animals have mild to severe gastritis, clinical disease caused by gastritis and ulcers is relatively uncommon.

The histopathologic lesions of *Helicobacter* gas-

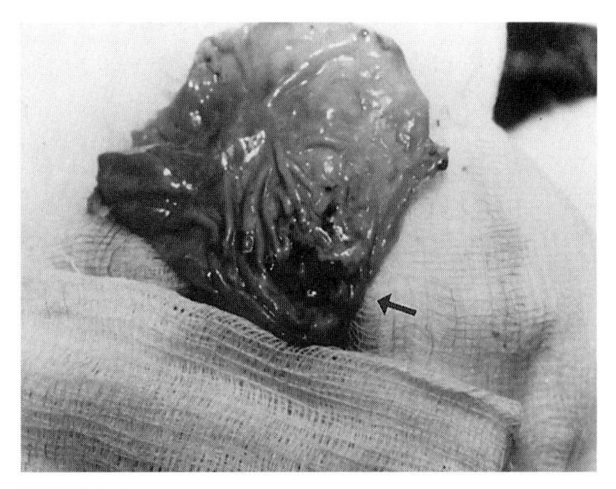

FIGURE 4–1
Single large ulcer (arrow) in the pyloric area of a ferret's stomach.

tritis are similar in humans and ferrets, consisting of mucus depletion, gland loss and regeneration, and leukocyte infiltration.[3] The organism can be observed in silver-stained histologic sections of affected human and ferret gastric mucosa. Ferrets that die of this disease usually have a single large pyloric ulcer or many small ones, and the stomach and intestinal tract contain dark-colored digested blood and mucus (Fig. 4–1).

Clinical Signs of *Helicobacter mustelae* Gastritis with Ulcers

Illness occurs most often in ferrets 12–20 weeks of age that are sufficiently stressed by a combination of factors such as rapid growth, dietary changes or inadequacy, and concurrent diseases. Ferrets with severe *H. mustelae* gastritis and ulcers are lethargic and anorexic and rapidly become emaciated. They are often moderately to severely dehydrated and may be moderately anemic. Black, tarry fecal material often stains the fur of the tail and perineal region.

PROLIFERATIVE BOWEL DISEASE

PBD in ferrets is associated with an intracellular organism (formerly known as "*Campylobacter*-like organism") that has not yet been cultured on artificial media. A morphologically similar and antigenically related organism is found in proliferative ileitis of pigs and hamsters.[4, 5] The intracellular organism associated with PBD of ferrets was recently identified by molecular techniques as a *Desulfovibrio* species with a ribonucleic acid sequence most closely related to that of *D. desulfuricans*.[4] Subsequently, the agent of porcine proliferative enteropathy was assigned a new genus and species name, and is known as *Lawsonia intracellularis*.[9] *L. intracellularis* is believed to be the cause of PBD in swine, ferrets, hamsters, and other affected species. *Campylobacter* species, particularly *C. jejuni,* have been cultured from ferrets,[5] pigs, and hamsters[8] with PBD; however, they are not isolated from all affected animals[2] and do not reproduce the disease when test animals are inoculated.[1]

In ferrets, the colon or the ileum, or both, may be affected. On examination, the bowel feels firm, appears grossly thickened, and is often discolored on the serosal surface. Ridges of proliferated tissue distinct from adjacent normal tissue are obvious on the mucosal surface (Fig. 4–2). Occasionally, perforation of the affected bowel causes fatal peritonitis. On histologic examination, the lesion demonstrates epithelial proliferation with hypertrophy of the muscularis and infiltration of the bowel wall with either monocytic or granulocytic inflammatory cells, or with both. On silver-stained sections, *L. intracellularis* can be found inside enterocytes lining crypts or

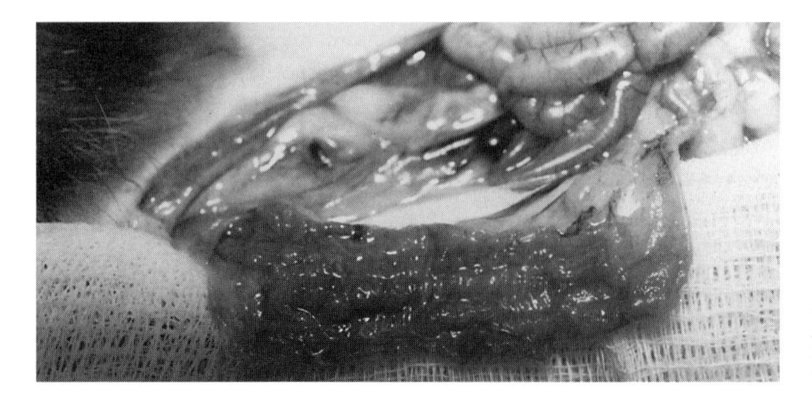

FIGURE 4–2
Ridges of proliferated tissue with adjacent areas of normal bowel mucosa in the colon of a ferret with proliferative colitis.

glands. The normal architectural pattern of the mucosa is lost. Normally, straight tubular glands are covered evenly with enterocytes and numerous goblet cells. In proliferative colitis, this pattern is replaced by irregular, branching, proliferative glands that lack goblet cells and by an accumulation of necrotic debris in the crypts. Severe glandular hyperplasia resembles neoplasia, and it may metastasize to extraintestinal sites.[6]

Clinical Signs of Proliferative Bowel Disease

PBD causes chronic diarrhea that may vary from dark, liquid feces streaked with bright red blood to scant, mucoid stool, often with bright green mucus. PBD is a disease of younger ferrets (typically less than 14 months of age). Many affected ferrets have continuous or intermittent prolapse of rectal tissue (Fig. 4–3). The fur of the tail and perineal area is usually stained and wet with fecal material. In males, the preputial area is often wet with urine that has dripped during straining to defecate. Affected animals moan or cry while straining. Some continue to eat but lose weight at an alarming rate. A ferret that originally weighed 800 g may weigh 400 g in less than 2 weeks if not appropriately treated. These animals are moderately to severely dehydrated and may be hypoalbuminemic.

Ferrets with PBD are more susceptible to other infectious diseases because of their general debility. They may have upper respiratory infections that do not affect other, healthy ferrets housed with them. Ferrets with PBD often develop clinical gastritis or ulcers (see later in chapter).

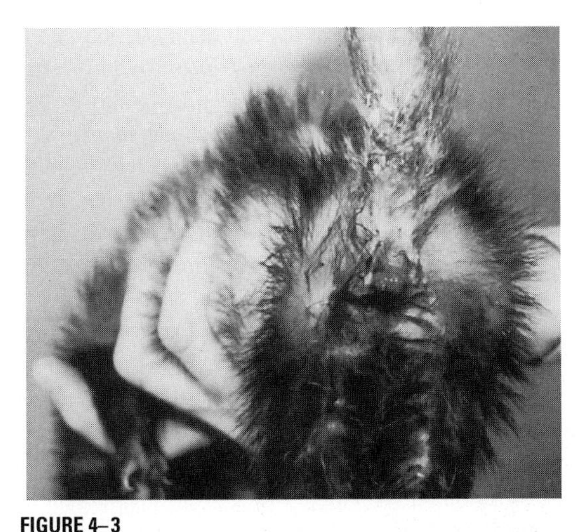

FIGURE 4–3
Prolapsed rectum and hair matted with fecal material in a wasted ferret with proliferative colitis.

EOSINOPHILIC GASTROENTERITIS

This is a rare disease in ferrets as in other animals. In all reported cases, the ferrets have been older than 6 months of age; however, because of the small number of reports available, the possibility of finding this disease in a younger animal cannot be absolutely ignored. No specific causative agent has been found in ferrets,[11] dogs,[12] or humans,[13] but an allergic or immunologic reaction to foods or parasitic migration is believed to initiate the eosinophilic response. Peripheral eosinophilia is a common but not a constant finding in affected dogs and humans[13] but has occurred in all of the relatively few ferrets diagnosed with this disease.[11] Food allergy is implicated in most human patients and in some dogs. No reports of food elimination testing in affected ferrets have been published.

The lesion of eosinophilic gastroenteritis in ferrets, as in other animals and humans, is a mild to extensive infiltration of the mucosa, submucosa, and muscularis of the stomach and small intestine by eosinophils. Focal eosinophilic granulomas are found in the mesenteric lymph nodes of ferrets.[11] No pathogens have been observed in or isolated from the lesions of affected ferrets.

Clinical Signs of Eosinophilic Gastroenteritis

Affected animals typically have chronic diarrhea, with or without mucus and blood, and severe weight loss. Vomiting, anorexia, and dehydration are variable signs.

DIFFERENTIATION OF WASTING DISEASES

PBD and *H. mustelae* gastritis may occur independently, sequentially, or concurrently in the same animal. PBD is a sufficient stressor for the induction of clinical gastritis in a ferret colonized with *H. mustelae.* Although these two diseases are most common in ferrets 12–16 weeks of age, sufficiently stressed mature ferrets may also be affected. Although eosinophilic gastroenteritis has so far been confirmed only in adults, it may be occurring and undiagnosed in younger animals; therefore, age is not a reliable indicator with which to differentiate the wasting diseases. However, the veterinarian may arrive at a presumptive diagnosis without results from complex or expensive laboratory workup. See Table 4–1 for a summary of the characteristics of the three wasting diseases already discussed. Other important differential diagnoses for diarrhea and wasting in domestic ferrets include the presence of a gastrointestinal foreign body, lymphoma, and Aleutian disease.

STEPS IN DIAGNOSIS

When presented with a lethargic, anorexic ferret with diarrhea that has suddenly lost weight, question the owner carefully about changes in the ferret's diet or feeding schedule and ask whether water has been inadvertently restricted. The stressor most commonly associated with wasting diseases is restriction of food for any reason. This may include self-denial of food. Ferrets resist changing to a food different in flavor and texture from the one to which they are accustomed and may fast for several days rather than eat the new food. Such ferrets lose weight and fat stores while they fast. Do not confuse this situation with the loss of muscle mass associated with the wasting diseases. If water is inadvertently withheld, ferrets cannot eat dry food pellets (they usually consume about three times as much water as dry food). Food hoppers may be easily blocked by some dietary pellets with unusual shapes, and an owner may not realize that a ferret is not able to get its food. Occasionally, new owners try to give their ferrets inappropriate foods, such as dog food or poor-quality cat food. Rapidly growing young animals with inadequate nutrition are much more susceptible to all infectious diseases. Exposure to extremes of temperature, particularly heat, is very stressful to ferrets. Animals may be stressed during inclement weather if they are housed outdoors without adequate protection from wind and rain and especially if their food is of poor quality or subject to wetting, caking, and molding. Question an owner carefully if the affected pet is the household's first ferret. You may identify stressors that the owner would not have taken into consideration.

Palpate the abdomen of a wasted ferret. PBD and eosinophilic gastroenteritis cause a grossly thickened gut that can usually be palpated. A focal area of pain in the abdomen is more typical of the presence of a gastrointestinal foreign body. Although rectal prolapse is not absolutely pathognomonic for PBD, it is safe to assume this diagnosis in a ferret with diarrhea and wasting. Coccidiosis may be associated with rectal prolapse in young ferrets with diarrhea but is not usually associated with significant weight loss. Both Aleutian disease and lymphoma usually are insidious; thin ferrets will have lost body condition over a period of weeks or months and may not have diarrhea.

Radiography is the most useful tool for detecting a gastrointestinal foreign body. Collect a blood sample for a complete blood count to help rule out lymphoma and eosinophilic gastroenteritis. Ferrets with eosinophilic gastroenteritis have consistently shown dramatic eosinophilia (10–35% eosinophils, compared with 3–5% in normal ferrets). Ferrets with lymphoma may not be leukemic, and further

TABLE 4–1

DIFFERENTIATION OF THREE DISEASES THAT CAUSE DIARRHEA AND WASTING IN DOMESTIC FERRETS*

Clinical findings common to PBD,* H. mustelae *gastritis, and EG
Wasting
Diarrhea
Clinical findings variably associated with PBD,* H. mustelae *gastritis, and EG
Green mucus in stool
Vomiting
Anorexia
Leukocytosis
Hypoalbuminemia
Clinical findings common to PBD and EG
Palpably thickened areas of intestine
Palpably enlarged mesenteric lymph nodes
Clinical findings indicative of PBD
Prolapsed rectum
Tenesmus
Clinical findings indicative of* H. mustelae *gastritis with ulcers
Black, tarry stool
Significant anemia
Clinical findings indicative of EG
Peripheral eosinophilia

Abbreviations: PBD = proliferative bowel disease; EG = eosinophilic gastroenteritis.

*Other differential diagnoses for diarrhea and wasting include the presence of a gastrointestinal foreign body, lymphoma, Aleutian disease, and intestinal mycobacteriosis.

tests such as peripheral lymph node biopsy and examination are necessary for confirmation of this diagnosis. PBD often causes leukocytosis with neutrophilia and a shift to the left. Ferrets with bleeding ulcers usually are anemic (normal hematocrit, 40–55% [lower in jills in estrus]). Dehydration may mask mild anemia and hypoproteinemia in wasted animals; therefore, repeat a complete blood count after rehydration. Aleutian disease may cause diarrhea, anemia, leukocytosis, and wasting. Serologic tests for Aleutian disease virus are available, but many ferrets with positive test results show no clinical signs of the disease. Do not assume that any illness in ferrets positive for the Aleutian disease virus is caused by the virus.

Any of the wasting diseases can be diagnosed on the basis of biopsy results, but often a presumptive diagnosis can be based on a clinical examination, data from a complete history, and complete blood count. Confirm the diagnosis by the affected ferret's response to appropriate treatment.

TREATMENT FOR PROLIFERATIVE BOWEL DISEASE

The agent that causes PBD is sensitive to chloramphenicol. No other antibiotic consistently resolves this problem.[7] Give affected animals 50 mg/kg q12h, either by IM or SC injection (chloramphenicol sodium succinate) or PO. A palatable chloramphenicol suspension of appropriate concentration can be made by a compounding pharmacist (see Chapter 33). A ferret with colitis of recent onset improves quickly with this treatment and gains 50–100 g/d within a few days of the first dose. Repair of rectal prolapse with a pursestring suture is rarely necessary because, as the colon heals, the prolapse usually disappears spontaneously. It may appear intermittently for weeks but causes no apparent distress. If a pursestring suture is used, the owner must closely monitor the ferret to make sure that it can defecate, especially when the stool regains its normal consistency.

TREATMENT FOR *HELICOBACTER MUSTELAE* GASTRITIS WITH ULCERS

Chloramphenicol has no effect on *H. mustelae*.[10] The most effective treatment for *H. mustelae* gastritis and ulcers is a combination of three drugs—amoxicillin, metronidazole, and bismuth subsalicylate—that must be given concurrently q12h for at least 2 weeks (see Table 4–2 for dosages). *H. mustelae* is sensitive to either amoxicillin or metronidazole, but drug resistance quickly develops unless the two agents are given simultaneously. Metro-

TABLE 4–2

SUMMARY OF TREATMENT REGIMENS FOR PROLIFERATIVE BOWEL DISEASE, *HELICOBACTER MUSTELAE* GASTRITIS, AND EOSINOPHILIC GASTROENTERITIS*

Disease	Drugs	Drug Form and Route	Dosage Frequency
Proliferative bowel disease	Chloramphenicol	Sodium succinate, injectable, IM, SC	50 mg/kg q12h
		Palmitate,† oral suspension, PO	50 mg/kg q12h
Helicobacter mustelae gastritis with ulcers	Amoxicillin	Oral suspension, PO	10 mg/kg q12h
	Metronidazole	Tablet (crushed), PO	20 mg/kg q12h
	Bismuth subsalicylate‡	Oral suspension, PO	17 mg/kg (1 mL/kg) q12h
Eosinophilic gastroenteritis	Prednisolone	Oral suspension, PO	1.25–2.5 mg/kg q24h
	Ivermectin	Injectable preparation, SC or PO	0.4 mg/kg once; repeat 2 wk later

Abbreviations: IM = intramuscular; SC = subcutaneous; PO = peroral.

*Parenteral administration preferred for sick ferrets, if possible.

†Chloramphenicol palmitate is no longer commercially available but can be prepared by compounding pharmacists (see Chapter 33).

‡For example, Pepto-Bismol (Procter & Gamble, Cincinnati, OH).

nidazole is not available in liquid form, but a suspension may be prepared with a combination of pulverized tablets and a sweet-tasting syrup. Compounding pharmacists can prepare a palatable metronidazole suspension (see Chapter 33). Cimetidine (10 mg/kg q8h) or other H_2 receptor blockers may be helpful in very sick animals that are bleeding from extensive gastric ulceration. Cimetidine and home-made metronidazole suspension are very bitter, and ferrets resist their dosing. When administering either drug, scruff the ferret firmly and use a soft eye dropper or plastic dose syringe. Oral veterinary or pediatric amoxicillin suspensions are palatable and well accepted by most ferrets.

TREATMENT FOR EOSINOPHILIC GASTROENTERITIS

Eosinophilic gastroenteritis in humans, dogs, and cats is usually responsive to steroid treatment. Because the disease in ferrets resembles that in other species, prednisone administration has been the treatment of choice.[11] Remission has occurred in ferrets treated with dosages of prednisone from 1.25 to 2.5 mg/kg q24h given PO for the first week and q48h thereafter until the ferret is clinically normal. Immediate recovery also followed removal of an enlarged mesenteric lymph node in one ferret and treatment with ivermectin (0.4 mg/kg) in another. Ivermectin is a safe drug in ferrets, even at a dose of 0.5 mg/kg. When eosinophilic gastroenteritis is a response to the presence of a parasite, elimination of the parasite is a more logical approach to the problem than is the administration of corticosteroids for a longer period of time to relieve the symptoms.

TREATMENT REGIMENS FOR WASTED FERRETS WITH DIARRHEA

Rehydrate sick ferrets with either subcutaneously or intravenously administered balanced electrolyte solutions. These animals are often very weak and may allow the insertion of a jugular or cephalic catheter with little resistance. One advantage of giving intravenous fluids is that glucose can be administered by this route. However, subcutaneously administered fluids are well and rapidly absorbed. Give oral supplements such as Nutri-Cal (EVSCO Pharmaceuticals, Buena, NJ) or Liquical (The Butler Company, Dublin, OH) immediately and frequently to supply calories and amino acids until the sick ferret begins to eat. Hospitalize an emaciated, dehydrated ferret until it has more normal electrolyte and energy balance. When the life-threatening episode is over, the owner will probably be willing and able to give the tender loving care needed to restore the ferret to health.

While waiting for results of diagnostic tests for other diseases, assume that all wasted ferrets with diarrhea that do not have a gastrointestinal foreign body or eosinophilia have both ileitis/colitis and *H. mustelae* gastritis with ulcers. If a ferret is treated for only one disease when it has both, the time required for determining whether the treatment is inadequate may be the factor that ultimately decides whether the ferret will survive or not. Unfortunately, the effective drugs used for treating the two diseases are different, and therapy necessitates multiple daily doses of several drugs for a period of at least 2 weeks. Long-term administration of broad-spectrum antibiotics does not cause diarrhea in ferrets as it does in most animals and in humans because the gut flora of ferrets is very simple and has no vital role in digestion.

Wasted animals that die usually have either very extensive gastric ulcers or severe ileitis, each of which drastically reduces the absorption of essential nutrients. These emaciated animals have no energy reserve and should receive intensive care. Offer the ferret a smorgasbord of premium cat foods and ferret diets. Some animals do not eat their regular diet of dry pellets but do accept the same food mixed with water and heated in a microwave until it develops a porridge-like consistency. Some ferrets eat baby food meats, especially liver and chicken, and most drink milk. Milk causes loose stool in normal ferrets and in those with colitis, but it is very palatable. If milk fat is increased to 10–20% with cream, it appears to be absorbed well and contributes to weight gain even though diarrhea continues. Most sick ferrets accept Nutri-Cal or Liquical at numerous times during the day. Many ferrets like the human food supplement Ensure Plus (Abbott Laboratories, Ross Products Division, Columbus, OH), particularly the strawberry-flavored variety, and they sometimes eat softened pellets mixed with this product when they refuse pellets alone. Use concentrated supplements as their sole source of nutrition for weeks at a time, if necessary. Calculate a minimum daily intake of 400 kcal per kilogram of body weight. Sick ferrets may not make the effort to get up and drink from a water bottle but do usually drink from a dish. Provide fresh food and water several times daily if the ferret is hospitalized; this is because the animal often takes a few mouthfuls of every new offering but never goes back to it for more. The first 2 days are critical for an animal that has lost 40–50% of its body weight, and no amount of care is wasted.

When animals with PBD or ulcers regain their appetites within 48 hours of the first doses of medication and the diarrhea has resolved significantly, some owners are tempted to stop treatment. However, relapses often occur in ferrets treated for less than 2 weeks, and some ferrets need antibiotic therapy for an additional 2 to 3 weeks if they are to make a complete recovery. Ferrets with eosinophilic gastroenteritis that do not respond to ivermectin require longer periods of monitoring and prednisone therapy. Most ferrets with these wasting diseases can be saved with aggressive and persistent treatment.

REFERENCES

1. Bell JA, Manning DD: Evaluation of *Campylobacter jejuni* colonization of the domestic ferret as a model of proliferative colitis. Am J Vet Res 1991; 52:826–832.
2. Fox JG, Ackerman JI, Taylor NS, et al: *Campylobacter jejuni* in the ferret: a model of human campylobacteriosis. Am J Vet Res 1987; 48:85–90.
3. Fox JG, Correa P, Taylor NS, et al: *Helicobacter mustelae*–associated gastritis in ferrets: an animal model of *Helicobacter pylori* gastritis in humans. Gastroenterology 1990; 99:352–361.
4. Fox JG, Dewhirst FE, Fraser GJ, et al: Intracellular *Campylobacter*-like organism from ferrets and hamsters with proliferative bowel disease is a *Desulfovibrio* sp. J Clin Microbiol 1994; 32:1229–1237.
5. Fox JG, Lawson GHK: *Campylobacter*-like omega intracellular antigen in proliferative colitis of ferrets. Lab Anim Sci 1988; 38:34–36.
6. Fox JG, Murphy JC, Otto G: Proliferative colitis in ferrets: epithelial dysplasia and translocation. Vet Pathol 1989; 26:515–517.
7. Krueger KL, Murphy JC, Fox JG: Treatment of proliferative colitis in ferrets. J Am Vet Med Assoc 1989; 194:1435–1436.
8. McOrist S, Boid R, Lawson GHK, et al: Monoclonal antibodies to intracellular *Campylobacter*-like organisms of the porcine enteropathies. Vet Rec 1987; 121:421–422.
9. McOrist S, Gebhart CJ, Boid R, Barns SM: Characterization of *Lawsonia intracellularis* gen. nov., sp. nov., the obligately intracellular bacterium of porcine proliferative enteropathy. Int J Syst Bacteriol 1995; 45:820–825.
10. Otto G, Fox JG, Wu P-Y, et al: Eradication of *Helicobacter mustelae* from the ferret stomach: an animal model of *Helicobacter pylori (Campylobacter)* chemotherapy. Antimicrob Agents Chemother 1990; 34:1232–1236.
11. Palley LS, Fox JG: Eosinophilic gastroenteritis in the ferret. *In* Kirk RW, Bonagura JD, eds: Kirk's Current Veterinary Therapy 11: Small Animal Practice. Philadelphia, WB Saunders, 1992, pp 1182–1184.
12. Sherding RG: Diseases of the small bowel. *In* Ettinger SJ, ed: Textbook of Veterinary Internal Medicine: Diseases of the Dog and Cat. 3rd ed. Vol 2. Philadelphia, WB Saunders, 1989, pp 1365–1366.
13. Talley NJ, Shorter RG, Phillips SF, et al: Eosinophilic gastroenteritis: a clinicopathological study of patients with disease of the mucosa, muscle layer and subserosal tissues. Gut 1989; 31:54–58.

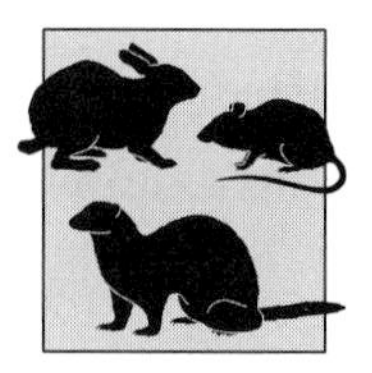

CHAPTER 5

Urogenital Diseases

Elizabeth V. Hillyer, DVM

Urogenital diseases are not common in pet ferrets. Renal diseases, including renal cysts, hydronephrosis, and renal failure, are uncommon, as are urolithiasis and cystitis. Estrogen toxicity secondary to prolonged estrus is encountered rarely now that most female ferrets are spayed at an early age. However, the incidence of prostatic cysts (and urinary blockage secondary to the formation of these cysts), which usually occur in association with adrenocortical tumors, appears to be increasing, reflecting the high prevalence of adrenal disease in ferrets and our improving ability to diagnose this condition.

RENAL CYSTS

Renal cysts are a relatively frequent finding in ferrets at necropsy.[1, 10] At one institution, they were seen in 10–15% of ferrets necropsied.[12] In my experience, however, renal cysts, although not uncommon, are not a frequent finding in clinical practice. The cysts can be single or multiple; present on one or both kidneys; and clinically silent or associated with renal insufficiency. The cause of renal cysts in ferrets is uncertain; however, they are not reported in association with hepatic or biliary cysts, and there is no documented hereditary basis for their formation as is the case for some forms of polycystic renal disease in humans.

Renal cysts in ferrets are usually detected as an incidental finding either during physical examination (as one or more smooth masses on the surface of the kidney or kidneys) or during abdominal ultrasound (as one or more hypoechoic areas with smooth walls in the kidneys). Cysts may be noted incidentally during abdominal surgery as translucent swellings visible through the renal capsule.

Occasionally, a ferret presents in renal failure secondary to disruption of normal renal architecture because of the presence of multiple cysts (Fig. 5–1). Perform a complete blood count (CBC), a serum chemistry workup, and urinalysis to evaluate renal function in all ferrets with cysts, even those not showing clinical signs. Ultrasound is a noninvasive means of evaluating the architecture of the kidneys. Intravenous pyelography might be useful for evaluating renal function in some affected ferrets.

One case report describes a 3-year-old neutered male ferret that presented for multiple seizures over 12 hours. At necropsy, the ferret was found to have multiple renal cysts.[6] Although a serum chemistry workup was not performed in this case, it is possible that the ferret had seizures because of uremic encephalopathy. Histopathology of the kidneys revealed multiple cystic spaces of various sizes lined by cuboidal epithelium. Fibrosis of the intervening renal tissue was present with multifocal infiltration of lymphocytes. Normal glomeruli and tubules were found in many areas between cysts.

There is no specific treatment for renal cysts. Monitor affected ferrets with periodic palpation, ultrasound, and, if possible, serum chemistry workup and urinalysis. In humans, pain and hematuria are the most common clinical manifestations of renal cysts.[11] If a cyst becomes very large or painful, unilateral nephrectomy is an option; however, before taking this approach, be sure that the contralateral kidney is functioning adequately.

HYDRONEPHROSIS

I have seen one ferret with hydronephrosis; also, one case of this disease in a ferret has been reported.[19] Both ferrets were young spayed females that presented for progressive abdominal distention without other clinical signs. Abdominal radiographs showed a large fluid density in the abdomen; on abdominal exploratory examination, the density was found to be a grossly enlarged, fluid-filled kidney (Fig. 5–2). In both ferrets, hydronephrosis had occurred secondary to inadvertent ligation of a ureter during ovariohysterectomy. A third ferret with hydronephrosis has been reported; however, the cause of the condition was not presented.[1]

If you suspect hydronephrosis, perform a CBC, serum chemistry evaluation, and urinalysis as part of the medical workup. Abdominal ultrasound or pyelography can be used to characterize the swelling further. Fine-needle aspiration of the fluid-filled abdominal mass should reveal a transudate. Secondary infection may be present. The treatment for hydronephrosis is unilateral nephrectomy, and the prognosis is good if the function of the remaining kidney is normal.

RENAL DISEASE AND RENAL FAILURE

Clinically significant renal disease other than cysts is not common in ferrets. However, many ferrets older than the age of 4 years necropsied at one institution showed varying degrees of chronic interstitial nephritis.[12] Possible conditions affecting the kid-

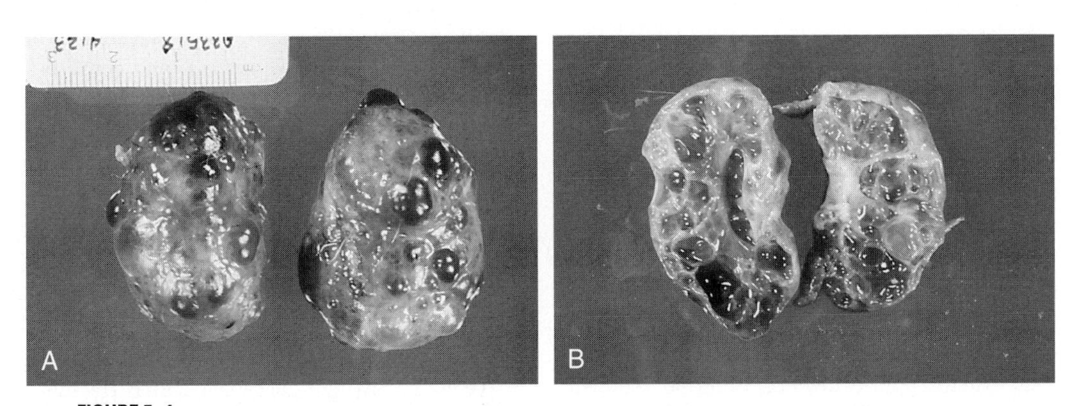

FIGURE 5–1
Polycystic kidney. *A*, Capsular aspect. *B*, Cut surface. This 3-year-old female ferret presented with acute renal failure.

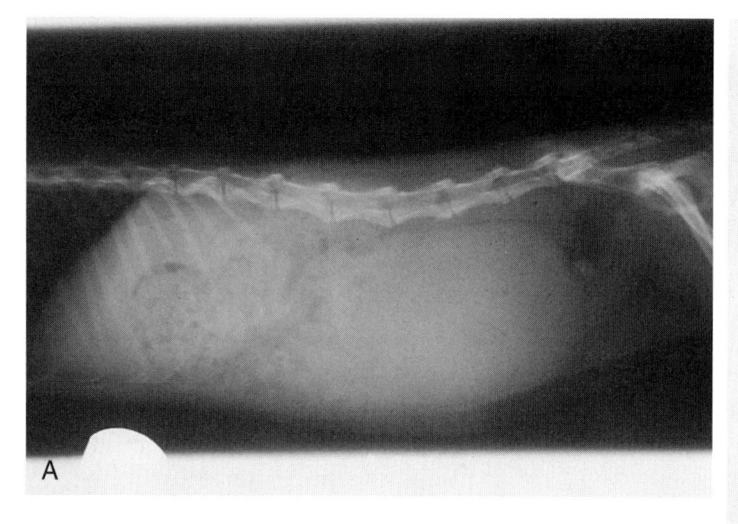

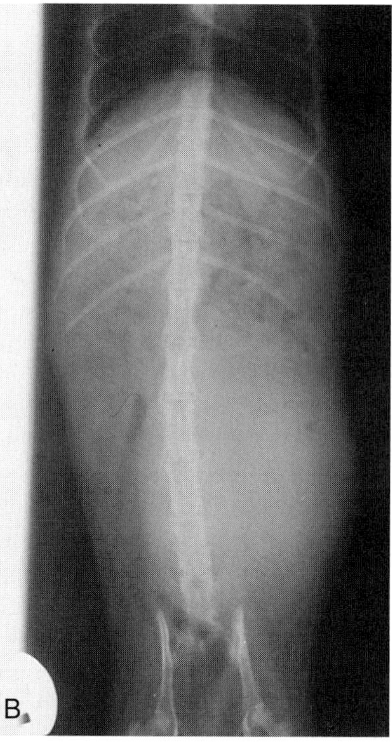

FIGURE 5–2
Abdominal radiographs showing a hydronephrotic kidney (*A*, lateral projection; *B*, ventrodorsal projection). This 2-year-old spayed female ferret did well after unilateral nephrectomy. Hydronephrosis occurred secondary to inadvertent ligation of a ureter during ovariohysterectomy.

neys, all uncommon to rare in pet ferrets from a clinician's perspective, include pyelonephritis, chronic interstitial nephritis, glomerulonephropathy secondary to Aleutian disease or other causes, and neoplasia. Primary renal neoplasia is rare; a renal pelvic transitional cell carcinoma has been reported in one ferret,[3] and a renal carcinoma in another (see Chapter 10). Lymphoma can occasionally involve the kidneys.

Diagnosis and Treatment

The approach to the diagnosis and treatment of renal disease in ferrets is the same as for other companion animal species. Clinical signs of renal disease in ferrets can include depression, lethargy, inappetence, weight loss, oral ulcers, polyuria and polydipsia, melena, and rear leg weakness. Findings on physical examination can include cachexia, dehydration, and pallor. Palpate the kidneys carefully to evaluate kidney size and to feel for irregularities. Perform a CBC, serum chemistry workup, and urinalysis. Microscopic evaluation of urine sediment may be helpful in characterizing renal disease. Abdominal radiographs may show disparity in the size of the kidneys, and abdominal ultrasound can be used to evaluate renal architecture. Pyelography is useful as an evaluation of renal function.

Results of a CBC may show nonregenerative anemia in ferrets with advanced renal disease. Normal urine specific gravity has not been reported for ferrets; however, isosthenuria in conjunction with dehydration is suspicious for renal dysfunction.

Interpretation of serum chemistry results is somewhat unusual in ferrets with renal disease. Preliminary findings at several veterinary hospitals suggest a species-specific feature—namely, elevation of serum creatinine does not parallel elevation of blood urea nitrogen (BUN) in ferrets with renal failure. Kawasaki[12] described two ferrets with histopathologically confirmed severe renal disease; both ferrets had a creatinine level of 1.1 mg/dL in conjunction with BUN values of 140 and 320 mg/dL, respectively (urine specific gravity was not reported). In an informal survey of other clinicians, the consensus is that BUN levels rise quite high in renal failure; however, creatinine elevations are relatively modest (less than 2–3 mg/dL).

There are two possible explanations for this phenomenon.[8] The reported normal mean creatinine level (0.4–0.6 mg/dL) is lower and the range for creatinine level (0.2–0.9 mg/dL) is narrower in ferrets than in dogs and cats.[9, 14, 26] Therefore, an elevation in creatinine level for a ferret may be substantially lower than that in a dog or cat. Alternatively, other mechanisms, such as renal tubular secretion or enteric degradation, may play a relatively larger role in creatinine excretion in ferrets than in other species.

Other serum chemistry abnormalities seen in ferrets with renal disease include hyperphosphatemia, hypocalcemia, and reduced total carbon dioxide.

Endogenous creatinine, exogenous creatinine, and inulin clearance tests have been used for evaluating glomerular filtration rate in ferrets. Mean 24-hour endogenous creatinine clearance was 2.55 mL/min per kilogram in 26 healthy ferrets (24 female, 2 male) aged 9 months to 7 years.[8] In the same study, the mean exogenous creatinine clearance was 3.32 and the mean inulin clearance 3.02 mL/min per kilogram in 12 female ferrets. The mean inulin clearance was significantly higher for 1-year-old ferrets (3.65 mL/min per kilogram) than for ferrets aged 4 to 6 years (2.29 mL/min per kilogram).

If you confirm renal disease, try to identify the cause with ultrasound and, if necessary, ultrasound-guided renal biopsy (as for cats). Treatment should be aimed at the primary cause.

Other treatment for ferrets with renal disease includes fluid therapy, supportive care, and treatment with an antibiotic if infection is suspected or documented. Select the antibiotic on the basis of culture and sensitivity results, when available, and on its pharmacologic properties—most importantly, tissue distribution, route of excretion, and safety in renal failure. Follow basic guidelines for treatment of renal failure in dogs and cats. The prognosis for ferrets with renal failure depends on laboratory findings and response to therapy.

UROLITHIASIS

Urolithiasis in ferrets can be characterized by solitary or multiple renal or cystic calculi or by the presence of sandy material in the bladder and urethra. Magnesium ammonium phosphate (struvite) uroliths are most common, and urinary tract infection may or may not be present concurrently. Other types of uroliths occur rarely in ferrets; however, this discussion focuses primarily on struvite urolithiasis. See Chapter 6 for a discussion of struvite urolithiasis in pregnant jills.

Although the cause of struvite urolithiasis in ferrets is unknown, several features of the disease suggest that dietary factors play a role in its pathogenesis. In my experience, affected ferrets have been fed dog food or a low-quality cat food. Urolithiasis is rare in ferrets fed a high-quality feline diet containing protein from animal sources. Moreover, urolithiasis seems to be less common in ferrets now than when I first began working with them. The diets offered to pet ferrets also have improved over this time, with higher protein and more meat-based protein diets being available.

Struvite tends to precipitate in alkaline urine; its solubility increases greatly when urine pH is 6.6 or less.[22] In turn, urine pH is greatly influenced by diet—specifically the source of protein in the diet. Metabolism of a diet containing animal protein tends to produce an acidic urine, whereas that of a diet containing plant protein tends to produce an alkaline urine, which promotes struvite crystallization. The normal reported range for urine pH in ferrets is 6.5 to 7.5.[27] However, like that in dogs and cats, urine pH in ferrets can vary according to diet. The normal urine pH should be approximately 6.0 in ferrets on a high-quality, meat-based diet.*

Although the nutritional requirements of ferrets have not been fully determined, it seems likely that poor-quality, plant protein–based diets may predispose to urolithiasis.[2] In one report, 6 of 43 (14%) ferrets necropsied had renal or cystic calculi.[20] Interestingly, these ferrets were maintained on a commercial pelleted dog food diet (source of protein not specified), an inappropriate diet for ferrets because of its insufficient protein content.

Other factors that may predispose to the formation of struvite uroliths include infection with urease-producing bacteria, particularly *Staphylococcus* and *Proteus* species, and metabolic or genetic factors.

Diagnosis

Clinical signs of urolithiasis in ferrets are similar to those in dogs and cats and include dysuria, frequent urination, wet fur in the perineal area, frequent licking of the perineum, urine dribbling, and hematuria. Ferrets with urethral obstruction may strain violently or cry when attempting to urinate. Occasion-

*Bell J: Personal communication, 1995.

ally, a ferret with blockage presents with lethargy and inappetence without having shown obvious signs of being unable to urinate. If not corrected, urinary obstruction can result in severe metabolic disturbances, coma, and death. Urethral obstruction is most common in male ferrets; however, females also can become obstructed.

The diagnosis of urolithiasis is often made on the basis of findings on physical examination. Cystic calculi and sand are usually palpable in ferrets without obstruction, whereas a distended bladder is readily palpable in obstructed ferrets. Obtain a complete history, including dietary history, from the owner.

Abdominal radiographs are the most important diagnostic tool, both for evaluating the entire urinary tract for uroliths (struvite calculi are radiodense) and for ruling out other possible causes of urinary obstruction, the most important of which are prostatic cysts and abscess. Calculi lodged at the os penis in male ferrets can be difficult to detect. An abdominal ultrasound may be helpful in delineating and identifying any abnormal structures, including radiolucent calculi, which may occur. Perform a packed cell volume (PCV) and rapid test for BUN (Azostix, Miles, Inc., Shawnee, KS) or, ideally, a full CBC and serum chemistry workup to evaluate the ferret's metabolic status. If the ferret does not have urethral obstruction, obtain a urine sample for a urinalysis and urine culture by cystocentesis.

Treatment

Parenteral fluid therapy and supportive care are important for ferrets with urolithiasis, whether or not they have a urethral obstruction. Correct metabolic and acid-base disturbances. Begin antibiotic therapy if you suspect infection, which is more common in females than in males, and after surgical removal of calculi. When possible, base your choice of antibiotic on the results of culture and sensitivity testing. Choose a broad-spectrum antibiotic that reaches high levels in the urinary tract, such as amoxicillin, a trimethoprim-sulfa combination, or enrofloxacin.

If the ferret does not have urethral obstruction, surgical removal of cystic calculi should be scheduled when the ferret is stable. Renal calculi can often be managed medically with changes in diet (i.e., to a meat protein–based diet; see later in this chapter) and the use of antibiotics; however, surgical removal may be necessary, depending on the clinical signs.

Treatment of urinary obstruction in male ferrets often is a challenge because a urinary catheter can be very difficult to pass in males (see Chapter 2), particularly when they have urethral obstruction. Moreover, the opening of the urethra may be difficult (or impossible in some ferrets with blockage) to visualize. Female ferrets are easier to catheterize (see Chapter 2). In one study, a technique that involves the use of a 3.5-French red rubber urinary catheter has been described for urinary catheterization of ferrets.[16] However, only two male ferrets were used in this study; they did not have urethral obstruction, and the opening of the urethra was located by expressing urine from the bladder (impossible in blocked ferrets). When attempting urinary catheterization, place the ferret under isoflurane anesthesia to obtain skeletal muscle relaxation. If isoflurane is not available, administer halothane or an injectable sedative, preferably avoiding or using with great caution ketamine and tiletamine hydrochloride, both of which are excreted by the kidneys.

If attempts at urinary catheterization are unsuccessful, two alternatives remain: emergency cystotomy with anterograde flushing of the urethra, or cystocentesis for decompression of the bladder followed by further attempts to flush the urethra. To decompress the bladder by cystocentesis, use a 22- to 25-gauge needle and, as for cats, remove most but not all of the urine, leaving some urine to protect against needle trauma.[21] Even cystocentesis can be difficult in some ferrets with sludgy, turbid urine. Submit urine for urinalysis and culture and sensitivity testing. Then, place a catheter inside the prepuce and pinch the prepuce firmly closed as you flush. In theory, the urethra is the path of least resistance for the fluid, and it may be possible to flush calculi retrograde into the bladder in this manner.* Alternatively, pass a feline metal urinary catheterization needle or other catheter as far as you can into the distal urethra and flush from there.

An emergency cystotomy is often the most expeditious and effective alternative to urinary catheterization (see Chapter 13). In rare instances, blockage is so severe that anterograde flushing of the urethra via the cystotomy is not possible; in such cases, an emergency perineal urethrostomy is necessary. In

---

*Jenkins J: Personal communication, 1995.

addition to submitting a calculus for stone analysis, submit crushed calculi and a piece of bladder mucosa for culture and sensitivity testing.

Long-term management of urolithiasis involves antibiotic therapy for 10 to 14 days (or longer, depending on the results of urinalyses and repeat urine culture and sensitivity tests) and gradual conversion of the ferret to an animal protein–based diet. Urinary acidifiers are usually not necessary if the ferret receives a high-quality, meat-based diet because the urine pH of a ferret on such a diet is about 6.0. Addition of phosphoric acid (H_3PO_4) to a diet at a level of 0.9% (dry matter basis) phosphorus and 0.6% calcium increased urine volume and maintained urine pH at a mean of 6.02–6.11 in a group of six male ferrets, creating conditions favorable for preventing the formation of or for dissolving struvite calculi.[7] However, this kind of dietary adjustment is impractical in clinical practice.

Medical management of cystic calculi has been attempted infrequently and has not been successful in ferrets, in part because the struvite-dissolving diet (Prescription Diet Feline s/d, Hill's Pet Products, Topeka, KS) is not palatable for some ferrets and contains insufficient protein for this species.

Consider a perineal urethrostomy for male ferrets with persistent problems (see Chapter 13). Fortunately, recurrence of urolithiasis is uncommon after successful therapy and management changes.

CYSTITIS

Cystitis without urolithiasis is uncommon in ferrets. Clinical signs can include pollakiuria, dysuria, crying with urination, urine staining of the perineum, and hematuria. The bladder wall may feel thickened on palpation. Perform a cystocentesis to obtain urine for urinalysis and culture and sensitivity testing. Consider a CBC and serum chemistry workup, particularly if the ferret is older than the age of 3 years or if it shows systemic signs of illness. Abdominal radiographs and ultrasound may be indicated for ruling out renal involvement and other causes of dysuria, including urolithiasis, bladder neoplasia, the presence of an abdominal mass, or prostatic enlargement in males.

Treat the ferret with a broad-spectrum antibiotic until the culture results are back; then, adjust the antibiotic therapy accordingly and continue it for a minimum of 2 weeks, as indicated on the basis of results of urinalyses and repeat urine cultures. Administer fluid therapy and supportive care as necessary and be sure that the ferret is receiving a high-quality, meat protein–based diet (as for ferrets with urolithiasis).

TESTICULAR NEOPLASIA

Both interstitial cell and Sertoli cell tumors have been found in ferrets. These tumors cause enlargement of the affected testicle. Although not reported in ferrets,[18] feminization or androgenization can occur with these tumors in other species. I have treated one ferret with Sertoli cell tumor that had total body alopecia and severe pruritus, presumably secondary to hyperestrogenism. Castration is curative.

PROSTATIC DISEASES

Ferrets can develop sterile or infected prostatic cysts in association with adrenal disease. Prostatic abscesses have also been reported in association with transitional cell tumor of the bladder.[5] Neither of these conditions is common; however, prostatic enlargement causes urethral obstruction more commonly than does urolithiasis. Histologically, prostatic cysts appear as large keratin-filled cysts resulting from squamous metaplasia of prostatic glands. The cysts impinge on the urethra, causing urethral obstruction, which is the most common presenting sign.

Perform a full medical workup in these ferrets, remembering that adrenal disease is usually the primary disease (see Chapter 9). On abdominal radiographs, prostatic enlargement may appear as a mass dorsal to the urinary bladder and displacing the bladder ventrally. Ultrasound is usually needed for confirmation of the diagnosis and examination of the architecture of the prostate.

Treatment involves management of urethral obstruction and adrenalectomy when adrenal disease is present (also see Chapter 13). Simple cystic hypertrophy of the prostate shrinks within days after removal of a hormone-producing adrenal tumor. Grossly enlarged or infected prostates may require surgical debulking or drainage or, at the worst, marsupialization. Perform culture and sensitivity testing on infected tissue. Provide postoperative supportive care and antibiotics as necessary.

ESTROGEN TOXICITY

Fortunately, estrogen toxicity has become uncommon since the large ferret breeding farms began to spay ferrets routinely before sale. Female ferrets are induced ovulators, and roughly one half of estrous females remain in estrus (during which time estrogen levels are high) if they are not bred or artificially stimulated to ovulate. Ferrets, like dogs, are very susceptible to estrogen-induced toxicity of hematopoietic tissue. In one study, 8 of 20 nonbred estrous females remained in estrus and subsequently died or were euthanized because of bone marrow hypoplasia caused by hyperestrogenism.[25] The first deaths occurred about 2 months after and the last death about 6 months after the onset of estrus. The 12 remaining ferrets went into anestrus. In spayed females, an estrogen-secreting ovarian remnant or adrenal tumor can also be associated with estrogen toxicity, the latter rarely and typically after long-standing disease has remained untreated.

Hematologic findings in ferrets during prolonged estrus consist of an initial thrombocytosis and neutrophilia followed by thrombocytopenia, neutropenia, eosinopenia, and normocytic normochromic or macrocytic hypochromic anemia.[25] Lymphopenia was noted in one study[25] but not in another.[13] Hemorrhage secondary to thrombocytopenia is usually the cause of death. Infections may occur secondary to granulocytopenia. Gross findings at necropsy include pale tissues, light red–to–pale pink bone marrow, and hemorrhages in the skin, buccal mucosa, gastrointestinal tract, abdominal organs, and, occasionally, under the dura. Histopathologic findings include bone marrow hypoplasia affecting all cell lines, decreased splenic extramedullary hematopoiesis, mild-to-moderate hepatic centrilobular fatty degeneration, and hemosiderosis in multiple organs.[25]

Diagnosis

Prominent vulvar enlargement is an external indication of estrus in ferrets. Although rarely necessary for evaluation because a swollen vulva is such an obvious marker of estrus, vaginal cytology has been described for domestic ferrets.[28] Cytologic samples were collected by vaginal lavage. Blunted pipette tips were introduced approximately 1.0–1.5 cm into the vagina until meeting slight resistance; then, 0.05–0.1 mL of sterile physiologic saline was flushed and aspirated several times. During proestrus, which lasted 2–3 weeks, the percentage of superficial epithelial cells increased as the vulva began to enlarge; however, there was no clear marker for the start of proestrus. Superficial cells constituted more than 90% of cells during estrus. These cells were mostly keratinized and anucleate after days 4 to 6 of estrus. During anestrus, superficial cells constituted up to 30% of cells and were mostly intermediate and superficial-intermediate cells. Neutrophils were common during all stages of the estrous cycle. However, bacteria were uncommon except during estrus, when they were seen in association with superficial cells. Vaginal cytologic findings in females in prolonged estrus was characterized by numerous bacteria, neutrophils, cellular debris, and some erythrocytes.

Any ferret in estrus for longer than 1 month is at risk for developing hyperestrogenism. Early in the course of disease, affected ferrets have a swollen vulva, thrombocytosis, and neutrophilia. Anemia develops gradually; therefore, ferrets initially tend to compensate for the reduced red blood cell volume, and clinical signs may be subtle until disease becomes advanced. The onset of estrogen toxicity associated with an adrenal tumor, when it occurs, appears to be much slower, often occurring over 1–2 years.

Clinical signs and physical findings in ferrets with advanced hyperestrogenism include swollen vulva, vulvar discharge, depression, inappetence, weakness, pale mucous membranes, soft systolic murmur, subcutaneous and mucosal petechiae or ecchymoses, melena, and bilaterally symmetric thinning or loss of hair on the hindquarters or trunk (Fig. 5–3). Neurologic signs can occur in ferrets with subdural hemorrhages. Some animals may develop hydrometra or pyometra.[4]

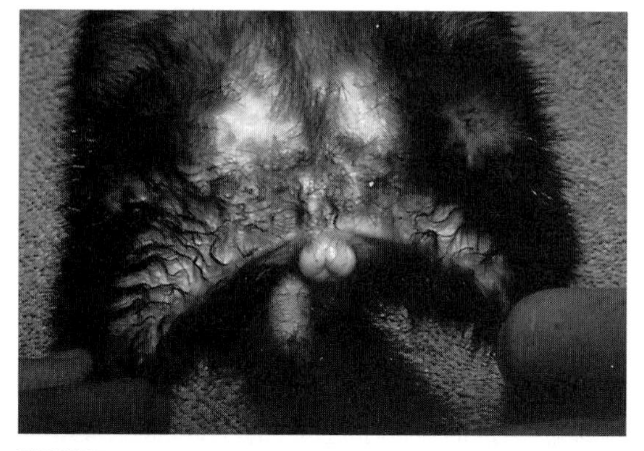

FIGURE 5–3
Caudoventral abdomen of a ferret with hyperestrogenism. Note the swollen vulva, ecchymoses in the skin, and hair loss on the tail.

At a minimum, obtain a CBC and a platelet count if you suspect hyperestrogenism. Thrombocytosis and neutrophilia may be evident at the onset of bone marrow suppression and are followed by a decrease in the number of platelets and other peripheral blood cells.

Treatment

The goal of treatment is to bring the ferret out of estrus and provide supportive care until the bone marrow again becomes functional (this can take days to weeks). The ideal and definitive method for terminating estrus is ovariohysterectomy; however, many affected ferrets are too anemic and thrombocytopenic to withstand surgery. Hormonal stimulation of ovulation is almost equally effective. Use 100 IU (or 1000 USP units) of human chorionic gonadotropin (hCG) IM; repeat the dose 1 week later if vulvar swelling has not begun to regress within 3 or 4 days. Alternatively, give gonadotropin-releasing hormone (GnRH) at a dose of 20 μg IM or SC; repeat administration 1–2 weeks later if necessary.

Perform an ovariohysterectomy when you believe that the ferret is stable, ideally when anemia and thrombocytopenia have resolved. If surgery becomes necessary before this time, administer a fresh ferret blood transfusion immediately preoperatively to provide fresh platelets.

In spayed females showing signs consistent with estrogen toxicity, the medical workup consists of a search for a remnant ovary (most common) or adrenal tumor (see Chapter 9). Hormonal stimulation of ovulation from an ovarian remnant may be effective and, therefore, can be used to distinguish between this condition and an estrogen-producing adrenal tumor. An abdominal exploratory surgery may be necessary for a definitive diagnosis.

Supportive care includes fluid therapy, hand-feeding, iron and B vitamin supplementation, and a broad-spectrum antibiotic for the prevention of secondary infection. The ferret should be confined to a cage to reduce the possibility of trauma and subsequent hemorrhage. Administer fresh ferret blood transfusions as indicated by the status of the patient and the PCV. Ferrets can receive up to three (and probably more) transfusions from the same donor because no blood groups have been identified in this species.[15]

Therapy and prognosis for ferrets with hyperestrogenism can be estimated and categorized on the basis of the ferret's PCV on presentation. If the PCV is more than 25%, the prognosis is good and termination of estrus is usually the only treatment required. If the PCV is 15–25%, the prognosis is guarded because the PCV typically decreases further after termination of estrus. If the PCV is less than 15%, then the prognosis is poor, and aggressive supportive care is indicated, including multiple blood transfusions until bone marrow function is restored. Ryland[23] described successful treatment of a ferret with estrus-associated anemia. This ferret presented with a PCV of 7%. Treatment included ovariohysterectomy, supportive care, and 13 blood transfusions over a 5-month period.

Prevention of estrogen toxicity caused by persistent estrus is with routine spaying of all female ferrets not intended for breeding. Hormonal stimulation of ovulation with hCG or GnRH can be used for females that are to be bred at a later date. However, hormonal methods are not effective until a ferret has been in estrus for at least 10 days, a second injection may be necessary, and not all ferrets will ovulate. In one study, 95% of estrous females (n = 152; day of estrus not defined) ovulated after administration of a single dose of 100 IU hCG given intraperitoneally.[17] Be sure to confirm that vulvar swelling regresses after you administer hCG or GnRH. Theoretically, another method for stimulating ovulation without fertilization is breeding estrous females with a vasectomized male.[24]

PYOMETRA

Pyometra is uncommon in clinical practice because most female pet ferrets are spayed. The diagnosis and management of pyometra are the same as for dogs and cats. Surgical removal (ovariohysterectomy) is the treatment of choice (also see section on metritis in Chapter 6). Occasionally, a ferret with adrenal disease develops a stump pyometra. Treatment of this condition involves adrenalectomy and surgical excision of the infected stump, along with appropriate antibiotic therapy and supportive care (see Chapter 13).

REFERENCES

1. Andrews PLR, Illman O, Mellersh A: Some observations of anatomical abnormalities and disease states in a population of 350 ferrets *(Mustela furo L.)*. Z Versuchstierkd 1979; 21:346–353.
2. Bell J: Management of urinary obstruction in the ferret. Proceedings of the North American Veterinary Conference, Orlando, January 1993.
3. Bell RC, Moeller RB: Transitional cell carcinoma of

the renal pelvis in a ferret. Lab Anim Sci 1990; 40:537–538.
4. Bernard SL, Leathers CW, Brobst DF, Gorham JR: Estrogen induced bone marrow depression in ferrets. Am J Vet Res 1983; 44:657–661.
5. Brown SA: Ferrets. *In* A Practitioner's Guide to Rabbits and Ferrets. Denver, The American Animal Hospital Association, 1993, pp 43–111.
6. Dillberger JE: Polycystic kidneys in a ferret. J Am Vet Med Assoc 1985; 186:74–75.
7. Edfors CH, Ullrey DE, Aulerich RJ: Prevention of urolithiasis in the ferret *(Mustela putorius furo)* with phosphoric acid. J Zoo Wildl Med 1989; 20:12–19.
8. Esteves MI, Marini RP, Ryden EB, et al.: Estimation of glomerular filtration rate and evaluation of renal function in ferrets *(Mustela putorius furo)*. Am J Vet Res 1994; 55:166–172.
9. Fox JG: Normal clinical and biologic parameters. *In* Fox JG, ed.: Biology and Diseases of the Ferret. Philadelphia, Lea & Febiger, 1988, pp 159–173.
10. Fox JG: Systemic diseases. *In* Fox JG, ed.: Biology and Diseases of the Ferret. Philadelphia, Lea & Febiger, 1988, pp 255–273.
11. Gabow PA: Cystic disease of the kidney. *In* Wyngaarden JB, Smith LH, Bennett JC, eds.: Cecil Textbook of Medicine. 19th ed. Philadelphia, WB Saunders, 1992, pp 608–612.
12. Kawasaki TA: Normal parameters and laboratory interpretation of disease states in the domestic ferret. Semin Avian Exotic Pet Med 1994; 3:40–47.
13. Kociba GJ, Caputo CA: Aplastic anemia associated with estrus in pet ferrets. J Am Vet Med Assoc 1981; 178:1293–1294.
14. Lee EJ, Moore WE, Fryer HC, Minocha HC: Haematological and serum chemistry profiles of ferrets *(Mustela putorius furo)*. Lab Anim 1982; 16:133–137.
15. Manning DD, Bell JA: Lack of detectable blood groups in domestic ferrets: implications for transfusion. J Am Vet Med Assoc 1990; 197:84–86.
16. Marini RP, Esteves MI, Fox JG: A technique for catheterization of the urinary bladder in the ferret. Lab Anim 1994; 28:155–157.
17. Mead RA, Joseph MM, Neirinckx S: Optimal dose of human chorionic gonadotropin for inducing ovulation in the ferret. Zoo Biol 1988; 7:263–267.
18. Meschter CL: Interstitial cell adenoma in a ferret. Lab Anim Sci 1989; 39:353–354.
19. Nelson WB: Hydronephrosis in a ferret. Vet Med 1984; 79:516–521.
20. Nguyen HT, Moreland AF, Shields RP: Urolithiasis in ferrets *(Mustela putorius)*. Lab Anim Sci 1979; 29: 243–245.
21. Osborne CA, Kruger JM, Lulich JP, Polzin DJ: Feline lower urinary tract diseases. *In* Ettinger SJ, Feldman EC, eds.: Textbook of Veterinary Internal Medicine. 4th ed. Philadelphia, WB Saunders, 1995, pp 1805–1832.
22. Rich LJ, Kirk RW: The relationship of struvite crystals to urethral obstruction in cats. J Am Vet Med Assoc 1969; 154:153–157.
23. Ryland LM: Remission of estrus-associated anemia following ovariohysterectomy and multiple blood transfusions in a ferret. J Am Vet Med Assoc 1982; 181:820–822.
24. Ryland LM, Lipinski E: A technique for vasectomizing male ferrets. Canine Pract 1994; 19:25–27.
25. Sherrill A, Gorham J: Bone marrow hypoplasia associated with estrus in ferrets. Lab Anim Sci 1985; 35:280–286.
26. Thornton PC, Wright PA, Sacra PJ, Goodier TEW: The ferret, *Mustela putorius furo,* as a new species in toxicology. Lab Anim 1979; 13:119–124.
27. Williams CF: Ferret. *In* Practical Guide to Laboratory Animals. St. Louis, CV Mosby, 1976, pp 65–71.
28. Williams ES, Thorne ET, Kwiatkowski DR, et al.: Comparative vaginal cytology of the estrous cycle of black-footed ferrets *(Mustela nigripes),* Siberian polecats *(M. eversmanni),* and domestic ferrets *(M. putorius furo)*. J Vet Diagn Invest 1992; 4:38–44.

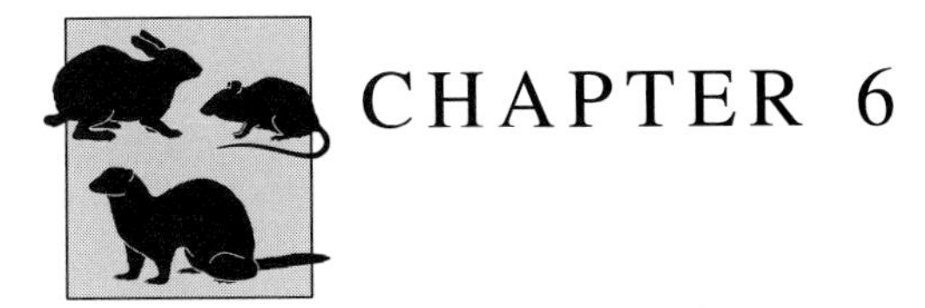

CHAPTER 6

Periparturient and Neonatal Diseases

Judith A. Bell, DVM, PhD

Well-fed and well-managed jills give birth to litters of 8–10 kits and lose about 1 kit per litter before weaning. Greater losses may stem from problems that begin before breeding and can be prevented with proper nutrition, housing, and management. Pregnancy toxemia, urolithiasis in pregnant jills, lactation failure, low conception rate, and small litter size mainly result from inadequate nutrition and management and can be virtually eliminated by improvements in diet, care, housing, and breeding techniques. Dystocia, mastitis, metritis, and neonatal kit diseases may also be reduced with improvement of management practices; however, because many variables are involved, a low frequency of these problems can be expected in any group of breeding ferrets.

GENERAL PRINCIPLES

Nutrition for Breeding Ferrets

The most important single factor in keeping any ferret healthy is nutrition. Feed male and female kits intended for breeding the highest quality diet available at weaning and throughout their entire productive life. Select a ration containing 35–40% protein and 18–20% fat, with meat listed as the first ingredient. Jills come in heat for the first time at 4 months of age if they are exposed to light for longer than 12 hours per day. If bred at this age, they must have an excellent diet that enables them to sustain both growth and pregnancy.

There are several serious sequelae to feeding an inadequate diet to breeding ferrets. Multiparous jills fed poor-quality cat foods have small litters, and primiparous jills on such diets are very susceptible to pregnancy toxemia. Failure to conceive or, more commonly, small litter size can be the result of several factors, including poor nutrition. Primiparous jills should have at least eight kits. Smaller litters result from the use of a hob of low fertility, breeding at the wrong time or only once during estrus, breeding of a jill and hob of an unusual color phase that carry lethal recessive genes, and the feeding of an inadequate diet. If the diet does not contain at least 35% protein and 15% fat, suggest that the owner use a higher plane of nutrition for both the jill and hob as the first step in improving production.

The first ingredient in a diet suitable for ferrets should be meat or poultry meal. Food products vary in quality and may have a high proportion of bone and indigestible tissue. The price of the food is a good indicator of its protein quality. Some older ferrets refuse to change to a different diet; offer them a smorgasbord of premium cat and ferret foods so that they can make their own selection. Some foods labeled as ferret diets were developed from commercial mink rations. They contain poorly processed fish that is unpalatable to ferrets that have not been raised on them. Although fish is a natural diet for mink, it is not for ferrets. They prefer chicken or other meats, which are the usual ingredients in premium cat foods and diets formulated specifically for ferrets. Mink rations, premium cat foods, and high-quality ferret diets all can provide more than adequate nutrition for breeding ferrets; however, if a jill refuses to eat the diet, it obviously has no nutritional value for her.

Increase dietary fat levels to 30% for lactating jills 2–3 weeks post partum if the litter is of normal size. Even if they are provided with a concentrated meat-based diet, lactating jills become thin if they feed litters of more than 10 kits. Moreover, if bred on every estrous cycle, jills fed very high-calorie diets between litters do not become fat enough to have obesity-related reproductive problems.

Management for Breeding Ferrets

Place a pregnant jill's cage in a quiet area well before parturition. This is particularly important for primiparous jills, which are more likely to settle down and care for their kits if they are not disturbed. A plastic dishpan with rolled edges makes a good nest box. Place the dishpan directly inside the cage or, ideally, drop it through an opening in the cage bottom so that the upper edge of the pan is level with the cage floor. The jill must be able to easily enter and exit the nesting box without risking trauma to the mammary glands. The kits should not be able to climb out of the nesting box. Shredded aspen or corn husks make good bedding for whelping nests. In small breeding operations, small terry cloth towels are a practical alternative for bedding material. Do not use large terry towels because kits can get lost in them. Also, avoid using coarse wood shavings and shredded newspaper (the latter clumps in a solid mass when wet).

For the jill's comfort, the room temperature should be lower than 21.1°C (70°F). Place a heat lamp over part of the nesting box so that the jill and kits can select warmth as necessary. Be sure that food and water are readily accessible to the jill so that she can eat and drink without leaving the kits. Place a clip-on food dish and a water bottle on the edge of the nest box so that the jill can eat and drink even while lying down.

Breeding Pet Ferrets

Discourage owners of single ferrets from trying to raise a litter from their pets unless they are prepared to devote most of their time for several weeks to observation and care of the periparturient jill. Breeding ferrets and raising kits successfully requires constant supervision during gestation, parturition, and lactation; if not prevented or promptly treated, unattended problems can lead to fatality.

PROBLEMS OF PERIPARTURIENT JILLS

Pregnancy Toxemia

Pregnancy toxemia is a life-threatening disease caused by negative energy balance in late gestation. It is most common in primiparous jills carrying average litters and fed an adequate diet when an accidental fast occurs during the last week of gestation. This sometimes happens when owners try to replace the normal ration with a higher quality diet that the jills refuse to eat. Occasionally, pregnancy toxemia occurs in well-fed primiparous jills that conceive 15 or more kits. In the presence of this many fetuses, nourishment of the dam and kits is compromised because there is barely room in the abdomen for both the gravid uterus and a sufficient quantity of even a concentrated diet.

Warn owners to guard against accidental fasts during pregnancy. Owners must make palatable food and water available 24 hours a day. Provide both a bottle and a dish of water. Most jills prefer to drink from a dish and use the bottle secondarily. Ferrets drink about threefold the volume of water that they eat of dry pellets, and when deprived of water they soon stop eating. Even one overnight fast can induce toxemia in a jill with a large litter. Owners should place several small food dishes in the cage so that accidental spillage or contamination does not restrict the jill's intake at this critical time. Most ferrets are tenderly cared for by their owners, but it is essential to emphasize the importance of providing constant access to an excellent diet during late gestation. Recommend that owners provide high-calorie nutritional supplements such as Nutri-Cal (EVSCO Pharmaceuticals, Buena, NJ) or Ensure Plus (Abbott Laboratories, Ross Products Division, Columbus, OH) to jills that appear to be carrying very large litters.

Pregnancy toxemia should be suspected in a jill that suddenly becomes lethargic just before her due date. Question the owner about the ration and its availability and about any recent changes in the food or feeding schedule. A toxemic jill is dehydrated, feels "doughy," and may have black, tarry stools. If the jill is severely dehydrated, the outline of the uterus and, sometimes, the individual kits can be seen on her abdomen. Her hair falls out in handfuls, her blood glucose may be very low (<50 mg/dL), and she may be ketonuric and azotemic. A toxemic jill is cold but does not attempt to curl up or crawl into a warm spot. Instead, she lies flat on her abdomen with open, glazed eyes. The prognosis for such an animal is poor, even if she is given excellent care.

An immediate cesarean section is necessary if the life of the jill is to be saved, but success of the procedure depends on the extent of liver damage. During surgery, use gas anesthesia, and, if possible, administer IV fluids containing glucose. Some jills are so dehydrated that catheter insertion is very difficult, but SC fluids are well absorbed if the jill is warm. If IV glucose is not given, offer or force-feed a preanesthetic dose of oral glucose or a high-calorie supplement. These jills must be kept warm; however, because ferrets are so susceptible to heat prostration, the use of a heating pad during or after surgery is risky. During surgery, place the jill on a circulating warm water heating pad or a warmed terry cloth towel.

Perform the cesarean section as quickly as possible. A midline incision gives best access to both uterine horns. Rapidly remove all kits through an incision made midway along each horn.

Postsurgical care includes frequent force-feeding of small amounts of high-calorie supplements and maintaining hydration as well as keeping the jill warm and comfortable. Position the heat source so that the jill can move away from the heat when she wants. Toxemic ferrets usually do not make the effort to climb over or out of anything, even when fully conscious. Continue intensive care as long as the jill looks lethargic and until she begins to eat significant quantities on her own. Offer her favorite food (softened with warm water if she prefers it) at frequent intervals and allow free access to drinking water at all times. Sometimes, the owner is better able than veterinary hospital staff to care for a ferret on a continuous basis. The jill can be seen twice daily by someone who can assess hydration, determine blood glucose level (if desired), and administer parenteral fluids when required. The first 24 hours after surgery are critical, and ferrets that survive this period usually recover. Those that die have clay-colored fatty livers and are anemic; they may also have gastritis or gastric ulcers.

If the kits have no foster mother or if they are born at less than 40 days' gestation, they are best euthanized because hand-rearing ferret kits from birth is extremely difficult.[2] The toxemic jill will have no milk, even if she survives.

Struvite Urolithiasis in Pregnant Jills

In a large colony, 5–10% of pregnant jills on a diet containing mainly plant protein will develop struvite bladder stones. Pregnant jills are particularly susceptible to urolithiasis because they constantly mobilize minerals; however, any ferret on a diet having ground yellow corn as its primary ingredient can develop this life-threatening problem. Magnesium ammonium phosphate (struvite) crystallizes when urine pH rises above 6.4. The mineral content of the food is not as important a consideration as the protein source when a diet to prevent urolithiasis is chosen. Ferrets are obligate carnivores with a normal urine pH of about 6. Metabolism of cystine and methionine in animal proteins produces an acid urine, whereas metabolism of the organic acids in plant protein produces an alkaline urine that promotes struvite crystallization. Moreover, when the pH is from 6 to 7, stones form to some extent in the pregnant ferret on a corn-based diet but not in one on a meat-based diet.[1]

Jills are not as likely as hobs to develop complete urinary obstructions. However, straining eventually causes rectal or vaginal prolapse (or both), which may lead to self-mutilation and severe, possibly fatal hemorrhage. When a jill in the last trimester of gestation or the first week of lactation presents with straining, carefully palpate for stones, which are often large and usually easy to feel (Fig. 6–1). If necessary, use radiography to confirm the diagnosis. When urolithiasis is diagnosed, undertake preparation for a cystotomy as soon as possible (see also Chapter 13). A cesarean section is performed before the cystotomy if the jill is due within 24 hours; this prevents the jill from putting strain on the fresh suture line while giving birth to the kits. Jills that receive good postoperative care will nurse their kits normally.

Although gas anesthetics are ideal for use in uremic animals, IM ketamine (35 mg/kg) with xylazine (5 mg/kg), reversed with IV yohimbine (0.11 mg/kg) after surgery, is also safe for both the jill and the unborn kits. Start IV or SC fluid administration before surgery.

The bladder is palpable and often visible in the lower abdomen when the jill is anesthetized. Carefully make an incision directly over the largest part of the bladder, allowing it to be pulled through the incision, folded back to expose its dorsal surface, and packed off. The bladder wall is often very thick and vascular. Make an incision in a relatively avascular area, and, after removing the stones from the bladder, make a careful search for smaller stones far down in the urethra that may have caused the observed tenesmus. If these are not removed, the jill will strain violently as she recovers from anesthesia and may tear her sutures. After all stones are removed, swab the bladder mucosa for culture and sensitivity testing, then flush the bladder with an acidifying solution (e.g., saline) to remove mucus, blood, and "sand" before closure. Close the bladder with two rows of 5–0 sutures placed as close as possible to the wound edges in a continuous Cushing pattern. Even very thick bladder walls close well when this technique is used.

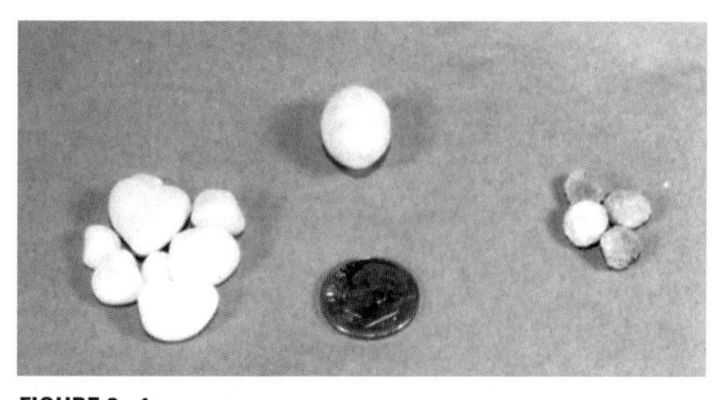

FIGURE 6–1
Struvite uroliths surgically removed from three pregnant ferrets that were fed a poor-quality diet.

Administration of flunixin (Banamine, Schering-Plough Animal Health Corporation, Kenilworth, NJ) at 2.5 mg (0.05 mL) IM before surgery and q12h for 1 or 2 days thereafter reduces inflammation and pain and prevents straining. If possible, the ferret should continue to receive IV or SC fluids for 24–48 hours postoperatively. Allow constant access to water in a dish. The use of urinary acidifiers slightly lowers the pH of urine but does not prevent the formation of more stones when the diet is poor. Trimethoprim-sulfa combination antibiotics (15–30 mg/kg q12h) are concentrated in urine and usually prevent postoperative bladder infection with urease producers such as *Staphylococcus* and *Proteus* species. These organisms raise urine pH rapidly, inducing struvite stone formation within hours. Perform antimicrobial culture and sensitivity testing on samples collected from the bladder during surgery to confirm the effectiveness of a trimethoprim-sulfa preparation in an individual animal.

An immediate improvement in diet must be made if recurrence of urolithiasis is to be prevented after surgery, but a drastic change in diet in late gestation can induce pregnancy toxemia. A safer approach is to mix several high-quality foods with the original diet; reduce the proportion of low-quality food until only a premium food is available at 1 week after surgery. Supplement the jill's diet with a high-calorie product that includes amino acids or with cow's milk with cream or egg yolk added until a final fat concentration of 20% is attained (such supplementation causes mild physiologic diarrhea that may disturb the owner).

Problems Associated with Small Litter Size

The gestation period for ferrets is 41–42 days; this period is slightly shorter for primiparous jills. Litters of one or two kits often are overdue, probably because the hormonal stimulus from the fetuses is inadequate to induce parturition. After the 43rd day, the kits die; however, until then they continue to grow and may cause dystocia if labor is induced.

If presented with a jill having only one palpable kit, induce labor on the 41st day of gestation. Give 0.5 mg (0.1 mL) IM of prostaglandin $F_{2\alpha}$ (Lutalyse, The Upjohn Company, Kalamazoo, MI), then administer 6 USP units of oxytocin IM 1–4 hours later. Most jills deliver 2–12 hours after this treatment. If the kit is not delivered within 24 hours, repeat the treatment or perform a cesarean section. Waiting another day rarely harms the jill, but her milk will dry up, and the kit's chances of survival are greatly decreased by the 43rd day.

Some jills do not produce milk for fewer than five kits even after spontaneous delivery, and the smaller litters starve unless fostered at a few days of age. Alternatively, if another jill whelps a large litter at the same time, some of her kits can be added to the small litter. Most jills accept kits of any size or age at any stage of lactation.

Other Causes of Dystocia

Dystocia occurs at a rate of about 1% in a large group of ferrets, including those with small litters that are not delivered. Some jills repeatedly have whelping problems. Common causes of dystocia are kits of very large size (14–20 g, as compared with the normal 8–10 g), deformed fetuses with bent necks, or anasarcous fetuses. Delayed parturition is associated with kits with congenital head deformities.

Cesarean Section

An average parturition in ferrets occurs over 2–3 hours, with approximately five kits born per hour; however, some jills take longer than others to whelp. A good mother is attentive to the first-born kits before the births of subsequent kits, although she seldom settles down long enough to let them nurse. Progress should be steady and without distress on the part of the jill. Do not hesitate to perform a cesarean section on a jill that has been in labor for longer than 24 hours or on one in distress for a much shorter time. Jills recover well from surgery and usually nurse the litter uneventfully. The kits recover well even when the jill has had an injectable anesthetic; however, the best choice for cesarean section is a gas anesthetic. If injectable anesthetics must be used, a good combination is ketamine (35 mg/kg) plus xylazine (5 mg/kg) IM because it can be partially reversed with IV yohimbine (0.11 mg/kg). Preanesthetic administration of atropine reduces the cardiovascular depressant effects of xylazine. Jills will be able to walk 10 minutes after the yohimbine is given but should not be returned to their kits for at least 1 hour.

Keep the kits warm by placing them on a heating pad or a circulating warm water pad after a cesarean delivery, but check often for overheating. Kits that are very overdue are not active and may be very dehydrated. Kits with a gray pallor at birth are not viable. Those that look cyanotic usually are able to breathe with manual stimulation and benefit from a few minutes in an oxygen-rich environment.

Poor Mothering of Kits

Experienced jills rarely reject their kits, but primiparous jills often do. They may not mother their litter for several days, which is too late for many kits that are not aggressive enough to follow the jill and nurse. The more privacy these jills have, the more likely they are to bond with the litter. Handling of the kits does not cause the jills to reject their litter, but unusual noise and confusion nearby do. Ferrets get very excited and may bury the kits in the bedding or put them in a pile in a corner of the enclosure or in food or water containers. Some jills cannibalize the first few or all of their kits as they are born.

If a primiparous jill rejects but does not cannibalize her kits, place her and the litter inside a very small container, such as a dishpan, with a wire lid that allows air circulation but not exit by the jill. Offer moist food frequently and attach a water bottle. Letting the jill out to eat her favorite snack and satisfy her appetite and then replacing her in the container with the kits sometimes helps her to concentrate, allowing her to accept the litter immediately. Once she accepts the kits, the jill can be allowed to move around more freely; however, some young jills get out to play and seem to forget their young.

If the room temperature is too warm (over 21.1°C [70°F]), the jill may be reluctant to stay in the nest. To avoid accidental chilling of the kits, place a heat lamp near but not directly over the nest so that the jill can move away from it when she becomes too warm.

Lactation Failure

Jills that fail to produce enough milk to feed their kits may be genetically incapable of doing so. Before this conclusion is made, at least four variables should be examined: management, nutrition, systemic diseases of the jill, and chronic mastitis.

Primiparous jills or older jills that are poorly managed at whelping time may never settle down with their newborn kits and quickly dry up when the stimulus from nursing is inadequate. Make sure the jill is housed away from unaccustomed noisy activity, and, until the litter is more than 5 days old, discourage visits by people unfamiliar to the jill. A good mother rarely leaves the nest for the first few days after whelping. Inadequate access to food and water limit the jill's ability to make milk. Low dishes of food and water should be placed close enough to the nest that the jill can reach them without leaving her kits.

Nutrition determines the difference between adequate and outstanding milk production. Jills fed a maintenance diet raise slow-growing kits with poor coats that are more susceptible to infectious diseases than well-nourished kits. Three-week-old kits that are doing poorly benefit from milk and moist food supplements, but nothing ensures that kits will be healthy and robust as much as a steady and plentiful supply of ferret milk. Offer the best quality diet available to lactating jills; the dietary fat level should be 25–30% at 2–3 weeks after parturition. Also, jills need access to water at all times. Question owners of ferrets that have consistently small litters and poor kits about their ferrets' diet, and suggest upgrading to a premium food.

Postparturient jills with serious systemic diseases stop producing milk. Their kits look thin and are noticed crying and moving around instead of nursing or lying quietly next to the jill. The common reasons for a sudden reduction in milk production are mastitis and metritis. Other diseases that may appear during the postparturient period include bladder infections, urolithiasis, and lymphosarcoma.

If acute infections are promptly treated, the jill usually continues lactating; however, if she is very ill for a few days early in lactation, she will probably dry up. Feed the litter of a sick jill at least four times a day when their mother has little milk, but leave them with her so that as soon as she is able to produce milk the stimulus of nursing will induce lactation. Later in lactation, the jill has a lesser tendency to dry up immediately when sick or dehydrated. Whenever a lactating jill is ill, encourage her to take as much nourishment as possible by frequently offering high-calorie treats such as Nutri-Cal or Ensure Plus as well as her regular food mixed with warm water.

Acute Mastitis

Acute mastitis usually appears either soon after whelping or after the third week of lactation, when the kits begin to demand very great quantities of milk (stressing the dam) and have teeth that can damage the nipples. The affected glands are swollen, firm, red or purple, and painful to the jill. The milk may not appear grossly discolored. Common organisms cultured are *Staphylococcus* species and coliforms. Acute mastitis often becomes gangrenous only hours after it is first noticed (Fig. 6–2*A*). The skin turns black, and the jill becomes very ill and dehydrated.

Immediate aggressive treatment is needed to save the jill with acute mastitis. Trim the necrotic tissue away with a scalpel; no anesthetic or sedation is necessary because the gangrenous tissue is insensitive. This alone improves the jill's chances for survival. Administer broad-spectrum antibiotics such as chloramphenicol, 50 mg/kg IM or SC q12h, or amoxicillin with clavulanate (Clavamox Drops, SmithKline Beecham Animal Health, Exton, PA), 18.75 mg per ferret q12h (combined dosage of amoxicillin and clavulanate; equal to 0.3 mL of the oral suspension). Avoid gentamicin in ferrets. It causes renal damage, particularly in dehydrated animals, and it is responsible for deafness in some ferrets (see Chapter 33, Formulary). To be sure of the sensitivity of the specific organism, culture the milk before giving the first dose of antibiotic.

Jills are reluctant to let their kits nurse because of the pain of acute mastitis, and the toxins released by

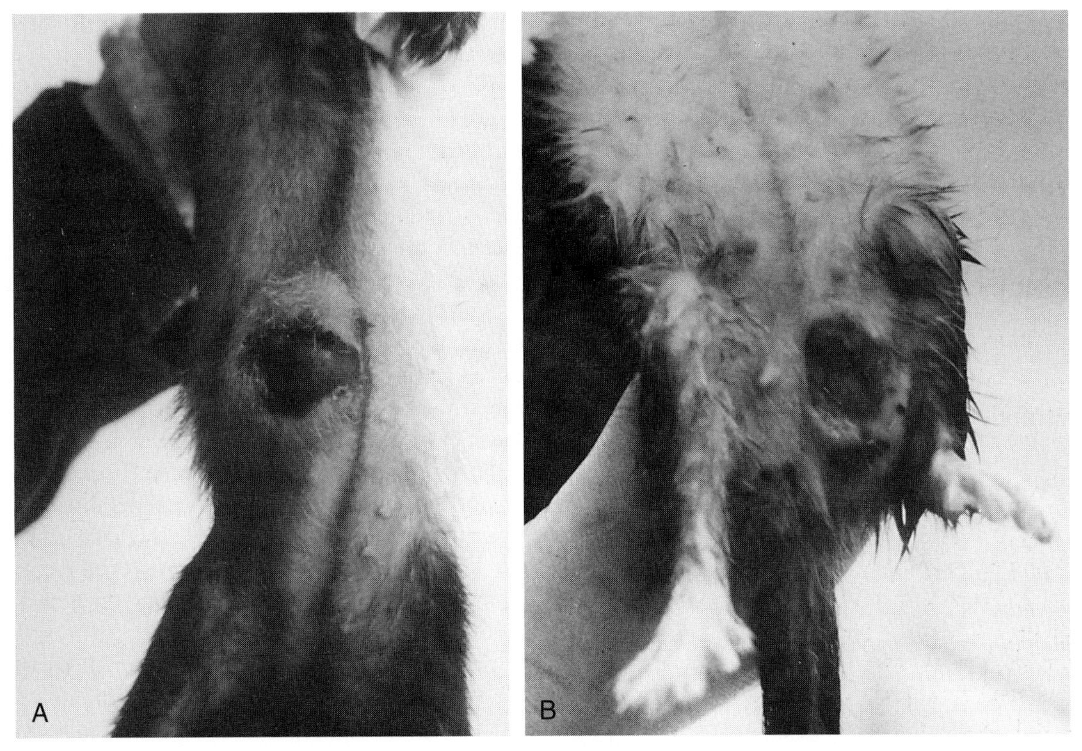

FIGURE 6–2
A, Acute gangrenous mastitis in a ferret with a single gland affected. *B,* "Crater" resulting from necrosis caused by acute gangrenous mastitis in a ferret.

the necrotic tissue make them very ill. Flunixin relieves pain, reduces inflammation and toxemia, and is safe in ferrets, saving jills that would not survive with antibiotics alone. Give 2.5 mg (0.05 mL) IM q12h as required. Also administer SC electrolyte solutions as needed. Be sure that soft, palatable food is available or give high-calorie supplements.

If treatment is instituted rapidly, the jill continues to lactate, although the kits might need supplementation with a milk replacer for a few days. Avoid fostering the kits even temporarily because they commonly infect the foster mother with the organism that caused mastitis in their dam. Those handling the infected jill should wash their hands before handling another lactating ferret. Occasionally, the infected milk causes diarrhea in the kits. Twice daily administer orally to the kits a few drops of the same antibiotic used in the mother.

Jills that have acute mastitis may heal completely but more often lose the gland (Fig. 6–2*B*) or have recurrent mastitis. Loss of a single gland has little effect on the ability of a well-producing jill to raise an average litter; however, if several glands are affected, her kits will not do well. A valuable jill can be synchronized with another dam that can take some extra kits when both whelp.

Chronic Mastitis

Chronic mastitis is so subtle it can be missed by the owner. The glands are firm but not painful or discolored. They appear to be full of milk, but most of the milk-producing tissue has been replaced by scar tissue. The organism that is usually responsible, *Staphylococcus intermedius,* is commonly found on the skin of normal ferrets. Although it may be sensitive to several antibiotics in vitro, these agents rarely have an effect in vivo. The jills with chronic mastitis are never able to nurse kits again. This type of mastitis is very contagious, and affected jills should be culled and kept separate from other breeders.

Chronic mastitis may follow acute mastitis, but it usually appears insidiously when the kits are 3 weeks of age. At this time, the jill ordinarily reaches peak production. If lactation regresses instead of peaking, the kits continue growing in stature but stop gaining weight. They look long and thin and have rough coats. To reduce the rate of infection to foster mothers, bathe the kits and keep them away from both jills for a few hours until their intestinal tracts empty of the infected milk. Treat them with an appropriate oral antibiotic. Neither this therapy nor treatment of the foster mother with antibiotic entirely prevents transmission of mastitis. Kits that are left with a jill with chronic mastitis need to be fed as much warm milk replacer as they will take at least 3 times daily (see Supplemental Feeding).

Metritis

A jill with metritis may not have excessive vaginal discharge. Palpate the abdomen. If the uterus is distended, induce uterine contraction with prostaglandin $F_{2\alpha}$, 0.5 mg (0.1 mL) IM, and initiate antibiotic therapy. A trimethoprim-sulfa combination drug is a good choice because it is concentrated in urine and helps prevent ascending bladder infection and subsequent urolithiasis. Treat jills that have a red, sticky discharge without uterine distention with trimethoprim-sulfa or other antibacterial agent plus flunixin to make the jill more comfortable and to reduce toxemia. Flunixin is a prostaglandin antagonist and should not be given in conjunction with prostaglandin $F_{2\alpha}$.

The kits look better within 24 hours, after the appropriate treatment has improved the jill's milk production. Continue treatment with antibacterial drugs for at least 5 days, but stop flunixin therapy earlier because prolonged use can cause gastritis or stomach ulcers in some animals.

PROBLEMS OF NEONATAL KITS

Ferret kits are altricial and have little ability to maintain their body temperature for the first 2 weeks of life. Normal kits weigh about 8–10 g at birth, 30 g at 1 week, 60–70 g at 2 weeks, and 100 g at 3 weeks of age. Their eyes usually open at 30–35 days of age, although in some they open as early as 25 days of age.

Healthy, normal litters lie quietly and close to the jill and nurse or sleep except when the jill leaves the nest. By 3 weeks of age, even though their eyes are still closed, kits begin to explore and nibble on soft food, such as the regular diet moistened with water. Ferrets are weaned at 6–8 weeks of age.

Fostering and Supplemental Feeding of Nursing Kits

It is extremely difficult to hand-rear ferret kits from birth without a good supply of ferret milk and 24-hour-a-day attention.[2] If the jill is unable to care for her offspring, they should be fostered to another lactating jill if possible. Most jills accept kits of any size or age at any stage of lactation.

Supplementing milk for the kits is often the best alternative when the jill's milk production is reduced because of illness after parturition. Leave the kits with her so that the stimulus of nursing induces lactation as she improves. Supplement neonatal kits with puppy or kitten milk replacer enriched with cream until the fat content is 20% (e.g., three parts dog milk replacer to one part whipping cream). Kits drink much more if the milk is warm. Feed them as much as they will take at least four times a day from a dropper or plastic pipette.

Kits that have reached 3 weeks of age can survive on supplemental feedings of milk, with no milk from the jill, until they are old enough to subsist on solid food. Use the same formula as that for neonatal kits, and offer as much as they will take at least three times daily. Feed 3-week-old kits individually with a plastic pipette or dropper because at this age they crawl into milk in a dish and get wet and cold. Older kits drink well from a dish after a few lessons. A low flat dish is preferable to a saucer because ferrets put their feet on the dish when they eat or drink. Kits cannot live on solid food without milk until they are over 4 weeks old, and they do poorly on an adult diet before 5 weeks of age.

Medical Care of Neonatal Kits

If the jill is sick or a poor mother and the nest area is not sufficiently warm, the kits can become chilled. They chill quickly and do not attempt to nurse when they are cold or hypoglycemic. Hold chilled kits in warm water or place them on a heating pad until they are active. If they have been extremely cold, give a few drops of glucose solution orally. Dehydrated neonatal kits rapidly absorb 0.5–1 mL of SC fluids warmed to body temperature.

When antibiotic therapy is necessary for neonatal kits (see later), the dose is only one or two drops of most antibiotics q12h. Amoxicillin with clavulanate must be diluted 4:1 with water so that a dose sufficiently low for a baby kit is obtained. Chloramphen-

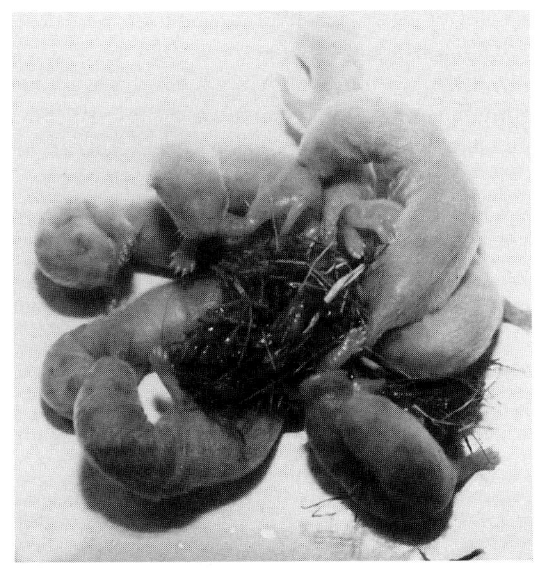

FIGURE 6–3
A ball of newborn kits bound together by tangled umbilical cords.

icol formulated for IV use is effective orally in neonatal kits.

Entangled Umbilical Cords

Occasionally, kits in large litters are born so rapidly that the dam is unable to chew the attached placenta off each one, and as a result a mass of kits is found bound together by their umbilical cords (Fig. 6–3). These kits cannot nurse and become hypoglycemic and hypothermic because the jill cannot curl around them. Very coarse or sharp-edged shavings are typically associated with entangled placentas.

It may be difficult to separate the ball of kits without injuring any of them. Soften the placentas with warm water if they have dried and pull out as much of the shavings as possible; then, gently cut the umbilical cords with blunt scissors as far from the kits' abdomens as possible. It may be necessary to sacrifice one kit to release the rest if they have been tangled for more than a few hours. To prevent umbilical cord tangling, owners should closely supervise births, picking up kits as they are born and shortening the umbilical cords. Shredded aspen, corn husks, or small terry cloth towels make good bedding for whelping nests.

Diarrhea of Neonatal Kits

Diarrhea of neonatal kits may be caused by rotavirus alone, secondary bacterial agents, or bacteria alone. Ferret rotavirus is not identical to rotaviruses of human infants, pups, calves, and pigs.[3] It is carried by adult ferrets and may affect even unstressed litters that have no passive immunity. Rotavirus diarrhea is life-threatening in kits 1–7 days of age. Older kits may not require treatment.

Kits with rotavirus diarrhea look wet and the hair on their heads and necks is slicked down (Fig. 6–4). Because the jill licks away all evidence of diarrhea, the owner may not recognize the problem. Neonatal kits with severe enteritis dehydrate rapidly. Most survive if treated with SC electrolyte solutions (0.5–1.0 mL per kit several times a day) and oral antibiotics for 4–5 days for the prevention of secondary bacterial enteritis. Useful antibiotics include spectinomycin, amoxicillin, amoxicillin with clavulanate, chloramphenicol, and trimethoprim-sulfa drug combinations. The kits are anorexic early in the

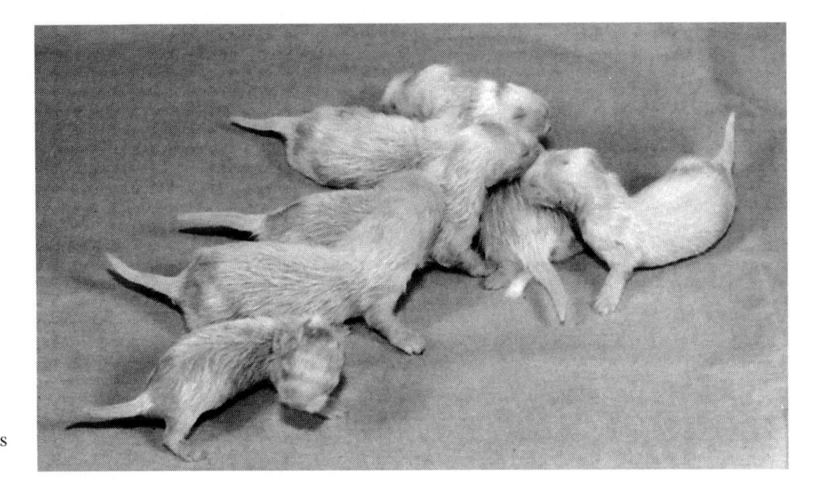

FIGURE 6–4
Litter of "sticky kits" with rotavirus diarrhea.

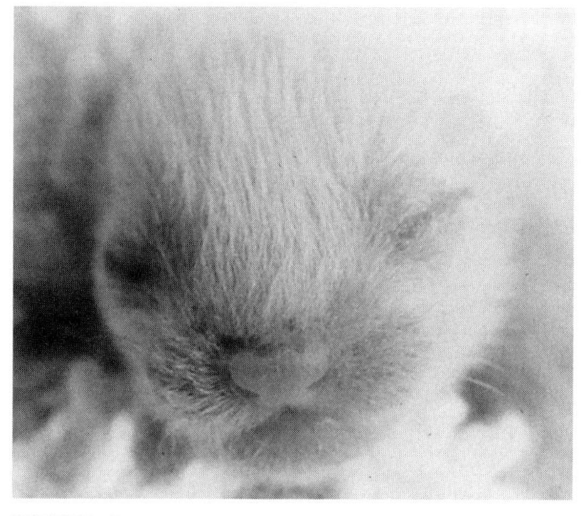

FIGURE 6–5
A baby kit with a swollen eye. Note the encrusted material on the eyelid suture line.

disease and allow pressure in the jill's mammary glands to build up, causing mastitis or inhibiting lactation.

Ophthalmia Neonatorum

Kits a few days to 3 weeks of age sometimes develop infections in their unopened eyes. Pus accumulates in the conjunctival sac until it bulges obviously and is noticed by the owner (Fig. 6–5). Usually, these kits have empty stomachs, probably because nursing causes pain. A variety of skin flora are cultured from these eyes, but their route of infection has not been determined.

Cut along the natural suture line of the eyelids with a scalpel or 25-gauge needle bevel to drain the pus. One or two treatments with broad-spectrum ophthalmic antibiotic ointment eliminates the infection. The eye remains open if the kit is older than 3 weeks of age but will seal up if it is younger, and the infection may recur. Carefully re-examine the litter twice daily because several littermates are usually affected.

REFERENCES

1. Buffington CAT: Nutritional diseases and nutritional therapy. *In* Sherding RG, ed.: The Cat: Diseases and Clinical Management. 2nd ed. Vol. 1. New York, Churchill Livingstone, 1994, p 167.
2. Manning DD, Bell JA: Derivation of gnotobiotic ferrets: perinatal diet and hand-rearing requirements. Lab Anim Sci 1990; 40:51–55.
3. Torres-Medina A: Isolation of an atypical rotavirus causing diarrhea in neonatal ferrets. Lab Anim Sci 1987; 37:167–171.

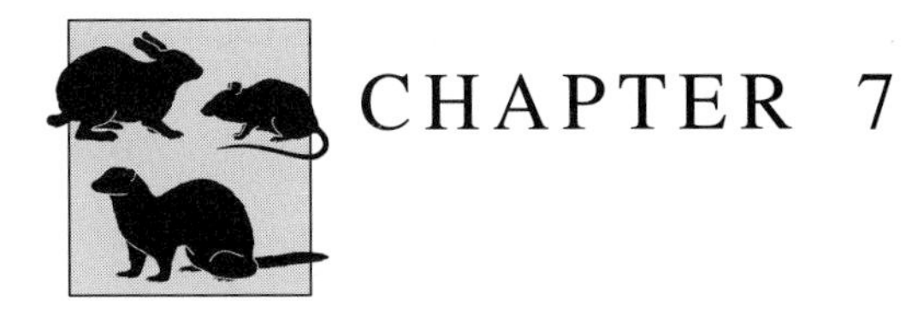

CHAPTER 7

Cardiovascular Diseases

Mark E. Stamoulis, DVM, Michael S. Miller, DVM, and Elizabeth V. Hillyer, DVM

PART I

Mark E. Stamoulis, DVM, and Michael S. Miller, DVM

CARDIAC DISEASE*

Cardiac disease is relatively common in ferrets; however, few papers have been published on this subject, and these are all single-case reports.[8, 12, 16] No published clinical studies have included more than one ferret with heart disease. In this chapter, we describe our experience in clinical practice and recommend an approach for the diagnosis and treatment of cardiac disease in this species. In clinical practice, cardiac disease usually is seen in middle-aged to older ferrets, and the most commonly observed disease entity is dilated cardiomyopathy.

General Principles

History

Ferrets with cardiac disease may have a history of inappetence, weight loss, lethargy, and difficulty in walking. Rear leg weakness is a common sign. Owners may report an elevated respiratory rate or progressive abdominal enlargement, which occurs secondary to ascites. Emesis and coughing are uncommon. In some ferrets, cardiac disease is discovered as an incidental finding; these ferrets are "asymptomatic" either because they have compen-

*The section on Cardiac Disease has been adapted with permission from Stamoulis ME: Cardiac disease in ferrets. Semin Avian Exotic Pet Med 1995; 4:43–48.

sated for early cardiac insufficiency or because the owner did not notice a decrease in activity.

Physical Examination

In ferrets, the heart extends from the sixth rib to the caudal border of the seventh or eighth rib ; therefore, perform cardiac auscultation more caudad than you would in cats, in which the heart lies between the third and fifth ribs (Fig. 7–1). On physical examination, the normal heart rate averages 180–250 beats per minute. A pronounced sinus arrhythmia is common. In normal ferrets, the heart rate may momentarily slow quite dramatically during auscultation.

Ferrets with cardiac disease have physical examination indicators that are detected on inspection, auscultation, and palpation. On inspection, affected ferrets may show cyanosis, prolonged capillary refill time, and jugular venous distention or pulsation. Pulse deficits may be palpable at the femoral artery. Findings on auscultation can include tachycardia, left-sided holosystolic murmur, or gallop rhythm (third or fourth heart sounds) and, less commonly, right-sided murmurs, pulmonary crackles, and muffled heart or lung sounds. An S_3 gallop occurs secondary to dilation of the left ventricle, and an S_4 gallop occurs secondary to accentuated atrial contraction filling a hypertrophied, noncompliant left ventricle.

On palpation, the precordial heart beat may be irregular and stronger or weaker than normal. Femoral arterial pulses may be weak or irregular, or both, and a pulse deficit may be noted.

Ferrets in cardiac failure are usually tachypneic or dyspneic. Ascites is relatively common, and there may be palpable hepatomegaly and splenomegaly. Other findings on physical examination can include hypothermia, depression, dehydration, and rear leg or generalized weakness.

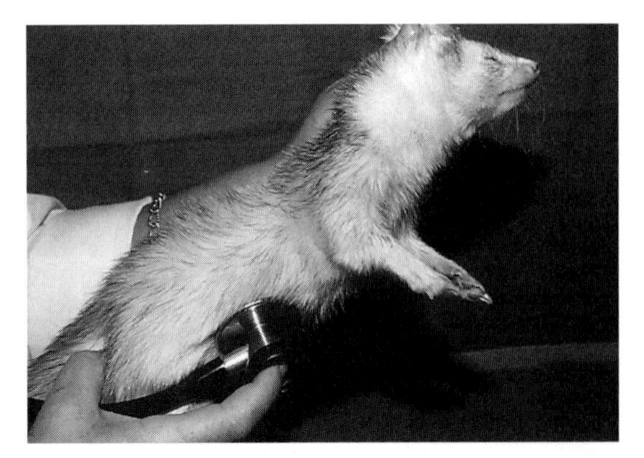

FIGURE 7–1
Auscultation of the heart in a ferret. Note the relatively caudal position of the heart.

Diagnosis

Diagnosis of symptomatic or asymptomatic cardiac disease is based on consistent integration of the data from the clinical history and physical examination, thoracic radiography, electrocardiography, and, when possible, echocardiography. On the basis of the initial test results, consider additional tests, including complete blood count (CBC) and biochemical profile, microfilaria test, occult heartworm test, and thoracocentesis or abdominocentesis with fluid analysis. Perform thoracocentesis and abdominocentesis as in cats. Thoracocentesis cranial to the heart is often productive in ferrets with pleural effusion.

It is important to remember that middle-aged and older ferrets with cardiac disease often have one or more concurrent diseases, such as insulinoma, adrenal tumor, and lymphoma.

RADIOGRAPHY. Ferrets have a long, narrow thorax, relatively large bronchi, a compliant rib cage, and lungs that are large relative to body weight. Always include the entire thorax on radiographs to check for anterior mediastinal masses that may develop in ferrets with lymphoma.

Thoracic radiographs often demonstrate a globoid cardiac silhouette in ferrets with cardiac disease. Other possible abnormal findings include pleural effusion, pulmonary venous congestion, and a diffuse interstitial pattern suggestive of pulmonary edema (see Chapter 31). Findings on abdominal radiographs can include hepatomegaly, splenomegaly, and ascites.

ELECTROCARDIOGRAPHY. The electrocardiogram (ECG) is critical for the diagnosis of arrhythmias and conduction disorders but findings must be correlated with the entire data base. Recording an ECG without sedation is preferred whenever possible; however, ferrets often object to the metal clips that are used with many ECG machines and do not remain still. Adapt the metal clips for ferrets by hammering out the teeth or by using gauze strips to cushion them (Fig. 7–2). You can distract some ferrets by offering them Nutri-Cal (Evsco Pharmaceuticals, Buena, NJ) from a syringe while recording the ECG. Alternatively, for a short procedure, consider the administration of isoflurane and oxygen by face mask.

The ECG has been described in normal ferrets.[4, 10, 29] Ferret ECGs differ from those of dogs and cats: in lead II, the P waves are small like those of

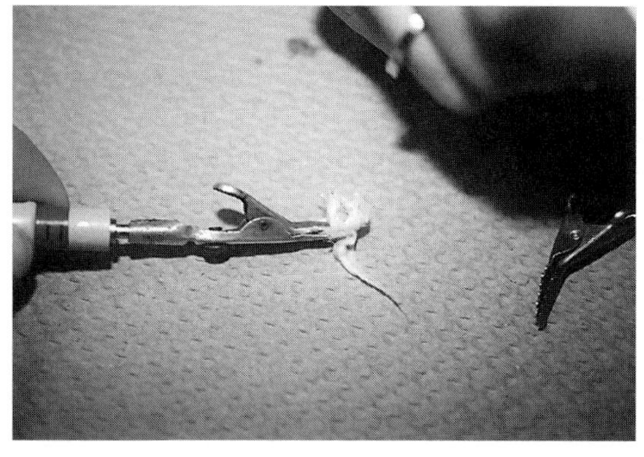

FIGURE 7–2
ECG clips adapted for use in ferrets by flattening of the teeth. (Courtesy of Heidi Hoefer, DVM.)

cats, whereas the R waves are large like those of dogs (Fig. 7–3, and Table 7–1). The normal mean electrical axis shows little variation between individual animals, with values for the frontal mean electrical axis ranging from +69° to +97° in one study[29] and from +79.6° to +90° in another[4] (all ferrets were males aged 3–20 months). A short QT interval and an elevated ST segment are often seen in normal ferrets.

Ferrets with cardiac disease may present in sinus rhythm, although sinus tachycardia appears to be more common. Atrial or ventricular premature complexes are also recorded. Sinus bradycardia and conduction disturbances, including second-degree and third-degree atrioventricular block, are rarely associated with primary cardiac disease; however, when these changes are present, the underlying process is usually extensive and difficult to treat. Other reported ECG changes include tall R waves, prolonged QRS complexes, and ST segment depression.[29] Right axis deviation was not observed among 20 adult male ferrets with experimentally induced right-sided ventricular hypertrophy.[29]

ECHOCARDIOGRAPHY. Echocardiography is the most sensitive and specific diagnostic test for characterizing cardiomyopathy and other types of cardiac disease. Most ferrets tolerate echocardiography without sedation if they are held in lateral recumbency by the neck scruff and around the hips.

Two-dimensional echocardiography enables objective assessment of chamber size, shape, and function. Pleural or pericardial effusion and masses within the heart or anterior mediastinum are easily detected. M-mode echocardiography allows quantitation of chamber size and wall thickness as well as assessment of indices of systolic function. Mean echocardiographic measurements for 34 normal ferrets are shown in Table 7–2. Color flow Doppler imaging illustrates direction of blood flow and detects turbulence, which is often associated with valvular insufficiency. Pulsed wave or continuous wave Doppler echocardiography can be added for verification and quantitation of the velocity of blood flow.

Mild aortic valvular insufficiency has been observed in several ferrets during Doppler studies.*

*Bond B: Personal communication, 1995.

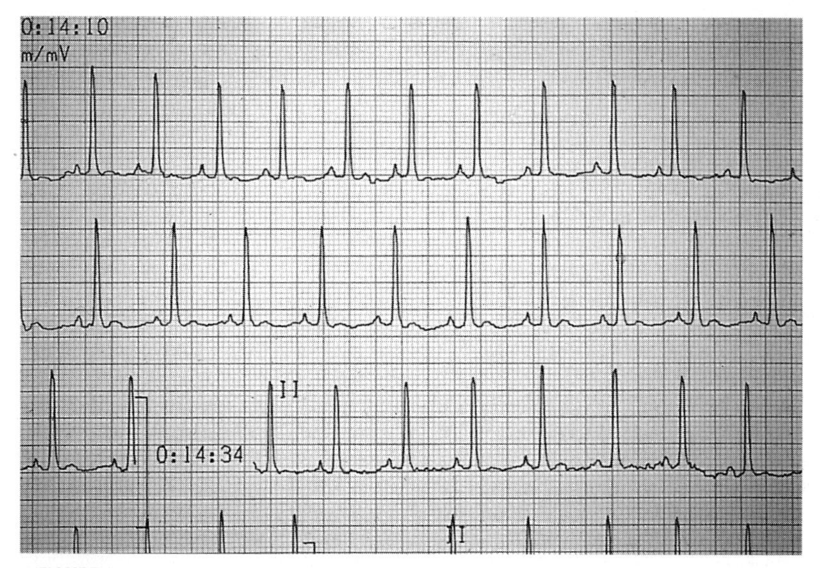

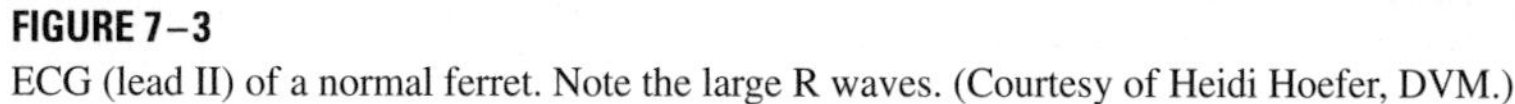

FIGURE 7–3
ECG (lead II) of a normal ferret. Note the large R waves. (Courtesy of Heidi Hoefer, DVM.)

TABLE 7–1

ELECTROCARDIOGRAPHIC DATA FOR 52 CLINICALLY NORMAL FERRETS*

Parameter	Mean ± SD (Range)† (n = 25)	Value‡ (n = 27)
Age (mo)	10–20	average, 5.2
Male : female ratio	All male	1.25
Body weight (kg)	1.4 ± 0.2	NA
Heart rate (beats/min)	196 ± 26.5 (140–240)	233 ± 22
Rhythm		
Normal sinus	NA	67%
Sinus arrhythmia	NA	33%
Frontal plane MEA (degrees)	+86.13 ± 2.5 (79.6–90)	+77.22 ± 12
Lead II		
P amplitude (mV)	NA	0.122 ± 0.007
P duration (s)	NA	0.024 ± 0.004
PR interval (s)	0.056 ± 0.0086 (0.04–0.08)	0.047 ± 0.003
QRS duration (s)	0.044 ± 0.0079 (0.035–0.06)	0.043 ± 0.003
R amplitude (mV)	2.21 ± 0.42 (1.4–3)	1.46 ± 0.84
QT interval (s)	0.109 ± 0.018 (0.08–0.14)	0.12 ± 0.04

Abbreviations: NA = not available; MEA = mean electrical axis.

*All ferrets were sedated with ketamine-xylazine.

†Data from Bone L, Battles AH, Goldfarb RD, et al: Electrocardiographic values from clinically normal, anesthetized ferrets (*Mustela putorius furo*). Am J Vet Res 1988; 49:1884–1887.

‡Data adapted from Fox JG: Biology and Diseases of the Ferret. Philadelphia, Lea & Febiger, 1988, p 170, and Edwards J: Unpublished data, 1987.

None of these ferrets showed clinical signs associated with aortic insufficiency although some had other cardiac disease. In humans, physiologic pulmonary valvular regurgitation, dubbed "trivial" regurgitation,[13] is common and is not considered to be of pathologic significance in healthy persons. Physiologic pulmonary valvular regurgitation was found on Doppler echocardiography in 43–100% of normal adult subjects in two studies; aortic insufficiency was less common, occurring in 6–8% of normal adult subjects.[13, 17] Physiologic valvular regurgitation also occurs in dogs. In one study of 20 normal beagle dogs, the prevalence of pulmonary, mitral, and aortic valvular regurgitation was 75%, 15%, and 10%, respectively; tricuspid valvular regurgitation was not detected.[21] At the time of this writing, the clinical significance of aortic insufficiency in ferrets is not known.

TABLE 7–2

MEAN ECHOCARDIOGRAPHIC VALUES FOR 34 NORMAL ADULT FERRETS

Parameter	Mean Value
Left ventricle, end-diastolic	11.0 mm
Left ventricle, end-systolic	6.4 mm
Left ventricular posterior or free wall	3.3 mm
Fractional shortening	42%
End-point septal separation	None

From Sitinas N, Beeber N, Skeels M: Unpublished data, 1992.

Treatment

Most treatment regimens for ferrets with cardiac disease are based on canine or feline regimens—that is, similar indications call for the use of similar drugs. When in doubt of the dosage for a new drug, use the feline dosage. Ferrets tolerate furosemide well; the dosage is 1–4 mg/kg q8–12h PO, IV, IM, or SC. Thiazide diuretics (feline dosages) can be used in combination with furosemide if necessary.

Published dosages for digoxin elixir in ferrets range from 0.01 mg/kg PO q24h[28] to 0.01 mg/kg PO q12h.[16] We usually start with the administration of digoxin once daily and adjust the frequency from once every other day to twice daily, depending on the ferret's clinical progress and serum digoxin levels. Calculate the dose based on lean body weight; as for dogs, assume a normal 15% body fat and watch for potential side effects, such as cardiac arrhythmias, inappetence, vomiting, and diarrhea.[30] There are no published pharmacokinetic studies of digoxin in ferrets. To evaluate the dosage, measure serum digoxin 8 hours after drug administration; therapeutic serum concentrations, as extrapolated from dogs and cats, are 0.8–2 ng/mL.[30] Contraindications for digoxin in dogs, such as moderate to severe azotemia or hypokalemia, or frequent ventricular arrhythmias, apply to ferrets.

Ferrets appear to be sensitive to the hypotensive effects of angiotensin-converting enzyme inhibitors and can become lethargic and inappetent 1 to several days after the start of angiotensin-converting enzyme inhibitor therapy. Always start with a low dosage—for example, enalapril (Enacard, Merck Agvet Division, Rahway, NJ) at 0.5 mg/kg PO q48h. If the ferret shows no side effects, increase the dosage slowly to the target dosage of 0.5 mg/kg q24h.

The presence of concurrent disease can complicate therapy for cardiac disease. Ferrets with lymphoma or insulinoma may be receiving prednisone, which can cause water and salt retention, which in turn aggravates cardiac failure. Follow these animals closely.

Diseases

Dilated (Congestive) Cardiomyopathy

Dilated cardiomyopathy is the most commonly reported cardiac disease in ferrets.[8, 12, 16] The cause of this disorder is not known. The usual clinical presentation is a middle-aged or older ferret with lethargy, weight loss, anorexia, and respiratory distress. Physical examination findings can include hypothermia, tachycardia, a systolic murmur, moist rales, muffled heart and lung sounds, ascites, and rear leg weakness.

Possible radiographic changes include an enlarged cardiac silhouette, pleural effusion, increased pulmonary radiodensity, ascites, hepatomegaly, and splenomegaly. Myriad ECG changes may be recorded. Echocardiographic changes are similar to those reported in other species for dilated cardiomyopathy.[5, 20, 33] Diagnostic features include increased left ventricular end-diastolic and end-systolic dimensions, depressed indices of systolic function (namely, fractional shortening), left atrial enlargement, and right ventricular dilation (Fig. 7–4).[11] Pulsed wave or continuous wave Doppler echocardiography usually shows mitral regurgitation and occasionally tricuspid regurgitation and decreased aortic forward flow.

Gross pathologic findings include dilation of both

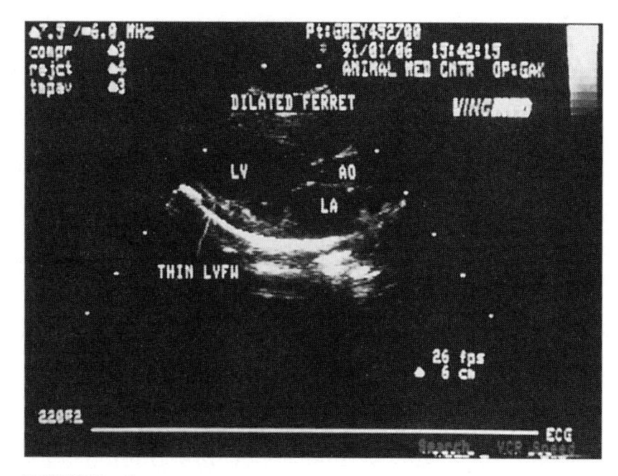

FIGURE 7–4
Two-dimensional echocardiogram of a ferret with dilated cardiomyopathy. Note the thin left ventricular free wall (LVFW). The left atrium (LA) is enlarged when compared with the aorta (AO). (From Stamoulis ME: Cardiac disease in ferrets. Semin Avian Exotic Pet Med 1995; 4:43–48.)

atria and ventricles. The ventricular walls are abnormally thin. Histologically, multifocal myocardial degeneration, myocardial necrosis, and replacement fibrosis are observed.[16]

Pharmacologic therapy for dilated cardiomyopathy is designed to manipulate the heart rate and rhythm, preload, afterload, and contractility.[14] If acute fulminant heart failure is present, place the ferret in an oxygen-enriched environment and administer furosemide (2–4 mg/kg SC or IM q8–12h). If the amount of pleural effusion is large, remove the fluid by thoracocentesis when the ferret is stable enough to be handled. Submit pleural fluid for cytologic evaluation, especially if the cranial thorax is obscured on radiography, because mediastinal lymphoma is a differential diagnosis.

The venous dilator nitroglycerin (2% ointment; ⅛ inch applied to skin q12–24h) reduces preload and aids in controlling pulmonary edema during the initial management of heart failure (beware of hypotension). Provide positive inotropic therapy with digoxin (0.01 mg/kg PO q24h) to stimulate the failing myocardium and to depress atrioventricular nodal conduction in the presence of supraventricular tachyarrhythmias. Continue furosemide therapy (1–4 mg/kg PO, IV, IM, or SC q8–12h) to reduce edema and effusion. The angiotensin-converting enzyme inhibitors, or balanced vasodilators, are a recent adjunct to therapy. These drugs reduce arteriolar and venous tone, thereby improving cardiac output and decreasing edema formation, respectively. Start with enalapril, 0.5 mg/kg PO q48h. If the ferret tolerates this dosage, try increasing to once daily administration; if the ferret seems hypotensive (lethargic and limp) with this dosage, decrease frequency of administration to once every third day.

A low-salt diet and exercise restriction are difficult to institute but theoretically could be beneficial. Taurine supplementation reverses dilated cardiomyopathy in cats; however, it has not been of benefit in ferrets with this disease.

Monitor the effects of therapy with periodic ECGs, radiography, echocardiography, and serum digoxin assays. Monitor blood urea nitrogen, creatinine, and potassium levels. Ferrets with dilated cardiomyopathy tend to respond better to treatment than do dogs with similar echocardiographic findings. If the disease is diagnosed at an early stage, the prognosis is fair for months of good-quality life.

Hypertrophic Cardiomyopathy

Hypertrophic cardiomyopathy is seen in ferrets; however, this disease has been insufficiently studied to allow a characteristic clinical description. Left ventricular hypertrophic disease secondary to hypertension or hyperthyroidism, as seen in cats, has not been recognized in ferrets.

In our experience, the clinical signs of hypertrophic cardiomyopathy range from none to sudden death. A systolic murmur may be detected on auscultation (usually left-sided or sternal in origin). Echocardiography is the most sensitive technique for evaluating hypertrophy (Fig. 7–5). The interventricular septum and left ventricular free walls are abnormally thickened, and internal dimensions are decreased; left atrial enlargement is common. Systolic function may be normal to hyperdynamic. Doppler echocardiographic evaluation usually shows mitral regurgitation.

Gross pathologic findings include an abnormally thickened interventricular septum and left ventricular free wall. Histologically, fibrous connective tissue is evident throughout the myocardium.

Therapy is based on the improvement of diastolic function and the reduction of congestion. Beta-adrenergic blocking drugs (e.g., atenolol, 6.25 mg PO q24h) or calcium channel antagonists (e.g., diltiazem, 3.75–7.5 mg PO q12h) are useful for reducing heart rate, improving diastolic filling, and relaxing the noncompliant myocardium. Start with a low dosage and monitor the ferret for possible side effects, which are similar for diltiazem and atenolol and include arrhythmias (especially heart block), lethargy, and inappetence. Follow the guidelines for diuretic therapy and therapeutic monitoring outlined in the previous sections.

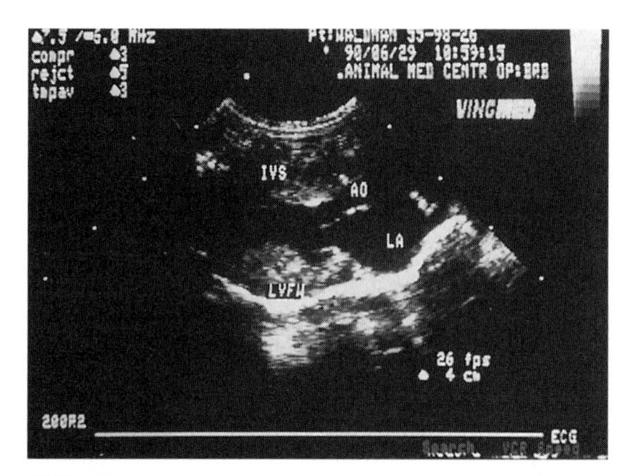

FIGURE 7–5

Two-dimensional echocardiogram of a ferret with hypertrophic cardiomyopathy. Note the abnormally thickened interventricular septum (IVS) and LVFW. The LA is enlarged as well. (From Stamoulis ME: Cardiac disease in ferrets. Semin Avian Exotic Pet Med 1995; 4:43–48.)

Valvular Heart Disease

Valvular heart disease is being recognized with increasing frequency, most commonly in middle-aged ferrets. Clinical signs are variable. The most consistent finding is a holosystolic heart murmur usually heard at the left apical region. Moist rales may also be heard on auscultation.

Radiographic and ECG signs are variable. Echocardiography demonstrates left or right atrial enlargement and mild dilation of the affected ventricle. Systolic function is normal to hyperdynamic. Mitral or tricuspid regurgitation, or both, are noted during Doppler echocardiographic studies.

Abnormally thickened valves and dilated atria are observed on gross pathologic examination. Histologically, myxomatous degeneration of the affected valve is noted; this degeneration is similar to that observed in dogs with endocardiosis.*

Treatment with furosemide and enalapril reduces regurgitant volume and congestion. Institute inotropic therapy with digoxin in later stages when systolic function is impaired or if there are supraventricular arrhythmias.

Myocarditis

Myocardial involvement with infectious disease is reported in ferrets. Infection with *Toxoplasma*-like organisms resulted in multifocal necrosis of the myocardium.[32] Aleutian disease, a parvoviral infection, can cause fibrinoid necrosis and mononuclear

---

*Williams B: Personal communication, 1993.

cell infiltration in arterioles of the heart.[7] Inflammatory lesions have been observed in the hearts of ferrets with sepsis.*

Ventricular arrhythmias without significant cardiomegaly or myocardial failure are clinical findings suspicious for myocarditis.

Congenital Disease

No reports of congenital heart disease in ferrets have been published. An informal survey of veterinary cardiologists and pathologists failed to uncover a single case, and none have been seen at a large ferret breeding farm over the past 5 years.† One of the editors (EVH) has treated a 10-month-old spayed female ferret with a large septal defect diagnosed on echocardiography. The ferret responded to medical therapy for 2 months and then died in fulminant cardiac failure. A necropsy was not performed.

Neoplasia

A recent survey did not report a single case of primary cardiac, intracardiac, or pericardial neoplasia in ferrets.[2] Lymphoma, one of the most common neoplastic diseases in ferrets, often involves the anterior mediastinum in younger ferrets. These animals typically present with marked dyspnea secondary to pleural effusion and the presence of the mediastinal mass. Use ultrasound and order cytologic evaluation of pleural fluid (or of a specimen from the mass collected on fine-needle aspiration) to differentiate between lymphoma and cardiac disease.

Heartworm Disease

Natural and experimental infections with the canine heartworm, *Dirofilaria immitis*, are reported in ferrets.[3, 6, 19, 23] The disease in ferrets resembles that in dogs; however, because of the ferret's small size, the presence of even one adult worm in the heart can be lethal. Reported adult worm burdens range from 1 to 10. Ferrets that live in or originate from areas endemic for heartworm are the most likely to be infected.

Clinical signs include lethargy, coughing, dyspnea, pulmonary congestion, and ascites.[19, 23] Melena was seen in three heartworm-infected ferrets.[23] Sudden death can occur because of occlusion of major pulmonary arteries by worms. Severe pleural effusion may be noted on radiographs (Fig. 7–6). No echocardiographic findings have been published; however, expected findings include enlargement of the right atrium, right ventricle, and main pulmonary artery.

Post mortem, adult worms are found in the right ventricle (Fig. 7–7), cranial vena cava, and main pulmonary artery. Histologically, villous endarteritis is seen.

Diagnosis of heartworm disease in ferrets is based on evaluation of clinical signs, findings on radiography with or without echocardiography, results of a microfilaria test, and results of testing for circulating heartworm antigen. Peripheral microfilaremia is uncommon in ferrets with heartworm disease. Testing for *Dirofilaria* antigen appears to be much more useful. Specifically, one enzyme-linked immunosorbent assay (ELISA)–based test (Snap Heartworm Antigen Test Kit, IDEXX Laboratories, Inc., Westbrook, ME), which has been approved for use in dogs and cats, has proved useful in detecting infected ferrets.‡

Successful treatment of heartworm disease in ferrets depends on early diagnosis and long-term antithrombotic therapy in conjunction with adulticide therapy. The protocol recommended here is based on the experience of a clinician in Florida who has treated 30 ferrets with this disease and necropsied many more who had died suddenly secondary to heartworm infection. She was not able to save any infected ferrets (all died with pulmonary emboli 2–12 weeks after treatment) until she altered the treatment protocol to include antithrombotic therapy. Since this change, she has successfully treated 10 of 14 ferrets with heartworm disease.‡

The current recommended treatment protocol is as follows: administer thiacetarsemide (Caparsolate, 2.2 mg/kg IV q12h for 2 days) by a cephalic catheter, using the same precautions as you would with dogs. Begin heparin therapy at the same time (heparin, 100 U SC q24h for ferrets weighing 0.45–1.35 kg) and continue it for 21 days. In addition, administer treatment for cardiac failure as indicated by clinical signs and results of diagnostic tests. The ferret should be confined to a cage and not be allowed exercise or unrestricted play during this time. After 3 weeks of heparin administration, change the heparin to aspirin (¼ of a 65- or 81-mg children's aspirin, or 22 mg/kg PO q24h) for 3 months. Perform a followup ELISA test for heart-

*Williams B: Personal communication, 1994.
†Bell JA: Personal communication, 1995.
‡Kemmerer D: Personal communication, 1995.

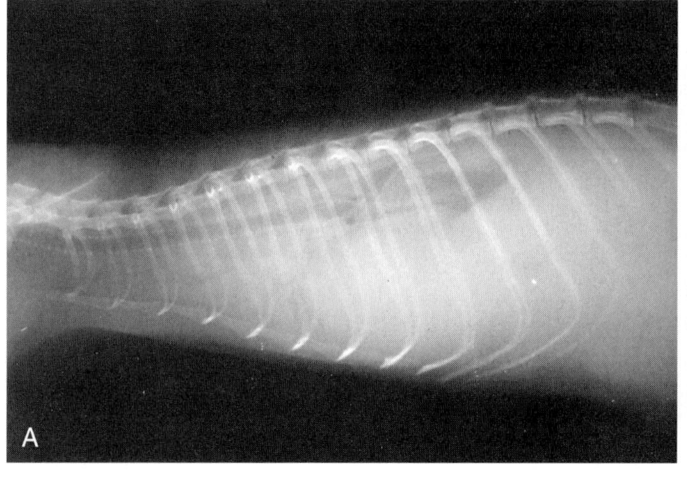

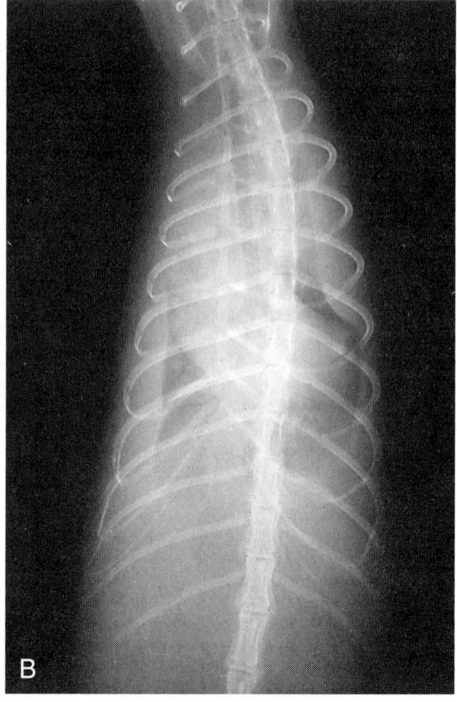

FIGURE 7–6
Lateral *(A)* and ventrodorsal *(B)* radiographs of a ferret in cardiac failure secondary to heartworm disease. This ferret, a 3-year-old spayed female, presented to a New York clinic for lethargy, inappetence, and coughing. It was severely dyspneic on physical examination. The ferret had been in Florida for several months the previous year.

worm antigen at 3 months after adulticide therapy and at monthly intervals thereafter until the ELISA results are negative. Most ferrets become seronegative at about 4 months after successful heartworm therapy. Begin heartworm prevention 1 month after adulticide treatment.

The use of prednisolone in place of standard antithrombotic therapy is a promising alternative. Two ferrets with heartworm disease were successfully treated according to the regimen as described except that they received prednisolone, 2.2 mg/kg q24h PO for 3 months instead of heparin and aspirin.*

All ferrets in heartworm endemic areas should be kept on preventive treatment year-round. Administer oral ivermectin once per month. One quarter of the smallest tablet (68 μg × 0.25 = 17 μg) of oral ivermectin (Heartgard-30, Merck Agvet Division, Rahway, NJ) is adequate for ferrets. An accurate dose can be given in this way because the drug is evenly distributed throughout the tablets. However, the drug deteriorates once the pill is broken; thus, the remaining pill should be discarded. Alternatively, make a liquid ivermectin preparation by mixing 0.3 mL of injectable ivermectin (Ivomec 1% Injection for Cattle, Merck Agvet Division, Rahway, NJ) in 28 mL (1 oz) of propylene glycol. This yields an ivermectin suspension of 0.1 mg/mL. Administer 0.2 mL/kg PO (0.02 mg/kg) once per month. Place the suspension in an amber bottle with a 2-year expiration date (assuming that the undiluted ivermectin had an adequate expiration date) and instruct the client to keep it in a dark place. Diethylcarbamazine (canine dosage) can be used also, although few clients are willing to administer a daily pill when a monthly medication is equally effective.

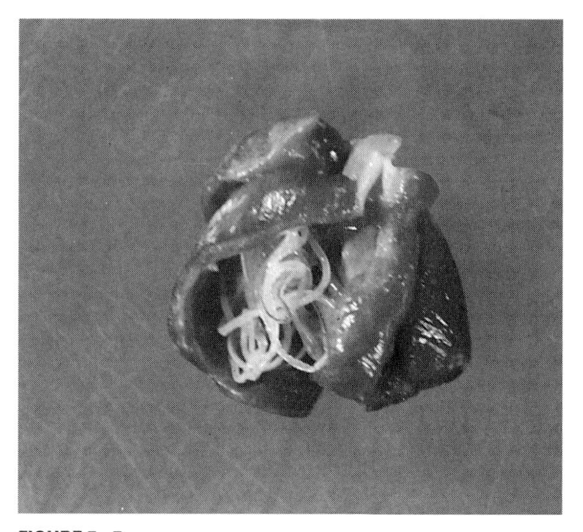

FIGURE 7–7
Adult *Dirofilaria immitis* in the heart of a ferret.

*Kemmerer D: Personal communication, 1995.

PART II

Elizabeth V. Hillyer, DVM

OTHER DISEASES

Aleutian Disease

Aleutian disease (AD) is caused by a parvovirus. It was first reported in ranch-bred mink *(Mustela vison)* in the 1950s and was named after mink homozygous for the Aleutian gene, which typically develop the most severe forms of the disease. Ferrets can be experimentally infected with mink strains of AD virus, and there is at least one ferret-specific strain of AD virus.[27] The infection in both ferrets and mink is characterized by viral persistence associated with non-neutralizing antibody.[15, 26] However, ferrets infected as adults usually do not develop AD virus–associated disease.[26, 27]

The classic form of AD in mink is an immune complex–mediated disease. Affected mink show severe hypergammaglobulinemia, glomerulonephritis, arteritis, plasmacytosis, and progressive wasting. Death usually occurs within 5 months of infection in Aleutian mink, which are susceptible to all strains of the virus.[24, 25] Depending on viral strain and host genotype and immune status, non-Aleutian mink may clear the AD virus, become inapparent carriers, or develop progressive disease similar to that seen in Aleutian mink. Decreased fertility, abortion, and neonatal interstitial pneumonitis may also be associated with AD virus infection in this species.[1] Ranch mink are regularly screened for AD; there is no vaccine for the disease.

Ferrets that are experimentally infected with mink strains of AD virus develop virus-specific antibody and show evidence of persistent infection for up to 180 days. However, they do not usually develop the severe disease seen in mink when they are inoculated with either ferret or mink strains of AD virus.[15, 27] In clinical practice, ferrets can be seropositive for AD virus without developing signs of the disease. Brown* screened over 500 shelter ferrets in Illinois during the 1980s and found that approximately 10% tested seropositive on counterimmunoelectrophoresis. Only two of these animals went on to develop signs of disease consistent with AD.

*Brown S: Personal communication, 1995.

Diagnosis

AD typically manifests as a wasting disease in ferrets. Weight loss, lethargy, pallor, hepatomegaly, splenomegaly, melena, rear leg or generalized weakness, and neurologic signs are all possible findings. A presumptive diagnosis of AD in ferrets is based on the presence of the typical clinical signs in conjunction with hypergammaglobulinemia and a positive antibody titer. Hypergammaglobulinemia is usually pronounced, with gamma globulins representing more than 20% of total protein, and serum protein electrophoresis shows a monoclonal spike (Fig. 7–8).

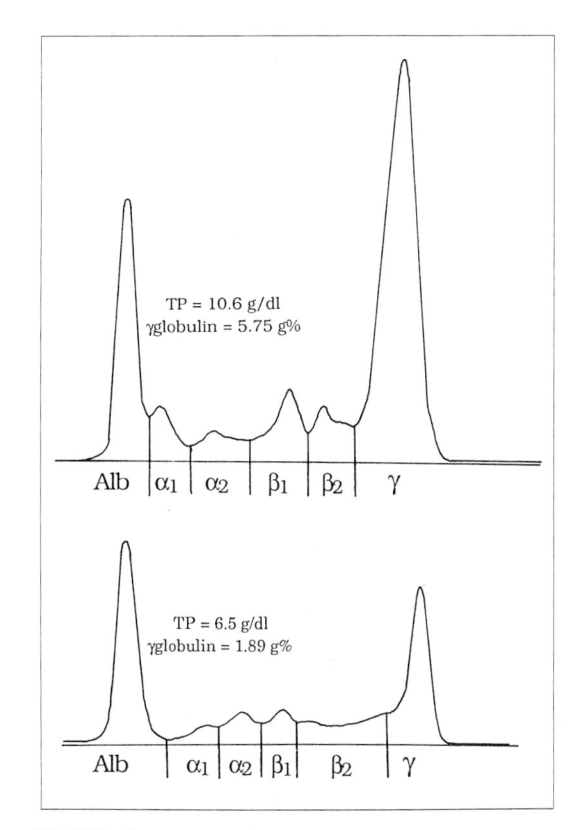

FIGURE 7–8

Serum protein electrophoretograms from two ferrets with parvovirus-associated syndromes (Aleutian disease). *Top,* Ferret 1: Notice the pronounced hypergammaglobulinemia. The gamma globulin fraction is equivalent to 54% of the total protein. *Bottom,* Ferret 2: The gamma globulin fraction is equivalent to 29% of the total protein. Hypergammaglobulinemia is the hallmark of Aleutian disease virus infection. Abbreviations: TP = total protein; Alb = albumin. (From Palley LS, Corning BF, Fox JG, et al: Parvovirus-associated syndrome (Aleutian disease) in two ferrets. J Am Vet Med Assoc 1992; 201: 100–106.)

The two most common tests for AD virus antibody are counterimmunoelectrophoresis and immunofluorescent antibody tests. Counterimmunoelectrophoresis is used for screening mink and is rapid, highly specific, and inexpensive.* The immunofluorescent antibody test may be more sensitive than counterimmunoelectrophoresis.[22]†

Two case reports describe naturally occurring AD in ferrets. In one report, four ferrets aged 2 years or older developed a chronic, wasting disease; mild hepatomegaly and splenomegaly were present at necropsy.[7] Histologic findings varied in severity but included splenic reticuloendothelial cell hyperplasia, lymphocytic-plasmacytic infiltration in hepatic portal areas, periportal fibrosis, bile duct hyperplasia, and membranous glomerulonephritis.

The second case report describes AD in two 2-year-old castrated male ferrets, both of which had positive AD virus antibody titers on both counterimmunoelectrophoresis and immunofluorescent antibody testing.[22] Clinical and necropsy findings in these two animals illustrate the spectrum of disease possible in association with AD virus. The first ferret showed anorexia, cachexia, hypochromic microcytic anemia, progressively increasing hyperglobulinemia, and tarry feces. Histologic evaluation at necropsy revealed a mild-to-severe inflammatory infiltrate composed mostly of plasma cells interspersed with lymphocytes in multiple organs, including the meninges, choroid plexus, liver, thyroid gland, heart, salivary glands, common bile duct, pancreas, kidneys, lungs, and lymph nodes. The second ferret presented for posterior paresis; laboratory testing revealed hypoalbuminemia and hypergammaglobulinemia. Clinical signs that developed in this animal included intermittent head tremor, diarrhea, and fecal and urinary incontinence. On histopathologic examination, infiltrations of plasma cells and lymphocytes were found in the duodenum, stomach, salivary gland, liver, thyroid gland, lungs, and right atrium; disseminated, nonsuppurative, lymphoplasmacytic encephalomyelitis was present.

*Contact United Vaccines, Inc., 2826 Latham Drive, P.O. Box 44220, Madison, WI 53744-4220; tel.: 1-(608)-277-2030.

†Contact the diagnostic laboratory at the Division of Comparative Medicine, Massachusetts Institute of Technology, Building 45, 37 Vassar Street, Cambridge, MA 02139-4307; tel.: 1-(617)-253-9472.

Treatment and Prevention

There is no specific treatment for ferrets with AD. Instruct the owner how to provide supportive care and be sure that the ferret is on a good diet. The course of disease is typically chronic. Remember that infected animals can serve as a potential source of infection for other ferrets. There is no vaccine for this disease.

Splenomegaly

The distinction between splenomegaly and hypersplenism is very important because splenomegaly is extremely common in ferrets, whereas hypersplenism is rare (see next section). The clinical approach to these two conditions is different. *Splenomegaly* simply means an enlarged spleen. *Hypersplenism* is a condition in which one or more cytopenias, including anemia, leukocytopenia, and thrombocytopenia, are present as a result of excessive splenic destruction; the spleen is usually, but not always, enlarged.

Splenomegaly may be found in clinically normal ferrets and in ferrets with almost any conceivable, seemingly unrelated disease, including insulinoma, adrenal disease, upper respiratory infection, presence of a gastrointestinal foreign body, enteritis, dental disease, and cardiomyopathy. Often, but not always, the clinical significance of the enlarged spleen, per se, is minor.

Histopathologic examination of enlarged spleens in ferrets usually reveals nonspecific findings, typically extramedullary hematopoiesis or congestion, or both. In my experience, disease directly involving the spleen, most commonly lymphoma and occasionally a myeloid tumor, occurs in approximately 5% of ferrets with splenomegaly. Primary splenic neoplasms are rare: three splenic hemangiosarcomas and one hemangioma were reported in one review.[2] Splenomegaly has also been reported in ferrets with AD virus infection and idiopathic hypersplenism.[7,9]

Diagnosis

Perform a full medical workup in ferrets with splenomegaly. The medical workup is necessary both for identification of the primary disease and for evaluation of the spleen itself. Do not assume that splenomegaly is the primary medical problem or even part of the medical problem.

Ferrets with splenomegaly usually present for clinical signs of the primary disease, which is rarely the enlarged spleen. For example, ferrets with insulinoma present for signs of hypoglycemia; ferrets with adrenal disease typically present for hair loss; ferrets with a gastrointestinal foreign body typically present for anorexia and lethargy; and ferrets with cardiomyopathy present with signs of heart failure. Ferrets with lymphoma can present for a variety of clinical signs. (See the appropriate chapters of this book for further information about these diseases.)

Obtain a complete history from the owner and perform a complete physical examination. An enlarged spleen is readily palpable in most ferrets except perhaps those with severe peritoneal effusion. The size of the spleen does not correlate with severity of disease. Ferrets with advanced lymphoma sometimes have mild to no splenomegaly, whereas ferrets with early insulinoma sometimes have massive splenomegaly. Be alert for clinical signs and physical findings suggestive of the primary diagnosis. A minimum workup for ferrets with splenomegaly includes a CBC and platelet count for screening for lymphoma and hypersplenism (see next section; also see Chapter 10). In animals 3 years of age or older, determine blood glucose level after a short fast (2–4 hours) to screen for insulinoma, which is very common. If possible, perform a full serum chemistry workup and urinalysis, and obtain whole-body radiographs for older animals. The results of initial tests dictate appropriate further testing.

Occasionally, you may detect splenomegaly on routine physical examination of an otherwise healthy ferret. If initial diagnostic tests are normal and the ferret shows no signs of illness, note splenic enlargement in the medical record; then, perform a complete physical examination and assessment of splenic size annually. If the spleen is very enlarged, perform a physical examination, CBC, and platelet count two or more times a year to monitor the ferret for subclinical lymphoma or hypersplenism.

Methods of evaluating the spleen itself include gentle palpation for detection of irregularities, abdominal ultrasound for evaluation of size and density, splenic fine-needle aspiration for cytologic analysis, and splenic biopsy. Splenic fine-needle aspiration is easily performed in most ferrets without sedation (see Chapter 2). However, the usefulness of splenic cytologic examination is controversial, particularly in the diagnosis of lymphoma. This is because of the multifollicular architecture of the spleen and the possibility of aspirating actively dividing lymphocytes in the center of a follicle or, conversely, missing a focus of malignant lymphocytes. Nonetheless, the technique has minimal attendant morbidity and may be useful in some animals, particularly if abdominal exploratory surgery is impractical. Always obtain an aspirate from two different sites.

If you suspect insulinoma, adrenal tumor, or other intra-abdominal disease, an abdominal exploratory surgery with splenic biopsy is a useful diagnostic tool (see Chapter 13). Surgery whose sole purpose is obtaining a splenic biopsy is rarely indicated unless other diagnostic tests have yielded negative results or primary splenic disease is likely. A total splenectomy is also rarely indicated (see below). As mentioned previously, histopathologic examination of the spleen usually shows extramedullary hematopoiesis and congestion.

Treatment

The management of ferrets with splenomegaly is aimed at treating the primary disease, whether it be insulinoma, cardiomyopathy, lymphoma, or another disorder. Splenomegaly itself does not require specific treatment unless the spleen is so large that it causes discomfort or appears in danger of rupturing. Indications for splenectomy in other species also apply to ferrets and include hypersplenism, splenitis, and splenic neoplasia, torsion, rupture, and abscess. Lymphoma is the most common indication for splenectomy in ferrets. Splenectomy may also be indicated in some ferrets with insulinoma because the spleen is a possible, although uncommon, site for metastasis. No studies comparing the course of insulinoma in ferrets with or without splenectomy have been published. The possible sequelae of splenectomy, including altered immune function and decreased resistance to hemorrhagic shock, have not been investigated in ferrets.

Occasionally, a ferret presents for lethargy and inappetence with no attendant physical or laboratory abnormalities other than a gross enlargement of the spleen (idiopathic splenomegaly). Although most ferrets do not seem bothered by splenomegaly, a very enlarged spleen can cause significant discomfort in some animals, and splenectomy may be curative in these cases. Perform a splenectomy only after having ruled out all other possible causes of lethargy and inappetence.

Idiopathic Hypersplenism

As mentioned in the previous section, hypersplenism is a condition in which deficiency of one or more of the peripheral blood elements (red blood cells, leukocytes, or platelets) occurs as a result of excessive destruction by the spleen. The bone marrow may be normal or hypercellular, and splenomegaly (namely, enlargement of the spleen) may or may not be present. By definition, idiopathic hypersplenism is reversed by splenectomy.

Hypersplenism is uncommon, if not rare, in ferrets. Nonetheless, ferrets with splenomegaly should always be evaluated for hypersplenism (see previous section). Perform a complete medical workup if you suspect hypersplenism. A CBC, platelet count, and bone marrow aspiration provide the minimum data needed. Whole-body radiography and a serum biochemistry workup are helpful for ruling out other diseases. The presence of one or more cytopenias, in association with normal to hypercellular bone marrow, and no evidence of infection, neoplasia, or other cause of cytopenia provide presumptive evidence of hypersplenism.

Splenectomy is the treatment of choice for hypersplenism. Indeed, clinical improvement after splenectomy completes the diagnostic definition of idiopathic hypersplenism. Administer other therapy, including blood transfusions (see Chapter 2), B vitamins, a broad-spectrum antibiotic for the prevention of secondary infection, and supportive care, as indicated for the individual animal. A fresh ferret blood transfusion just before surgery as a source of platelets may help in minimizing intraoperative and postoperative bleeding.

One case report describes the successful treatment of hypersplenism in a 3-year-old spayed female ferret.[9] This animal presented for an abdominal mass, polyuria, polydipsia, and polyphagia of 2 weeks' duration, and pallor, weight loss, and decreased activity of 1 week's duration. It had pale mucous membranes and splenomegaly. Laboratory testing revealed anemia, leukopenia, and profound thrombocytopenia. Splenectomy was performed on day 12 of hospitalization because of evidence of responsive anemia, the massive size of the spleen, and lack of improvement with supportive care and medical therapy consisting of administration of tetracycline, corticosteroids, iron dextran, and B vitamins. A fresh ferret blood transfusion was administered just before surgery. The ferret did well after splenectomy.

Anemia

There are many causes of anemia in ferrets, as in other species. In the past, the most common cause of anemia in female ferrets was bone marrow suppression caused by hyperestrogenism secondary to persistent estrus (see Chapter 5). Estrogen toxicity is now uncommon because of the current practice of spaying female ferrets before their sale as pets. The other possible causes of anemia are many (see Table 1 in Appendix) and can be divided, as for other species, into regenerative and nonregenerative anemias.

Regenerative anemia typically occurs as the result of blood loss or hemolysis. Causes of blood loss in ferrets include gastrointestinal blood loss secondary to the presence of a foreign body, gastroduodenal ulcers, gastroenteritis, or colitis; trauma; fleas; hemorrhage secondary to thrombocytopenia; and AD virus-associated hemorrhage. Theoretically, hemolytic anemia could occur because of heavy metal poisoning, immune-mediated disease, or, as in mink, in association with AD virus infection. Immune-mediated disease would be difficult to diagnose definitively in ferrets because of the lack of ferret-specific reagents.

Nonregenerative anemia occurs because of disruption of hematopoiesis in the bone marrow. Possible causes include bone marrow infiltration by neoplastic cells, anemia of chronic disease, and hyperestrogenism associated with persistent estrus, an ovarian remnant, or an adrenal tumor.

Diagnosis and Treatment

The approach to the diagnosis and treatment of anemia in ferrets is very similar to that in other species; therefore, apply basic principles from companion animal medicine when you are unsure how to proceed. The normal adult ferret PCV is high, typically 45–60%, relative to the PCV in other species; therefore, a PCV of 35% in an adult ferret represents a mild anemia.

Ferrets with anemia usually present for nonspecific signs, such as weakness, lethargy, and inappetence. The owner may report melena. Mucous membrane pallor is evident on physical examination, and subcutaneous petechial or ecchymotic hemorrhages may be evident in ferrets with concomitant thrombocytopenia. Female ferrets with hyperestrogenism have a swollen vulva. Question the owner about possible foreign body or toxin ingestion. Perform a complete physical examination and proceed with a medical workup as you would for other companion animals with possible anemia.

If you suspect anemia, obtain a small volume of blood for determination of PCV before you draw more blood. If the PCV is low (normal range, 45–60%, and up to 63%), take the minimal amount of blood necessary to perform a CBC, reticulocyte count, platelet count, and, if indicated, serum chemistry. (Remember that a given amount of blood taken from an anemic animal produces relatively more plasma or serum than that from a nonanemic animal.) The reticulocyte count, presence or absence of polychromasia, and cytologic assessment of erythrocytes are useful in determining whether the anemia is regenerative or nonregenerative. The reported normal mean reticulocyte count in albino ferrets is 4% (range, 1–12%) and 5.3% (range, 2–14%) for males and females, respectively.[31] Obtain a bone marrow sample if the anemia is nonregenerative to evaluate bone marrow morphology (see Chapter 2 for technique).

Treatment of ferrets with anemia consists of supportive care, the use of hematinics, and therapy specific for the cause of the anemia. Evaluate the need for a blood transfusion (see Chapter 2) on the basis of the ferret's clinical status and the PCV. Usually a transfusion is not necessary until the PCV falls below 15%. Ferrets do not have detectable blood groups; therefore, a fresh ferret blood transfusion can be administered without cross-matching.[18]

ACKNOWLEDGMENT

We would like to thank Dr. Nick Sitinas for his contributions to the section on cardiac diseases.

REFERENCES

1. Alexandersen S: Pathogenesis of disease caused by Aleutian mink disease parvovirus. Acta Pathol Microbiol Immunol Scand Suppl 1990; 98:1–32.
2. Beach JE, Greenwood B: Spontaneous neoplasia in the ferret *(Mustela putorius furo)*. J Comp Pathol 1993; 108:133–147.
3. Blair LS, Campbell WC: Suppression of maturation of *Dirofilaria immitis* in *Mustela putorius furo* by single dose of ivermectin. J Parasitol 1980; 66:691–692.
4. Bone L, Battles AH, Goldfarb RD, et al: Electrocardiographic values from clinically normal, anesthetized ferrets *(Mustela putorius furo)*. Am J Vet Res 1988; 49: 1884–1887.
5. Calvert C, Brown J: Use of M-mode echocardiography in the diagnosis of congestive cardiomyopathy in Doberman pinschers. J Am Vet Med Assoc 1986; 189:293–297.
6. Campbell WC, Blair LS: *Dirofilaria immitis*: experimental infections in the ferret *(Mustela putorius furo)*. J Parasitol 1978; 64:119–122.
7. Daoust PY, Hunter DB: Spontaneous Aleutian disease in ferrets. Can Vet J 1978; 19:133–135.
8. Ensley PK, Van Winkle T: Treatment of congestive heart failure in a ferret *(Mustela putorius furo)*. J Zoo Anim Med 1982; 13:23–25.
9. Ferguson DC: Idiopathic hypersplenism in a ferret. J Am Vet Med Assoc 1985; 186:693–695.
10. Fox JG: Normal clinical and biologic parameters. *In* Fox JG, ed.: Biology and Diseases of the Ferret. Philadelphia, Lea & Febiger, 1988, pp 159–173.
11. Fox PR: Feline myocardial disease. *In* Fox PR, ed.: Canine and Feline Cardiology. New York, Churchill Livingstone, 1988, pp 439–466.
12. Greenlee PG, Stephens E: Meningeal cryptococcosis and congestive cardiomyopathy in a ferret. J Am Vet Med Assoc 1984; 184:840–841.
13. Jobic Y, Slama M, Tribouilloy C, et al: Doppler echocardiographic evaluation of valve regurgitation in healthy volunteers. Br Heart J 1993; 69:109–113.
14. Keene BW: Canine cardiomyopathy. *In* Kirk RW, ed.: Current Veterinary Therapy 10. Philadelphia, WB Saunders, 1989, pp 240–251.
15. Kenyon AJ, Kenyon BJ, Hahn EC: Protides of the Mustelidae: immunoresponse of mustelids to Aleutian mink disease virus. Am J Vet Res 1978; 39:1011–1015.
16. Lipman NS, Murphy JC, Fox JG: Clinical, functional and pathologic changes associated with a case of dilatative cardiomyopathy in a ferret. Lab Anim Sci 1987; 37: 210–212.
17. Macchi C, Orlandini SZ, Orlandini GE: An anatomical study of the healthy human heart by echocardiography with special reference to physiological valvular regurgitation. Anat Anz 1994; 176:81–86.
18. Manning DD, Bell JA: Lack of detectable blood groups in domestic ferrets: implications for transfusion. J Am Vet Med Assoc 1990; 197:84–86.
19. Miller WR, Merton DA: Dirofilariasis in a ferret. J Am Vet Med Assoc 1982; 180:1103–1104.
20. Moise NS, Dietze AE, Mezza LE, et al: Echocardiography, electrocardiography, and radiography of cats with dilation cardiomyopathy, hypertrophic cardiomyopathy, and hyperthyroidism. Am J Vet Res 1986; 7:1477–1485.
21. Nakayama T, Wakao T, Takiguchi S, et al: Prevalence of valvular regurgitation in normal beagle dogs. J Vet Med Sci 1994; 56:973–975.
22. Palley LS, Corning BF, Fox JG, et al: Parvovirus-associated syndrome (Aleutian disease) in two ferrets. J Am Vet Med Assoc 1992; 201:100–106.
23. Parrott TY, Greiner EC, Parrott JD: *Dirofilaria immitis* infection in three ferrets. J Am Vet Med Assoc 1984; 184:582–583.
24. Porter DD: Aleutian disease: a persistent parvovirus infection of mink with a maximal but ineffective host humoral immune response. Prog Med Virol 1986; 33: 42–60.
25. Porter DD, Larsen AE, Porter HG: Aleutian disease of mink. Adv Immunol 1980; 29:261–286.
26. Porter DD, Porter HG, Larsen AE: Aleutian disease parvovirus of mink and ferrets elicits an antibody response to a

second nonstructural viral protein. J Virol 1990; 64: 1859–1860.
27. Porter HG, Porter DD, Larsen AE: Aleutian disease in ferrets. Infect Immun 1982; 36:379–386.
28. Rosenthal K: Ferrets. Vet Clin North Am Small Anim Pract 1994; 24:1–21.
29. Smith SH, Bishop SP: The electrocardiogram of normal ferrets and ferrets with right ventricular hypertrophy. Lab Anim Sci 1985; 35:268–271.
30. Snyder PS, Atkins CE: Current uses and hazards of the digitalis glycosides. *In* Kirk RW, Bonagura JD, eds.: Kirk's Current Veterinary Therapy 11: Small Animal Practice. Philadelphia, WB Saunders, 1992, pp 689–693.
31. Thornton PC, Wright PA, Sacra PJ, et al: The ferret, *Mustela putorius furo,* as a new species in toxicology. Lab Anim 1979; 13:119–124.
32. Thornton RN, Cook TG: A congenital *Toxoplasma*-like disease in ferrets *(Mustela putorius furo).* N Z Vet J 1986; 34:31–33.
33. Uretsky BF: Diagnostic considerations in the adult patient with cardiomyopathy or congestive heart failure. Cardiovasc Clin 1988; 19:35–56.

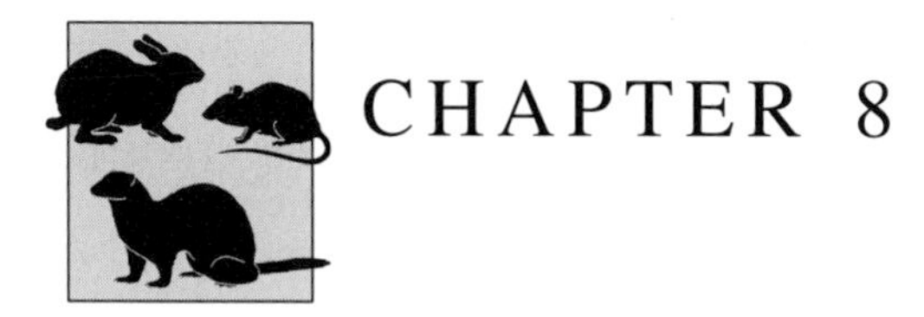

CHAPTER 8

Respiratory Diseases

Karen L. Rosenthal, DVM

CANINE DISTEMPER VIRUS

Canine distemper virus (CDV) is a ribonucleic acid virus in the family Paramyxoviridae.[24] Different strains of the virus vary in virulence, but canine distemper is typically a fatal disease in ferrets. Ferrets risk being exposed to this disease because it is ubiquitous. It is the most prevalent viral disease of dogs.[24] Reservoirs of CDV include members of the families Canidae, Mustelidae, and Procyonidae.

Transmission of the virus is most commonly accomplished by aerosol exposure.[1] Direct contact with conjunctival and nasal exudates, urine, feces, and skin also causes infection.[9] Ferrets shed virus in all body excretions, and shedding begins about 7 days after exposure.[1] Fomites are also implicated in transmission because virus on gloves is viable for up to 20 minutes.[9] Once in a ferret's body, the virus appears to spread by viremia.[18] The incubation period in ferrets is 7–10 days.[9]

History and Physical Examination

CDV infection should be suspected in any unvaccinated, exposed ferret showing compatible clinical signs. Unvaccinated ferrets of any age are equally susceptible to this disease. In dogs, pyrexia is noted 3–6 days after infection with CDV and is soon followed by anorexia and a serous nasal discharge.[1] A serous ocular discharge then appears; this discharge quickly becomes mucopurulent.

Often, the first sign of disease in a ferret is a rash on the chin. The skin around the lips and chin becomes swollen and then crusty. These changes can be accompanied by a dermatitis on the anus and inguinal area (Fig 8–1).[9] Some ferrets have an orange-tinged dermatitis. Other clinical signs include anorexia, depression, pyrexia, photophobia, blepharospasm, and abundant mucopurulent ocular and nasal discharge. Brown crusts may form on the face, and the eyelids may adhere to each other. Hyperkeratosis of the footpads is common (see Fig. 8–1). Vomiting and diarrhea, which are seen in dogs with CDV,[24] are not common in ferrets.

Coughing may then ensue. The respiratory system is the preferred site of replication for CDV.[18] The secondary bacterial infections that are responsible for many of the severe respiratory signs and death are caused by the immunosuppressive effects of the canine distemper virus.[24]

In dogs with CDV infection, seizures and blindness are common,[24] and nervous signs may be noted without previous systemic signs.[1] Nervous signs such as incoordination, torticollis, nystagmus, and incoordination are all noted in ferrets with advanced CDV infection.[1]

Diagnosis

Diagnosis of CDV infection is based on history of exposure to the virus, observation of clinical signs, a positive result on fluorescent antibody testing, and histopathologic results. Nonspecific test results can include a leukopenia on complete blood count (CBC) and lung congestion or consolidation on radiographs.[1, 24]

Perform a fluorescent antibody test on conjunctival smears, mucous membrane scrapings, or blood smears to identify CDV antigen in cells.[9, 24] This test is useful only in the first few days of disease, and false-negative results are possible. The modified live viral strains used for vaccination do not interfere with this testing method.[24]

CDV and influenza virus infections are usually distinguishable on the basis of information in the history, observation of clinical signs, and findings on physical examination. Clinical signs of CDV initially may resemble those of influenza; however,

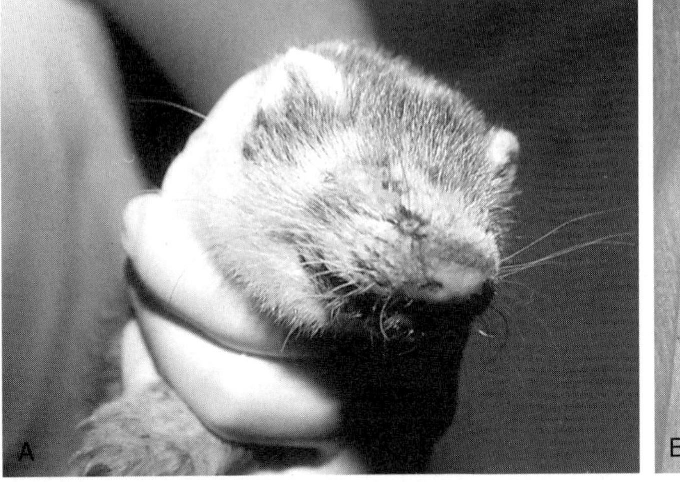

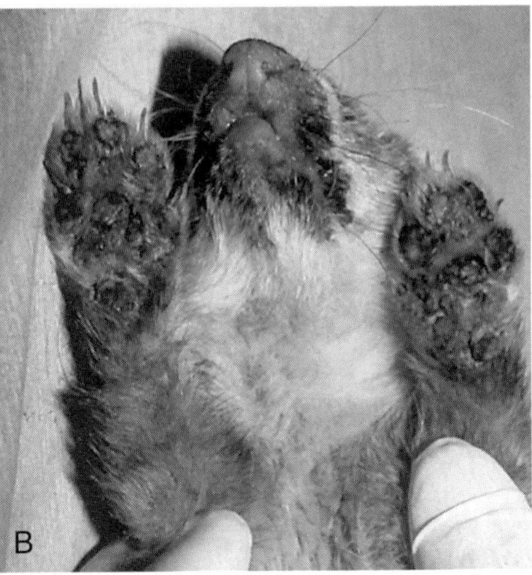

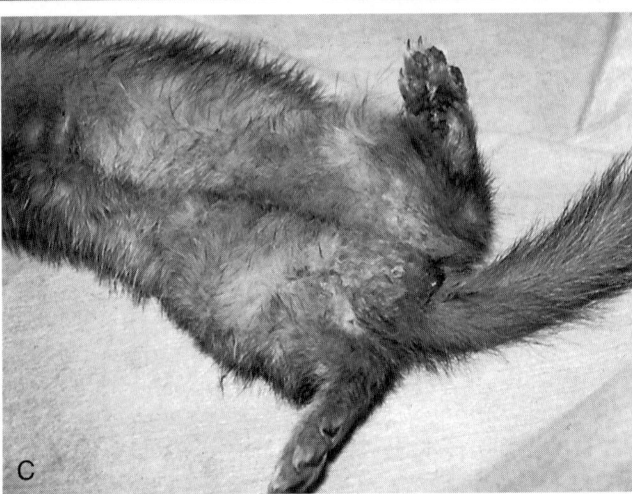

FIGURE 8–1
Young ferret with CDV infection. *A,* The eyes are encrusted shut with mucopurulent exudate. *B,* Dermatitis, excoriations, and crusting around the lips and chin; hyperkeratosis of the footpads. *C,* Dermatitis in the inguinal area.

TABLE 8–1

CLINICAL DISTINCTIONS BETWEEN CANINE DISTEMPER VIRUS AND INFLUENZA VIRUS INFECTIONS

Clinical Findings	Canine Distemper Virus	Influenza
Nasal and ocular discharge	+++ (Mucopurulent)	++ (Mucoserous)
Sneezing	+	+++
Coughing	+	+++
Pyrexia	+++ (>40°C)	++†
Dermatitis (chin, lips, inguinal)	+++	—
Footpad hyperkeratosis	++	—
Central signs	+*	—
Outcome	Almost 100% fatal	Self-limiting‡

Key to frequency of clinical signs: + = may be present; ++ = common; +++ = the usual presentation; – = absent.
*Central nervous system signs seen in advanced stages of disease (rarely the only signs).
†Pyrexia occurs early in the course of disease and may be resolved by the time of presentation.
‡Influenza virus infection can be fatal in neonates.

within 1–2 days, serous nasal and ocular discharge turns mucopurulent, and a dermatitis that is pathognomonic for CDV infection (when seen in conjunction with the other usual findings) develops around the chin and lips. Ferrets with CDV tend to be much sicker than those with influenza infection. Further distinctions are made in Table 8–1.

A positive postmortem diagnosis can be made with fluorescent antibody staining of imprints from lymph nodes, the bladder epithelium, and the cerebellum.[1] Histopathologic examination of affected cells can also confirm the disease. CDV inclusion bodies are usually intracytoplasmic but can be intranuclear. They are generally found in the epithelial cells of the trachea, urinary bladder, skin, gastrointestinal tract, lymph nodes, spleen, and salivary glands.[9] Diffuse, interstitial pneumonia is reported. In the central nervous system, inflammatory cell invasion with demyelination is observed.[1]

Treatment

No treatment is available for CDV infection in ferrets, and the mortality rate is almost 100%. Until such time as treatment becomes available for CDV, euthanasia of affected ferrets is usually the most humane route. If euthanasia is not an option, palliative treatment consists of the use of antibiotics for secondary infections as well as supportive care.

Prevention

Vaccination is the best way to prevent CDV infection in ferrets. Start vaccinations at 6 or 8 weeks of age for kits from nonimmune or immune dams, respectively, and then continue vaccinating every 3–4 weeks until the kits are 14 weeks old. Revaccinate yearly.

A modified live vaccine is recommended for protection from CDV. Killed vaccines do not offer reliable long-term protection. Use a vaccine derived from non-ferret cell lines, because ferrets vaccinated with ferret cell line–derived vaccines can develop the disease. Avoid multivalent canine vaccines, which can be associated with adverse effects (see Chapter 2).

If an outbreak occurs in a group of susceptible ferrets, all clinically affected animals should be removed, and healthy ferrets should be vaccinated immediately. However, vaccination of unvaccinated ferrets in the face of an outbreak may not stop infection and mortality.[9]

CDV is relatively labile, and its infectivity is destroyed by heat, drying, detergents, and disinfectants.[24] Routine cleaning and disinfection procedures are effective in destroying CDV on hard surfaces.

INFLUENZA

Several strains of human influenza virus, from the family Orthomyxoviridae, can infect ferrets.[5,16] Influenza in ferrets, as in people, mainly causes upper respiratory disease. The different strains of influenza virus have varying degrees of virulence, which account for the difference in severity of clinical signs.[22]

Transmission is readily accomplished by inhalation of aerosol droplets from ferret to ferret and from human to ferret. Ferrets can even transmit this disease back to people.[16] Ferrets transmit the virus, starting at the height of pyrexia and continuing for the next 3–4 days.[23]

History and Physical Examination

Ferrets contract this disease after being exposed to infected people or other infected ferrets. All ferrets are susceptible to influenza, although neonates typically develop a more severe form of the disease than do older ferrets.

After a short incubation period, body temperature increases and then decreases approximately 48 hours later.[5, 9, 16, 21] Bouts of sneezing and eye watering and a mucoid or mucopurulent nasal discharge are common clinical signs and can appear within 48 hours of exposure.[5, 16] Lethargy and inappetence are common.[23] Photophobia and conjunctivitis may be present.[9] Neonates may develop a much more severe upper respiratory infection than do adults, and death may ensue secondary to lower airway obstruction.[4, 22]

Lower respiratory tract signs are less common than upper respiratory tract signs. Lower respiratory tract infection is usually confined to the bronchial epithelium[22] and is usually the result of secondary bacterial infections. Deaths are reported following secondary pulmonary infection with Lancefield group C hemolytic streptococci.[16] Neonates are more likely than older ferrets to develop bronchiolitis and pneumonia,[5] and neonates are more likely to die from the lower respiratory tract infection than are adults.[22]

Influenza can establish an infection in the intestinal mucosa and cause a limited enteritis.[10] The potential for hepatic dysfunction has been described in ferrets infected experimentally with influenza.[15] Hearing loss has been associated with influenza infection in ferrets.[20]

Diagnosis

Diagnosis of influenza is made on the basis of observation of clinical signs, history of exposure to infected individuals, isolation of virus from nasal secretions, and increasing antibody titer.[16] See Table 8–1 for the differences in presentation of influenza and canine distemper. Experimentally, it has been shown that an enzyme-liked immunosorbent assay (ELISA) test can detect antibodies against influenza A and can be used to establish a serologic diagnosis rapidly.[3] Antibodies to influenza infection have been shown to be present within 3 days after infection.[17]

A transient leukopenia can be seen with this disease. Elevations in blood urea nitrogen, creatinine, alanine aminotransferase, potassium, and albumin levels with influenza infection have been reported, but usually the results of the biochemistry profile are within normal limits.[15]

Treatment

Influenza has a 7- to 14-day course and is associated with a low mortality rate in adult ferrets. Most affected ferrets can be treated at home. Instruct owners to offer favorite foods and to encourage their ferrets to eat and drink. If necessary, use a pediatric cough suppressant without alcohol (at the pediatric dosage on a per weight basis) or an antihistamine, such as diphenhydramine (0.5–2 mg/kg PO q8–12h), or both, for symptomatic therapy.

Experimentally, the antiviral medication amantadine (6 mg/kg administered as an aerosol q12h) has been shown to be efficacious in the treatment of this disease.[9] Antibiotics can be used to control secondary respiratory bacterial infections. Deaths in neonates are typically the result of secondary bacterial infections; therefore, mortality in neonates can be reduced with the use of antibiotics.[12]

The use of aspirin to control fever is of questionable merit because fever is an important host defense mechanism. Ferrets given aspirin have a lowered body temperature, but they shed more virus and their viral levels decrease less rapidly than in ferrets not treated with an antipyretic; this suggests that fever is instrumental in restricting the severity of infection.[13, 22]

Prevention

Control of influenza rests mainly on prevention of exposure of susceptible ferrets to infected individuals. Newborn ferrets are completely protected from disease by milk-derived antibodies in immunized mothers.[14] Experimentally, ferrets are resistant to infection from the same influenza strain 5 weeks after primary infection.[9]

Vaccination of ferrets against influenza virus is not generally recommended for a number of reasons. Influenza is commonly a relatively benign disease in ferrets. The wide antigenic variation of the virus makes vaccination difficult, and vaccination seems to confer only short-term immunity.[9] However, if giving a vaccine, use live rather than inactivated vaccines. Live vaccines induce a greater protective effect and are more likely to stimulate local antibody production.[7]

PNEUMONIA

Pneumonia is not a common diagnosis in ferrets. It is usually associated with CDV or influenza virus infection. Respiratory syncytial virus has been shown to cause rhinitis and infection in the lungs of ferrets, but clinical signs of pneumonia have not been seen.[19] Bacterial pneumonia is a common sequela of megaesophagus in ferrets.

Reported primary bacterial pathogens causing pneumonia in ferrets include *Streptococcus zooepidemicus, S. pneumoniae,* and groups C and G streptococci. Gram-negative bacteria such as *E. coli, Klebsiella pneumoniae,* and *Pseudomonas aeruginosa* have been isolated from ferrets.[8] Other bacteria that have been isolated from the lungs of ferrets include *Bordetella bronchiseptica* and *Listeria monocytogenes*. Bacterial pneumonia is characterized by a suppurative inflammatory process that affects the bronchial tree or the lung lobes, or both.

Pneumocystis carinii is known to infect the lungs of ferrets. Latent infections can become active with immune suppression.[2] Diagnosis is based on identification of the organism in a tracheal or lung wash.[11] Treatment recommendations for *P. carinii* pneumonia include pentamidine isethionate or trimethoprim-sulfamethoxazole.[11]

History and Physical Examination

Affected ferrets exhibit clinical signs typical of a mammal with pneumonia. Labored breathing, dyspnea, cyanotic mucous membranes, increased lung sounds, nasal discharge, fever, lethargy, and anorexia are all possible clinical signs. Fulminant pneumonia leading to sepsis and death has been reported.[8, 11]

Diagnosis

The diagnosis of pneumonia in ferrets is made on the basis of observation of clinical signs, CBC results, culture and cytologic findings, and radiographic signs. The CBC may show a leukocytosis with a neutrophilia and a leftward shift.[11]

Radiographs at first reveal an interstitial pattern that changes to an alveolar pattern if pneumonia progresses (Fig. 8–2). If aspiration pneumonia is present, the primary involvement of dependent lung lobes is present. Marked bronchial patterns are suggestive of primary airway disease.[11]

Microbial cultures of a tracheal wash or lung wash are invaluable for establishing diagnosis and treatment of pneumonia. Perform both bacterial and fungal cultures. Along with cultures, cytologic analysis of the collected fluid and debris is instrumental for diagnosing the cause of the pneumonia. Cytologic assessment of a tracheal wash from a ferret with pneumonia typically reveals septic inflammation and degenerating neutrophils.[11] The results of the tracheal wash or lung wash reflect the degree, category, and chronicity of disease.

Treatment

Treatment of ferrets with pneumonia comprises good supportive care, including fluid therapy and force-feeding, as well as antimicrobial therapy tailored according to test results. First-line antibiotics to consider before culture results are known include a trimethoprim-sulfa drug combination, chloramphenicol, and the cephalosporins.[11]

The prognosis for pneumonia in ferrets depends on the response to treatment. Most ferrets with bacterial pneumonia respond to antibiotic therapy.

PULMONARY MYCOSES

Pulmonary mycoses are uncommon in pet ferrets. It is not likely for ferrets reared indoors to be exposed to mycotic spores, which are mainly found in the soil. These spores are responsible for mycotic pneumonia.

History and Physical Examination

Not all animals with mycoses exhibit signs consistent with pulmonary disease. If lesions develop in the lungs, coughing is frequently observed. Other signs consistent with a mycotic infection include wasting,

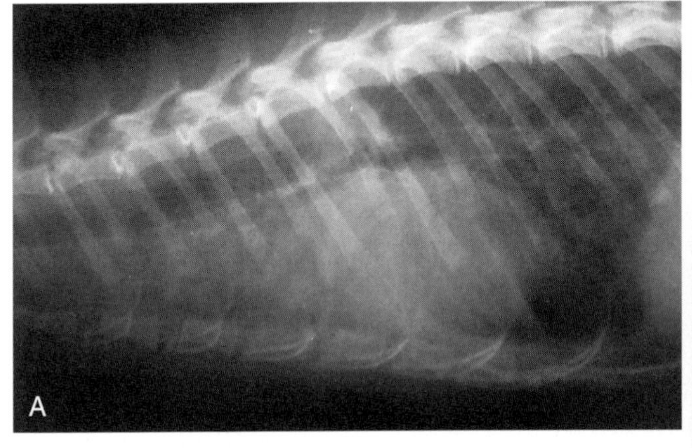

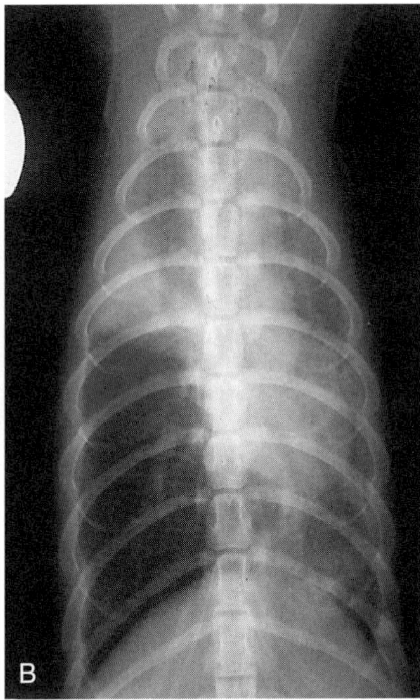

FIGURE 8–2
A, Lateral and *B,* ventrodorsal radiographs of a ferret with bacterial pneumonia. An alveolar pattern with air bronchograms is evident in the cranial lobe of the right lung and in all of the lobes of the left lung.

lethargy, anorexia, lymph node enlargement, lameness, ocular and nasal discharge, and draining tracts unresponsive to antibiotics.[6, 25] The prognosis for ferrets with pulmonary mycoses is poor.

Blastomycosis

Blastomycosis caused by *Blastomyces dermatitidis* is endemic in the southeastern United States, the Mississippi River Valley, and the Ohio River Valley.[25] Experimentally, the incubation period is 5–12 weeks in dogs. The mycelial phase is found in the soil, and the yeast form is found in the tissues. Diagnosis is made on the basis of a history of travel to an endemic region, observation of signs, results of cytologic assessment, positive periodic acid–Schiff reaction, or culture of *B. dermatitidis.* Recommended treatment includes the use of amphotericin B and ketoconazole.[25]

Coccidioidomycosis

Coccidioides immitis is the cause of coccidioidomycosis. It is endemic in the southwestern United States and parts of Latin America. Primary infection develops after inhalation of the mycelia. In the host, the spherules are formed and then produce endospores.[6, 25] Pulmonary signs are present 1–3 weeks following infection. Diagnosis is based on identification of the spherules on cytologic examination; these appear as refractile, double-walled bodies.[25] Recommended treatment, which is based on that for cats with coccidioidomycosis, includes the use of amphotericin B and ketoconazole.[6, 25]

OTHER CAUSES OF RESPIRATORY SIGNS

Differential diagnoses for tachypnea, dyspnea, and respiratory distress are listed in Appendix 1. After the history and physical examination, chest and abdominal radiography is the most important tool for differentiating the causes of lower respiratory signs. The recommended diagnostic approach to dyspnea is presented diagramatically in Figure 8–3.

Ferrets that have been hit by a car or experienced a fall can develop pneumothorax or diaphragmatic hernia. Approach these animals as you would a dog or cat with the same condition. See Chapter 13 for a description of the surgical repair of diaphragmatic hernia.

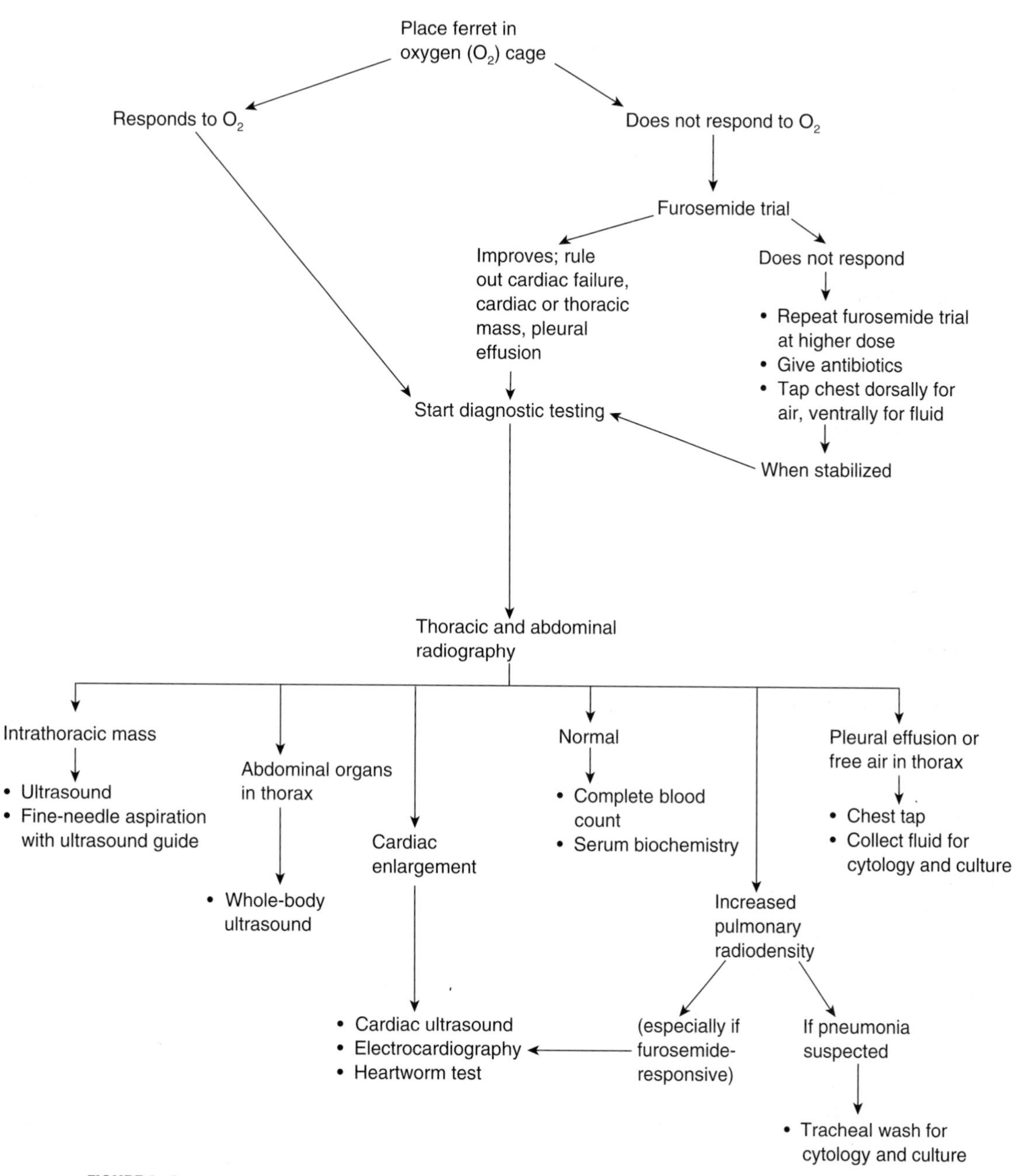

FIGURE 8–3

Diagnostic approach to dyspnea. The approach recommended here is the most conservative one. It often is possible to obtain chest radiographs (even one view can be very helpful) with the use of supplemental oxygen by facemask, with or without isoflurane for stress reduction, before the ferret is fully stabilized. Use your clinical judgment in determining the best time to perform radiography.

REFERENCES

1. Appel M: Canine distemper virus. *In* Appel M, ed.: Virus Infections of Carnivores. New York, Elsevier Science Publishers, 1987, pp 133–159.
2. Bauer NL, Paulsrud JR, Bartlett MS, et al: *Pneumocystis carinii* organisms obtained from rats, ferrets, and mice are antigenically different. Infect Immunol 1993; 61: 1315–1319.
3. Boer GFD, Back W, Osterhaus ADME: An ELISA for detection of antibodies against influenza A nucleoprotein in humans and various animal species. Arch Virol 1990; 115:47–61.
4. Collie MH, Rushton DI, Sweet C, Smith H: Studies of influenza virus infection in newborn ferrets. J Med Microbiol 1980; 13:561–570.
5. Doggart L: Viral disease of pet ferrets: Part II. Aleutian disease, influenza, and rabies. Vet Technol 1988; 9:384–389.
6. DuVal-Hudelson KA: Coccidioidomycosis in three European ferrets. J Zoo Wildl Med 1990; 21:353–357.
7. Fenton RJ, Clark A, Potter CW: Immunity to influenza in ferrets: XIV. Comparative immunity following infection or immunization with live or inactivated vaccine. Br J Exp Pathol 1981; 62:297–307.
8. Fox JG: Bacterial and mycoplasmal diseases. *In* Fox JG, ed.: Biology and Diseases of the Ferret. Philadelphia, Lea & Febiger, 1988, pp 197–216.
9. Fox JG, Pearson RC, Gorham JR: Viral and chlamydial diseases. *In* Fox JG, ed.: Biology and Diseases of Ferrets. Philadelphia, Lea & Febiger, 1988, pp 217–234.
10. Glathe H, Lebhardt A, Hilgenfeld M, et al: Untersuchungen zur enteralen Influenzainfektion bei Frettchen. Arch Exp Vetinarmed 1984; 38:771–777.
11. Hawkins EC, Ettinger SJ, Suter PF: Lower respiratory tract (lung) and pulmonary edema. *In* Ettinger SJ, ed.: Textbook of Veterinary Internal Medicine. 3rd ed. Philadelphia, WB Saunders, 1989, pp 816–866.
12. Husseini RH, Collie MH, Rushton DI, et al: The role of naturally-acquired bacterial infection in influenza-related death in neonatal ferrets. Br J Exp Pathol 1983; 64:559–569.
13. Husseini RH, Sweet C, Collie MH, Smith H: Elevation of nasal viral levels by suppression of fever in ferrets infected with influenza viruses of differing virulence. J Infect Dis 1982; 145:520–524.
14. Husseini RH, Sweet C, Overton H, Smith H: Role of maternal immunity in the protection of newborn ferrets against infection with a virulent influenza virus. Immunology 1984; 52:389–394.
15. Kang ES, Lee HJ, Boulet J, et al: Potential for hepatic and renal dysfunction during influenza B infection, convalescence, and after induction of secondary viremia. J Exp Pathol 1992; 6:133–144.
16. Marini RP, Adkins JA, Fox JG: Proven or potential zoonotic diseases of ferrets. J Am Vet Med Assoc 1989; 195: 990–994.
17. McLaren C, Butchko GM: Regional T- and B-cell responses in influenza-infected ferrets. Infect Immunol 1978; 22:189–194.
18. Pearson RC, Gorham JR: Viral disease models. *In* Fox JG, ed.: Biology and Diseases of the Ferret. Philadelphia, Lea & Febiger, 1988, pp 305–314.
19. Prince GA, Porter DD: The pathogenesis of respiratory syncytial virus infection in infant ferrets. Am J Pathol 1976; 82:339–352.
20. Rarey KE, DeLacure MA, Sandridge SA, Small PA: Effect of upper respiratory infection on hearing in the ferret model. Am J Otolaryngol 1987; 8:161–170.
21. Ryland LM, Gorham JR: The ferret and its diseases. J Am Vet Med Assoc 1978; 173:1154–1158.
22. Smith H, Sweet C: Lessons for human influenza from pathogenicity studies in ferrets. Rev Infect Dis 1988; 10:56–75.
23. Squires S, Belyavin G: Free contact infection in ferret groups. J Antimicrob Chemother 1975; 1(Suppl):35–42.
24. Swango LJ: Canine viral diseases. *In* Ettinger SJ, ed.: Textbook of Veterinary Internal Medicine. Philadelphia, WB Saunders, 1989, pp 298–311.
25. Wolf AM, Troy GC: Deep mycotic diseases. *In* Ettinger SJ, ed.: Textbook of Veterinary Internal Medicine. Philadelphia, WB Saunders, 1989, pp 341–372.

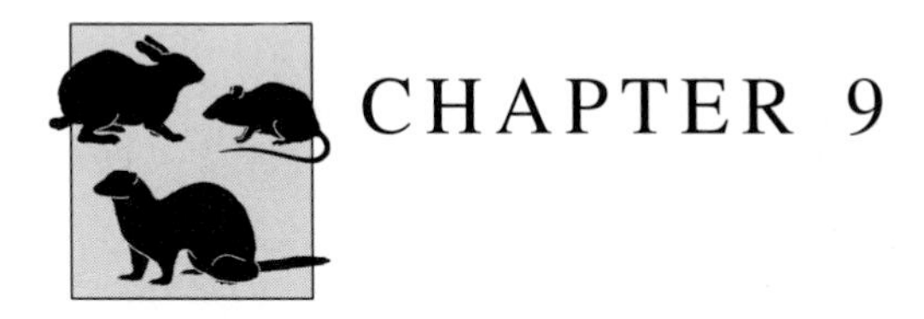

CHAPTER 9

Endocrine Diseases

Katherine E. Quesenberry, DVM
and Karen L. Rosenthal, DVM

PART I

Katherine E. Quesenberry, DVM

INSULINOMA

Insulinomas are pancreatic islet cell tumors of the beta cells and are one of the most common tumors that occur in middle-aged to older ferrets. These tumors produce an excessive amount of insulin, resulting in hypoglycemia. The clinical signs associated with hypoglycemia commonly prompt ferret owners to seek veterinary care.

Pathophysiology

Pancreatic beta cell tumors cause an increase in basal insulin secretion. Additionally, the tumor cells fail to respond to normal inhibitory stimuli and release excessive amounts of insulin in response to normal provocative stimuli.[20] Continuous hyperinsulinemia sustains the metabolic effects of insulin. Hepatic gluconeogenesis and glycogenolysis are inhibited, and peripheral uptake of glucose by tissue cells is increased. In normal animals, low blood glucose concentrations trigger the glucoreceptors in the hindbrain and hypothalamus, inducing the release of glucagon, cortisol, epinephrine, and growth hormone.[13] These hormones act to increase the blood glucose concentration by stimulating gluconeogenesis and glycogenolysis in the liver and by inhibiting peripheral use of glucose. This feedback mechanism is inoperative in animals with insulinomas; the hyperglycemic effects of glucagon, epinephrine, cortisol, and growth hormone are inhibited, and blood glucose concentrations continue to decrease.[13, 23]

Clinical signs of hypoglycemia are correlated to the rate of decline and concentration of blood glucose and to the duration of hypoglycemia.[13] Clinical signs can be categorized as neuroglucopenic manifestations or adrenergic manifestations, or as a combination of both. Neuroglucopenic signs result from the effect of hypoglycemia on the central nervous system, as glucose is the primary energy source for these tissues. Uptake of glucose occurs by diffusion and is not insulin dependent.[22] Glucose deprivation of the cells of the nervous tissues results in clinical signs of hypoglycemia, including mental dullness, confusion, seizures, and coma. Adrenergic manifestations occur when blood glucose concentrations decrease rapidly, resulting in catecholamine release and increased sympathetic tone. Adrenergic signs include tachycardia, hypothermia, tremors, nervousness, and irritability.[13] Prolonged, severe hypoglycemia can result in cerebral hypoxia and, possibly, irreversible cerebral lesions.[22]

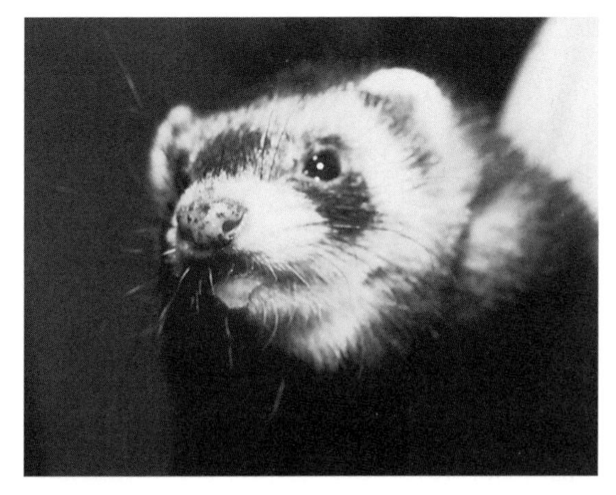

FIGURE 9–1
Typical glassy eyed appearance and hypersalivation in a ferret experiencing hypoglycemia.

History and Physical Examination

Insulinomas are usually seen in ferrets between the ages of 3 and 8 years, but they are most common in ferrets 4 to 5 years of age. Both male and female ferrets are affected, and there is no apparent sex predilection.

The history varies from an acute onset of clinical signs to a chronic course of weeks to many months. An owner may describe an acute episode of collapse during which the ferret is depressed, minimally responsive, and recumbent. The episode may last from several minutes to several hours and ends with a spontaneous recovery or after administration of an oral sugar solution or syrup by the owner. Ferrets are occasionally presented for examination while in this collapsed state. Owners may notice increased salivation, and many describe the eyes as appearing "glazed" during these episodes (Fig. 9–1). The number of episodes of collapse varies from one to several over a period of days to months; episodes may be isolated occurrences or increase in frequency over time.

Another common presentation involves a gradual onset of weakness and lethargy over weeks to months. The appetite may be normal or decreased, and weight loss may be noted. Often, the owner notices ataxia or pronounced weakness, particularly in the hind legs. Clinical signs are often intermittent, with normal activity and demeanor between periods of weakness. Ferrets often show hypersalivation and paw at the mouth, signs that may indicate nausea, caused by hypoglycemia, during these episodes.

Some ferrets with insulinomas have no discernible clinical signs. In these animals, insulinoma is diagnosed during surgery for other problems, most commonly adrenal neoplasia. During routine examination of other abdominal organs at surgery, one or more pancreatic nodules are noted and are then excised and confirmed on histologic examination as pancreatic tumors.

Physical examination findings are variable in ferrets with insulinoma. Some ferrets have no abnormalities noted at the time of examination, although most have varying degrees of splenomegaly (see Chapter 7). Clinical findings consistent with other disease problems (e.g., hair loss or thinning, skin masses, and cardiac arrhythmias) are often present. Adrenal neoplasia, lymphoma, various skin tumors, and cardiomyopathy are common concurrent problems.

Clinical Pathology and Diagnostic Testing

Blood Glucose and Insulin Concentrations

A presumptive diagnosis of insulinoma is based on clinical signs and laboratory evidence of hypoglycemia. More than one blood sample or a carefully monitored fast (4–6 hours is sufficient) may sometimes be necessary for documenting hypoglycemia. The presence of an elevated blood insulin concentration coupled with hypoglycemia further supports the diagnosis, although normal blood insulin concentration coupled with hypoglycemia is also suggestive of insulinoma. In dogs with insulinomas, serum insulin concentrations are often normal.[3] If the serum insulin concentration is below detectable limits with a low blood glucose concentration, insulinoma is unlikely. Other less common differential diagnoses for hypoglycemia in ferrets include starvation, liver disease, and sepsis.

Absolute insulin concentrations are used by many clinicians as the basis for presumptive diagnosis of insulinoma. The insulin/glucose, glucose/insulin, and amended insulin/glucose ratios are sometimes used for distinguishing normal animals from those with disease. The amended insulin/glucose ratio is most commonly used in veterinary medicine and gives fewer false-negative results than the criteria of increased serum insulin concentration. However, in dogs the amended insulin/glucose ratio is less specific and does give false-positive results in animals without insulinomas.[13, 19] Results do not differentiate definitively between hypoglycemic dogs with and those without insulin-secreting tumor.[3] False-positive results may occur in dogs with liver disease, sepsis, and non–islet cell tumors, especially in the presence of hypoglycemia.[13] Because of the lack of specificity of insulin and glucose ratios and the possibility of normal serum insulin concentration, serum glucose testing is the most reliable method of establishing a tentative diagnosis of insulinoma in dogs.[3] Surgical exploration of the pancreas and histopathologic examination of neoplastic tissue is needed for definitive diagnosis of insulinoma.

In other species, if the results of resting blood tests or those taken after short-term or prolonged fasting do not support the presumptive diagnosis of insulinoma with low blood glucose and increased insulin concentrations, provocative tests are sometimes used. These tests include administration of glucagon, glucose, leucine, tolbutamide, or calcium, which acts a secretogogues.[13] However, severe and prolonged hypoglycemia may result, and these tests must be used with extreme caution.[13, 22] To my knowledge, these tests have not been used in ferrets.

Check the blood glucose concentration at the initial physical examination with either a strip glucose measurement method (Chemstrip bG, Boehringer Mannheim, Gaithersburg, MD) or a digital glucose meter such as the One Touch II (Lifescan, Inc., Milpitas, CA) or the Accu-Chek III (Boehringer Mannheim, Gaithersburg, MD). These glucose meters are manufactured for use by human diabetic patients and are very convenient and easy to use. If the blood glucose concentration is not measured immediately, then the reported glucose value on the serum chemistry analysis may be difficult to interpret because of artifact. The initial blood glucose concentration can be confirmed by analysis of blood collected into sodium fluoride (gray top tube); however, because of the limited volume of blood that can be collected from a ferret, this is not usually feasible if other blood tests are also required.

Ferrets with blood glucose concentrations lower than 70 mg/dL are suspected of having insulinoma. In one study of 49 ferrets with confirmed insulinoma, all had blood glucose concentrations lower than 60 mg/dL.[2] Ferrets that present profoundly weak or comatose commonly have blood glucose concentrations in the range of 20–40 mg/dL. The reference range for resting blood glucose concentration in ferrets is 94–207 mg/dL; normal fasting blood glucose is 90–125 mg/dL (see Table 2–2).

In one study, the mean blood glucose concentration after a 4-hour fast in six ferrets with confirmed insulinoma was 44 mg/dL, and the mean fasting insulin concentration was 416 pmol/L (58 μU/mL).[18]

Submit a sample for measurement of blood insulin concentration at the time of the initial examination. In our laboratory, the reference values for serum insulin concentrations in normal ferrets are 35–250 pmol/L (4.88–34.84 μU/mL; see Table 9–1). Reference intervals for insulin previously reported in ferrets are 33–311 pmol/L (4.6–43.3 μU/mL) with a mean of 101 pmol/L (14.1 μU/mL).[17] (Values expressed as picomoles per liter [pmol/L] in Système International [SI] units can be converted to microunits per milliliter [μU/mL] by dividing by the conversion factor 7.175.[15]) However, reported reference values for insulin concentrations should not be used indiscriminately for comparison, as observed values depend on the type of commercial radioimmunoassay used for insulin measurement.[17] Ferrets with suspected insulinomas may have insulin concentrations ranging from within the reference range up to 2000 pmol/L (278.7 μU/mL). Reported insulin values in ferrets with insulinomas have ranged from 772.7–12,470 pmol/L (107.7 to 1738 μU/mL).[5, 9, 10, 16] Reported reference intervals for the insulin/glucose ratio in

TABLE 9–1
REFERENCE VALUES FOR TESTS OF THE ENDOCRINE SYSTEM IN FERRETS

Hormone	Sex	Values
Insulin*		35–250 pmol/L (4.9–34.8 μU/mL)
Cortisol† (nmol/L)		25.9–235 (mean ± SEM, 73.8 ± 7)
Thyroxine‡ (μg/dL)	♂	1.01–8.29 (mean, 4.5)
	♀	0.71–2.54 (mean, 1.38)
Tri-iodothyronine‡ (ng/mL)	♂	0.45–0.78 (mean, 0.61)
	♀	0.29–0.73 (mean, 0.53)
Mean thyroxine§ (μg/dL)	♂	2.53 at 0 h, 3.37 at 2 h, 3.97 at 4 h, and 3.45 at 6 h

*Reference range for Vet Research Laboratories, Farmingdale, NY.

†Administration of cosyntropin, 1 μg/kg intramuscularly, generally caused a three- to fourfold increase in plasma cortisol concentration in this study (see reference 26).

‡Data from Garibaldi BA, Pequet-Goad ME, Fox JG: Serum thyroxine (T_4) and tri-iodothyronine (T_3) radioimmunoassay values in the normal ferret. Lab Anim Sci 1987; 37:544–547.

§Mean T_4 at baseline (0 h) and 2, 4, and 6 h after administration of thyroid-stimulating hormone, 1 IU intravenously (n = 8 intact males). Data from Heard DJ, Collins B, Chen DL, Coniglario J: Thyroid and adrenal function tests in adult male ferrets. Am J Vet Res 1990; 51:32–35.

ferrets are 4.6–44.2 pmol/mmol or 3.6–34.1 μU/mg.[17]

If a ferret with suspected insulinoma has a normal insulin concentration, repeat the insulin assay at a later date or serially measure blood glucose concentrations to demonstrate a consistent pattern of hypoglycemia. Alternatively, measure the blood glucose and insulin concentrations after a 4-hour fast.

Hematology and Serum Chemistry Analysis

Submit blood samples for a complete blood count (CBC) and serum biochemical analysis in any ferret suspected of having an insulinoma. Increases in alanine aminotransferase (ALT) and aspartate aminotransferase (AST) levels are commonly seen and may reflect hepatic lipidosis secondary to chronically low blood glucose concentration or liver metastasis. Hematologic abnormalities that are sometimes present include leukocytosis, neutrophilia, and monocytosis.[2]

Radiography and Ultrasound Examination

Radiographic results are usually unremarkable except for splenomegaly. Lung metastases have not been seen in ferrets with insulinoma. Abdominal ultrasound is sometimes helpful in the diagnosis and management of ferrets with insulinomas. Discrete insulinomas are rarely detected by ultrasound because of their small size, but ultrasound is useful from a prognostic standpoint and in presurgical evaluation. Hepatic lipidosis or hepatic infiltrates, which may indicate liver metastasis, are sometimes detected by ultrasound. If any abnormalities are detected, do a liver biopsy at surgery.

Other Diagnostic Tests

If any clinical signs of concurrent disease are present, do appropriate diagnostic tests to confirm the diagnosis. This is especially critical in ferrets with cardiomyopathy, as these ferrets are often poor anesthetic risks.

Management

Ferrets with insulinomas can be managed medically or surgically. The choice of therapy depends on the severity of clinical signs, the age of the ferret, and the owner's preference. Medical therapy to alleviate clinical signs of hypoglycemia can begin once a presumptive diagnosis of insulinoma has been made.

Medical Management

Medical therapy can effectively control clinical signs of hypoglycemia but does not stop progression of the insulinoma. Prednisone and diazoxide are used singly or in combination, depending on the severity of clinical signs, in conjunction with dietary management. Prednisone acts to increase peripheral blood glucose concentrations by inhibiting glucose uptake of peripheral tissues and increasing hepatic gluconeogenesis. Ferrets with mild to moderate clinical signs of hypoglycemia can usually be controlled with prednisone therapy alone, in peroral (PO) dosages ranging from 0.5 to 2 mg/kg q12h. Begin at the lowest dosage and increase the dosage gradually as needed to control clinical signs. Prescribe either the oral suspension of prednisolone or the 1-mg tablets of prednisone, depending on the owner's preference. Make sure that the oral suspension is not a generic form that contains alcohol, which can cause unwanted side effects.

Diazoxide (Proglycem, Baker Norton Pharmaceuticals, Inc., Miami, FL) is a benzothiadiazine derivative that acts by inhibiting insulin release from the pancreatic beta cells, by promoting glycogenolysis and gluconeogenesis by the liver, and by decreasing the cellular uptake of glucose. Add diazoxide (5–10 mg/kg q12h PO) to the therapeutic protocol when clinical signs of hypoglycemia cannot be controlled with prednisone alone; at this time, the prednisone dosage can often be lowered to 1–1.25 mg/kg q12h PO. The diazoxide dosage can be gradually increased to a maximum of 60 mg/kg/q24h divided q8h–12h if lower dosages do not effectively control clinical signs. Side effects associated with diazoxide treatment include vomiting and anorexia.[13] The major disadvantage of diazoxide therapy is the expense of the commercial suspension. Compounding pharmacists can make suspensions of diazoxide from tablets, but the concentration of the resultant suspension cannot be guaranteed.

Instruct owners of ferrets with insulinomas to feed their animals frequently and to avoid prolonged periods without food. Recommended diets include meat-based, high-protein cat or ferret food. Avoid foods with a high sugar or carbohydrate (cereal) content, including canine or feline semi-moist diets. Unless ferrets show signs of hypoglycemia, instruct owners not to give simple sugars such as honey or corn syrup because these foods can stimulate insulin secretion, precipitating a hypoglycemic episode soon thereafter.

Somatostatin, a natural polypeptide hormone secreted by the pancreas, suppresses insulin secretion. Octreotide, a somatostatin analogue (Sandostatin, Sandoz Pharmaceuticals Corp., East Hanover, NJ), is sometimes used in dogs for the treatment of insulinoma.[24] We have used somatostatin in the treatment of one ferret with equivocal results.

Medical management is usually effective in controlling clinical signs for periods of 6 months to 1.5 years. Ferrets treated medically commonly show progressive severity of clinical signs, and gradually increasing doses of medications are usually needed. Older ferrets (>6 years of age) and ferrets with concurrent complicating diseases such as cardiomyopathy or lymphosarcoma are the primary candidates for medical therapy. Owners sometimes elect medical therapy over surgical therapy for other reasons (e.g., because of the expense of or their opposition to surgery).

Treatment of a Hypoglycemic Episode

Mild to moderate hypoglycemic episodes can often be treated successfully at home. Owners of ferrets with insulinoma should always have honey, corn syrup, or other liquid sugar product readily available. Instruct owners how to recognize the signs of hypoglycemia and how to administer the sugar product with a syringe. If the ferret has collapsed, instruct the owner to rub honey or corn syrup on the gingiva, taking care not to be bitten. If the ferret is having seizures, instruct the owner not to place hands or objects in the ferret's mouth because of the danger of being bitten. Once the ferret has improved, the owner should feed the ferret some of its regular diet and schedule a veterinary visit as needed.

Ferrets that have hypoglycemic episodes that do not respond to home therapy or that result in continuous seizures require hospital treatment. Administer a slow intravenous (IV) bolus of 50% dextrose (0.5–2 mL) until the ferret responds. If the ferret remains comatose or is having seizures, establish an IV catheter, give shock therapy with IV fluids and corticosteroids, and begin a continuous infusion of 5% dextrose.

It is important to give IV 50% dextrose slowly and at the minimal amount to control clinical signs. A rapid increase in blood glucose concentration can cause overstimulation of the tumor, resulting in the release of massive amounts of insulin and subsequent severe hypoglycemia; this then requires treatment with more IV dextrose. This can become a vicious cycle, with progressive worsening of rebound hypoglycemia.[22] Therefore, we emphasize that the goal of therapy is the correction of clinical signs, not the correction of hypoglycemia. Once the ferret is conscious again, initiate enteral feedings and prednisone therapy as necessary.

Ferrets that seizure or are comatose usually must be monitored closely as critical patients for 1 to 2 days. Rarely, anticonvulsant therapy (e.g., diazepam 1–2 mg IV titrated to effect; repeat as necessary up to 5 mg) is necessary for the control of seizures until supportive therapy becomes effective. Follow anticonvulsant protocols as for dogs and cats in status epilepticus, making sure that the correction of hypoglycemia is the first priority.

Surgical Therapy

We currently recommend surgical therapy for ferrets younger than 6 years of age or for those suspected of having concurrent adrenal disease. Surgical therapy is usually not curative but may stop or slow progression of the insulinoma. Surgical therapy has been shown to prolong the life span of dogs with insulinoma, compared with dogs that are treated with medical management alone.[13] In dogs with pancreatic beta cell tumors, greater preoperative insulin concentrations were associated with significantly shorter survival times[3]; however, this finding has not been confirmed in ferrets. In a recent study, the mean survival time of 49 ferrets undergoing surgical excision of tumor nodules was 462 days (range, 14–1207 days).[2]

Preoperative considerations include placement of an indwelling IV catheter before fasting and the infusion of maintenance fluids with added 5% dextrose. Fluid therapy is needed before and during surgery for the maintenance of systemic blood pressure and pancreatic perfusion and, thus, for decreasing the risk of pancreatitis.[24] Fast ferrets minimally (3–10 hours) before surgery to prevent severe hypoglycemia; in our hospital, we fast ferrets after midnight, and surgery is first on the schedule the following day. Continue the infusion of fluids with 5% dextrose during surgery, and check the blood glucose concentration with a rapid measurement test before and immediately after surgery. Begin prophylactic treatment with a parenteral antibiotic before surgery; we routinely use ampicillin.

Usually, one or two pancreatic nodules are found at surgery, but as many as seven to nine nodules may be present. Nodulectomy or partial pancreatectomy, or both are done, depending on the number and location of the pancreatic nodules (see Chapter 13). Routinely do a liver biopsy in ferrets with insulinoma to check for liver metastasis. Biopsy the spleen and any lymph nodes if they are enlarged or appear abnormal, and examine the adrenal glands carefully for abnormalities, as concurrent adrenal disease is common.

Ferrets usually recover quickly from surgery, and, unlike in dogs, complications related to pancreatic surgery are rare. Withhold food and water for 12 hours after surgery in routine cases. Continue antibiotic therapy, changing to oral administration once the ferret is eating. Maintain fluid administration with 5% dextrose until the ferret is euglycemic or eating.

Monitor the blood glucose concentration at least two to three times daily after surgery while the ferret is hospitalized. Many ferrets become euglycemic immediately after surgery, whereas others remain hypoglycemic or are borderline euglycemic. Rarely, a ferret may become hyperglycemic after insulinoma surgery. This also occurs in a small percentage of dogs postoperatively and is attributed to the suppression of normal beta cells by tumor insulin, which results in loss of insulin production.[3, 13] Hyperglycemia is typically transient in these ferrets, resolving within 2–3 weeks, and usually does not require treatment. Monitor blood glucose concentrations in these ferrets periodically until hyperglycemia resolves.

Most ferrets that have been treated surgically require medical management for hypoglycemia within 2–6 months after surgery. In one study, only 14% of ferrets remained euglycemic postoperatively.[2] Therefore, recheck the blood glucose concentration in any ferret that has had surgery for insulinoma 7–14 days after surgery and at 2- to 3-month intervals thereafter. Repeat measurements of serum insulin concentrations are also recommended.

Histopathology

Insulinomas in ferrets are usually malignant,[2] as they are in dogs.[19] On histopathologic examination of pancreatic tissue, beta cell carcinoma is usually found, sometimes in combination with beta cell hyperplasia or adenoma. In dogs, the morphology of endocrine neoplasms does not reflect their malignancy,[19] and malignancy is determined by the presence or absence of metastasis.[3]

In ferrets, metastasis at the time of surgery is uncommon; however, when it does occur, it is usually to regional lymph nodes, the spleen, or the liver.[2, 5, 18] Immunocytochemical staining can be done on biopsied specimens to demonstrate insulin-, glucagon-, or somatostatin-positive cells. In one study of immunocytochemical staining of pancreatic tumors from three ferrets, the authors concluded that pancreatic beta cell tumors in ferrets are similar to those in dogs.[5]

PART II

Karen L. Rosenthal, DVM

ADRENAL GLAND DISEASE

Adrenocortical disease has recently been recognized as a common malady affecting pet ferrets in the United States.[6, 8, 14, 21, 25, 27] It is seen typically in middle-aged to older ferrets and is characterized by hair loss in both sexes and by vulvar enlargement in female ferrets. Clinical signs of adrenocortical disease in ferrets differ from those of classic Cushing's disease in dogs; moreover, serum cortisol concentrations are rarely elevated in ferrets. Instead, the levels of one or more of the plasma androgens, estradiol, or 17-hydroxyprogesterone may be elevated as a result of adrenocortical hyperplasia, adenoma, or adenocarcinoma.

The underlying cause of the pathologic changes in these ferrets' adrenal glands is unknown. It is tempting to speculate that premature neutering has a role. In support of this, studies in some strains of mice have shown that gonadectomy at an early age can lead to adrenocortical nodular hyperplasia or to the formation of tumors of one or both adrenal glands that hypersecrete estrogens or androgens.[4, 12, 29] Ovaries and adrenal glands develop in close anatomic relation to one another during embryologic development. Both arise in intimate association in the urogenital ridge.[1] Small nests of gonadal cells may be carried with the adrenal glands during migration and come to rest under the adrenal gland capsule. With appropriate stimulation (i.e., gonadectomy with resultant unopposed pituitary gonadotropin activity), these undifferentiated gonadal cells in the adrenal gland may be transformed into cells that are functionally similar to the cells of gonadal tissue.

Like mice that are gonadectomized during the first few days of life, most commercially raised ferrets in the United States are ovariohysterectomized or castrated before they are 6 weeks of age. Therefore, it is possible that adrenocortical hyperplasia and tumors may develop in ferrets as a result of metaplasia of undifferentiated gonadal cells in the adrenal capsule.

Speculation regarding other causes of adrenal gland disease in ferrets may be based on a comparison of the husbandry of ferrets in the United States with that of ferrets in other countries—specifically, in Great Britain, where adrenal gland disease of ferrets is rare. Ferrets in the United States are typically fed prepared food (e.g., cat food), whereas ferrets in England eat whole prey. Also, ferrets in the United States are mostly kept indoors, whereas ferrets in England are often kept outdoors and thus are exposed to natural photoperiods. Finally, the ferret population in the United States is more inbred than that in England.

History and Physical Examination

Progressive alopecia is the most common historical finding. Hair loss typically begins in the late winter or early spring and may continue until the affected ferret is partially or completely bald. Occasionally, a ferret may regrow a full hair coat during the following fall. Commonly in this case, alopecia begins again in the winter or spring. This sequence has been reported to recur over a period of 2–3 years. At some point, the hair does not regrow. Spayed female ferrets with adrenocortical disease frequently have a history of vulvar enlargement, with or without a mucoid discharge. Male ferrets may have a history of dysuria or urinary blockage, or of both.

The majority of ferrets reported with adrenocortical disease are female. This may be because many owners are aware that an enlarged vulva in a female is a cause for concern. Vulvar enlargement occurs during estrus, and prolonged estrus can result in estrogen-induced bone marrow toxicity (see Chapter 5). Thus, although more females than males are reported to have this disease, the predilection may be due to a presentation bias rather than to an actual difference in incidence rate.

At our hospital, the average age at which signs of adrenal disease are first noted by ferret owners is approximately 3.5 years. A small study has reported an older age distribution for this disease.[25]

Alopecia is the most common clinical manifestation of adrenocortical disease and occurs in both male and female ferrets (Fig. 9–2). Over 90% of ferrets with adrenal disease have some extent of hair loss. The hair can be epilated easily. Alopecia is usu-

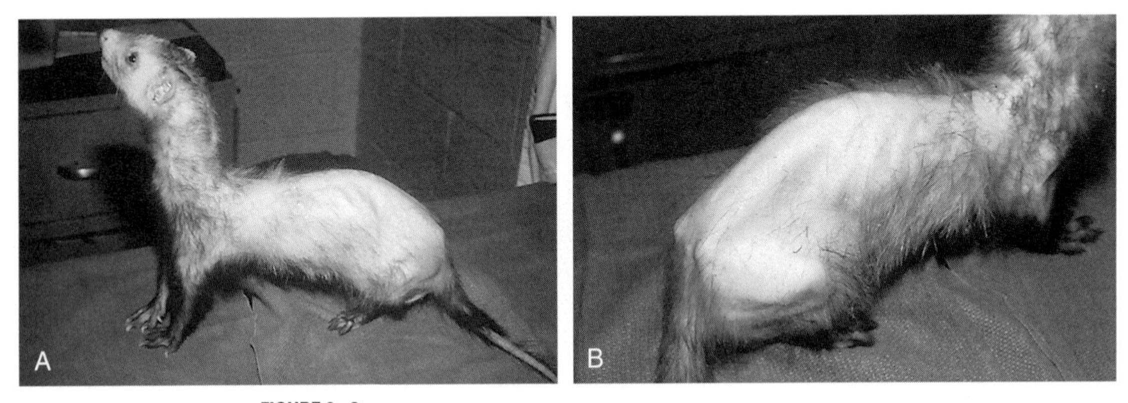

FIGURE 9–2
A and B, Typical pattern of hair loss in ferret with an adrenocortical tumor.

ally symmetric, beginning on the rump, the tail, or the flanks and spreading to the sides, dorsum, and ventrum. Areas of alopecia should be well documented in the record for comparison as the disease progresses.

Over one third of ferrets with adrenal gland disease are pruritic. Usually, the pruritus is accompanied by hair loss (Fig. 9–3), but we have seen a few ferrets in which pruritus was the only sign of adrenal gland disease. Pruritus is most frequently observed on the dorsum between the shoulder blades. The skin tends to be erythematous in pruritic areas.

Over 70% of female ferrets with adrenal gland disease have an enlarged vulva (Fig. 9–4). The vulva can range in size from slightly enlarged to grossly enlarged, appearing as a turgid and edematous structure resembling the vulva of a female ferret in estrus. A seromucoid discharge may be present, and local vaginitis may be diagnosed on cytologic examination. The perivulvar skin may appear dark and seem bruised.

Partial or complete urinary blockage in male ferrets is occasionally seen in association with adrenal cortical disease. Hyperplasia or cystic change, or both, occur in tissue in the region of the prostate (possibly originating from hormone-responsive cells) and cause urethral narrowing (see Chapter 5). Affected ferrets have difficulty urinating and are seen to have stranguria. It is difficult to pass a urinary catheter in these ferrets.

On physical examination, enlarged adrenal glands may be palpated. Enlargement of the left adrenal gland is more easily identified than that of the right. The left adrenal gland is usually found engulfed in a large fat pad cranial to the left kidney. It may feel like a small, firm round mass. The right adrenal gland is more difficult to palpate because it has a more cranial location and is under a lobe of the liver. Enlarged intra-abdominal lymph nodes are a possible finding.

Abdominal palpation may reveal an enlarged spleen, which usually has smooth borders and is not painful. In some instances, the spleen has an irregular texture and is knobby. Many older ferrets have an

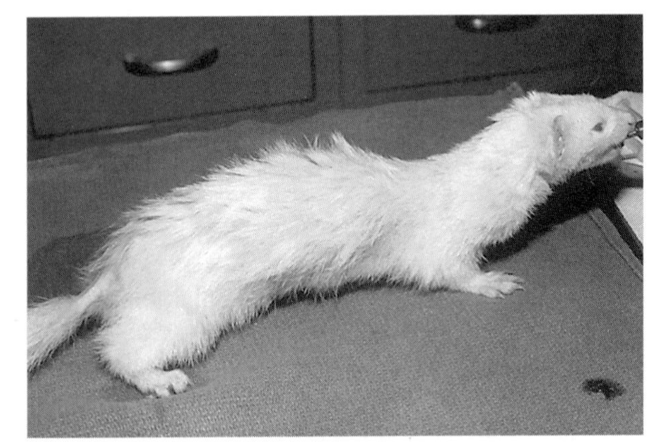

FIGURE 9–3
Ferret with thinning of the hair and severe pruritus. A left adrenocortical tumor was found at surgery. Clinical signs resolved after adrenalectomy.

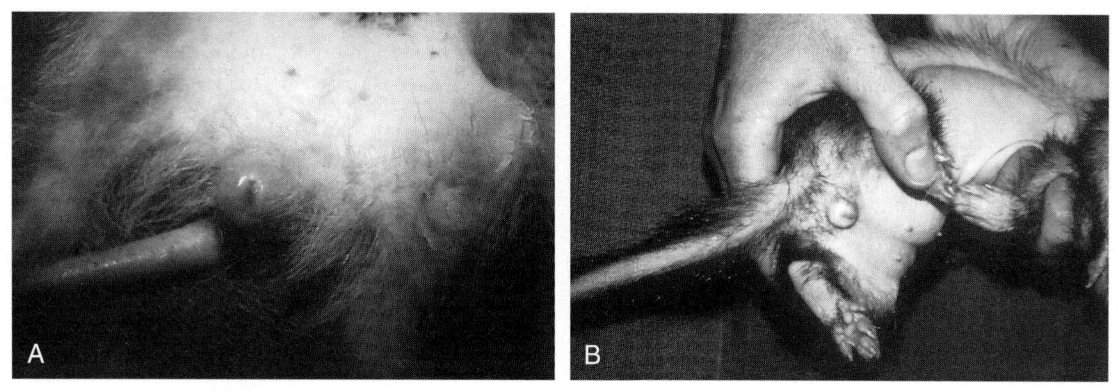

FIGURE 9–4
A and B, Enlarged vulva and hair loss in two female ferrets with adrenocortical disease.

enlarged spleen, which is an incidental finding on physical examination (see Chapter 7); enlargement of the spleen with adrenal disease may be coincidental.

Clinical Pathology and Diagnostic Testing

The diagnosis of adrenal gland disease is based on history, clinical signs, imaging diagnostics, steroid hormone assay, and confirmation at surgery.

The CBC is usually within normal limits. In rare instances, adrenocortical disease is associated with anemia. If disease is severe, pancytopenia is present. The anemia or pancytopenia, or both, mimic that found in ferrets with estrogen-induced bone marrow toxicity (see Chapter 5). A packed red blood cell volume (PCV) less than 15% carries a grave prognosis.

The biochemistry panel is also usually within normal limits. Occasionally, the level of ALT is elevated. Hypoglycemia due to a pancreatic beta cell tumor (insulinoma) may be present. Insulinomas are common in older ferrets and may be coincidentally present with adrenocortical disease.

Radiographs are not generally helpful in diagnosing this disease. Adrenal gland enlargement that causes radiographically visible displacement of other organs is uncommon. Because it is also unusual for an abnormal adrenal gland to calcify, adrenal gland mineralization is not usually seen on radiographs. Radiography is a useful screening tool for evaluating concurrent conditions such as heart disease and splenomegaly.

Abdominal ultrasound is useful for detecting enlarged adrenal glands. The size, the side of enlargement, and the architecture can often be determined. Abdominal ultrasound is also useful for detecting concurrent diseases, such as renal or liver disease, metastasis from a pancreatic insulinoma, and enlargement of the lymph nodes. Thoracic ultrasound examination is used for detecting and characterizing heart disease.

Computed tomography of the abdomen of ferrets can demonstrate adrenal gland abnormalities. In practice, however, it is rarely performed.

Ancillary Diagnostic Tests

An adrenocorticotropic hormone (ACTH) stimulation test cannot be used to establish a diagnosis of this disease. Both normal ferrets and those with adrenal gland disease respond equally as well to an ACTH stimulation test. In a study performed at our hospital, ferrets with confirmed adrenal gland disease had normal cortisol responses to an ACTH stimulation test.

The dexamethasone suppression test also does not appear to be helpful in diagnosing this disease, although further research is necessary for evaluating both this test and the urinary cortisol/creatinine ratio. In one study, urinary cortisol/creatinine ratios were elevated in 12 ferrets with adrenocortical tumors when compared with 51 clinically normal ferrets.[7] In dogs, the urinary cortisol/creatinine ratio is a sensitive but not a specific indicator of hyperadrenocorticism. Further studies are needed to evaluate urinary cortisol/creatinine ratios in ferrets with diseases other than hyperadrenocorticism.

The measurement of certain plasma steroids may be a reliable means of diagnosing adrenal gland disease. In ferrets with adrenal gland disease, the levels of one or more of the following compounds may be elevated: dehydroepiandrosterone sulfate, andro-

TABLE 9–2
MEAN PLASMA STEROID HORMONE CONCENTRATIONS IN NORMAL FERRETS AND FERRETS WITH ADRENOCORTICAL DISEASE

Steroid	Normal	Diseased
Androstenedione (nmol/L)	6.6	67
Dehydroepiandrosterone sulfate (μmol/L)	0.01	0.03
Estradiol (pmol/L)	106	167
17-hydroxyprogesterone (nmol/L)	0.4	3.2

stenedione, 17-hydroxyprogesterone, and estradiol.* In a normal, neutered ferret, these steroids are found in minute quantities. Table 9–2 shows the mean values for these steroids in normal ferrets and in ferrets with adrenal gland disease.

Differential Diagnosis

An intact female ferret in estrus or one with an ovarian remnant may display an enlargement of the vulva and a limited amount of alopecia, resembling a ferret with adrenal gland disease. A number of methods are used for differentiating active ovarian tissue from adrenal gland disease. An intramuscular (IM) injection of 100 IU of human chorionic gonadotropin is administered and then repeated in 7–10 days. If the ferret is intact or if an ovarian remnant is present, this measure should cause the vulva to decrease in size. Alternatively, steroid hormone measurement may help differentiate the two problems. If the levels of androgens such as androstenedione, dehydroepiandrosterone sulfate, or 17-hydroxyprogesterone are elevated, then an adrenal tumor may be present. If only the level of estradiol is elevated, then either condition may be present. An ultrasound examination of the abdomen may differentiate between an adrenal tumor and an intact genital tract in a female ferret. Surgery is the definitive method for confirming the presence of ovarian tissue or an abnormal adrenal gland.

Seasonal alopecia of the tail is observed in some ferrets. The hair typically regrows after several weeks. This condition does not appear to be related to an adrenal tumor.

Possible Concurrent Abnormalities

Pancreatic beta cell tumors are common in older ferrets. Because adrenal gland disease is also seen in older ferrets, it is possible to find these diseases concurrently. It is not known whether a correlation exists between the two diseases. An insulinoma is diagnosed on the basis of clinical signs in conjunction with a low blood glucose concentration and the finding of pancreatic disease at surgery (see section on insulinomas at the beginning of this chapter). Blood insulin concentrations are usually elevated but may be normal.

Older ferrets commonly have splenic enlargement. Histopathology of the spleen usually shows extrameduallary hematopoiesis. Infrequently, neoplasia, including lymphoma and hemangiosarcoma, causes splenic enlargement. Nodular hyperplasia is also seen. Perform a percutaneous aspirate of the spleen or biopsy it during abdominal exploratory surgery for adrenalectomy. Splenectomy is rarely necessary unless neoplasia is present in the spleen or the spleen is so grossly enlarged that it interferes with the ferret's movement (see Chapter 7).

Older ferrets frequently have heart disease, which can be clinical or subclinical (see Chapter 7). Evaluate all older ferrets preoperatively for subclinical heart disease because of the possibility of decompensation that can accompany the stress of surgery or fluid administration.

Lymphoma is a common neoplasia of ferrets and may be found incidentally during a physical examination or an abdominal exploratory operation. Biopsy or perform an excisional biopsy of any abnormal lymph nodes.

Management

There are two treatment modalities for adrenocortical tumors: medical management and surgical removal or debulking of an affected adrenal gland or glands. Surgical removal is the preferred treatment for ferrets, as it is for dogs with adrenocortical tumors.[11] Medical management with the drugs currently available is usually unsuccessful and may be accompanied by dangerous side effects.

*Plasma steroid assays are performed at the Clinical Endocrinology Laboratory of the Department of Comparative Medicine at the University of Tennessee. Before collecting samples, call the laboratory at (615) 974-5638 to obtain instructions on sample submission.

Surgical Therapy

Preoperative testing can include a CBC, biochemical analysis, abdominal and thoracic radiography, and abdominal and cardiac ultrasound examination. Keep the ferret off food for 8–12 hours before surgery. Placement of an IV catheter during the preoperative period is optional unless the ferret is known to have an insulinoma. Do not fast a ferret with an insulinoma without providing fluid support with added dextrose.

Adrenalectomy techniques are described in Chapter 13. Place an IV catheter during induction if one is not already present. Identify the adrenal glands during a routine abdominal exploratory examination, and fully explore the abdomen. Visualize and palpate both adrenal glands because bilateral adrenal gland disease can be present. Compare the adrenal glands with each other. Other structures to be examined include the liver, the lymph nodes, the pancreas, the kidneys, and the spleen.

Perform a unilateral adrenalectomy when only one adrenal gland is diseased. If both glands are diseased, then consider a bilateral surgical procedure. Completely remove one adrenal gland and perform a subtotal adrenalectomy on the other gland. The decision of which to remove completely is based on the degree of abnormality. Because of the relative ease of removal, the left adrenal gland is usually removed outright, and the right adrenal gland is partially removed.

After surgery, give the ferret maintenance and replacement fluids as needed. If there are no other complications and the gastrointestinal tract has not been entered, feed the ferret 6–12 hours after surgery. We rarely give postoperative corticosteroid replacement therapy. A study performed at our hospital showed that ferrets still had the ability after adrenalectomy to respond to an ACTH challenge with cortisol release. We do give sodium dexamethasone phosphate at 4 mg/kg IV once if the ferret appears lethargic after surgery for no apparent reason or if both adrenal glands are biopsied.

Medical Management

MITOTANE

Mitotane, or *o,p'*-DDD (Lysodren, Bristol-Myers Squibb Oncology, Princeton, NJ), is most effective in dogs for treating pituitary-dependent hyperadrenocorticism, which has not been recognized in ferrets. This may explain why treatment with mitotane is rarely successful in ferrets with adrenocortical tumors. In my experience, mitotane treatment does not reliably produce resolution of clinical signs in ferrets with adrenocortical tumors; moreover, if clinical signs do resolve, they typically recur when mitotane is discontinued.

Be careful when administering mitotane and in warning owners of potential side effects associated with the drug. The primary danger associated with mitotane administration in ferrets is the possible development of severe hypoglycemia after several days of therapy in animals with concurrent insulinoma. We have seen this occur even in ferrets that had shown no clinical signs or laboratory results suggestive of insulinoma. Perhaps mitotane causes sufficient lowering of endogenous cortisol concentrations to result in decompensation in ferrets with subclinical insulinoma. Instruct owners how to recognize the signs and to treat an episode of hypoglycemia (see section on insulinomas at the beginning of this chapter). Dispense prednisone to be used as "rescue" therapy if needed.

Mitotane treatment, although not curative, may be palliative and therefore useful in certain instances. Consider mitotane for the treatment of older ferrets that are poor surgical candidates, ferrets with bilateral adrenal disease that could not be totally resected, and ferrets whose owners cannot afford surgery. The mitotane dosage that has been used for ferrets is 50 mg PO once daily for 1 week, followed by a maintenance dosage of 50 mg every 3 days. A compounding pharmacist can prepare 50-mg capsules of mitotane. The capsules can be difficult to administer. Offer the ferret a small amount of Nutri-Cal (Evsco Pharmaceuticals, Buena, NJ) or Linatone (Lambert Kay, Cranbury, NJ) immediately after capsule administration to encourage swallowing.

Monitor the effects of treatment by following progression or regression of clinical signs. The effects of mitotane on adrenal cortisol production can be evaluated with the ACTH stimulation test. Administer cosyntropin (Cortrosyn, Organon Inc., West Orange, NJ), a synthetic subunit of ACTH, at 1 μg/kg IV or IM and measure plasma cortisol concentration at baseline (preadministration or 0 minutes) and 60 minutes after administration. In normal ferrets, cosyntropin causes plasma cortisol concentrations to increase to levels three- to fourfold greater than resting concentrations. Resting plasma cortisol concentrations measured six times in eight normal ferrets (n = 48) ranged from 25.9 to 235 nmol/L (mean $\pm$ SEM = 73.8 $\pm$ 7.0 nmol/L; see Table 9–1).[26]

The ACTH stimulation test can be used for monitoring the depression in adrenal cortisol output; however, it cannot be used for tracking the effectiveness of mitotane therapy. We use this test after 1 week of mitotane therapy to determine whether the loading dose has been effective.

KETOCONAZOLE

In our experience, ketoconazole is not helpful in diminishing the signs of this disease in ferrets. Ketoconazole is used in adrenocortical disease of other species because of its ability to inhibit the steroid biosynthetic pathway at several steps.[28]

Managing Concurrent Insulinoma

As previously discussed, one of the more common complications with adrenal gland disease is a concurrent insulinoma. The administration of medications (prednisone and diazoxide) for the control of the signs of insulinoma does not appear to interfere with adrenal gland disease. During surgery for adrenal gland disease, debulking of the pancreatic beta cell tumors can take place (see Chapter 13). This is another reason for performing abdominal exploratory surgery if you suspect adrenal disease. Remember that the administration of mitotane can cause severe hypoglycemia in ferrets with insulinoma.

Adrenal Histopathology

Adrenal gland disease has been described on histopathologic assessment as adrenocortical hyperplasia, adrenocortical adenoma, and adrenocortical carcinoma. At our hospital, adenoma is most common. Metastasis in ferrets seen in our hospital is rare; however, some tumors show local invasion of the vena cava.

Prognosis

The prognosis with surgical treatment is good. In the majority of ferrets, once the diseased adrenal gland has been removed, the associated clinical signs resolve (Fig. 9–5). The later complications with surgical treatment include recurrence of adrenal tumor due to metastasis (very rare) or the appearance of an adrenocortical tumor in the other adrenal gland.

The prognosis with medical treatment is unpredictable because the results of medical treatment are equivocal. If no treatment is undertaken and if the effects of the adrenal tumor are only cosmetic (alopecia), then the prognosis for life is good. The prognosis worsens if bone marrow suppression, urinary tract obstruction, tumor-related mechanical interference with the vena cava, or metastasis occurs.

DIABETES MELLITUS

History and Physical Examination

Diabetes mellitus is uncommon in ferrets. Most ferrets with diabetes develop it secondary to surgery for debulking of a pancreatic beta cell tumor. Rarely do ferrets develop spontaneous hyperglycemia.

Hyperglycemic ferrets show clinical signs similar to those of other species with hyperglycemia. The

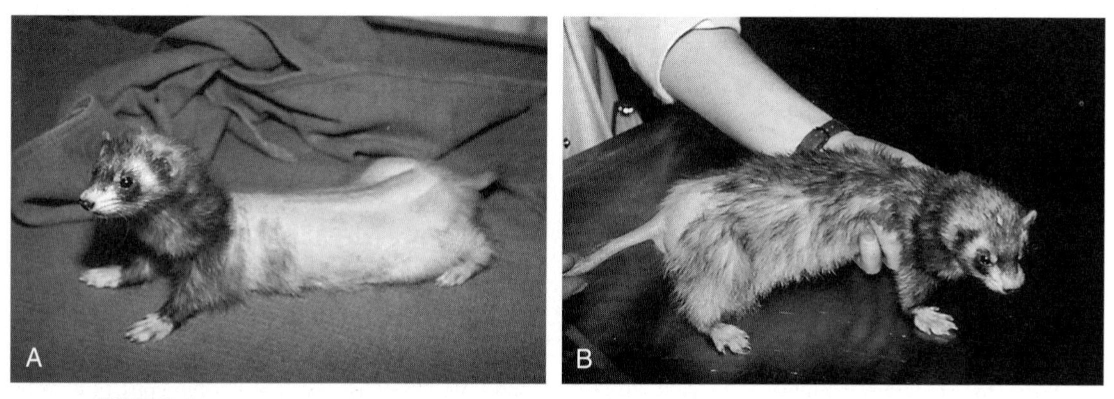

FIGURE 9–5

A, Four-year-old spayed female ferret with a left adrenocortical tumor. *B*, The same ferret 2 months after left adrenalectomy. Hair regrowth is almost complete except on the feet, rump, and tail. The hair never fully returned on the tail.

severity of signs depends on the severity and chronicity of the disease. Affected ferrets are polyuric/polydipsic and may lose weight in the presence of a good appetite. They may appear lethargic, especially if there is metabolic derangement such as ketoacidosis.

The findings on physical examination are often unremarkable. Ferrets may be thin and have a distended urinary bladder.

Clinical Pathology and Diagnostic Testing

The diagnosis of diabetes mellitus in ferrets is dependent on some or all of the following: clinical signs (polyuria/polydipsia), history of recent insulinoma surgery, high blood glucose concentration, low blood insulin concentration, and normal to high blood glucagon concentration.

The CBC is usually unremarkable. The white blood cell count may be elevated if a concurrent bladder infection is present. A profound hyperglycemia is usually present in ferrets with diabetes. A blood glucose concentration consistently greater than 400 mg/dL is suspicious for diabetes. In uncomplicated diabetes, the rest of the biochemistry profile is usually normal. In severe diabetes, the same metabolic derangements that are present in other mammals might be expected to be seen in ferrets.

A consistent glycosuria is present. In severe cases, ketones are detected. As with other animals with diabetes, ferrets with diabetes can have an active urine sediment.

Radiography and ultrasound are not useful for diagnosing diabetes mellitus. They can be used to screen for other conditions such as splenomegaly, hepatic enlargement, and cardiac disease.

Ancillary Diagnostic Tests

Glucagon concentration is an important indicator to measure in ferrets with hyperglycemia. Diabetes mellitus due to a lack of insulin or to a glucagonoma causes an increase in the blood glucose concentration. Unfortunately, the routine measurement of glucagon concentration is difficult because it must be done in a laboratory that has validated the assay for ferrets.

Measurement of insulin concentration should be done by a diagnostic laboratory that has validated the test for ferrets. A low insulin concentration in conjunction with hyperglycemia confirms the diagnosis of diabetes mellitus. A normal or high insulin concentration could represent either an insulin-resistant state or the presence of a glucagonoma.

Treatment

Treatment of diabetes mellitus depends on the severity of hyperglycemia and of other metabolic disturbances. In our hospital, we institute treatment with insulin in ferrets with blood glucose concentrations consistently greater than 300 mg/dL, following the treatment principles used for dogs and cats. We have had limited success in tightly regulating the blood glucose concentrations of these ferrets. In the hospitalized ferret, we measure serial blood glucose concentrations while administering insulin injections twice daily. We use NPH (neutral protamine Hagedorn) insulin, starting it at an empirical dosage of 0.1 unit of insulin per ferret twice daily. We monitor the urine for the presence of glucose and ketones. The insulin dose is increased or decreased as dictated by the blood glucose concentration.

Once the blood glucose concentration is stabilized below 200 mg/dL, we discharge ferrets to their owners with a prescribed insulin regimen. Some ferrets receive Ultralente insulin, which may have a longer period of action than NPH insulin, in an effort to give injections only once per day. Instruct owners to check for the presence of ketones and glucose in the urine at home with urine dipsticks. If no glucose is present in the urine, instruct the owner not to give insulin. If trace amounts of glucose are found, the insulin dose is not changed. If the amount of glucose in the urine is large, then the insulin dose is slightly increased. We have found it difficult to regulate most diabetic ferrets. Realistically, our goal is to have negative ketones in the urine and a small amount of spillage of glucose in the urine.

Prognosis

Ferrets that develop hyperglycemia immediately after insulinoma surgery may be transient diabetics, and their prognosis as it relates to diabetes is good because the hyperglycemia usually normalizes without treatment during the first 1–2 weeks after surgery. The prognosis is worse, or at best unpredictable for ferrets with diabetes mellitus that occurs spontaneously or is detected weeks to months after insulinoma surgery. Blood glucose is usually difficult to regulate in these animals.

THYROID DISEASE

Hyperthyroidism and hypothyroidism have not been reported in ferrets, nor have I seen these conditions in practice. Normal resting values for thyroxine (T_4) and tri-iodothyronine (T_3) and results for the thyroid-stimulating hormone test in one study of normal intact male ferrets are presented in Table 9–1.

REFERENCES

1. Arey LB: Developmental Anatomy. 7th ed. Philadelphia, WB Saunders, 1965, pp 321–324.
2. Caplan ER, Peterson ME, Mullen HS, Quesenberry KE: Surgical treatment of insulin-secreting pancreatic islet cell tumors in 49 ferrets. ACVS Abstract. Vet Surg 1995; 24:422.
3. Caywood DD, Klausner JS, O'Leary TP, et al: Pancreatic insulin-secreting neoplasms: clinical, diagnostic, and prognostic features in 73 dogs. J Am Anim Hosp Assoc 1988; 24:577–584.
4. Fekete E, Woolley G, Little CC: Histological changes following ovariectomy in mice: dba high tumor strain. J Exp Med 1941; 74:1–8.
5. Fix AS, Harms CA: Immunocytochemistry of pancreatic endocrine tumors in three domestic ferrets *(Mustela putorius furo).* Vet Pathol 1990; 27:199–201.
6. Fox JG, Pequet-Goad ME, Garibaldi BA, Wiest LM: Hyperadrenocorticism in a ferret. J Am Vet Med Assoc 1987; 191:343–344.
7. Gould WJ, Reimers TJ, Bell JA, et al: Evaluation of urinary cortisol:creatinine ratios for the diagnosis of hyperadrenocorticism associated with adrenal gland tumors in ferrets. J Am Vet Med Assoc 1995; 206:42–46.
8. Hillyer EV: Ferret endocrinology. *In* Kirk RW, Bonagura JD, eds.: Current Veterinary Therapy 11: Small Animal Practice. Philadelphia, WB Saunders, 1992, pp 1185–1188.
9. Jergens AE, Shaw DP: Hyperinsulinism and hypoglycemia associated with pancreatic islet cell tumor in a ferret. J Am Vet Med Assoc 1989; 194:269–271.
10. Kaufman J, Schwarz P, Mero K: Pancreatic beta cell tumor in a ferret. J Am Vet Med Assoc 1984; 185:998–1000.
11. Kintzer PP, Peterson ME: Mitotane treatment of 32 dogs with cortisol-secreting adrenocortical neoplasms. J Am Vet Med Assoc 1994; 205:54–61.
12. Krishna Murthy AS, Brezak MA, Baez AG: Postcastrational adrenal tumors in two strains of mice: morphologic, histochemical, and chromatographic studies. J Natl Cancer Inst 1970; 45:1211–1222.
13. Leifer CE, Peterson ME, Matus RE: Insulin-secreting tumor: diagnosis and medical and surgical management in 55 dogs. J Am Vet Med Assoc 1986; 188:60–64.
14. Lipman NS, Marini RP, Murphy JC, et al: Estradiol-17beta-secreting adrenocortical tumor in a ferret. J Am Vet Med Assoc 1993; 203:1552–1555.
15. Lundberg G, Iverson C, Radulescu G: Now read this: the SI units are here. JAMA 1986;255:2329–2339.
16. Luttgen PJ, Storts RW, Rogers KS, Morton LD: Insulinoma in a ferret. J Am Vet Med Assoc 1986; 189:920–921.
17. Mann FA, Stockham SL, Freeman MB, et al: Reference intervals for insulin concentrations and insulin:glucose ratios in the serum of ferrets. J Small Exotic Anim Med 1993; 2:79–83.
18. Marini RP, Ryden EB, Rosenblad WD, et al: Functional islet cell tumor in six ferrets. J Am Vet Med Assoc 1993; 202:430–433.
19. Mehlhaff CJ, Peterson ME, Patnaik AK, Carrillo JM: Insulin-producing islet cell neoplasms: surgical considerations and general management in 35 dogs. J Am Anim Hosp Assoc 1985; 21:607–612.
20. Meleo K: Management of insulinoma patients with refractory hypoglycemia. Probl Vet Med 1990; 2:602–609.
21. Mor N, Qualls CW, Hoover JP: Concurrent mammary gland hyperplasia and adrenocortical carcinoma in a domestic ferret. J Am Vet Med Assoc 1992; 201:1911–1912.
22. Nelson RW: Insulin-secreting islet cell neoplasia. *In* Ettinger SJ, Feldman EC, eds.: Textbook of Veterinary Internal Medicine. 4th ed. Philadelphia, WB Saunders, 1995, pp 1501–1509.
23. Nelson RW, Foodman MS: Medical management of canine hyperinsulinism. J Am Vet Med Assoc 1985; 187:78–82.
24. Nelson RW, Salisbury SK: Pancreatic beta cell neoplasia. *In* Birchard SJ, Sherding RG, eds. Saunders Manual of Small Animal Practice. Philadelphia, WB Saunders, 1994, pp 257–262.
25. Neuwirth L, Isaza R, Bellah J, et al: Adrenal neoplasia in seven ferrets. Vet Rad Ultra 1993; 34:340–346,
26. Rosenthal KL, Peterson ME, Quesenberry KE, Lothrop CD Jr: Evaluation of plasma cortisol and corticosterone responses to synthetic adrenocorticotropic hormone administration in ferrets. Am J Vet Res 1993; 54:29–31.
27. Rosenthal KL, Peterson ME, Quesenberry KE, et al: Hyperadrenocorticism associated with adrenocortical tumor or nodular hyperplasia in ferrets: 50 cases (1987–1991). J Am Vet Med Assoc 1993; 203:271–275.
28. Saadi HF, Bravo EL, Aron DC: Feminizing adrenocortical tumor: steroid hormone response to ketoconazole. J Clin Endocrinol Metab 1990; 70:540–543.
29. Sharawy MM, Liebelt AG, Dirksen TR, et al: Fine structural study of postcastrational adrenocortical carcinomas in female CE-mice. Anat Rec 1980; 198:125–133.

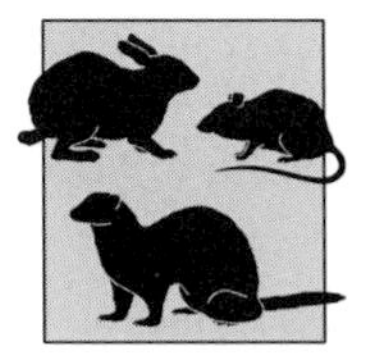

CHAPTER 10

Neoplasia

Susan A. Brown, DVM

The probability is excellent that a ferret in the United States will develop one or more neoplastic diseases by the time it reaches 5 years of age. In a 1993 article, over 50 different neoplasms in ferrets were reported.[3] In no other country where ferrets are kept as pets has such an overwhelming incidence of cancer in ferrets been reported.

Ferrets may be afflicted with neoplasia in essentially any organ of the body and at any age, although some neoplasms are more common in ferrets 3 years of age and older. Neoplasia is not a new problem in ferrets. Several authors have reported numerous neoplastic diseases, particularly in colonies of laboratory ferrets.[3, 14] However, the overall incidence of neoplasia in the general pet population appeared small, according to the literature. Over the last 10 years, ferrets have increased in popularity as pets. The majority of the ferrets in the pet market today are supplied by large ferret breeding facilities that are producing ferrets by the thousands. The fact that the number of ferrets kept as pets has increased and that the sources of ferrets have been consolidated may have played a role in the increased incidence of neoplasia in this species.

ETIOLOGY

There is no current consensus on the cause of the neoplasia problem in domestic ferrets in the United States. A number of theories have been proposed, and it is likely that the problem is a combination of one or more of these theories or of causes yet to be determined. I emphasize that none of the theories listed here has been conclusively proven to date. A great deal of research is needed for determining whether any or all of these theories may be involved.

1. *Genetic predisposition.* The gene pool of ferrets in this country may contain factors that predispose our ferrets to neoplasia. Some of the large ferret breeding facilities have closed colonies to minimize exposure to infectious disease. This might result in the inadvertent "recycling" of genetic factors that result in neoplastic disease. Ferrets in Europe and Australia are not produced in this manner, possibly because the demand for ferrets as pets or laboratory animals is not as great as it is in the United States.
2. *Early neutering of ferrets at 5–6 weeks of age.* This is a common practice within the pet industry in the United States for preventing the occurrence of hyperestrogenism and fatal anemia in the unspayed female and for making the ferret more marketable in the pet trade. Some speculate that early neutering may interfere with normal endocrine system development (see Chapter 9). Preadolescent neutering is not performed in Europe or Australia.
3. *Lack of natural photoperiod or exposure to natural sunlight.* Ferrets are very sensitive to the photoperiod, particularly with respect to their reproductive cycle.[13] The long-term effects of keeping ferrets indoors and under artificial lighting with varying light cycles and light intensity are unknown. Interestingly, it appears from my conversations with veterinarians and ferret owners that the majority of ferrets kept as pets in Europe and Australia are still housed outdoors all year. In the United States, it uncommon to encounter ferrets that are housed outdoors.
4. *Diet.* Ferrets in the United States are fed primarily a processed dry cat food or ferret food diet. Although the number of studies undertaken within the pet industry on the nutritional requirements of ferrets has increased, whether a processed diet provides all their needs and whether chemical factors used in the food's processing may create disease is still questioned. In all fairness, the quality of the cat and ferret foods available now is far superior to what it used to be, and, as research into ferret nutritional requirements continues, perhaps we can exclude diet as a consideration in determining the cause of cancer. In Europe and Australia, many ferret owners continue to feed their ferrets whole prey animals, such as rabbits, mice, and rats.
5. *Infectious agent.* At least in the case of lymphoma, some evidence suggests a viral cause.[12] No infectious agent has yet been shown to be a factor in other neoplasia of ferrets.

According to a recent survey that I did on histopathology reports of neoplasia in ferrets at our hospital over a 5-year period (from 1990 to 1994), the most common neoplasm found among 301 cases was insulinoma, followed by lymphoma, adrenocortical carcinoma, and various skin neoplasms (Tables 10–1 through 10–4). (The number of skin neoplasms I have encountered is actually much greater than that reported because histopathologic examination of skin masses was often not authorized.) Multiple neoplastic disease also is common. In 57 cases, two or more neoplastic diseases were present in a patient simultaneously. The most common combination (33 of the 57 cases, representing 58%) was insulinoma with adrenal cortical carcinoma.

Insulinoma and adrenal neoplasia are discussed in detail in Chapter 9; neoplasia of the skin is covered in Chapter 11, although this subject is discussed briefly in the present chapter as it relates to metastatic disease and chemotherapy.

It is best to give a guarded prognosis in all cases of neoplasia in ferrets. Many of the neoplasms discussed in this chapter have the potential for metas-

TABLE 10–1
BIOPSY RESULTS FOR FERRETS, 1990–1994*

Total Number of Animals with Histopathology Reports	429
Non-neoplastic	128 (30%)
Neoplastic	301 (70%)
Males	157
Females	124
Sex unknown	20
Ages of Ferrets with Neoplasia	
<1 y	3
1 y	9
2 y	29
3 y	53
4 y	40
5 y	58
6 y	24
7 y	10
8 y	3
9 y	2
Unknown age (adults)	70

*Data from Midwest Bird and Exotic Animal Hospital, Westchester, IL.

TABLE 10–2

HISTOPATHOLOGICALLY CONFIRMED NEOPLASMS IN 301 FERRETS, 1990–1994*,†

Tumor Type‡	Site	Number of Tumors
Adenoma, benign cystic	Face	2
	Perineum	1
	Perivulvar and tail	1
Adenoma, sebaceous gland	Skin	10
Adrenocortical adenoma		22
Adrenocortical carcinoma		75
Metastasis to the spleen		1 of 75
Dermatofibroma, benign	Prepuce	1
	Skin, behind ear	1
	Shoulder	1
	Trunk	1
Carcinoma and adenocarcinoma	Popliteal lymph node (metastatic and probably of endocrine origin)	1
	Epithelial (skin)	1
	Ocular globe	1
	Prostate	1
	Pancreas	1
	Pancreas with omental metastasis	1
	Mammary gland, cystic	1
	Multicentric (liver, intestine, omentum)	1
	Salivary gland	1
	Prepuce	3
Chondroma (possibly misdiagnosed chordoma)	Tail	2
Fibroma	Skin	1
Fibrosarcoma	Bone	1
	Mouth	1
	Multicentric abdominal	2
	Cervical vertebrae, subcutaneous	1
Hemangioma	Digit	1
	Mesentery	1
	Skin, trunk	4
Hemangiosarcoma	Liver	1
Histiocytoma	Skin	1
Insulinoma		114
Metastasis to the liver		8
Metastasis to local lymph nodes and mesentery		2
Lymphoma		88
Mast cell tumor	Skin	14
	Lung	1
	Lymph node (popliteal)	1
	Multicentric (liver, lymph node, lung, gallbladder)	1
Metastatic endocrine neoplasia (unknown origin)	Liver	1
	Lung	1
Sarcoma	Skin	1
Schwannoma (neurilemoma)	Leg	1
Squamous cell carcinoma	Lip	2
Transitional cell carcinoma	Bladder	1
Undifferentiated carcinoma	Ovarian stump	1

*Data from Midwest Bird and Exotic Animal Hospital.

†Many ferrets had more than one neoplasm concurrently (see Table 10–4); therefore, the total number of neoplasms is greater than the number of animals.

‡Other neoplasms found before 1990 and not included in this table: seminoma (testicle), lipoma (subcutaneous tissue), uterine adenoma, melanoma (skin), granulosa cell tumor (ovarian), leiomyoma (ovarian), leiomyoma (subcutaneous), adenocarcinoma (pylorus), lymphoma (skin, prepuce), and renal carcinoma.

TABLE 10–3
LYMPHOMA IN 88 FERRETS, 1990–1994

Males	54 (62%)
Females	34 (38%)
Age at Time of Diagnosis	
<1 y	3
1 y	5
2 y	15
3 y	10
4 y	7
5 y	10
6 y	6
7 y	1
8 y	2
9 y	1
Unknown age (adults)	28
Sites	
Popliteal node	50
Abdominal lymph node	8
Bone marrow	7
Mandible	4
Pleural fluid	4
Mediastinum	1
Colon	1
Small intestine	1
Multifocal, including pancreas, liver, adrenal glands, lung, kidney, lymph nodes, intestine, and spleen	12

*Data from Midwest Bird and Exotic Animal Hospital.

tasis. Thoracic radiography is recommended before the removal of any tumors in ferrets, including benign-appearing skin masses. In addition, it may be necessary to perform other diagnostic tests and blood work, as indicated by the condition of the pet and the nature of the disease.

LYMPHOMA

Lymphoma is among the most common neoplasms in ferrets, and it is probably the most common neoplasm in young ferrets. Occasionally, siblings or several cohabiting ferrets are affected.[10] Preliminary transmission data suggest that a viral agent may be involved.[12]

Manifestations of lymphoma in ferrets vary with the age of the ferrets and with the location (or locations) of the neoplasia. In the present neoplasia survey (see Table 10–3), a greater incidence of the disease was noted in males (62%); however, no predilection by sex was noted in other studies.[9–12]

Lymphoma can involve numerous tissues, most often including peripheral and visceral lymph nodes, spleen, liver, intestine, mediastinum, bone marrow, lung, and kidney and, less often, the nervous system, stomach, pancreas, and adrenal glands. The skin is sometimes involved.[23]

Hemogram data may range from completely normal to mild anemia, mild to moderate lymphocytosis, lymphopenia, or neutropenia.[9, 21] A white blood cell (WBC) count greater than $10,000/mm^3$ is more often associated with lymphoma than with bacterial disease, although lymphoblastic leukemias are observed in fewer than 25% of ferrets with lymphoma.[11, 21] An elevated lymphocyte count may be an early indication of lymphoma. However, many older ferrets with chronic disease become lymphopenic with time.

Tissues with neoplastic lymphoid infiltrates usually have white nodules or streaks throughout the parenchyma on macroscopic examination. A soft dark brown or tan necrotic center that is indicative of necrosis is common in larger masses.

TABLE 10–4
MULTIPLE SYSTEM INVOLVEMENT WITH NEOPLASIA IN FERRETS, 1990–1994*

Tumor Type	Number of Animals
Insulinoma, adrenocortical carcinoma	33
Insulinoma, adrenocortical adenoma	8
Insulinoma, lymphoma	6
Insulinoma, adrenocortical carcinoma, lymphoma	2
Insulinoma, mast cell tumor (skin)	2
Insulinoma, adrenocortical carcinoma, mast cell tumor (lung)	1
Insulinoma, adrenocortical carcinoma, mast cell tumor (skin)	1
Insulinoma, adrenocortical carcinoma, prostatic carcinoma	1
Insulinoma, hemangioma (mesentery)	1
Adrenocortical carcinoma, mast cell tumor (skin)	1
Adrenocortical adenoma, mast cell tumor (skin)	1
Total ferrets with multiple neoplasms	57

*Data from Midwest Bird and Exotic Animal Hospital.

Histologically, diffuse small noncleaved cell and immunoblastic or immunoblastic polymorphic lymphomas are most common. Diffuse small lymphocytic lymphomas are also common in older ferrets. Aleutian disease, a lymphoproliferative disease induced by a parvovirus, may manifest similar histologic lesions.

Animals of any age with lymphoma may be completely without clinical signs or abnormalities on laboratory testing other than a mild to moderate lymphocytosis, which is defined as more than 3500 lymphocytes/mm^3 (or more than 60% lymphocytes in the differential count), that is observed incidentally on a complete blood count (CBC). Immature ferrets younger than 6 months of age may have a naturally occurring lymphocytosis.[18]

History and Physical Examination

Lymphoma in Young Ferrets

In young animals, the disease may be rapidly progressive. Peripubescent ferrets, some as young as 4 months of age, typically present with nonspecific signs, including anorexia, weight loss, acute weakness, and lethargy. Dyspnea, coughing, and tenesmus with mild rectal prolapse are occasionally observed. A mediastinal mass and pleural effusion may be noted on radiographs. Hind limb paresis may occur because of generalized weakness.

Young ferrets (younger than 1 year of age) may present with classic signs of gastric foreign body: anorexia, wasting, occasional vomiting, depression, and dehydration. A mass may be palpable in the area of the cranial abdomen, representing a grossly enlarged gastric or mesenteric lymph node (Fig. 10–1*A*). These ferrets frequently have multicentric lymphoma in abdominal lymph nodes, the liver, the stomach, and other organs.

Animals that are chronically affected may present with recurring signs of upper respiratory infection or gastrointestinal disease that respond briefly to antibiotics probably because of control of secondary bacterial infections. Treatment with corticosteroids may cause more dramatic improvement that lasts as long as the corticosteroids are administered. Therefore, consider lymphoma in the differential of chronically ill patients that respond well, at least initially, to corticosteroid therapy. Splenomegaly and enlarged peripheral and visceral lymph nodes may be seen (see Fig. 10–1*B* and *C*). Although most

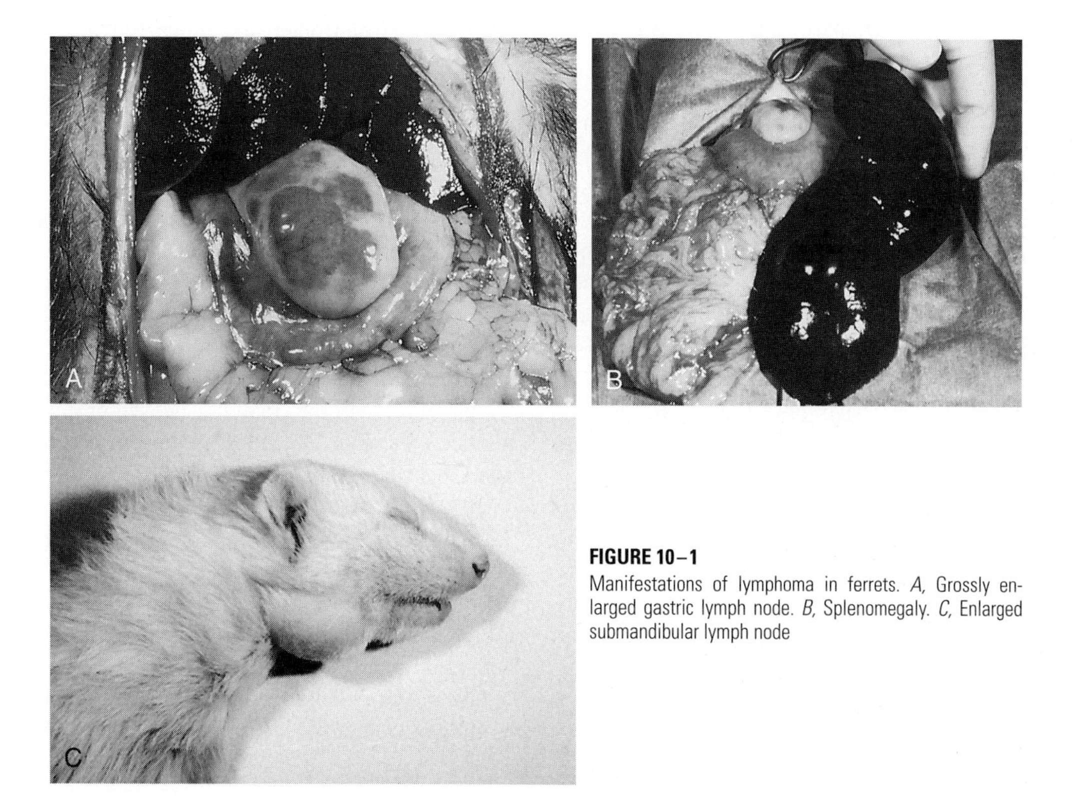

FIGURE 10–1
Manifestations of lymphoma in ferrets. *A,* Grossly enlarged gastric lymph node. *B,* Splenomegaly. *C,* Enlarged submandibular lymph node

common in hematopoietic and lymphatic organs, lesions have been noted in virtually every tissue of the body, including the central nervous system, eyes, skeletal muscle, intestine, and gonads.

Lymphoma in Adult Ferrets

Disease in adults is highly variable and, in many cases, chronic. Presenting signs are often nonspecific. The history may include cycles of inappetence, lethargy, and weight loss that alternate with spontaneous recovery periods that last for years. As in the young ferrets with lymphoma, adult ferrets may respond temporarily but dramatically to therapies that include corticosteroids. Other possible signs include peripheral lymphadenopathy that may be generalized or localized, chronic diarrhea or vomiting, mild to severe dyspnea (which may be confused on radiography as cardiac disease), icterus, posterior paresis, splenomegaly, and palpable abdominal mass or masses. Splenic lymphoma is seen; however, splenomegaly with extramedullary hematopoiesis and without neoplastic foci in the spleen frequently accompanies lymphoma in ferrets. Be aware that splenic extramedullary hematopoiesis is a very common finding in ferrets and that it is not necessarily associated with neoplasia (see Chapter 7).

Some adult ferrets, particularly younger adults from 1–2 years of age, demonstrate a rapidly progressive malignancy similar to that observed in peripubescent ferrets. In general, adult ferrets present with peripheral or visceral lymphadenopathy, often with renal, adrenal, gastric, pancreatic, or hepatic involvement. Some ferrets present with slowly evolving peripheral lymphadenopathy without other findings. Unilateral lymphadenopathy has been observed. Hematologic parameters may be within normal limits, or a slight to moderate lymphocytosis with rare reactive lymphocytes may be noted.

Although reports have linked Aleutian disease virus and feline leukemia virus with lymphoma in ferrets, most ferrets that were tested for these viruses had negative results on indirect immunofluorescence antibody testing, enzyme-linked immunosorbent assay, and polymerase chain reaction.[10, 12] Cluster outbreaks and cell free transmission of lymphoma in ferrets along with in vitro findings suggest that a ferret retrovirus may be involved.[10, 12] The potential viral nature of certain lymphomas in ferrets is currently being investigated.

Diagnosis

Diagnosis of lymphoma is accomplished by a variety of methods, depending on the presentation of the disease. A CBC provides important baseline information. Analysis of specimens collected by fine-needle aspiration or biopsy of solitary masses establishes the definitive diagnosis. A word of caution: ferrets whose body condition is good may have a fair amount of fat surrounding their peripheral lymph nodes, and, unless a node is grossly enlarged, fine-needle aspiration may yield only adipose cells. Therefore, tissue biopsy is preferable to fine-needle aspiration. A peripheral lymphadenectomy is performed with relative ease on the most commonly enlarged nodes, which include the prescapular, submandibular, axillary, inguinal, and popliteal lymph nodes.

Lymphatic tissue from a variety of sites is sampled during abdominal exploratory surgery. I have noted that the gastric lymph node is frequently enlarged and hyperplastic, even in the absence of lymphoma. This finding may be due to subclinical gastritis, which results in a hyperplastic gastric lymph node. One entity that may cause this inflammation in the gastric mucosa is *Helicobacter* species. Therefore, do not select the gastric node as the only abdominal lymph node to be sampled. Take biopsies from at least one other abdominal lymph node as well. Remember that the lymph nodes do not have to be grossly enlarged to be positive for lymphoma.

Histopathology

Histologically, the lymphomas of younger ferrets can be classified according to the National Cancer Institute's Working Formulation as high-grade, diffuse, small noncleaved, or immunoblastic.[9] The mitotic index of the tissues is often very high (greater than 10 per high-power field). In adult ferrets, the lymphomas are of the small noncleaved or immunoblastic types, as in juveniles; the mixed cell immunoblastic variant; or the mature lymphocytic. The small noncleaved and immunoblastic lymphomas are more often seen in young adult ferrets but do occur in 5- and 6-year-olds as well. These lymphomas are multicentric and diffuse, and they have a high mitotic index; these features are associated with rapidly progressive disease.

The mixed cell lymphomas are most often seen in middle-aged or older ferrets.[9] The immunoblastic polymorphic type is a diffuse heterogeneous lymphoma with a moderate to high mitotic index. This mixed cell lymphoma comprises immunoblasts, lymphoblasts, and small cleaved lymphocytes. Often, a component of large bizarre lymphoid cells and binucleate Reed-Sternberg–type cells are seen. This lymphoid mixture is similar to hyperplasias and lymphomas associated with viral infections in other species. The immunoblastic polymorphic lymphoma in ferrets is frequently found with visceral lymphadenopathy and splenomegaly. Other concomitant neoplasms are common.

Hematology

On a CBC, the parameters suggestive of lymphoma are either an absolute lymphocyte count of 3500/mm^3 or more or a relative count of 60% or greater of the total WBC count. However, some older adult ferrets become lymphopenic after many months to years of disease.[9] The normal range for a total WBC count (see Chapter 2 for clinical pathology values) in the normal ferret is 3500 to 7000/mm^3. Ferrets with WBC counts of 10,000/mm^3 or more may have a relative lymphocyte count of about 45%; however, this still represents an absolute count of 4500/mm^3, which would be considered suspicious. In my practice, the most common disease associated with a WBC count of 10,000/mm^3 or more is lymphoma. I have seen WBC counts as high as 90,000/mm^3. Bacterial disease causing an elevation of the WBC count is a much rarer occurrence in the ferret and is normally associated with a relative neutrophilia of 85% or greater and the presence of bands. Kawasaki notes a similar finding in cases of bacterial septicemia in which the relative neutrophilia is 90% or greater.[21] I recommend that CBCs routinely be performed at least annually on all ferrets 1 year of age or older as a screening procedure for lymphoma.

Other Diagnostic Tests

Radiography is indicated for animals experiencing dyspnea. Be extremely cautious in handling dyspneic animals because they can expire under the stress of being restrained for radiography. Have oxygen available at all times. It may be necessary to use light sedation with isoflurane anesthesia in order to minimize stress to the patient. If pleural effusion is present, cytologic analysis of a thoracic aspirate is frequently diagnostic. This procedure is often necessary in helping to differentiate among cardiac disease, pyothorax, chylothorax, and lymphoma. In ferrets with ascites, collect an abdominal fluid aspirate for cytologic evaluation. If splenomegaly is present, splenic aspiration can be performed with little or no sedation (see Chapter 2). I find the assessment of splenic aspirates to be only occasionally diagnostic because, as has been mentioned, extramedullary hematopoiesis in splenomegaly is common and is not necessarily associated with other disease.

Ultrasound is useful in differentiating thoracic disease and in identifying abdominal masses. However, it is not conclusively diagnostic of lymphoma. Biopsies or aspiration still must be performed for a definitive diagnosis.

Perform a bone marrow aspirate in ferrets with leukemia, anemia, or circulating atypical lymphocytes. The femur is easily accessible, and the procedure is the same as that described for cats. Use a 20- to 22-gauge spinal or hypodermic needle and approach through the trochanteric fossa. A bone marrow aspirate is most helpful in cases in which atypical lymphocytes are present, and it is a necessary procedure for evaluating a patient before chemotherapy is begun. For ferrets that have a persistent relative or absolute lymphocytosis but are otherwise clinically asymptomatic, bone marrow aspiration is usually unrewarding diagnostically; a biopsy specimen from a peripheral lymph node is the preferred diagnostic sample.

The most valuable combination of tests for diagnosing lymphoma in the mature ferret (older than 6 months of age) that is either asymptomatic or has vague general signs is the CBC, used as a screening tool, and subsequent popliteal nodectomy. In at least 50% of cases, the popliteal nodes were not grossly enlarged in ferrets that were diagnosed with lymphoma in this manner.

If a ferret has a relative or absolute lymphocytosis and is otherwise asymptomatic, I recommend a recheck of the CBC in 3–4 weeks. If the lymphocytosis still persists at this time, perform a popliteal nodectomy, regardless of whether the node is enlarged. Twenty-three of 73 lymphadenectomies (32%) performed in my practice because of lymphocytosis were reported as lymphoid hyperplasia. Biopsies in 50 of 73 ferrets (68%) were identified as lymphoma. The cause or significance of persistent lymphoid hyperplasia in the ferret, in the absence of other clinical signs, is unknown. In other species, lymphoid hyperplasia can be associated with viral infections or chronic antigenic stimulus. In these cases, it may be beneficial to use a course of antibiotic therapy and to recheck CBCs periodically. In the short time that I have been following ferrets with persistent lymphoid hyperplasia, I have seen several ferrets develop lymphoma within 2 years of the original diagnosis but many that remained hyperplastic and asymptomatic. I recommend following these ferrets with physical examinations and CBCs twice a year. Lymphadenectomies (popliteal, inguinal, or axillary) may be performed once a year or less frequently as a followup, as dictated by specific circumstances.

Popliteal Lymphadenectomy

With a bit of practice, this procedure is simple to perform. After inducing general anesthesia, clip and scrub the caudal aspect of the thigh. Drape the area routinely. Then palpate the caudal aspect of the thigh and locate the distinct, fat-padded popliteal node that is located approximately midway between the acetabulum and the stifle. Grasping the tissue firmly, apply pressure from the cranial aspect toward the caudal aspect of the thigh and bring the fat mass up under the skin. Incise over the skin; the fat will protrude under the firm pressure of your grasp. Gently dissect through this fat, which should be very white in color. Look for a tan-colored, round to oblong tissue that is only slightly firmer than the surrounding fat. Bluntly resect the lymph node without ligation of its rather insignificant blood supply.

Close the incision with either skin sutures or subcuticular sutures. Healing is usually uneventful, although this is one of the few surgical areas that ferrets want to lick postsurgically. Apply an unpleasant tasting substance to the area; this usually solves the problem. Ferrets generally stop bothering the area once the sutures are removed.

Treatment

General Principles

Depending on the condition of the patient and the organs affected with lymphoma, chemotherapy may be useful. Lymphoma should be considered a systemic disease, even if only one mass is clinically evident, and chemotherapy is the most aggressive systemic treatment available. Surgical removal of solitary tumors may improve the success of chemotherapy.

Over the years, I have used a number of protocols with varying success. Ferrets have responded poorly or not at all to chemotherapy if they had lymphoma in the following sites: intestine, liver, solitary lymph node (most commonly, the mandibular nodes), abdominal organs (multifocally), and bone marrow (more than 50% of the marrow displaying neoplastic cells). In addition, patients with concurrent disease such as insulinoma and adrenal neoplasia present complications to therapy and therefore may not be suitable chemotherapy candidates. Ferrets that have been treated with moderate to high levels of corticosteroids for several weeks to months, as for an insulinoma, are also poor candidates. The lymphoid cells of animals that have received glucocorticoids for an extended period may develop resistance to the antitumoral effects of the steroids.[30] This may make these patients refractory to further chemotherapeutic treatment.

The ferrets that respond most favorably to chemotherapy are those in which the disease is focused primarily in one of the following sites: mediastinum, spleen, skin, and peripheral lymph nodes without obvious abdominal lymph node involvement. In ferrets with splenomegaly, treatment success may be enhanced by a splenectomy. If the spleen occupies 50% or more of the abdominal cavity, perform a splenectomy to maximize the potential for chemotherapeutic success and to ease the patient's abdominal discomfort.

The patients in which it is most difficult to assess whether chemotherapy will be successful are ferrets that are asymptomatic but that have a persistent lymphocytosis and a positive result on peripheral lymph node biopsy analysis. Because ferrets with lymphoma can be asymptomatic for years, it is difficult to judge whether chemotherapy has prolonged the period. Treatment of asymptomatic ferrets is determined on an individual basis and includes such considerations as client compliance, the age of the pet, and the presence of concurrent disease.

The age of the ferret does not seem significant in relation to the success of therapy. Clinically ill patients as young as 8 months and as old as 6 years of age have successfully undergone chemotherapy and entered varying periods of remission.

Prognosis

Do not assume that a ferret with lymphoma is ever "cured" by chemotherapy, but rather that it goes into a period of remission. Indeed, even the assumption that chemotherapy is responsible for a remission is difficult to assess because lymphoma may present with a cyclical nature, as discussed previously.

Signs of a remission include a marked improvement or return to normal in the clinical picture in those patients with obvious physical signs. An affected enlarged organ or mass may return to normal size. In ferrets with persistent lymphocytosis, the CBC values may return to normal. Repeat biopsies of peripheral nodes or other affected tissue may show the presence of disease even in the face of return to clinical normalcy. Repeat CBCs performed after therapy at 1- to 3-month intervals are useful indicators of the return of the disease in previously lymphocytic patients. Remissions, as best I have been able to determine with the methods discussed, have lasted from 3 months to as long as 5 years.

Chemotherapy

Before considering chemotherapy, evaluate the patient thoroughly. A CBC for baseline data is essential. A biochemistry profile is necessary for evaluating renal and hepatic function. Whole-body radiography determines whether thoracic lesions, heart disease, or other masses are present in the body. It is useful to have a baseline radiograph in cases of lymphoma-induced thoracic masses. Ultrasound is also useful in ferrets with thoracic disease or abdominal organ involvement for judging the success of treatment. Perform bone marrow aspiration to evaluate the ability of the bone marrow to sustain the serious damage that will be wrought by the chemotherapeutic drugs. Ferrets with a proportion of malignant cells greater than 50% in their bone marrow have a tremendously high risk of serious or fatal complications during treatment. Counsel owners thoroughly before the start of therapy to ensure that they understand all of the risks and potential shortcomings of the treatment. Client compliance with administration of medications, nutritional support, and patient monitoring is crucial to the success of therapy.

Ferrets that are considered good candidates for therapy—namely, those that have disease focused in the mediastinum, spleen, skin, or peripheral nodes and do not have concurrent systemic disease; whose proportion of normal WBCs in bone marrow is 50% or greater; and whose body condition is still good—generally tolerate chemotherapy well. Side effects include those also observed in other species and depend on the agents being used. The most common signs of chemotherapy toxicity in ferrets include lethargy, posterior paresis, anorexia, vomiting, mild hair loss (usually just the whiskers), dyspnea, and complete collapse. One ferret developed a necrosis of the tail, which proceeded to slough completely at the tail base for unknown reasons. Signs may appear within 1–2 days of administration of the drug or drugs or as late as 2 weeks thereafter, depending on the time of the agents' peak of activity.

When using chemotherapeutic drugs, follow the usual safety guidelines to protect staff, clients, and patients. Wear gloves when handling all these agents and the equipment in which they are housed. Administer intravenous chemotherapeutic drugs to ferrets under anesthesia (isoflurane is the anesthetic agent of choice). Before using any cytotoxic drug, place an indwelling catheter in the cephalic vein and flush it well to determine patency. If cytotoxic drugs are injected extravascularly, use normal therapeutic procedures that are appropriate for the drug being used. (Be prepared beforehand with any materials that you might need.)

Perform a CBC no sooner than 24 hours before each administration of a cytotoxic drug. Discontinue therapy with cytotoxic drugs if the WBC count decreases to 1500/mm^3 or less, if the packed cell volume drops below 30%, if the pet becomes clinically debilitated, or if any combination of these three events occurs. In affected ferrets, perform weekly or biweekly CBCs and platelet counts until the hematologic parameters improve. At that point, make a decision whether to continue therapy.

Numerous protocols have been used for the treatment of lymphoma in ferrets. One author used a combination of doxorubicin and orthovoltage radiation therapy.[19] Table 10–5 describes a protocol that I have been using with slight modifications since 1988.[4] Table 10–6 describes an alternative protocol.[29]

Doxorubicin may also be used for single-agent chemotherapy. It may be used as the initial and only therapy or as a rescue therapy for the two protocols described in Tables 10–5 and 10–6. (Rescue therapy is defined as therapy for disease that has recurred after a remission.) The dosage is 1 mg/kg intravenously every 21 days for a maximum of 5 treatments. Do not use heparinized saline as a flush solution because heparin may cause the precipitation of doxorubicin. Prednisone at the dosage of 1 mg/kg PO either q24h or divided q12h may be used concurrently.

The condition of the patient and client compli-

TABLE 10–5
CHEMOTHERAPY PROTOCOL I FOR LYMPHOMA*

Week	Day	Drug	Dose
1	1	Prednisone	1 mg/kg, PO, q12h and continued throughout therapy
	1	Vincristine	0.12 mg/kg, IV
	3	Cyclophosphamide	10 mg/kg, PO or SC
2	8	Vincristine	0.12 mg/kg, IV
3	15	Vincristine	0.12 mg/kg, IV
4	22	Vincristine	0.12 mg/kg, IV
	24	Cyclophosphamide	10 mg/kg, PO or SC
7	46	Cyclophosphamide	10 mg/kg, PO or SC
9		Prednisone	Start decreasing the dose gradually to zero over the next 4 wk

Key: IV = intravenously; PO = perorally; SC = subcutaneously

*CBCs should be checked weekly during therapy. After therapy is discontinued, continue to monitor CBCs and do physical examinations at 3-month intervals.

From Brown SA: Ferrets. *In* A Practitioner's Guide to Rabbits and Ferrets. Denver, American Animal Hospital Association, 1993, pp 87–89.

ance determine whether a second or third course of chemotherapy is warranted. It has been my experience that a second course of therapy, but not a third, occasionally is useful. Use a different protocol when readministering chemotherapy for a second or third time.

TABLE 10–6
CHEMOTHERAPY PROTOCOL II FOR LYMPHOMA*

Week	Drug	Dose
1	Vincristine	0.07 mg/kg, IV
	Asparaginase	400 IU/kg, IP
	Prednisone	1 mg/kg, PO, q24h and continued throughout therapy
2	Cyclophosphamide	10 mg/kg, SC
3	Doxorubicin	1 mg/kg, IV
4–6	As weeks 1–3 above but discontinue asparaginase	
8	Vincristine	0.07 mg/kg, IV
10	Cyclophosphamide	10 mg/kg, SC
12	Vincristine	0.07 mg/kg, IV
14	Methotrexate	0.5 mg/kg, IV

Key: IV = intravenously; IP = intraperitoneally; PO = perorally; SC = subcutaneously

*Protocol is continued in sequence biweekly after week 14.

From Rosenthal KE: Ferrets. Vet Clin North Am 1994; 24: 19–20.

Palliative and Adjunct Therapy

Many ferrets with lymphoma are unsuitable candidates for chemotherapy; however, some measures that may offer these ferrets a degree of relief from the disease are available. The use of glucocorticoids alone, particularly prednisone, can be very beneficial in alleviating some of the signs for periods ranging from weeks to months. Glucocorticoids are not myelosuppressive, and they actually can cause destruction of sensitive tumor cells.[30] This may result in the reduction in the size of tumor masses or in the alleviation of signs such as chronic upper respiratory disease or chronic diarrhea. Prednisone therapy is initiated at a dose of 0.5 mg/kg PO q12h and increased as needed to control the signs. Do not use glucocorticoids in ferrets in which the only sign of disease is a peripheral lymphocytosis because the patient may become refractory to this therapy later when it is really needed.

For all ferrets with lymphoma, nutritional and environmental support is vital. These patients should be provided a healthy diet that is rich in good quality meat protein and fat (see Chapter 1 for discussion of diet). Supplement the diet of ferrets undergoing chemotherapy and those with loss of body condition with hand-feedings of items such as strained meat baby foods, pulverized moistened cat or ferret food, or Prescription Diet Feline a/d (Hill's Pet Nutrition, Topeka, KS). High-calorie supplements such as Deliver 2.0 (Mead-Johnson Nutritionals, Evansville, IN) can be added to these meat-based foods at a ratio of 1:3 (Deliver:food) for promoting weight gain.

A variety of homeopathic, herbal, and vitamin supplements used in humans can also be used in ferrets. I have given a combination of vitamin C and Pau d'Arco in ferrets with lymphoma both with and without chemotherapy. Vitamin C is a powerful antioxidant and an antineoplastic agent in humans.[2] As an antioxidant, it protects the body from free radicals that are a byproduct of body metabolism. Vitamin C also increases interferon production and stimulates T-effector cell activity. Pau d'Arco is extracted from the inner bark of the tabebuia tree of South America. It is thought to be supportive of the immune system and has been shown clinically to contain a natural antibiotic agent.[2] This activity may be useful in minimizing secondary infections in the face of an immunosuppressive disease.

The dosage of vitamin C is 50–100 mg/kg PO q12h. Use the chelated, buffered, or ester form of vitamin C rather than plain ascorbic acid. The former bind the vitamin C to a mineral, minimizing gastrointestinal irritation. Vitamin C has a bitter taste, so use the powder from a capsule and mix it with a meat-based food such as strained meat baby food. If the patient develops diarrhea, reduce the dose to a level that can be tolerated. Pau d'Arco comes as either an alcohol-containing or alcohol-free extract. Use either form, as ferrets are not bothered by the bitterness of the alcohol. The dose is 3–5 drops PO q12h. Ferrets generally enjoy the taste of this product right from the bottle. These medications are given for the rest of the ferret's life. Ferrets that were clinically ill and received no other treatment improved markedly while receiving vitamin C and Pau d'Arco. Improvements were in the form of weight gain, increased activity level, improved hair coat quality, and reduced peripheral lymphocytosis. These medications do not represent cures for lymphoma but may be beneficial supplements to support the patient suffering from this disease.

Other treatments that I have tried include Essiac (a combination herbal formula), pycnogenol (also found in health food stores), and Acemannan Immunostimulant (Carrington Laboratories, Inc., Irving, TX). The number of ferrets that have been treated is small, and I am unable to state at this time if any real clinical improvement was derived. Undoubtedly, many more alternative therapies will be proposed for the treatment of lymphoma and for the general support of ferrets with this disease. All avenues should be investigated for their potential merit.

OTHER LYMPHOID AND HEMATOLOGIC NEOPLASMS

Multiple myeloma (plasma cell myeloma) is a malignant disease originating in blood-forming cells in the bone marrow.[30] It has been reported in three ferrets.[3, 14, 24] This neoplasm can occur in either single or multiple bones, including the vertebral column, pelvis, skull, and appendicular skeleton. Radiographic appearance is focal osteolysis with no bony sclerosis around the lesion.[30] Clinical signs can include pathologic fractures, pain, lameness, and limb paresis or paralysis.

Megakaryocytic myelosis has been reported in two ferrets.[7, 14]

CUTANEOUS AND SUBCUTANEOUS NEOPLASMS

After insulinoma, adrenocortical neoplasia, and lymphoma, the fourth most commonly encountered neoplasms in the survey in Table 10–2 were cutaneous neoplasms. Those observed (in order of occurrence out of a total of 46) include mast cell tumor of the skin (mastocytoma) (30%); sebaceous gland adenoma (22%); hemangioma (13%; Fig. 10–2); benign cystic adenomas (9%); adenocarcinomas of the

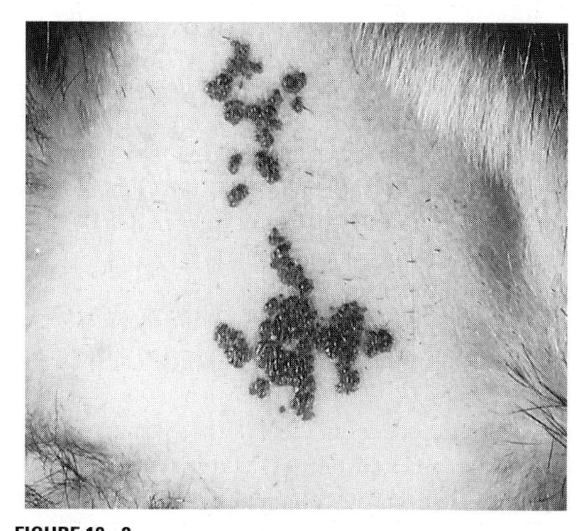

FIGURE 10–2
Benign cutaneous hemangiomas.

prepuce (7%); and dermatofibromas, carcinomas, fibromas, fibrosarcomas, histiocytomas, sarcomas, and squamous cell carcinomas (22%). Before this survey, I also encountered one case of melanoma and one case of cutaneous lymphoma involving the prepuce.

In one review, squamous cell carcinoma was the most commonly reported skin tumor, followed by sebaceous gland adenocarcinoma.[14] Another study of 57 cutaneous neoplasms in ferrets revealed a high incidence of basal cell tumor (58%), mastocytomas (16%), and fibromas (11%).[26] (See section on sebaceous epitheliomas in Chapter 11.) Cutaneous neoplasms may occur concurrently with other noncutaneous neoplasia (see Table 10–4).

Metastasis to distant sites is a high probability with adenocarcinoma. The prepuce was the most common subcutaneous site affected by adenocarcinoma in the present survey. In all three ferrets, neoplasia recurred at the same site within 2–5 months, even with aggressive surgical excision and resection. One case study reported limited success with the use of repeated radiation therapy in a recurrent adenocarcinoma of the prepuce of a ferret.[25] I used doxorubicin along with surgical resection without success for one ferret with adenocarcinoma of the prepuce.

Other cutaneous neoplasms that have the potential for metastasis are squamous cell carcinoma and fibrosarcoma. Mast cell tumors in ferrets usually are benign; however, I have seen three ferrets with visceral mastocytosis (in lung, in lymph node, and multicentric [see Table 10–2]); the one with pulmonary mastocytosis had had a cutaneous mast cell tumor removed the previous year.

Because of the potential for metastasis, do not adopt a "wait and see" attitude. Surgically remove skin masses as soon as possible. Perform a histopathologic examination to develop a prognosis. Electrocautery is especially suited for quick removal of many of the small skin masses that are encountered. (See Chapter 11 for a more detailed discussion of cutaneous neoplasms.)

ENDOCRINE AND EXOCRINE NEOPLASMS

Pancreatic endocrine neoplasms (insulinomas or pancreatic beta cell tumors) and adrenocortical tumors are the most commonly encountered neoplasms in ferrets in the United States and certainly in the present survey (see Table 10–2). A more detailed discussion of these neoplasms and their management can be found in Chapter 9. Pituitary, thyroid, and parathyroid neoplasms have not been reported in ferrets.

Pheochromocytomas are rare. Three ferrets with histologically confirmed pheochromocytoma have been seen at the Animal Medical Center in New York City.* One of these ferrets, a 4-year-old neutered male, presented for mild lethargy. He was tachycardic, and a walnut-sized midabdominal tumor was detected on physical examination. The tumor was shown on ultrasound to be at the cranial pole of a kidney and wrapped around the caudal vena cava. Surgical resection was impossible: the tumor was extremely vascular and entered the vena cava in many places. The ferret was treated with phenoxybenzamine and propranolol (feline dosages) and survived for 3 months after surgical debulking. In the two other ferrets, the pheochromocytomas were very large and nonresectable (see Chapter 13). Both tumors enveloped the abdominal aorta, and one also involved the caudal vena cava. Pheochromocytomas have not been previously reported in ferrets.

Pancreatic exocrine adenocarcinoma has been reported by several authors,[3, 14, 17, 22] and two ferrets with this neoplasm were seen in the present survey (see Table 10–2). Affected ferrets were of both sexes and 2 years of age and older. Presenting signs were nonspecific and included lethargy, anorexia, abdominal distention, and abdominal pain. This neoplasm tends to be very aggressive. In one ferret, it had metastasized to submucosal lymphatic vessels and mucosa of the duodenum and around vessels in the interstitial tissue of the lung, and osseous metaplasia was present within the primary tumor.[22] Pancreatic adenocarcinoma can metastasize to liver, omentum, abdominal lymph nodes, and gastric mucosa and can present as carcinomatosis, a condition in which tumors are disseminated throughout the abdominal cavity.[17] Abdominal ultrasound is very helpful in establishing a tentative diagnosis. Exploratory surgery with biopsy is necessary for establishing a definitive diagnosis. There is no treatment for pancreatic adenocarcinoma, and, by the time it is identified, it is likely to have already metastasized.

---

*Quesenberry K, Rosenthal K: Personal communication, April 1995.

REPRODUCTIVE TRACT NEOPLASMS

Although reproductive tract neoplasms are reported with frequency in the literature, they are encountered uncommonly in practice in the United States because most ferrets currently sold to the pet trade are neutered just after weaning. I rarely see sexually intact animals. In the present survey (see Table 10–2), one case each of carcinoma of the prostate, undifferentiated carcinoma of an ovarian stump, and cystic carcinoma of the mammary gland were reported. Before 1990, I encountered ferrets with a granulosa cell tumor, a leiomyoma, and a fibrosarcoma (all of ovarian remnant tissue); a uterine adenoma; and a seminoma.

Three older studies indicated that reproductive tract tumors were the first or second most commonly reported neoplasms.[3, 8, 14] Other reproductive neoplasms reported by other sources include ovarian thecoma, fibromyoma, carcinoma, leiomyoma, and arrhenoblastoma; uterine leiomyoma and teratoma; mammary gland papillary cystadenocarcinoma; testicular Sertoli cell tumor; and interstitial cell tumors.[3, 14] There was one report of an ovarian teratoma.[28] These neoplasms all occurred in animals older than 2 years of age. Some of the affected females had previously had normal pregnancies.[28]

Signs of disease are variable and depend on the tumor site and on whether sex hormone production is excessive. One ferret with fibrosarcoma of the ovarian remnant presented with a generalized alopecia and an enlarged vulva. The ferret had been previously ovariectomized. A large mass (2 cm) was palpable in the left upper abdominal quadrant. After removal of this mass, the hair regrew and the vulvar swelling regressed.

Although the most common cause of vulvar swelling and alopecia in the mature spayed female is adrenal disease, consider also the possibility of healthy or neoplastic ovarian tissue remnants, particularly if the ferret is younger than 2 years of age. Some of these affected ferrets may show no clinical signs, and the neoplasm may be found incidentally on palpation during a routine physical examination.[28]

Male ferrets with prostatic neoplasia may present with dysuria and hematuria. This is a rare tumor. I have seen one ferret with prostatic carcinoma; no others have been reported.

Treatment for reproductive tract neoplasms is surgical removal. It may be feasible to use chemotherapy or radiation therapy treatments, as described for canine and feline patients, if surgical therapy is impossible or unsuccessful.

GASTROINTESTINAL TRACT NEOPLASMS

In my experience, the most common tumor of the gastrointestinal tract (not including the pancreas) is metastatic neoplasia to the liver. Insulinoma was the most common metastatic neoplasm in the present survey (see Table 10–2). Pancreatic cancer may metastasize by direct extension because of its close proximity to the liver.[30] Other metastatic neoplasms to the liver include pancreatic adenocarcinoma and undifferentiated adenocarcinomas (of unidentified origin). Lymphoma can affect any area of the digestive tract, as discussed previously. Primary neoplasms that I have encountered in the gastrointestinal tract include hepatic hemangiosarcoma, oral fibrosarcoma, salivary gland adenocarcinoma, and pyloric adenocarcinoma.

Two studies reported that the most common gastrointestinal tract tumor was hepatic hemangiosarcoma.[3, 14] Other tumors reported in these two studies include bile duct cystadenoma, biliary carcinoma, and hepatic hemangioma. These neoplasms (other than lymphoma) occur primarily in mature animals older than 2 years of age. Signs of disease in the liver or intestine may include anorexia, cachexia, icterus, vomiting, diarrhea, melena, anemia, and abnormalities on a biochemical profile and CBC. Although ultrasound may be helpful, the diagnosis is ultimately based on endoscopic or exploratory abdominal examination and biopsy results.

Treatment for hepatic neoplasia (particularly metastatic) is futile unless the disease is confined to a focal area that can be surgically removed. The treatment for localized intestinal tumors is surgical resection.

Pyloric adenocarcinoma has been reported in a 3-year-old spayed female ferret that presented with severe depression, dehydration, and gastric distention with fluid.[27] I have encountered two cases of pyloric adenocarcinoma that had a presentation very similar to that of a chronic gastric foreign body. One ferret with pyloric adenocarcinoma responded favorably for a period of time to a pyloric myotomy. Before surgery, the ferret was cachectic and continually vomiting. After surgery, he was able to keep soft food down and eat on his own. He survived for another 12 months; at 12 months, the vomiting recurred, his condition deteriorated rapidly, and he was euthanized.

Fibrosarcoma of the oral mucosa appears as a firm, smooth mass in the mouth that rapidly advances to cover the teeth and interferes with mastication. All three cases I have observed have involved only the mucosa of the upper arcade and hard palate but not the tongue or lower arcade. I have attempted treatment of this tumor, using aggressive surgical resection with electrocautery, and Acemannan Immunostimulant injected both into the lesion and intraperitoneally. In all cases, both treatments resulted in only a temporary slowing in the growth of the tumor. The prognosis for fibrosarcoma of the oral mucosa is poor, and the tumor is usually quite advanced within 3 months of the initial diagnosis.

URINARY TRACT NEOPLASMS

Urinary tract tumors are relatively rare in ferrets. In the present survey (see Table 10–2), one ferret had transitional cell carcinoma of the bladder. Before 1990, I encountered two other ferrets with transitional cell carcinoma of the bladder and one ferret with renal carcinoma with pulmonary metastasis. Two reviews mention renal papillary cystadenoma.[3, 14] Urinary tract tumors occur primarily in mature animals.

Signs of transitional cell carcinoma may be very subtle initially and can be mistaken for a chronic cystitis. Clinical signs may include hematuria (resulting from the ulceration of the bladder mucosa) and some degree of dysuria. Ferrets may also be polyuric and develop incontinence. Abnormalities of the bladder are frequently not palpable. A urinalysis that reveals neoplastic cells can be diagnostic. Perform bladder washings to increase the probability of picking up abnormal cells. Survey radiography rarely demonstrates any abnormalities, and it is necessary to perform positive contrast imaging, pneumocystography, or double-contrast studies.[30] Ultrasound may be able to demonstrate a bladder lesion but is unable to differentiate neoplasia and inflammatory disease.[30] A biopsy of the bladder performed during exploratory surgery may be necessary for definitive diagnosis of the disease in some cases.

The prognosis is poor for ferrets with transitional cell carcinoma. Surgical excision may be attempted, but this neoplasm is usually diffuse and well infiltrated into the bladder at the time of surgery. In a recent retrospective study in dogs with transitional cell carcinoma of the bladder, it was noted that the systemic use of doxorubicin and cyclophosphamide provided the longest survival rate.[15] In addition, cisplatin was proposed as a possible helpful adjunct to this chemotherapy.

Renal carcinoma can easily be confused with renal cysts, which are seen in ferrets older than 3 years of age. A unilateral palpable kidney enlargement may be the only clinical abnormality noted unless both kidneys are affected or metastasis to other organs has occurred. Cytologic evaluation of urine may demonstrate neoplastic cells. Abnormalities are not noted in the biochemical profile unless the contralateral kidney is also affected. Ultrasound readily shows the difference between a fluid-filled renal cyst and a solid neoplastic mass. Treatment is surgical removal of the affected kidney. This neoplasm can metastasize quickly.

MUSCULOSKELETAL NEOPLASMS

Tumors involving the musculoskeletal system in the present survey (see Table 10–2) include chondroma of the tail and fibrosarcoma of the femur and cervical vertebrae. Before this study, I saw one ferret with subcutaneous leiomyoma in the thigh. Goad and Fox reported osteoma of the vertebral body, larynx, and head; chondroma of the intervertebral cartilage and caudal vertebrae; and chordoma of the caudal vertebrae.[14] Beach and Greenwood reported chondrosarcoma, chordoma, and osteomas in ferrets.[3] Leiomyosarcomas have also been reported in the ovary and subcutaneous tissue.[5] Musculoskeletal tumors occur primarily in the ferret older than 2 years of age.

Leiomyomas and leiomyosarcomas are of smooth muscle origin. Smooth muscle tumors found in the subcutaneous tissue may originate from tissue in vessel walls.[5] They are usually well circumscribed and firm in appearance. Surgically remove these tumors. There is a potential for recurrence if the excision is not complete.

An osteoma is an abnormally dense mass of mature bone tissue.[20] In other species, this neoplasm most commonly affects the flat bones of the head and rarely affects the appendicular skeleton. These tumors are benign in nature, tend to grow slowly, and are easily palpated. Signs of this tumor are based on the structures that are displaced by their growth. Radiographically, osteomas appear as dense bony masses.[30] Surgical removal is the treatment of choice.

Fibrosarcoma of the bone comes from either medullary or periosteal tissue.[30] Radiographically, this tumor appears similar to other bone neoplasms. A bone biopsy may be necessary to distinguish it from other bone disease. This tumor may metastasize rapidly to distant sites. Surgical removal is recommended, and amputation of a limb may be necessary if the tumor occurs in the appendicular skeleton. In cases in which surgical intervention is either impossible or unsuccessful, other forms of treatment such as chemotherapy or radiation therapy, as described for the canine and feline patient, can be attempted.

Chordomas are formed from the residual tissue of the notochord.[1, 16, 31] This tumor is frequently found on the tip of the tail and appears as a rounded, smooth, firm mass.[16] However, Williams and associates reported two cases of chordoma with no involvement of the tail: one involved the atlanto-occipital joint and resulted in hind limb paresis and cachexia; and the other involved the periosteum of the ventral aspect of C-2 and C-3 vertebrae, causing a ventral deviation of the trachea.[31] The tumor involving the cervical vertebrae recurred 4 months after surgical removal. In addition, evidence of metastasis to adjacent subcutaneous tissue, which is unusual in ferrets, was observed. Chordomas tend to grow slowly, and surgical removal is the treatment of choice. If the tumor occurs on the tip of the tail, remove that portion of the tail, including a wide margin of normal tissue. The prognosis is guarded because the potential for metastasis exists in the ferret as in other species.[16, 31]

Chordomas may be confused with chondrosarcomas on histologic examination.[16, 31] If special immunohistochemical staining or electron microscopy is not performed, it may be impossible to differentiate chondrosarcomas from chordomas.[16]

Two ferrets with nonresectable chondrosarcomas have been seen at the Animal Medical Center. One tumor involved the cervical vertebrae, and the other involved the ribs and sternum.

OTHER NEOPLASMS

Miscellaneous tumors reported in the present survey (see Table 10–2) include carcinoma of the ocular globe, hemangioma of the mesentery, and schwannoma (neurilemoma) in the hind leg. Tumors reported by other authors include mesothelioma and malignant mesenchymoma.[3, 8, 32]

Schwannomas originate from nerve tissue—specifically, from the nerve sheath or Schwann cells.[30] In other species, they are usually benign, but malignancy and local recurrence after surgical excision is possible. These tumors may occur anywhere in the body and appear as firm, encapsulated masses. Clinical signs are determined by the location of the tumor and the degree of nerve damage or compression that has occurred. Surgical removal should be attempted; however, in ferrets with large tumors, it may be difficult to excise all tissue, and recurrence is common.

Mesotheliomas are of mesodermal origin.[30] In other species, some evidence suggests a connection between exposure to asbestos and the development of mesothelioma on the pleural and peritoneal surfaces. Two cases of peritoneal mesotheliomas in ferrets have been reported by Williams and colleagues: one was in a 1.5-year-old intact male, and the other was in a 3-year-old spayed female.[32] Both had a primary complaint of a distended abdomen, which contained a large volume of serosanguineous abdominal fluid. In one case, reactive mesothelial cells were noted on cytologic examination of the abdominal fluid. The mesotheliomas appeared as multiple, small white nodules present throughout the omentum, mesentery, and serosal surface of the abdominal organs. Prognosis is very poor, and although these may be benign tumors, the extent of their involvement with the tissues on which they are growing make them life threatening. Surgical excision may be attempted. In humans, doxorubicin, cyclophosphamide, and radiation therapy have been attempted.[30] It is unknown whether this treatment would be useful in affected ferrets.

CONCLUSION

It is unfortunate that such a delightful pet as the domestic ferret has to suffer from such a plethora of neoplastic diseases, but unfortunately such is the case in the United States. Consider neoplasia in the differential diagnosis of disease, particularly in chronic disease of ferrets of all ages. Although many of the tumors that ferrets develop are treatable, the prognosis should always be guarded. Ferrets are prone to the development of multiple neoplastic processes as they age. I recommend frequent physical examinations (at least every 6 months) in ferrets 3 years of age and older, with diagnostic testing done at least annually. Such measures may not prevent disease, but they may help in the identification of neoplastic disorders early enough for them to be managed, making it possible to provide an increased life span and an improved quality of life for the patients.

ACKNOWLEDGMENT

A special thank-you to Dr. Stephen Badylak, DVM, PhD, MD of the Veterinary Professional Laboratory in West Lafayette, IN, for providing pathology services for the survey presented in Tables 10–1 through 10–4.

REFERENCES

1. Allison N, Rakich P: Chordoma in two ferrets. J Comp Pathol 1988; 98:371–374.
2. Balch JF, Balch PA. Prescription for Nutritional Healing. Garden Park City, NY, Avery, 1990, pp 18–19, 211–213.
3. Beach JE, Greenwood B: Spontaneous neoplasia in the ferret *(Mustela putorius furo)*. J Comp Pathol 1993; 108:133–147.
4. Brown SA: Ferrets. *In* A Pracitioner's Guide to Rabbits and Ferrets. Denver, The American Animal Hospital Association, 1993, pp 87–89.
5. Brunnert SR, Herron AJ, Altman NH: Leiomyosarcoma in a domestic ferret: morphologic and immunocytochemical diagnosis. Lab Anim Sci 1990; 40:208–210.
6. Chesterman FC, Pomerance A: Spontaneous neoplasms in ferrets and polecats. J Pathol Bacteriol 1965; 89:529–533.
7. Chowdhury KA, Shillinger RB: Spontaneous megakaryocytic myelosis in a four-year-old domestic ferret *(Mustela furo)*. Vet Pathol 1982; 19:561–564.
8. Dilberger JE, Altman NH: Neoplasia in ferrets: eleven cases with a review. J Comp Pathol 1989; 100:161–176.
9. Erdman SE, Brown SA, Kawasaki TA, et al: Clinical and pathological findings in ferrets with lymphoma: 60 cases (1982–1994). J Am Vet Med Assoc 1996; 208:1285–1289.
10. Erdman SE, Kanki PJ, Moore FM, et al: Clusters of malignant lymphoma in ferrets. Cancer Invest (in press).
11. Erdman SE, Moore FM, Rose R, Fox JG: Malignant lymphoma in ferrets: clinical and pathological findings in 19 cases. J Comp Pathol 1992; 106:37–47.
12. Erdman SE, Reimann KA, Moore FM, et al: Transmission of a chronic lymphoproliferative syndrome in ferrets. Lab Invest 1995; 72:1–8.
13. Fox JG: Reproduction, breeding and growth. *In* Biology and Diseases of the Ferret. Philadelphia, Lea & Febiger, 1988, pp 174–183.
14. Goad MEP, Fox JG: Neoplasia in ferrets. *In* Biology and Diseases of the Ferret. Philadelphia, Lea & Febiger, 1988, pp 274–287.
15. Helfand SC, Hamilton TA, Hungerford LL, et al: Comparison of three treatments for transitional cell carcinoma of the bladder in the dog. J Am Anim Hosp Assoc 1994; 30:270–275.
16. Herron AJ, Brunnert SR, Ching SV, et al: Immuno-histochemical and morphologic features of chordomas in ferrets *(Mustela putorius furo)*. Vet Pathol 1990; 27:284–286.
17. Hoefer HL, Patnaik AK: Pancreatic adenocarcinoma with metastasis in two ferrets. J Am Vet Med Assoc 1992; 201:466–467.
18. Hoover JP, Baldwin CA: Changes in physiologic and clinical pathologic values in domestic ferrets from 12 to 47 weeks of age. Comp Anim Pract 1988; 2:40–44.
19. Hutson CA, Kopit MJ, Walder EJ: Combination doxorubicin and ortho-voltage radiation therapy, single-agent doxorubicin, and high-dose vincristine for salvage therapy of ferret lymphosarcoma. J Am Anim Hosp Assoc 1992; 28:365–368.
20. Jenson WA, Myers RK, Liu CH: Osteoma in a ferret. J Am Vet Med Assoc 1985; 187:1375–1376.
21. Kawasaki T: Clinical pathology values in ferrets. Semin Avian Exotic Pet Med 1994; 3:44–45.
22. Kornegay JM, Morris JM, Cho D, Lozano-Alarcon F: Pancreatic adenocarcinoma with osseous metaplasia in a ferret. J Comp Pathol 1991; 105:117–121.
23. Li X, Fox JG, Erdman SE, Aspros DG: Cutaneous lymphoma in a ferret *(Mustela putorius furo)*. Vet Pathol 1995; 32:55–56.
24. Methiyapun S, Myers RK, Pohlenz JFL: Spontaneous plasma cell myeloma in a ferret *(Mustela putorius furo)*. Vet Pathol 1985; 22:517–519.
25. Miller TA, Denman DL, Lewis GC: Recurrent adenocarcinoma in a ferret. J Am Vet Med Assoc 1985; 187:839–841.
26. Parker GA, Picut CA: Histopathologic features and post-surgical sequelae of 57 cutaneous neoplasms in ferrets *(Mustela putorius furo* L.*)*. Vet Pathol 1993; 30:499–504.
27. Rice LE, Stahe SJ, McLeod CG. Pyloric adenocarcinoma in a ferret. J Am Vet Med Assoc 1992; 200:1117–1118.
28. Rodriquez JL, Martin de las Mulas J, Espinosa de los Monteros A, et al: Ovarian teratoma in a ferret *(Mustela putorius furo)*: a morphological and immunohistochemical study. J Zoo Wildl Med 1994; 25:294–299.
29. Rosenthal K: Ferrets. Vet Clin North Am 1994; 24:19–20.
30. Theilen GH, Madewell BR: *In* Veterinary Cancer Medicine. Philadelphia, Lea & Febiger, 1987.
31. Williams BH, Eighmy JJ, Berbert MH, Dunn DG: Cervical chordoma in two ferrets *(Mustela putorius furo)*. Vet Pathol 1993; 30:204–206.
32. Williams BH, Garner MM, Kawasaki TA: Peritoneal mesotheliomas in two ferrets *(Mustela putorius furo)*. J Zoo Wildl Med 1994; 25:590–594.

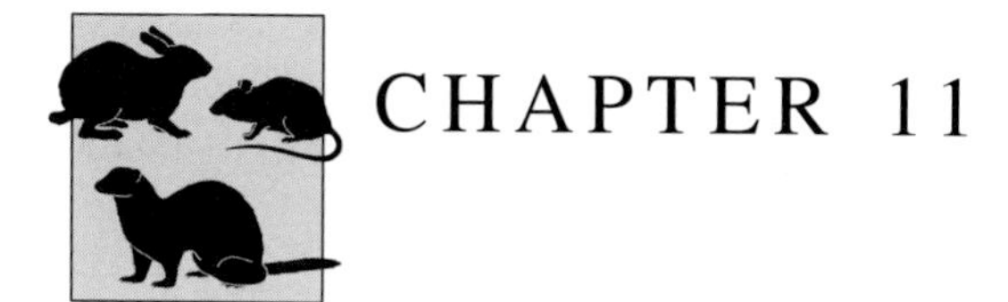

Dermatologic Diseases

Connie Orcutt, DVM

The initial approach to the examination of ferrets with dermatologic disease is very similar to that used for other domestic animals. The signalment (age, sex, and reproductive status) is important in forming the initial list of differential diagnoses. A thorough history should include information on the origin of the ferret, housing, diet, vaccinations, condition of cagemate (or cagemates), exposure to other animals, prior medical problems, and any skin problems affecting people in the household.

A complete physical examination is extremely important because certain skin conditions occur in conjunction with other clinical signs (e.g., pruritus and alopecia often accompany vulvar swelling in females with hyperadrenocorticism). The diagnostic tests performed depend on the refined list of differential diagnoses. Direct microscopic examination of skin scrapings and aural exudate are most helpful in diagnosing parasitic diseases. Fungal cultures of the hair and skin are performed when dermatophytosis is suspected. When dealing with wounds and abscesses, initial Gram's staining of exudate is helpful while awaiting the results of bacterial culture and sensitivity testing. Fine-needle aspiration and cytologic evaluation of an impression smear can be performed when cutaneous or subcutaneous masses are initially detected, but biopsy is the diagnostic modality of choice. With older ferrets, as well as with any ferret suspected of having systemic disease, a complete blood count, plasma biochemistry panel, and radiography are important. Other screening diagnostic tests may include abdominal ultrasound (e.g., if hyperadrenocorticism is suspected).

The clinical approaches to alopecia, pruritus, and skin masses in ferrets are depicted diagrammatically in Figures 11–1 through 11–3.

ANATOMY, PHYSIOLOGY, AND HUSBANDRY CONSIDERATIONS

The ferret's skin contains numerous sebaceous glands whose secretions sometimes cause the haircoat to have a greasy feel as well as a characteristic musky odor. Males have more of these glands than females do, and glandular production appears to be under androgenic control.[4, 7] Secretions may be so profuse that intact male albino ferrets can appear yellow and dirty. Ferrets do not have well-developed sweat glands and are predisposed to hyperthermia when ambient temperatures are high.[29]

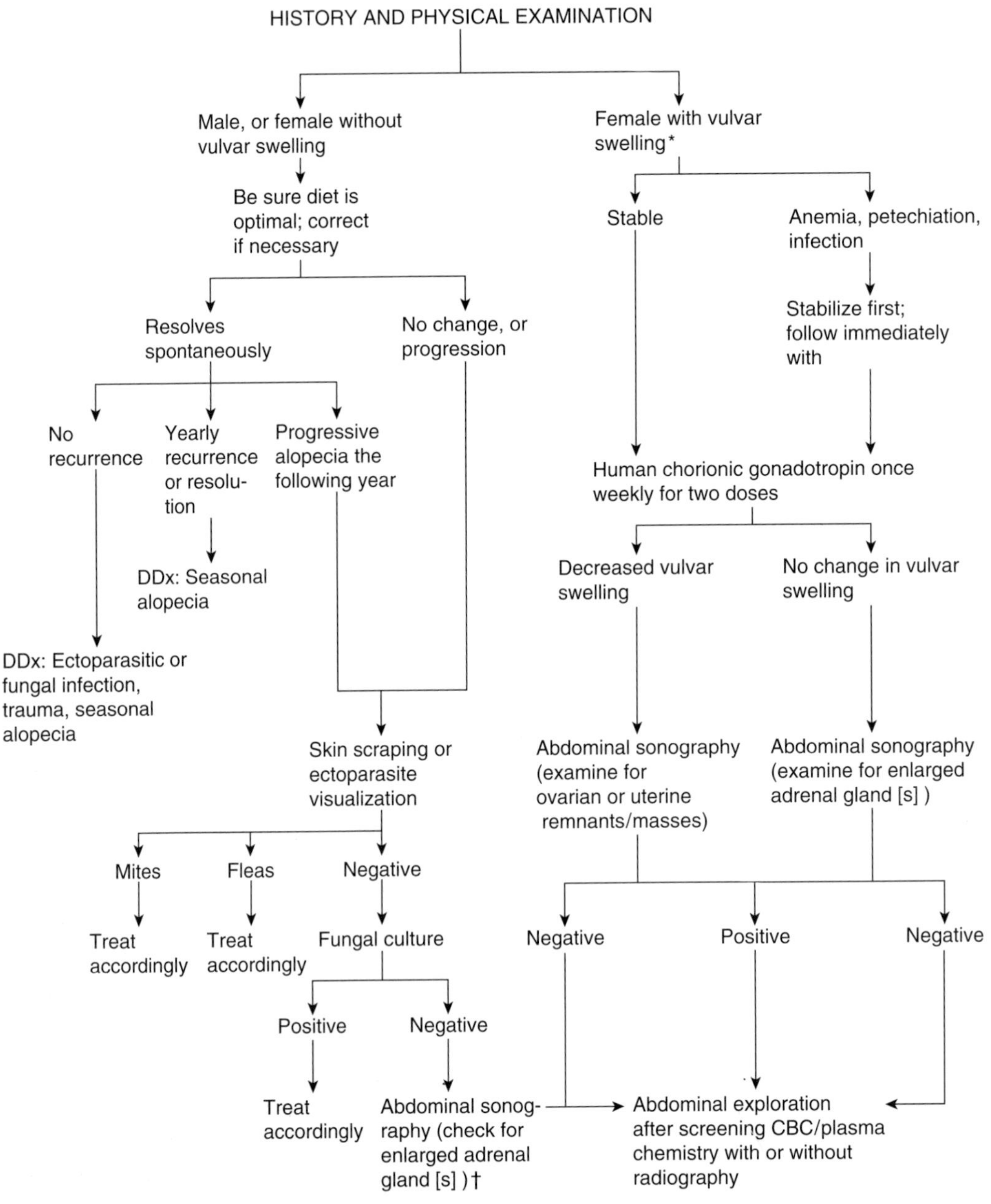

FIGURE 11–1
Clinical approach to hair loss and alopecia in a ferret. Abbreviations: DDx = differential diagnosis; CBC = complete blood count; * = see Chapters 5 and 9; † = see Chapter 9.

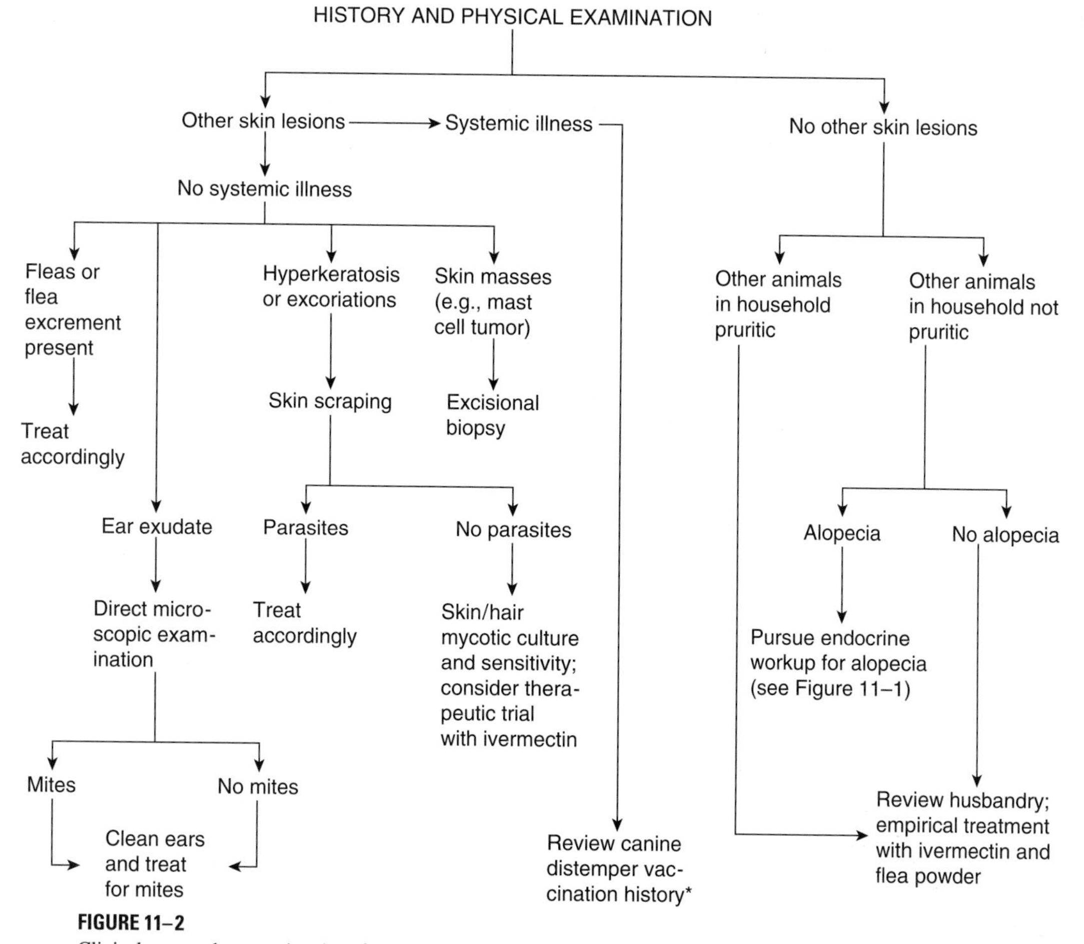

FIGURE 11–2

Clinical approach to pruritus in a ferret. *Note: Ferrets with anemia secondary to flea infestation or with severe sarcoptic mange may also show pruritus and systemic illness.

Paired musk-producing glands lateral to the anus store secretions that are released when ferrets are frightened, excited, or in estrus. It is uncommon for these glands to become impacted in ferrets, but if they do the treatment is the same as that for cats. Removal of the anal glands does not eliminate all scent because most of a ferret's body odor emanates from the dermal sebaceous glands.[4, 5] However, neutering does remove much of the skin odor because it reduces androgenic stimulation. Some clinicians do not recommend removal of the anal glands unless there is a specific problem.[4]

Ferrets generally have a thick, coarse haircoat, but a physiologic thinning of the coat ("pelt cycling") occurs in warm months.[30] A bilaterally symmetric alopecia of the tail, perineum, and inguinal area often occurs during the breeding season—generally, from March through August for females and from December through July for males.[5, 7] This seasonal alopecia is often more pronounced in females. The true cause of this process is unknown, but because even neutered animals experience thinning of the haircoat with an increase in the number of daylight hours and with warm temperatures,[5] it may be a result of the pineal and adrenal glands' response to changes in the photoperiod.[3] Usually, no obvious color change in the haircoat occurs between winter and summer, but reddish-brown, waxy deposits (possibly sebaceous secretions) or dark spots may be apparent on the skin during the period of hair thinning. Both sexes accumulate subcutaneous fat in winter, which is lost at the end of the breeding season.

If dietary requirements are not met, the haircoat can become dry and dull. Providing ferrets with a

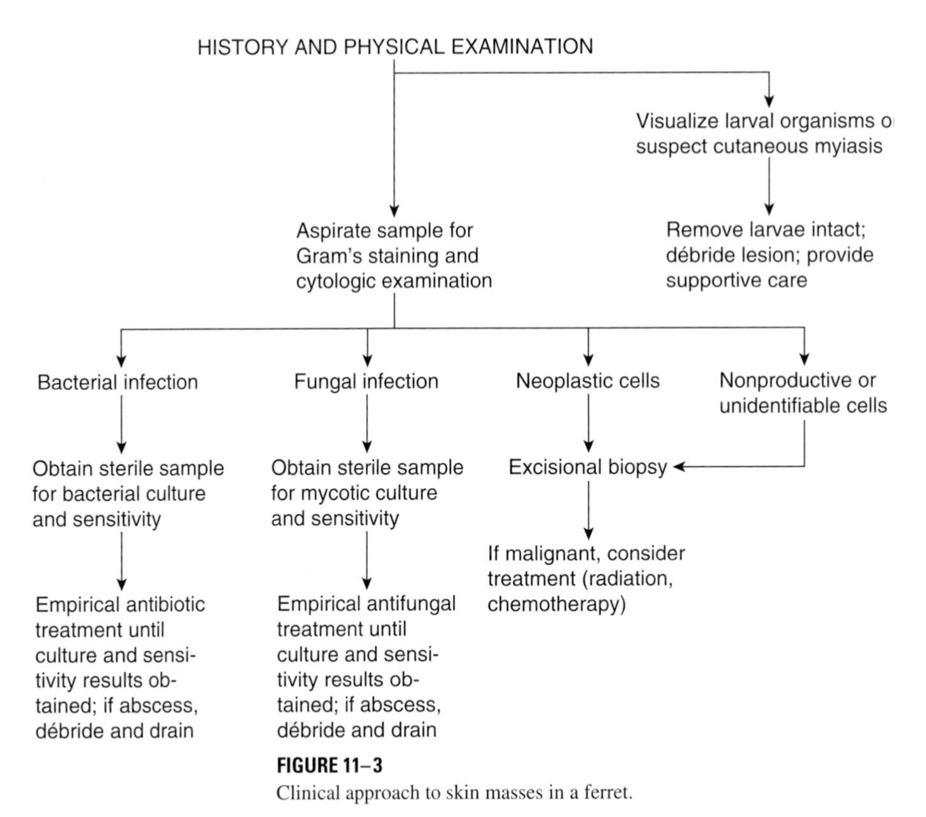

FIGURE 11–3
Clinical approach to skin masses in a ferret.

better diet, with or without short-term administration of a fat supplement, usually corrects this problem. Ferrets should be fed high-quality kitten, cat, or ferret foods (see Chapter 1).

With the exception of biotin deficiency, nutritional deficiencies are usually not a cause of alopecia.[3] Avidin, an enzyme found in raw egg white, binds biotin and has been reported to cause bilaterally symmetric alopecia in ferrets fed diets containing greater than 10% raw eggs.[7, 29]

Some skin and hair problems seen in ferrets are due to self-mutilation. Ferrets need privacy and should be provided with den boxes or artificial burrows. Facial abrasions in a ferret that has inadequate bedding, nesting, or hiding spots may be caused by rubbing of the face on the floor in an attempt to hide. Broken hair shafts can resemble those seen with dermatomycoses.[5] Intact females may pull hair from themselves to use as bedding material.[16] Ferrets can be quite rough during mating and playing and can inflict scratches and bite wounds.

Many ferrets come from large breeding farms where animals are tattooed at an early age after neutering. The tattoo is usually inside the pinna and appears as one or two gray or blue dots on the skin. On occasion, these dots have been mistaken for skin lesions.

DISEASES

In my experience, the most common dermatologic diseases in pet ferrets are hyperadrenocorticism, benign neoplasia, and ear mite infestation. Malignant skin neoplasms, fungal disease, viral disease, and sarcoptic mange are uncommon. Treatment protocols for dermatologic disease, including medication selection and dosing, are often extrapolated from those used for cats.

Ectoparasites

Ferrets are susceptible to most of the ectoparasites that affect dogs and cats.[29] However, other than fleas and ear mites, ectoparasites are rarely seen.

Fleas

Flea infestation is not uncommon in ferrets. *Ctenocephalides* species are involved as with dogs and cats.[15] Transmission is via direct contact with another animal or a flea-infested environment. Although some ferrets may be asymptomatic, clinical signs generally include mild to intense pruritus, especially on the dorsum near the nape of the neck.[7, 15, 33] With heavy infestations, alopecia may be appreciated on the dorsal thoracic and cervical areas. Identification of fleas or flea excrement confirms the diagnosis.

Treat the ferret as well as other animals in the household; concurrent treatment of the environment is also necessary. Treatment of the environment is the same as that used in the household with dogs and cats. On ferrets, use compounds that are approved for use in cats—for example, rotenone or pyrethrin powders or sprays. Dichlorvos-impregnated flea collars are not recommended because they can have toxic effects.[15] In fact, all organophosphates must be used with extreme caution because safe levels of these compounds have not been established for ferrets.[30] Lufenuron (Program, Ciba Animal Health, Greensboro, NC) may be effective for flea control in ferrets when given at dosages used in cats (scaled down for lower body weight).

Owing to the ferret's small body size, use caution when applying any topical medication. Ferrets can ingest sprays and powders while grooming. Be extremely cautious when using dips for small animals; some dips can be toxic with prolonged exposure, and ferrets need to be dried and kept moderately warm after dips.[33] When using sprays, first spray a cloth, and then rub the cloth on the ferret.

Mites

EAR MITES. Ear mites *(Otodectes cynotis)* are common in pet ferrets and also affect dogs and cats.[15] Transmission is via direct contact with other infested animals. Ferrets may shake their heads or scratch their ears; more commonly, they are asymptomatic. Other clinical signs vary from inflammation of the external ear canal with accompanying mild pruritus to severe pruritus with excoriations and crusting. A brown waxy aural exudate is often present; however, this also can be seen in some normal ferrets. Identification of the mite is confirmed on microscopic examination of the aural exudate. Although ear mites can reportedly colonize other parts of the body, specifically the perineum,[5] I have not seen this.

It has been reported that secondary otitis media with neurologic deficits is a common sequela to these infections[5]; however, this is not seen commonly in practice. I have seen one ferret with a head tilt that may have been the result of overzealous ear cleaning with subsequent damage to the tympanic membrane and middle ear. Clinical signs resolved completely within several months.

Treat all susceptible animals in the household to eliminate the problem. Gently clean the animals' ears before any treatment. The injection of ivermectin at a dose of 0.2–0.4 mg/kg subcutaneously once and repeated dosing every 2 weeks thereafter for three to four doses has proved successful.

A number of other treatments have been suggested for ferrets. Some clinicians treat a ferret's whole body with flea powder.[15] Topical treatments include massaging ivermectin into each ear at a dose of 0.5 mg/kg divided.[4, 28] A topical combination of thiabendazole, dexamethasone, and neomycin (Tresaderm, Merck Agvet Division, Rahway, NJ) also can be used.[15] However, topical treatments used alone can fail in ferrets for several reasons: the ear canal may be too narrow for the medications to penetrate, the ferret may resist treatment, or mites may be present on other areas of the body left untreated.[15] Do not use topical and parenteral ivermectin treatments concurrently because of the potential for toxicity.

SARCOPTIC MANGE. Infestation with *Sarcoptes scabiei,* which also affects dogs and cats, is not often seen in ferrets. Transmission of this zoonotic disease is by direct contact with the mite or by contact with fomites. Identification is usually made with a skin scraping; however, false-negative results are possible.

Two different clinical syndromes can be seen in ferrets with sarcoptic mange. In the generalized form, clinical signs include focal to generalized alopecia with intense pruritus.[2, 15, 28] The localized form of the disease, in which only the feet are affected, occasionally is seen. The paws become inflamed, swollen, and crusted and can be very pruritic. In severe cases, the nails may become deformed or even slough; if left untreated, the entire foot can be lost.[7] The layman's term for this form of the disease is *foot rot.*[15]

Treat affected ferrets with ivermectin at an initial dose of 0.2–0.4 mg/kg subcutaneously; repeat dosing every 7–14 days until the mites are gone. Ivermectin is the most reliable and rapidly effective agent. Alternatively, weekly dips in lime sulfur diluted to 1:40 for 6 weeks are very safe for animals of any age. Disadvantages of lime sulfur dips are discoloration of fur and the strong accompanying odor. In the past, weekly carbaryl (0.5%) shampoos[15, 22, 33] or organophosphate dips[30] were the recommended treatment; however, ivermectin is more effective and simpler to administer. It also is safer to use than organophosphates. Use topical or systemic antibiotics for secondary bacterial infections. Treat affected feet with warm water soaks and gentle débridement of crusts. Trim back diseased claws.

Treat all affected animals as well as those in contact with the ferrets, and thoroughly clean cages, bedding, and other materials the ferrets have touched.

Ticks

Ticks can be found on ferrets that are housed outdoors and reportedly are common in ferrets used for hunting (e.g., those in Great Britain).[5, 15] Remove ticks from ferrets as from other domestic animals by extracting the entire head from the skin. Use caution because ticks can carry zoonotic diseases. Wear gloves and use forceps. No cases of Lyme disease have been reported in ferrets.

Cutaneous Myiasis

Cuterebra species can be a cause of subdermal cysts in mustelids and have been uncommonly seen in ferrets.[15] In affected ferrets, the dipterid fly larvae generally are found in the subcutis of the neck; the moving larvae often can be seen through the open pore of the swollen area. Remove the larvae intact, if possible, in order to avoid leaving a nidus of infection or precipitating a systemic response. Débride the wound and use topical preparations with or without systemic antibiotics for the prevention or treatment of secondary bacterial infections. Allow the wound to heal by second intention.

Granulomatous masses in the cervical area caused by larval stages of *Hypoderma bovis* have been reported in ferrets but are not common.[15]

"Fly strike," or infestation by the flesh fly *(Wohlfahrtia vigil),* has been reported as a problem by commercial mink and ferret ranchers or by owners who keep ferrets outside. Mink kits are attacked during the summer months when 4–5 weeks old.[15] Eggs laid on the face, neck, or flanks of the kits bore into the skin and cause irritation. Larvae localized in subcutaneous tissues can produce abscess-like lesions. Remove the larvae, débride the wound, and provide supportive care for possible sepsis or shock, which can occur with any maggot infestation.

Viral Disease

Viral disease is a rare cause of dermatopathy in ferrets. Canine distemper virus (CDV) is the important exception. The skin lesions that are peculiar to the clinical syndrome seen with CDV in ferrets are described here. Other manifestations of the disease are more fully described in Chapter 8.

Paramyxovirus is the causative agent of canine distemper in dogs and in ferrets. Transmission of CDV occurs via direct contact, aerosol exposure, or contact with fomites. The virus begins to replicate in the skin and other organs about 1 week after infection. By 7–10 days after exposure to CDV, the ferret becomes anorexic and febrile and develops a mucopurulent ocular and nasal discharge. A characteristic erythematous skin rash develops under the chin, in the inguinal area, or in the perianal region within 10–15 days of exposure. A generalized orange-tinged dermatitis is sometimes appreciated. A secondary pyoderma may be present, and pruritus may be part of the syndrome.[2, 3, 17] Brown crusts develop around the face, and the chin, lips, and eyelids can swell.[3, 28] A characteristic clinical sign is swelling and hyperkeratosis of the footpads.[8] Rectal prolapse has also been described in conjunction with CDV.[3]

Definitive diagnosis of CDV is difficult ante mortem, although a presumptive diagnosis can be made on the basis of observation of distinctive clinical signs. Tests that use fluorescent antibodies against viral antigen can be performed on blood smears or conjunctival scrapings by the ninth day of the infection. Serum antibody titers can also be determined. The titer should not be high in an unvaccinated animal because natural immunity to this disease is not seen in ferrets.[8] Histopathologic examination reveals widespread eosinophilic cytoplasmic and intranuclear viral inclusions. These inclusions are present but fewer in skin epithelium and hair follicles.

CDV is a uniformly fatal infection in ferrets; death can occur from 12 to 22 days after exposure, with most ferrets dying by 1 week after the onset of clinical signs.[2, 8, 17] Owing to the untreatable and highly infectious nature of this disease, any ferret with a poor vaccination history or suspicious clinical signs should be isolated from other animals.

Fungal Disease

Dermatophytosis

Fungal disease involving the skin is uncommon in ferrets in my experience. Although superficial mycotic skin infection (ringworm) in ferrets is seen frequently by some clinicians,[5] others have not noted it to be a common problem.[2, 7] Perhaps this is because of the geographic variation in incidence, which depends on climate. Ferrets are susceptible to both *Microsporum canis* and *Trichophyton mentagrophytes*,[22] although the former is more often described.[2, 7, 29] *M. canis* can be transmitted by direct contact or via fomites and is reportedly associated with overcrowding and exposure to cats.[22] Dermatophytosis is a zoonotic disease.[14, 22] It is more common in kits and young ferrets, in which it can occur as a seasonal and self-limiting infection.[2, 7, 14, 29]

Superficial mycotic organisms have an affinity for cornified epidermis—that is, hair, horn, and nails. Skin and hair lesions are similar to those reported in other species.[5, 7] Dermatologic lesions can begin with small papules that spread peripherally.[14] These can lead to large circumscribed and sometimes circular areas of alopecia and inflammation that involve all parts of the body. The skin becomes thickened, erythematous, and hyperkeratotic with superficial crusts. Broken hair shafts may be appreciated. Accompanying pruritus leads to excoriation and, sometimes, secondary pyoderma.

Although clinical signs may be suspicious (especially if other animals or people in the household have skin lesions), definitive diagnosis of dermatophytosis is made on the basis of a mycotic culture from a skin and hair scraping. Fungal organisms can sometimes be appreciated on biopsy. *M. canis* in cats exhibits yellow-green fluorescence under Wood's ultraviolet lamp in fewer than 50% of cases, but *Trichophyton* species do not fluoresce.[5, 14] Although some clinicians describe microscopic visualization of fungal arthrospores in skin and hair scrapings that have been mixed with 10% potassium hydroxide,[14] others have not found this method useful.[5]

Shave off the hair around the lesions. Topical treatments include keratolytic shampoos, povidone-iodine scrubs, and antifungal medications. Griseofulvin, although rarely needed,[5] has been used at a dosage of 25 mg/kg orally q24h for 21–30 days.[7] Side effects with the use of griseofulvin in ferrets have not been reported, but idiosyncratic reactions have been implicated as a cause of leukopenia (neutropenia), anemia, lethargy, anorexia, ataxia, or depression in cats.[1] Gastrointestinal upsets and teratogenicity are reported side effects in dogs. Griseofulvin is not used in breeding dogs or cats and should not be used in breeding ferrets. As with cats, monitor the complete blood count every 2 weeks while the ferret is receiving treatment. Do not use corticosteroids in the treatment of fungal disease. Many authors report spontaneous remission of clinical signs of dermatophytosis in ferrets.[7, 14, 22]

Disinfect the entire environment to which the ferret was exposed to eliminate infectious spores, which remain contagious for up to 2 years. Methods of decontaminating the environment include application of dilute (1:10) bleach or chlorhexidine, steam cleaning of carpets, changing air conditioning filters, cleaning heating ducts, and vacuuming with prompt disposal of vacuum bags. Treat all animals in the household.

Other Fungal Infections

Systemic mycoses with skin manifestations have been infrequently reported in ferrets but should be included on a list of differential diagnoses for persistent draining tracts and skin eruptions that are not responsive to antibiotic therapy, especially if other systemic signs are evident (e.g., pneumonia, weight loss, or gastrointestinal signs).[28] *Blastomyces dermatitidis* was reported in a ferret with pneumonia and an ulcerated lesion in the metacarpal pad with a persistent draining tract.[20] Treatment included oral ketoconazole and intravenous amphotericin B. Infection with *Coccidioides* species was described in a ferret with pyrexia, pneumonia, and a persistent draining tract in the stifle that was nonresponsive to antibiotic therapy.[10] Treatment involved the use of oral ketoconazole. Mucormycosis, or infection with *Absidia corymbifera*, has been reported in ferrets raised for their fur in New Zealand.[14]

Bacterial Disease

Ferrets can incur bite wounds while playing, mating, or fighting and can sustain puncture wounds from chewing on objects. These can become infected and result in superficial or deep pyoderma, abscesses, or cellulitis. Causative organisms that have been reported most often include *Staphylococcus* and *Streptococcus* species[2, 7, 29]; others include

Corynebacterium, Pasteurella, and *Actinomyces* species as well as hemolytic *Escherichia coli.*[13] Abscesses usually wall themselves off, causing few systemic signs.[13]

A tentative diagnosis may be reached with Gram's staining of the discharge aspirated from an affected area. Definitive diagnosis is determined with bacterial culture and sensitivity testing of the exudate or infected tissue. Using sterile technique, lance, excise or débride, and flush abscesses. Place drains in the wound or stent bandages over the wound for wet-to-dry changes, if warranted. Start the ferret on a broad-spectrum systemic antibiotic (e.g., a cephalosporin) while awaiting culture results.

Actinomycosis, or "lumpy jaw," has been rarely reported in ferrets.[13] *Actinomyces* species are gram-positive, anaerobic to microaerophilic bacteria. Wounds to the oral mucosa or swallowing or inhaling the organism provide the portal of entry. Clinical signs include cervical masses with sinus tracts containing thick, yellowish-green, purulent material. Reportedly, masses occasionally become large enough to cause dyspnea. Similar clinical signs have been seen with mixed gram-negative bacterial populations isolated from submandibular abscesses.[2] A subcutaneous *Actinomyces*-related granuloma was reported in a ferret with lymphoma.[11] Actinomycosis is a common opportunistic infection associated with human and feline immunodeficiency virus and feline leukemia virus infections. Surgically débride and drain lesions, as with any abscessed area. Rely on specific bacterial culture and sensitivity test results for antimicrobial therapy. Empirical treatments that have been suggested for actinomycosis include the administration of high doses of penicillin or tetracycline.[13]

Neoplasia

Cutaneous neoplasms are the third most commonly reported form of neoplasia in ferrets[18, 25] (see Chapter 10 for results of a neoplasia survey conducted at Midwest Bird and Exotic Animal Hospital in Westchester, IL from 1990 to 1994). Although it has been reported that tumors of the skin and subcutaneous tissues in ferrets are most often malignant,[5] the majority of ferret skin tumors biopsied at The Animal Medical Center in New York and Angell Memorial Animal Hospital in Boston are benign. Perform an excisional biopsy when a mass is detected.

Sebaceous Epitheliomas

A study of 57 cutaneous neoplasms biopsied from ferrets from 1987 to 1992 reported a 58% incidence of basal cell tumors.[25] These tumors were composed of well-differentiated basaloid epithelial cells with varying degrees of sebaceous and squamous differentiation. These were benign tumors similar to those previously reported as basisquamosebaceous tumors[32] and as carcinomas containing basisquamous and sebaceous areas.[6, 7, 31] After reviewing the conclusions in this study and using established dermatopathologic criteria,[27, 34] I feel that these tumors may be better described as sebaceous epitheliomas rather than as simple basal cell tumors.

The previously mentioned study reported no specific site predilection for these tumors but indicated they were most commonly seen on the head, neck, shoulders, and feet.[25] The average age of an animal at detection was 5.2 years, and 70% of affected ferrets were females. The tumors were pedunculated or plaquelike in appearance. One ferret in the study had recurrence of a tumor excised from the tail, but no other recurrences or metastases were reported.

Sebaceous epitheliomas may be fast-growing and can become ulcerated.[9] Sebaceous adenomas, a subcategory, are commonly biopsied from ferrets at The Animal Medical Center. These tumors can be wartlike, ulcerated, or cystic.

Mast Cell Tumors

Mast cell tumors generally involve the skin and are benign in ferrets, being composed predominantly of well-differentiated mast cells and resembling cutaneous mastocytomas of domestic cats.[25, 29] Visceral involvement and malignant behavior of mast cell tumors are rare in ferrets (see Chapter 10).

In one study, cutaneous mast cell tumors represented 16% of all cutaneous neoplasms of ferrets submitted within a 5-year period.[25] The average age of detection was 4 years, and no sex predilection was noted. Although no site predilection was reported for these tumors, in practice they are most commonly observed over the neck, shoulders, and trunk. Mast cell tumors usually present as single or multiple raised, well-circumscribed, hairless nodules that can vary in size from 2 mm to 1 cm.[2, 9, 32] They are usually unpigmented but may be hyperemic (Fig. 11–4). Most of these tumors are intact, but they can become ulcerated with a black, crusty exudate.[12, 26, 28] In fact, some affected ferrets are

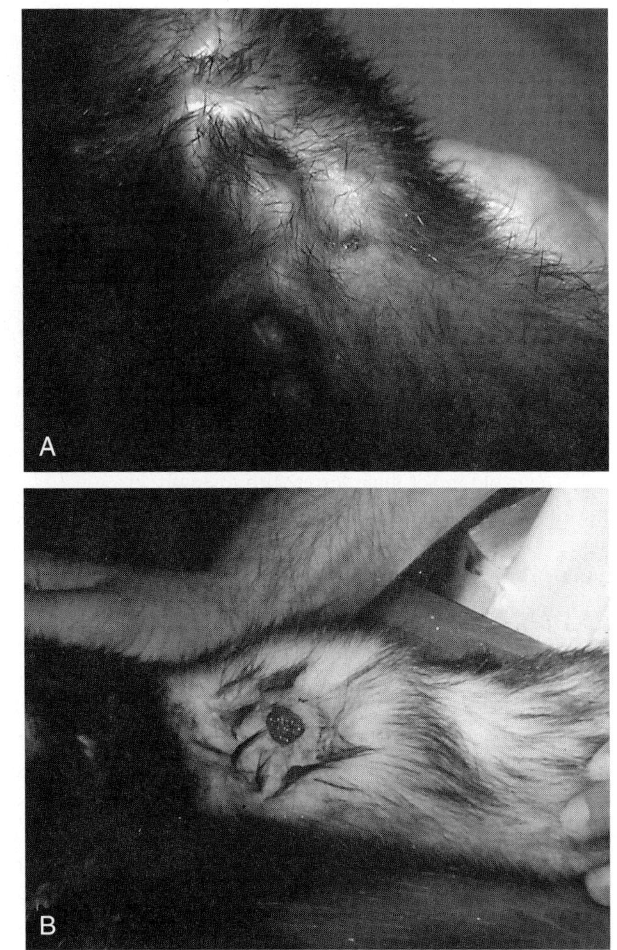

FIGURE 11–4
A and B, Mast cell tumors on two ferrets. The smaller one *(A)* is more typical of the gross appearance of these tumors.

presented because their owners notice the crumbly black exudate even though the tumor underneath is still very small and barely raised from the surface of the skin. Because they are sometimes associated with pruritus, the ulceration may be due to self-excoriation.

Surgical biopsy provides the definitive diagnosis, but analysis of an aspirate of the mass may reveal mature mast cells. Surgical resection is generally curative.[25, 28] One author has described spontaneous resolution and recurrence of lesions over a period of time.[2]

Squamous Cell Carcinoma

In the past, squamous cell carcinoma was reported to be the most common cutaneous tumor in ferrets.[18] However, tumors of this type are now uncommon in pet ferrets, and none were reported in a more recent study.[25]

Squamous cell carcinoma has been reported at a number of anatomic sites, including the cranium, lip, digit, tarsus, and footpads, and both discrete and metastatic forms have been reported in ferrets.[2, 7, 19, 24] These tumors tend to be firm and ulcerated. Vascular invasion is seen on biopsy, with subsequent metastasis to regional lymph nodes. I have seen a 5-year-old female, neutered ferret with a large, thickened, erythematous, ulcerated, nonresectable perianal squamous cell carcinoma. The ferret had a second mass in the right inguinal area with enlargement of the right inguinal lymph node.

Surgically excise masses whenever possible. Reports of resection with no recurrence of neoplasia after surgery have been published,[24, 31, 32, 35] but it is unclear how long some of the ferrets were followed. In other cases, tumors have recurred very quickly after excision.[19] Melphalan and bleomycin have been used unsuccessfully in the treatment of two ferrets with squamous cell carcinoma.[19, 24]

Adenocarcinoma

Several cases of adenocarcinoma involving adnexal structures of the skin have been reported in ferrets; however, this form of neoplasia is rare.[2, 25] Sebaceous and sweat gland adenocarcinomas have been diagnosed in geriatric, captive black-footed ferrets *(Mustela nigripes)*.[2] One report described a well-differentiated adenocarcinoma of sweat gland or preputial gland origin in a domestic ferret that presented with an acute, fluctuant swelling of the prepuce originally confined to the subcutis.[23] This tumor recurred fairly rapidly after each of multiple excisions as well as following radiation therapy, and metastasis to the inguinal area occurred. I have seen a 2.5-year-old intact male ferret with a slowly growing, broad-based, elevated skin mass on the lateral aspect of the tail. Excisional biopsy with partial tail amputation revealed a sweat gland adenocarcinoma with local infiltration. Within 2 months, the tumor had metastasized to the deep tissues of the right thigh and perianal area (Fig. 11–5), and a sublumbar mass (possible lymph node enlargement secondary to metastasis) was seen on radiographs. Two months later, the ferret died suddenly of unknown cause.

Two adenocarcinomas of apocrine gland origin have been reported.[25] One presented as an infiltrative cutaneous and subcutaneous mass over the anal gland of a 7-year-old castrated male ferret. This tumor was excised, and no recurrence or metastasis was reported. The second was a 2-cm mass surrounding the preputial orifice of a 6-year-old intact male ferret. The tumor was inoperable, and the ferret was euthanized. Adenocarcinomas of perianal gland origin have been reported.[18] A perineal adenocarcinoma with metastasis to an internal iliac lymph node has been described in a black-footed ferret.[25]

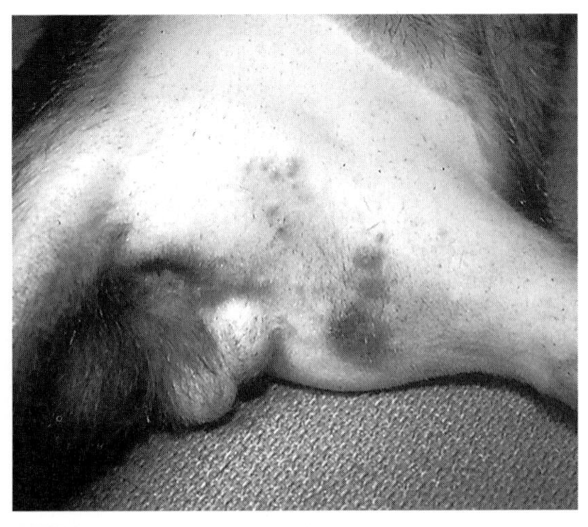

FIGURE 11–5
Sebaceous gland adenocarcinoma. This tumor recurred after resection and spread rapidly.

Other Neoplasms Involving the Skin or Subcutis

Malignant lymphoma rarely involves the skin or subcutis in ferrets. Cutaneous lymphoma was not observed in 19 ferrets with lymphoma[11] but has been reported to occur on the dorsum of a 5-year-old neutered male.[21] Lymphoma involving the prepuce was reported in a 6-year-old intact male ferret.[25] The tumor presented as a 2-cm ulcerated mass on the prepuce; the inguinal lymph node also was involved.

Hemangiomas have been reported in two middle-aged female ferrets.[25] One presented as a small black mass in the dorsal lumbar area, and the other as a small mass on the pinna. Both were well-circumscribed dermal masses, and no recurrence or metastasis of the masses was reported after resection (see also Chapter 10).

Six fibromas and two fibrosarcomas were described among 57 cutaneous neoplasms.[25] There was no site predilection, and the affected ferrets ranged in age from 10 months to 4.5 years. Both tumor types were identified as well-circumscribed dermal or subcutaneous masses on histopathologic examination. Neither recurrence nor metastasis of either type was reported in cases in which postoperative information was available.

Other reported cutaneous or subcutaneous tumors in ferrets include hemangiosarcoma,[25] rhabdomyosarcoma,[25] neurofibroma,[18, 25] neurofibrosarcoma,[18] histiocytoma,[9, 18] myxosarcoma of the subcutis,[18] myelosarcoma,[18] leiomyosarcoma,[28] and papillary cystadenoma.[9]

Endocrine Disease

Endocrine disease, primarily hyperadrenocorticism, is a very common cause of dermatopathy in ferrets. Hyperadrenocorticism is the most common cause of progressive and sustained alopecia, often with pruritus, in neutered ferrets. Other reported causes of alopecia in both intact and neutered ferrets include granulosa cell tumors, luteomas, and fibrosarcomas of an ovarian remnant.[3] Hyperestrogenism can be associated with alopecia in female ferrets during estrus.[3, 5] No cases of hypothyroidism in ferrets have been documented.

See Chapters 5 and 9 for discussions of hyperestrogenism and adrenal disease.

REFERENCES

1. Aronson AL, Aucoin DP: Antimicrobial drugs. *In* Ettinger SJ, ed.: Textbook of Veterinary Internal Medicine. 3rd ed. Vol. 1. Philadelphia, WB Saunders, 1989, p 402.
2. Besch-Williford CL: Biology and medicine of the ferret. Vet Clin North Am Small Anim Pract 1987; 17:1155–1183.
3. Brown SA: Commonly encountered non-neoplastic disorders of the domestic ferret. Proceedings of the Atlantic Coast Veterinary Conference, Atlantic City, NJ, October 1993.
4. Brown SA: Preventative health program for the domestic ferret. J Small Exotic Anim Med 1991; 1:6–11.
5. Burke TJ: Skin disorders of rodents, rabbits, and ferrets. *In* Kirk RW, Bonagura JD, eds: Kirk's Current Veterinary Therapy 11: Small Animal Practice. Philadelphia, WB Saunders, 1992, pp 1170–1175.
6. Chesterman FC, Pomerance A: Spontaneous neoplasms in ferrets and polecats. J Pathol Bacteriol 1965; 89: 529–533.
7. Collins BR: Dermatologic disorders of common small nondomestic animals. *In* Nesbitt GH, ed.: Topics in Small Animal Medicine: Dermatology. New York, Churchill Livingstone, 1987, pp 272–276.
8. Davidson M: Canine distemper virus infection in the domestic ferret. Compend Contin Educ Pract Vet 1986; 8:448–453.
9. Dillberger JE, Altman NH: Neoplasia in ferrets: eleven cases with a review. J Comp Pathol 1989; 100:161–176.
10. Duval-Hudelson KA: Coccidioidomycosis in three European ferrets. J Zoo Wildl Med 1990; 21:353–357.
11. Erdman SE, Moore FM, Rose R, et al: Malignant lymphoma in ferrets: clinical and pathological findings in 19 cases. J Comp Pathol 1992; 106:37–47.
12. Erik S, Robinette J, Basaraba R, et al: Mast cell tumors in three ferrets. J Am Vet Med Assoc 1990; 196:766–767.
13. Fox JG: Bacterial and mycoplasmal diseases. *In* Fox JG, ed.: Biology and Diseases of the Ferret. Philadelphia, Lea & Febiger, 1988, pp 197–216.
14. Fox JG: Mycotic diseases. *In* Fox JG, ed.: Biology and Diseases of the Ferret. Philadelphia, Lea & Febiger, 1988, pp 248–254.
15. Fox JG: Parasitic diseases. *In* Fox JG, ed.: Biology and Diseases of the Ferret. Philadelphia, Lea & Febiger, 1988, pp 241–247.
16. Fox JG: Reproduction, breeding and growth. *In* Fox JG, ed.: Biology and Diseases of the Ferret. Philadelphia, Lea & Febiger, 1988, pp 177–183.
17. Fox JG, Pearson RC, Gorham JR: Viral and chlamydial diseases. *In* Fox JG, ed.: Biology and Diseases of the Ferret. Philadelphia, Lea & Febiger, 1988, pp 217–234.
18. Goad MEP, Fox JG: Neoplasia in ferrets. *In* Fox JG, ed.: Biology and Diseases of the Ferret. Philadelphia, Lea & Febiger, 1988, pp 274–288.
19. Hamilton TA, Morrison WB: Bleomycin chemotherapy for metastatic squamous cell carcinoma in a ferret. J Am Vet Med Assoc 1991; 198:107–108.
20. Lenhard A: Blastomycosis in a ferret. J Am Vet Med Assoc 1985; 186:70–72.
21. Li X, Fox JG, Erdman SE, Aspros DE: Cutaneous lymphoma in a ferret *(Mustela putorius furo)*. Vet Pathol 1995; 32:55–56.
22. Marini RP, Adkins JA, Fox JG: Proven or potential zoonotic diseases of ferrets. J Am Vet Med Assoc 1989; 195:990–994.
23. Miller TA, Denman DL, Lewis GC: Recurrent adenocarcinoma in a ferret. J Am Vet Med Assoc 1985; 187:839–841.
24. Olsen GH, Turk MAM, Foil CS: Disseminated cutaneous squamous cell carcinoma in a ferret. J Am Vet Med Assoc 1985; 186:702–703.
25. Parker GA, Picut CA: Histopathologic features and postsurgical sequelae of 57 cutaneous neoplasms in ferrets (*Mustela putorius furo* L.). Vet Pathol 1993; 30:499–504.
26. Poonacha KB, Hutto VL: Cutaneous mastocytoma in a ferret. J Am Vet Med Assoc 1984; 185:442.
27. Pulley LT, Stannard AA: Tumors of the skin and soft tissues. *In* Moulton JE, ed.: Tumors in Domestic Animals. 3rd ed. Berkeley, CA, University of California Press, 1990, pp 58–66.
28. Rosenthal K: Ferrets. Vet Clin North Am Small Anim Pract 1994; 24:1–23.
29. Ryland LM, Bernard SL: A clinical guide to the pet ferret. Compend Contin Educ Pract Vet 1983; 5:25–32.
30. Ryland LM, Gorham JR: The ferret and its diseases. J Am Vet Med Assoc 1978; 173:1154–1158.
31. Symmers WStC, Thomson APD: A spontaneous carcinoma of the skin of a ferret (*Mustela furo* L.). J Pathol Bacteriol 1950; 62:229–233.
32. Symmers WStC, Thomson APD: Multiple carcinomata and focal mast-cell accumulations in the skin of a ferret (*Mustela furo* L.), with a note on other tumours in ferrets. J Pathol Bacteriol 1953; 65:481–493.
33. Timm KI: Pruritus in rabbits, rodents and ferrets. Vet Clin North Am Small Anim Pract 1988; 18:1077–1091.
34. Walder EJ, Gross TL: Sebaceous tumors. *In* Gross TL, Ihrke PJ, Walder EJ, eds.: Veterinary Dermatopathology. St. Louis, Mosby-Year Book, 1992, pp 374–385.
35. Zwicker GM, Carlton WW: Spontaneous squamous cell carcinoma in a ferret. J Wildl Dis 1974; 10:213–216.

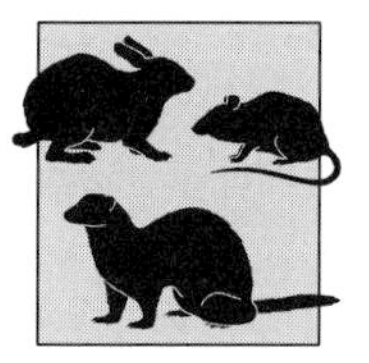

CHAPTER 12

Musculoskeletal and Neurologic Diseases

Natalie Antinoff, DVM

Primary neurologic and musculoskeletal disorders are not common in pet ferrets. Frequently, clinical signs that appear to be caused by primary neurologic disease, particularly posterior paresis, are instead manifestations of systemic illness. Therefore, a thorough and accurate history-taking and physical examination supported by radiography and laboratory testing are essential for establishing a diagnosis, treatment plan, and prognosis.

This chapter covers evaluation and treatment of ferrets showing neurologic signs, and the clinical approach to common neurologic and musculoskeletal disorders. Fracture management is covered in Chapter 30.

POSTERIOR PARESIS, ATAXIA, AND SEIZURES

Ferrets with neurologic disease or with other systemic disease may present with posterior paresis or ataxia, or both. *Posterior paresis* as used here is synonymous with rear leg weakness. Generalized weakness in ferrets is often more pronounced in the rear legs and may be mistakenly attributed to primary neurologic disease. A ferret that is weak loses the normal upward arch in its back, so that the long axis of its body becomes parallel to the ground when it is standing or walking.

The most common cause of posterior paresis or ataxia is hypoglycemia secondary to a pancreatic beta cell tumor, or insulinoma (see Chapter 9). Hypoglycemia can also result from food deprivation or anorexia, sepsis, neoplasia, severe hepatic disease, and other metabolic disorders.

Cardiac disease, hypoxia, anemia, and toxin ingestion can result in weakness, ataxia, or central nervous system (CNS) depression.[3, 28] Proliferative bowel disease can be associated with ataxia.[10] Discomfort caused by splenomegaly, caudal abdominal masses, cystic calculi, peritonitis, or urinary obstruction may mimic ataxia or posterior paresis when severe.

Primary neurologic problems reported as causing posterior paresis or ataxia in ferrets include intervertebral disc disease,[14] and plasma cell myeloma[23] and chordoma[31] involving the spinal column. Infection with Aleutian disease virus has been associated with posterior paresis, urinary incontinence, and tremors (see Chapter 7). Always also consider potential differential diagnoses for posterior paresis and ataxia in other species, such as thromboembolism and CNS trauma, infection, and other neoplasms. Spinal cord lymphoma is rare but can be associated with pathologic vertebral fracture (Fig. 12–1). Urine and fecal incontinence may accompany posterior paresis.

Seizures are not common in ferrets. Probably the most common cause is hypoglycemia secondary to insulinoma. Prolonged seizure activity can also result in hypoglycemia. Other potential causes of seizures include toxin ingestion; CNS infection, inflammation, trauma, or neoplasia; and metabolic disturbances such as hepatic or renal failure. Idiopathic epilepsy has not been reported in ferrets.

Diagnosis

Check the blood glucose concentration immediately in any animal presenting with seizures or ataxia. If the glucose level is below 60 mg/dL, give a slow intravenous bolus of 50% dextrose solution at a dose of 1–2 mL/kg, titrating to effect,[20] and begin a dextrose drip infusion adequate to maintain normoglycemia while further diagnostic testing is performed.

Record the medical history and perform a complete physical examination, auscultating carefully for cardiac murmurs or arrhythmias. Ferrets may normally have a respiratory sinus arrhythmia. Palpate for peripheral pulses to evaluate the strength of cardiac contraction and to determine presence of dropped or extra beats. Check mucous membranes for evidence of cyanosis. Palpate the abdomen carefully to check for discomfort, an abdominal mass, urinary calculi, or a distended urinary bladder.

Perform a complete neurologic and orthopedic examination if you suspect primary neurologic disease.[24] Characterize the signs as diffuse or focal, acute or chronic, progressive or static; localize the lesion to areas of brain or spinal cord.[21] Evaluate reflexes and palpate for spinal cord pain or hyperesthesia.

Evaluate a complete blood count and serum chemistry and electrolyte values in any ferret with neurologic signs to assess any metabolic or infectious component. Correct any underlying abnormalities and reassess the animal for changes in neurologic status. Perform whole-body radiography and, if you suspect cardiac disease, perform echocardiography.

If indicated, perform spinal radiography to look for possible fractures or bone abnormalities, such as proliferative or lytic lesions. Myelography may be useful for localizing lesions of the spinal cord and determining a site for surgical approach, if needed (see Fig. 12–1). Perform cerebrospinal fluid analysis to gain additional information. Sites for cerebrospinal fluid tap and myelography are the atlanto-occipital and lumbar (L5-L6) regions. Use a 22- or

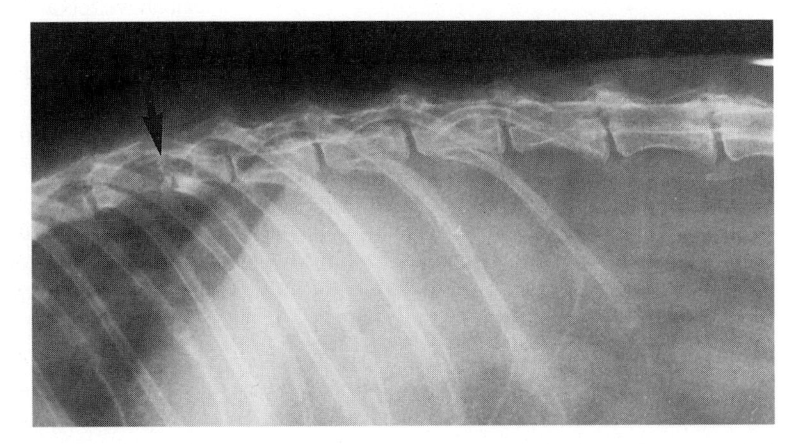

FIGURE 12–1

Lateral myelogram of a ferret showing thinning of the dye column at L1-L2 and a vertebral fracture with compression at T-11 *(arrow)*. This was a pathologic fracture associated with spinal cord lymphoma. The ferret had 14 thoracic vertebrae.

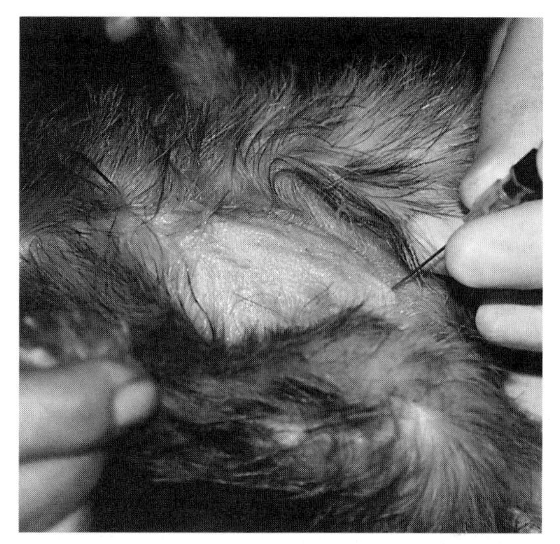

FIGURE 12–2
Lumbar cerebrospinal fluid tap in a ferret. The rear legs are extended forward in order to widen the intervertebral space.

20-gauge spinal needle as described for canine and feline myelography (Fig. 12–2); a suggested contrast medium is iohexol at 0.25–0.5 mL/kg.[30] Treatment with one IV dose of prednisolone sodium succinate, 30 mg/kg, may help in the prevention of seizures or further development of existing CNS edema.[4, 29] Some spinal lesions may be amenable to surgical resection or stabilization; many, however, carry a poor prognosis.

Treatment

Treatment of posterior paresis, ataxia, and seizures in ferrets is tailored to the diagnosis. Follow the standard treatment regimens used for dogs and cats when managing a similar condition in ferrets.

CANINE DISTEMPER

Canine distemper virus in the late stage affects the CNS of ferrets, although initial signs are usually localized to the respiratory and gastrointestinal tracts and to the skin.[12] Ferrets are highly susceptible to canine distemper virus and may seem to recover from the acute phase only to die later from the neurotropic form of the disease, presenting with salivation, muscle tremors, seizures, and coma.[12] The disease is nearly 100% fatal, and infected animals may be a source for infection of other ferrets.[12] See Chapter 8 for further discussion of canine distemper virus.

RABIES

Although reports of rabies in ferrets are rare, ferrets are susceptible to this disease. Clinical signs include anxiety, lethargy, and posterior paresis.[12] Suspect rabies in any unvaccinated ferret with clinical signs of neurologic disease and a history of exposure to rabid animals. A killed vaccine is approved for yearly use in ferrets (RM Imrab 3, Rhone Merieux, Inc., Athens, GA) but may not be considered protective if the vaccinated ferret bites a human. In most states, any ferret suspected of rabies and involved in a biting incident must be euthanized and tested appropriately. Be aware of local laws that may affect you or your clients, and educate ferret owners at the time of vaccination.

CHORDOMA AND CHONDROSARCOMA

Chordomas are tumors arising from remnants of notochord.[15] In ferrets, these tumors have been reported most commonly at the tip of the tail[1, 5, 6, 15, 17] but have also been described in the cervical region.[31] Ferrets with cervical chordoma have presented with posterior paresis and ataxia localizable to the area of the lesion.[31] Perform spinal radiography and myelography to identify a site for surgical approach. Depending on location, these tumors may be amenable to surgical resection; however, the only report of recurrence and metastasis of chordomas in ferrets was in a case of cervical chordoma that had been surgically removed.[31] Chordomas in the tail appear as lobulated, firm, nonencapsulated, ulcerated masses at or near the last caudal vertebra. Microscopically, these tumors are composed of lobules of physaliphorous cells with areas of well-differentiated bone or cartilage throughout.[6, 17, 31]

Chondrosarcoma of the tail has also been described in ferrets.[15, 16] Clinical and morphologic descriptions are nearly identical to those of chordoma. Differentiation must be made on the basis of immunohistochemical staining results, with positive uptake of low-molecular-weight cytokeratin occurring in chordoma but not in chondrosarcoma.[6, 17]

In ferrets with any distal tail mass, amputate several vertebrae proximal to the lesion. This is usually curative in cases of chordoma and chondrosarcoma. Recurrence has not been reported.

OSTEOMA

Osteomas of the skull arising from the zygomatic arch, parietal bone, and occipital bone have been reported in ferrets.[15, 18, 19, 27] Osteoma presents as a firm, dense, bony mass arising from one of the bones of the skull. Although benign, clinical signs are related to physical displacement or compression of normal structures.[18, 19, 25, 27] Obtain radiographs of any bony swelling to evaluate the extent of the lesion and the bone of origin. Biopsy may be difficult without surgical removal of the mass because of the extreme density of the tumor. The Jamshidi needle biopsy technique has been described.[26] Histopathologic evaluation generally reveals compact lamellar bone, bony trabeculae, and mild to moderate osteoblastic and hematologic activity.[18, 19, 27] Surgical removal is the treatment of choice and is usually curative if excision is complete.[19]

MISCELLANEOUS

Systemic mycoses, which may contribute to CNS depression and lethargy, have been reported in ferrets.[7, 8] *Cryptococcus* has been identified as a cause of meningitis in ferrets, including one who had died of congestive heart failure after being treated with steroids for intervertebral disc disease.[8] Blastomycosis has also been identified in ferrets, with multifocal granulomatous meningoencephalitis described in one ferret with systemic blastomycosis.[8, 22] Diagnose these diseases based on clinical signs, radiographic changes, and isolation of the organism. Impression smears of draining tracts or cerebrospinal fluid tap may be useful in identifying the organism.

A report of an eosinophilic granulomatous infiltrate in the choroid plexus of a ferret with diffuse eosinophilic gastroenteritis and multisystemic involvement has appeared in the literature.[11] Toxoplasmosis has been identified in ferrets, and it probably resulted from exposure to cat feces or raw meat.[2, 3, 9] Copper toxicosis has been reported and was believed to be congenital in two ferrets,[13] and iniencephaly in a litter of ferrets has also been described.[32] It is likely that other congenital anomalies exist, but they remain unreported at this time.

REFERENCES

1. Allison N, Rakich P: Chordoma in two ferrets. J Comp Pathol 1988; 98:371–374.
2. Bell JA: Parasites of domesticated pet ferrets. Compend Contin Educ Pract Vet 1994; 16:617–620.
3. Besch-Williford C: Biology and medicine of the ferret. Vet Clin North Am Small Anim Pract 1987; 17:1155–1183.
4. Dewey CW, Budsberg SC, Oliver JE: Principles of head trauma management in dogs and cats: part II. Compend Contin Educ Pract Vet 1993; 15:177–193.
5. Dillberger JE, Altman NH: Neoplasia in ferrets: eleven cases with a review. J Comp Pathol 1989; 100:161–176.
6. Dunn DG, Harris RK, Meis JM, Sweet DE: A histomorphologic and immunohistochemical study of chordoma in 20 ferrets. Vet Pathol 1991; 28:467–473.
7. DuVal-Hudelson KA: Coccidioidomycosis in three European ferrets. J Zoo Wildl Med 1990; 21:353–357.
8. Fox JG: Mycotic diseases. *In* Fox JG, ed.: Biology and Diseases of the Ferret. Philadelphia, Lea & Febiger, 1988, pp 248–254.
9. Fox JG: Parasitic diseases. *In* Fox JG, ed.: Biology and Diseases of the Ferret. Philadelphia, Lea & Febiger, 1988, pp 235–247.
10. Fox JG, Murphy JC, Ackerman JI, et al: Proliferative colitis in ferrets. Am J Vet Res 1982; 43:858–864.
11. Fox JG, Palley LS, Rose R: Eosinophilic gastroenteritis with Splendore-Hoeppli material in the ferret. Vet Pathol 1992; 29:21–26.
12. Fox JG, Pearson RC, Gorham JR: Viral and chlamydial diseases. *In* Fox JG, ed.: Biology and Diseases of the Ferret. Philadelphia, Lea & Febiger, 1988, pp 217–234.
13. Fox JG, Zeman DH, Mortimer JD: Copper toxicosis in sibling ferrets. J Am Vet Med Assoc 1994; 205:1154–1156.
14. Frederick MA: Intervertebral disc syndrome in a domestic ferret. Vet Med Small Anim Clin 1981; 76:835.
15. Goad MEP, Fox JG: Neoplasia in ferrets. *In* Fox JG, ed.: Biology and Diseases of the Ferret. Philadelphia, Lea & Febiger, 1988, pp 274–288.
16. Hendrick MJ, Goldschmidt MH: Chondrosarcoma of the tail of ferrets. Vet Pathol 1987; 24:272–273.
17. Herron AJ, Brunnert SR, Ching SV, et al: Immunohistochemical and morphologic features of chordomas in ferrets. Vet Pathol 1990; 27:284–286.
18. Jensen WA, Myers RK, Liu CH: Osteoma in a ferret. J Am Vet Med Assoc 1985; 187:1375–1376.
19. Jensen WA, Myers RK, Merkley DF: Diagnostic exercise: a bony growth of the skull in a ferret. Lab Anim Sci 1987; 37:780–781.
20. Kirk RW, Bistner SI, Ford RB: Metabolic Emergencies. *In* Handbook of Veterinary Procedures and Emergency Treatment. 5th ed. Philadelphia, WB Saunders, 1990, pp 133–145.
21. Lawes INC, Andrews PLR: The neuroanatomy of the ferret brain. *In* Fox JG, ed.: Biology and Diseases of the Ferret. Philadelphia, Lea & Febiger, 1988, pp 66–99.
22. Lenhard A: Blastomycosis in a ferret. J Am Vet Med Assoc 1985; 186:70–72.
23. Methiyapun S, Myers RK, Pohlenz JFL: Spontaneous plasma cell myeloma in a ferret. Vet Pathol 1985; 22:517–519.
24. Oliver JE, Lorenz MD: Handbook of Veterinary Neurologic Diagnosis. Philadelphia, WB Saunders, 1983.
25. Pool RR: Tumors of bone and cartilage. *In* Moulton J, ed.:

Tumors in Domestic Animals. 2nd ed. Los Angeles, University of California Press, 1978, pp 91–99.
26. Powers BE, LaRue SM, Withrow SJ, et al: Jamshidi needle biopsy for diagnosis of bone lesions in small animals. J Am Vet Med Assoc 1988; 193:205–210.
27. Ryland LM, Gogolewski R: What's your diagnosis? J Am Vet Med Assoc 1990; 197:1065–1066.
28. Rosenthal K: Ferrets. Vet Clin North Am Small Anim Pract 1994; 24:1–23.
29. Shores A: Spinal trauma: pathophysiology and management of traumatic spinal injuries. Vet Clin North Am Small Anim Pract 1992; 22:859–888.
30. Widmer WR, Blevins WE: Veterinary myelography: a review of contrast media, adverse effects, and technique. J Am Anim Hosp Assoc 1991; 27:163–176.
31. Williams BH, Eighmy JJ, Berbert MH, Dunn DG: Cervical chordoma in two ferrets. Vet Pathol 1993; 30:204–206.
32. Williams BH, Popek EJ, Hart RA, Harris RK: Iniencephaly and other neural tube defects in a litter of ferrets. Vet Pathol 1994; 31:260–262.

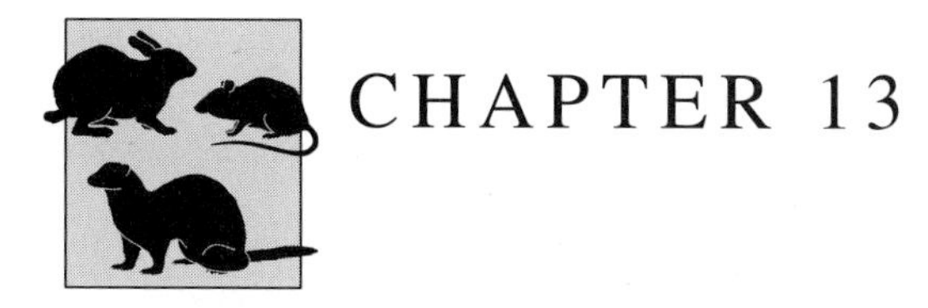

CHAPTER 13

Soft Tissue Surgery

Holly Mullen, DVM

The domestic ferret is a monogastric animal with anatomy and physiology that are similar to those of the dog and cat. Ferrets have a thick subcutis and a thin abdominal musculature. The linea alba is well defined. Most ferrets have significant deposits of intra-abdominal fat that can obscure the definition of structures such as the adrenal glands, ovaries, ureters, and lymph nodes.

Ferrets do not have a cecum. The division between the jejunoileum and the colon is indistinct. It can be identified histologically or visually because of the change in vasculature from the arcuate pattern of the small intestine to the linear vessels of the colon. Other than this difference, the anatomy of the abdominal viscera is like that of dogs and cats.

Anesthesia in ferrets is similar to anesthesia in cats. A circulating warm water heating pad should always be used, as ferrets are prone to hypothermia during anesthesia. Most ferrets are easily intubated despite their small size because they do not seem prone to laryngospasm. The endotracheal tube diameter required varies from 2.0 mm to 4.0 mm.

A variety of anesthetic agents are available for use in ferrets. Specific anesthetic agents are discussed in Chapter 32. I prefer to use chamber induction until the ferret is recumbant; then, I use mask induction while placing an indwelling IV catheter. The cephalic and saphenous veins are readily accessible; the jugular vein may also be used. Make a small skin puncture to the side of the vein with a No. 11 scalpel blade or a hypodermic needle. Puncture facilitates passage of an over-the-needle catheter through the skin and into the vein. After catheter placement, IV anesthetic agents may be used, if necessary, for endotracheal intubation. This is followed by maintenance anesthesia with an inhaled agent, preferably isoflurane.

ROUTINE OVARIOHYSTERECTOMY

Ovariohysterectomy (OHE) is commonly done in ferrets at large breeding farms when they are 5–7 weeks of age, before their delivery to pet stores. Intact female ferrets should be spayed by 6–8 months of age if they are not to be used for breeding. This prevents the development of the often fatal, estrogen-induced bone marrow hypoplasia, which occurs in more than half of estrual females that are not bred.[20]

The ferret uterus is bicornuate and resembles that of cats and dogs. I have seen uterus unicornus in a 1-year-old female presented for routine OHE. The left uterine horn and both ovaries were present.

The surgical procedure for OHE in a ferret is similar to that in a cat. Make a ventral midline abdominal incision over the midpoint between the umbilicus and the pubis. Large fat deposits may surround the ovaries, making identification of the ovarian vessels difficult. It is important to avoid the ureters when ligating the ovarian pedicles.

The suspensory ligament is usually slack and is easily torn. Doubly ligate the ovarian vascular pedicles, uterine arteries, and uterine body with 3–0 chromic gut suture, and transect and remove the ovaries and uterus as for a cat OHE. Close the linea with 4–0 absorbable or monofilamant nonabsorbable suture material. Close the subcuticular layer with 5–0 absorbable suture. Skin sutures are not necessary.

PYOMETRA

Occasionally, pyometra may develop in an intact female. In most cases of pyometra, a ferret is presented for a vaginal discharge noted by the owner. Some ferrets may be partially anorectic, lethargic, or depressed. Hyperestrogenism with bone marrow toxicity may occur concurrently. Be sure to screen for hyperestrogenism, especially if the ferret has a swollen vulva (see Chapter 5). Polyuria and polydipsia have not been reported. Laboratory values are usually normal; neutrophilic leukocytosis is the most common laboratory abnormality if the ferret is not pancytopenic. Unlike in dogs and cats, *Escherichia coli* does not appear to be the most common microorganism involved. Bacteria cultured from ferret pyometra include *E. coli* and *Staphylococcus, Streptococcus,* and *Corynebacterium* species.[7]

Stump pyometra is not reported in ferrets. I have seen one case in which a 1-year-old, spayed female ferret was presented with a swollen vulva unresponsive to human chorionic gonadotropin. On abdominal exploration, a stump pyometra 1 cm in diameter was discovered and excised. No ovarian remnant tissue was seen. The result of bacterial culture of the purulent material within the uterine stump was negative.

The surgical procedure for ferret pyometra is the routine OHE. Take care not to spill uterine contents in the abdomen. Leave a minimal amount of uterine body in the stump to decrease the potential for stump pyometra formation. Recovery is routine.

OVARIAN REMNANT SURGERY

A female ferret presented with a swollen vulva may show signs of estrus because of the retention of ovarian tissue from a prior OHE that was improperly performed. A swollen vulva may also indicate adrenal disease (see Chapter 9). Usually, vulvar swelling caused by an ovarian remnant occurs in young ferrets (1–2 years of age), whereas adrenal disease is uncommon before the age of 2–3 years. Intramuscular administration of 100 IU of human chorionic gonadotropin usually causes a decrease in size of a vulva that is enlarged secondary to an ovarian remnant. This treatment has no effect on vulvar enlargement that is secondary to adrenal neoplasia.[18]

Abdominal exploration is indicated for the identification and removal of retained ovarian tissue. Before surgery, perform a complete blood count and platelet count to determine whether the ferret has signs of bone marrow suppression from prolonged estrus. If results are abnormal, surgery usually must be delayed (see Chapter 5).

Make a ventral midline abdominal incision as for the OHE, extending it slightly more cranial to the umbilicus. A section of ovary torn during OHE may have been dropped and reimplanted anywhere within the abdomen. Improper removal is the most common cause of ovarian tissue retention. You will most likely find the remnant in the normal location of the ovary, caudolateral to the caudal pole of the kidney (Fig. 13–1). Remove the ovarian remnant as

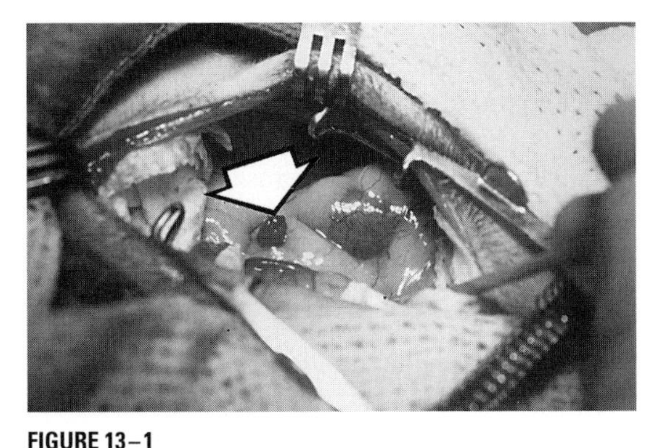

FIGURE 13–1
Retained left ovarian remnant *(arrow)* caudolateral to the caudal pole of the left kidney in a ferret.

you would remove an ovary. Always check for a second retained ovarian remnant.

Following removal of all ovarian remnant tissue, recovery is uneventful. Vulvar swelling begins to subside in 1–5 days.

ORCHIECTOMY

Orchiectomy (castration) should be done by 6–8 months of age. Castration reduces aggressive behavior and decreases the intensity of the odiferous musky odor produced by the sebaceous glands of the ferret's skin. Although rare, testicular neoplasia may develop in some older, intact male ferrets. Sertoli cell tumor and interstitial cell tumor are reported testicular tumors in ferrets.[8]

The testes are located caudoventrally in the scrotal sac, which is less furred than that of the cat. Some authors report a seasonal variation in location of the testes (subcutaneous in the caudoventral abdomen from January through June).[20] I have not observed this variation in practice in the northeastern United States.

Shave or pluck the scrotal sac. Make bilateral longitudinal incisions and perform either an open or closed castration technique, as for a cat. I prefer the open, "self-tie" procedure; however, the spermatic cord and vessels occasionally are too fragile for this, and ligature with 4–0 chromic gut is required. No sutures are placed in the scrotal incisions.

Ferrets may also be successfully vasectomized.[21] Vasectomy only alters fertility; it does not affect behavior or the odor produced by the scent glands. This procedure may not become popular in pet ferrets but would be very practical in a breeding colony. Sterile males can be used to breed with and induce ovulation in estrual females, thus avoiding the potential bone marrow suppression associated with prolonged estrus.

ANAL SACCULECTOMY

At ferret breeding farms, anal sacculectomy (popularly referred to as "descenting") is commonly done at an early age simultaneously with neutering. If not, it may be done when the older ferret is neutered, or at any time. Although the odiferous musk from the anal sacs is extremely strong and objectionable, removal of the anal sacs does not truly "descent" the animal because the sebaceous glands in the skin will continue to produce a less odorous musk.

The paired anal sacs are 10–20 mm in length and are located on either side of the anus in the 4 o'clock and 8 o'clock positions. Identify the ducts at the mucocutaneous junction of the anus and cannulate the opening with a tomcat urethral catheter. Circumferentially incise the skin 2–3 mm from the opening of the duct. Grasp the skin and catheter with a mosquito forceps and retract the duct while sharply dissecting the neck of the sac. The first 3–5-mm depth of tissue contains perianal glands and is firmly attached.[4] After this, a fascial plane around the sac is evident. Once the yellowish-white gland is visualized, bluntly dissect it from its position in the perianal tissues and anal sphincter (Fig. 13–2). Dis-

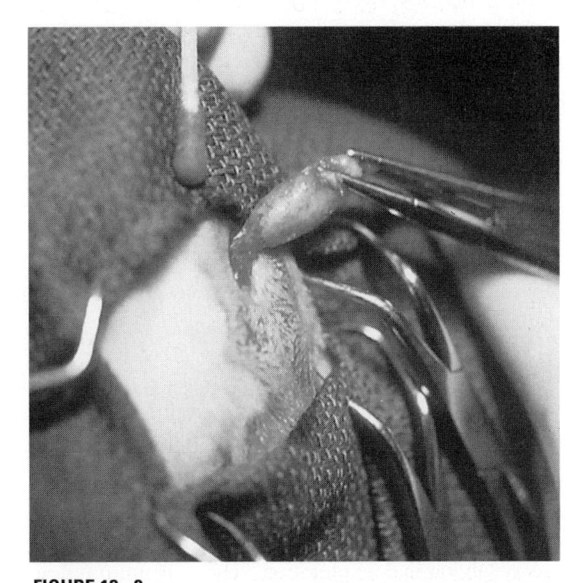

FIGURE 13–2
Anal sac excision in a ferret. Hemostats are on the neck of the gland.

section is facilitated by the use of sterile, cotton-tipped applicator swabs. Take care not to damage the anal sphincter.

A small vessel entering the caudal pole of the gland occasionally may need to be ligated. In most cases, this is the only significant bleeding encountered during anal sacculectomy.

Remove the anal sac intact, if possible. The incisions are left open to heal without sutures. A single 5–0 absorbable subcuticular suture may be used if the incision appears to gap excessively.

Rupture of the anal sac releases the musk. If rupture occurs, lavage the wound with sterile saline. Infection of the surgical site because of intraoperative anal sac rupture is uncommon. However, if the sac does rupture, the surgeon will be instantly reviled by all other persons present in the room!

Perianal draining tracts will form if an anal sac is incompletely removed. This can happen when the descenting is done by cautery at an early age, or if the anal sac ruptures during surgery and some sac wall is left in the tissues.

Carefully explore a perianal draining tract. The sac wall is identified by its mucosal appearance. Resect all abnormal tissue. Scar tissue associated with the fistula can make identification of retained sac lining difficult, but if all secretory lining is not removed, the draining fistula will reform. Fortunately, this is not a common problem.

Anal gland neoplasia is very rare in ferrets. Anal sac adenocarcinoma has been identified, but insufficient data are available for comment on the predilection or behavior of this tumor in ferrets. I have seen one neutered male ferret with a right anal sac adenocarcinoma that had metastasized to the inguinal lymph node. Resection of the enlarged inguinal node and the right anal sac mass was performed. The ferret had an uneventful recovery and was fecally continent. The owners declined further therapy, and the ferret was lost to followup.

LIVER BIOPSY

Liver biopsy is frequently performed during abdominal exploration. Hepatic lipidosis, lymphosarcoma, metastatic pancreatic insulinoma, and other hepatic diseases can be diagnosed from the liver biopsy. A good rule of thumb is to perform a liver biopsy on every abdominal exploration. There is minimal if any morbidity associated with this procedure.

If all lobes of the liver appear similar, choose any lobe as the biopsy site. The biopsy specimen should be no smaller than 5–7 mm^3. If a small section of the lobe protrudes, the guillotine method is appropriate. Encircle the protruding piece of liver tissue with 3–0 chromic gut and tighten the ligature until it closes firmly. Use three throws on the gut ligature. Trim away the isolated liver tissue for biopsy.

The transfixation biopsy method should be used when there are no convenient protrusions of liver tissue (most of the time). Place a 3–0 chromic gut suture through the liver parenchyma about 7 mm from the edge. Make the first throw and cinch it down at a 45° angle to one side (Fig. 13–3). Make a second throw and cinch it down at about 90° to the first throw. Tie a third throw to complete the knot on the chromic gut. With scissors, trim away the wedge-shaped liver biopsy. If necessary, a small piece of hemostatic gelatin sponge (Gelfoam, The Upjohn Company, Kalamazoo, MI) can be placed over the end of the biopsy site for the control of hemorrhage.

SPLENECTOMY AND SPLENIC BIOPSY

Primary splenic disease is uncommon in ferrets. Splenomegaly is very common and may be incidental or indicative of disease. Lymphoma, mast cell disease, insulinoma, Aleutian disease, and splenitis are some of the conditions associated with splenomegaly. Splenic biopsy is helpful in the diagnosis of splenomegaly or if the spleen appears abnormal during abdominal exploration.[9]

Most diseases involving the spleen do not require splenectomy. Lymphosarcoma and metastatic insulinoma are two of the more common indications for splenectomy. Idiopathic splenomegaly is sometimes seen in a sick ferret with an otherwise normal medical workup. Such a ferret may become clinically normal following splenectomy for the grossly enlarged spleen. No disease process has been identified with this condition.

The same guillotine and transfixation biopsy techniques used in the liver can be employed for splenic biopsy. Unlike the thin liver capsule, the splenic capsule is important in containing hemorrhage. Be careful to include splenic capsule in the biopsy ligatures, otherwise bleeding from the cut edge of the biopsy site will occur. Application of gelatin sponge and gentle pressure for 3–5 minutes stops the hemorrhage.

Splenectomy in ferrets is performed as it is in cats

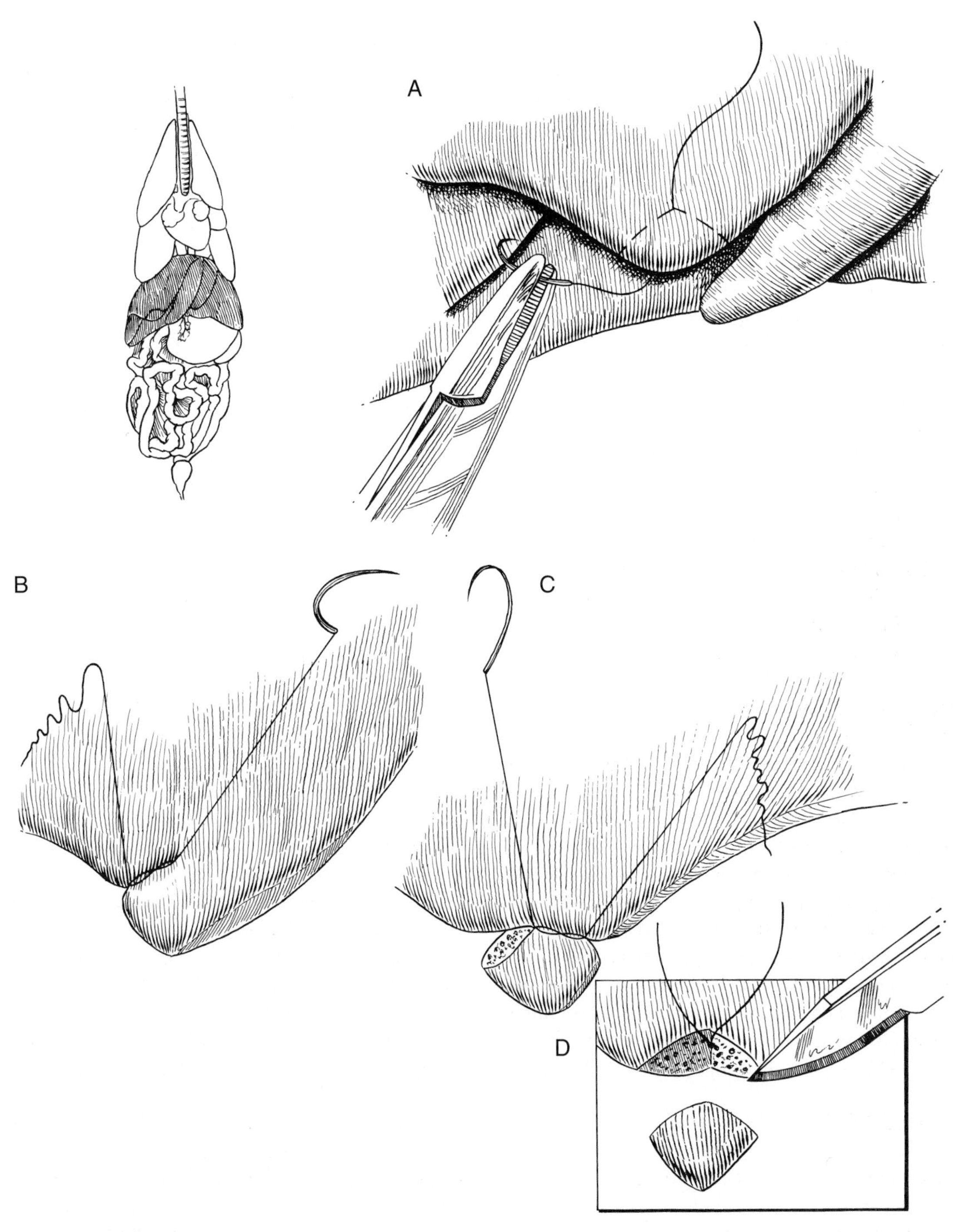

FIGURE 13–3

Transfixation liver biopsy technique. *A,* Pass suture through the liver 5–8 mm from the border. *B,* Place a ligature on one side of the transfixation. *C,* Place the second and third throws at an angle to the first and tighten to a knot. *D,* Remove the isolated liver biopsy specimen and trim the suture material's ends.

and dogs. Identify and ligate the main splenic artery and vein and all other smaller splenic vessels. Be careful not to damage the tip of the left limb of the pancreas, which may lie very close to the spleen. Absorbable 3–0 ligature or hemostatic metal clips may be used for ligatures. I find that the ligate-divide-staple devices used in dog and cat splenectomy, such as the Autosuture LDS (U.S. Surgical Corp, Norwalk, CT), place too large a staple on most of the small ferret's splenic vessels and thus should not be used.

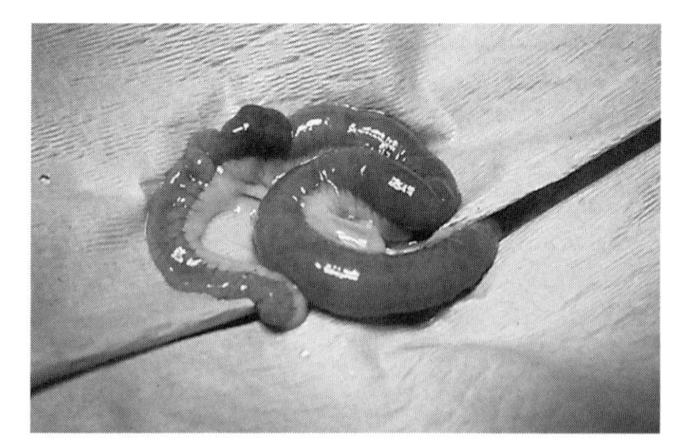

FIGURE 13–4
Intestinal foreign body in a ferret.

GASTROINTESTINAL FOREIGN BODY

Ferrets are very prone to ingestion of foreign bodies. For this reason, a ferret should not be allowed to have free range of the house without supervision. Toys made of foam rubber, rubber, or cork should not be given to ferrets, as they appear to prefer ingesting these materials. Grooming behavior may also result in the formation of trichobezoars, which are usually found in the stomach. Most ingested foreign bodies lodge in the small intestine.[16] Cases of esophageal foreign body in ferrets are rare but have been reported.[3, 16]

Presenting signs are similar to those in dogs and cats with a gastrointestinal (GI) foreign body, except that ferrets with foreign body do not often exhibit vomiting. Anorexia, lethargy, pawing at the mouth (a sign of nausea), weight loss, and diarrhea are the signs most frequently noted by the owner.

Physical examination may reveal dehydration. A palpable abdominal mass (the foreign body) is often present. Radiographs may show an obstructive gas or fluid pattern in the intestine. Occasionally, the foreign body may be radiographically visible.

The presence of a GI foreign body in all species indicates the need for emergency surgery. Although ferrets should be rehydrated and stabilized if necessary before surgery, the surgery should not be postponed until the next day.

Esophageal foreign body is rare. The foreign object may be removed surgically via thoracotomy and esophagotomy,[3] may be pushed into the stomach and retrieved via gastrotomy, or may be retrieved via endoscopy in large ferrets.

Abdominal exploration for GI foreign body begins with a ventral midline abdominal incision. Inspect the GI tract carefully because some ferrets have multiple pieces of foreign material present at one time. Gastrotomy, enterotomy, and intestinal resection are performed as for dogs and cats. Ferret intestinal tissue is thin and delicate and must be handled gently to prevent tearing or subsequent stricture (Fig. 13–4). Close a gastrotomy incision in two layers with 3–0 or 4–0 absorbable or nonabsorbable suture. Close an enterotomy with 4–0 or 5–0 monofilament, absorbable or nonabsorbable suture. As always, after an incision in the GI tract is closed, change gloves and instruments and flush the abdomen copiously with sterile saline to minimize intraoperative contamination. Abdominal closure is routine except that the subcutaneous tissues are also flushed well with saline after abdominal wall closure. This decreases incisional infection, which is the most common postoperative complication of enteric surgery.

Food and water are withheld for 12–24 hours after surgery. Administer maintenance fluids and antibiotics parenterally until the ferret is able to eat. Most ferrets eat well following removal of the foreign body and may be discharged by the second day after surgery. Instruct the owner to "ferret proof" the environment and to watch for signs of subsequent recurrence. Stenosis of the intestinal lumen may occur following enterotomy, making the ferret prone to intestinal obstruction by a piece of foreign material that was previously small enough to pass unimpeded.

PANCREATIC SURGERY FOR INSULINOMA

Insulinoma is frequently diagnosed in the middle-aged to older ferret.[11, 14] Signs include weakness, lethargy, ptyalism, collapse, and generalized seizures accompanied by hypoglycemia and hyperinsulinemia. Diagnosis and medical treatment for insulinoma is covered elsewhere in this text (see Chapter 9).

Surgical treatment of insulinoma is aimed at reducing tumor volume and making subsequent medical management more successful. Although all visible tumor is removed at surgery, the tumor has commonly already spread, and a surgical "cure" is unlikely.[17]

Keep the ferret NPO for 12 hours before surgery while administering a 2.5–5% dextrose and fluid solution IV to prevent hypoglycemia. Make a standard cranial ventral midline abdominal incision, and perform a routine abdominal exploration. Pay particular attention to the adrenal glands, as adrenal gland tumors are also common in middle-aged ferrets. It is not known whether there is actually an association between the two types of tumor in ferrets or whether both tumors are so common that it is reasonable to find them in the same ferret for unrelated reasons.

Inspect the spleen and liver carefully for metastatic nodules. Palpate the entire pancreas gently between two fingers to detect very small nodules. Tumor size may range from grossly invisible (but histologically identifiable) up to 2 cm^3 (Fig. 13–5). Nodules tend to "shell out" cleanly with blunt dissection. Place a small piece of gelatin sponge over a bleeding nodule bed to provide hemostasis without injuring the pancreas. Multiple nodules are often found; solitary tumors are less common. Tumors are found in the right and left limbs of the pancreas with equal frequency and may also be located in the body of the gland.

If several nodules are found at the right or left tip of the limbs, a partial pancreatectomy may be preferable to multiple nodulectomies. Dissect the pancreas free of adjacent structures (i.e., the duodenum on the right and the spleen on the left) and place a circumferential ligature of nonreactive absorbable or nonabsorbable suture material around it, crushing the pancreatic tissue and ligating the vessels and ducts within the gland. This will not cause clinically detectable pancreatitis. Delicate dissection of the pancreatic tissue to expose ducts and vessels for individual ligation is not necessary. Trim away the tip of the gland containing the tumors for biopsy. Lavage the pancreas after all nodules are removed to clear away pancreatic enzymes liberated by tissue handling. Abdominal closure is routine.

Check the blood glucose level immediately after surgery and at least every 6–12 hours until the ferret goes home. If substantial tumor volume has been removed, the blood glucose level should increase rapidly after surgery, and the dextrose drip infusion may be discontinued. A few ferrets may not have blood glucose level elevations until 1–3 days after surgery despite the successful removal of tumor. Ideally, the blood glucose level after surgery should be at least 60–80 mg/dL without the benefit of IV dextrose. Some ferrets may show partial response and may need to be maintained on medical therapy (prednisone, frequent feedings, and diazoxide) after surgery.

Food is offered within 12 hours after surgery. Pancreatitis is extremely rare following pancreatic surgery for insulinoma. Ferrets should not be kept NPO for long periods following insulinoma surgery simply because of fear of postoperative pancreatitis.

Recheck the ferret's blood glucose and insulin levels 10–14 days after surgery. These levels should be monitored periodically thereafter.

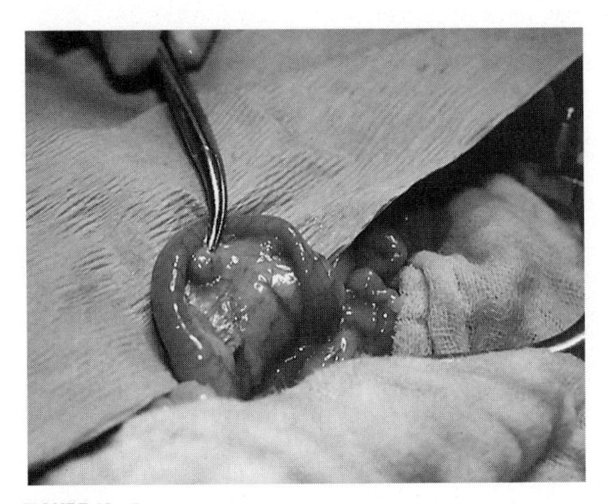

FIGURE 13–5
Pancreatic insulinoma at the tip of the right limb of the pancreas in a 5-year-old ferret.

ADRENAL GLAND SURGERY

Adrenal gland neoplasia is common in American pet ferrets. Tumor types include adenoma, adenocarcinoma, and cortical hyperplasia. The majority of reported cases occur in females. Signs include alopecia, pruritus, and vulvar enlargement in neutered females[18] (see Chapter 9). Some male ferrets may have strangury due to the cystic enlargement of tissue at the base of the bladder (see Paraurethral Cysts).

Adrenocortical disease in ferrets is very rarely (if ever) true Cushing's disease. Plasma cortisol level is almost never elevated; instead, elevations are seen in the concentrations of androgens, estradiol, and 17-hydroxyprogesterone.[13, 18, 19] The majority of ferrets with adrenal neoplasia have been neutered before the age of 6 weeks. Mice that have been gonadectomized in the first few days of life show an increase in predilection for adrenal tumors later in life.[19] The embryonic gonads and adrenal glands arise in close proximity to each other. Some gonadal cells may be carried with the developing adrenal gland during migration. Early neutering may stimulate the development of these undifferentiated gonadal cells in the adrenal capsule.

Pheochromocytoma of the adrenal glands is extremely rare. I have seen two cases, one in a male ferret and the other in a female ferret. These ferrets were presented for weight loss, anorexia, and lethargy. Neither ferret had tachycardia or cardiac arrhythmias on physical examination. Both ferrets had very large (4 × 6-cm and 8 × 4-cm), nonresectable abdominal masses that arose in the craniodorsal abdomen between the kidneys. Both masses encompassed the abdominal aorta, and one also involved the caudal vena cava. One ferret died during attempted resection, and the other was euthanized. Pheochromocytoma was confirmed by biopsy. These two tumors were much larger than the sex hormone–secreting adrenal tumor most commonly seen in ferrets.

Diagnosis of adrenal gland neoplasia is based on characteristic physical examination findings. Abdominal ultrasound shows adrenal enlargement in 50% or more of cases.[19] Serum chemistry values and blood counts are usually within normal limits. Rarely, estrogen suppression of bone marrow may be detected. Tumors may be unilateral (most commonly, left-sided) or bilateral.

Surgery is the definitive treatment for adrenal gland neoplasia.[12, 19] A lateral surgical approach to the adrenal glands has been described,[5] but this approach does not allow for exploration of the abdomen. Adrenal disease may be bilateral, or concurrent pancreatic insulinoma may be present; thus, a standard, ventral midline abdominal approach is best.

Examine the abdominal organs carefully, especially the pancreas. Palpate the adrenal glands thoroughly because they are often obscured by intra-abdominal fat. The normal adrenal glands are light pink in color, 6–8 mm in length, and 2–3 mm in thickness (very similar in size, shape, and texture to a cooked lentil bean). Irregular gross enlargement, "rounding up" of the gland into a pea size, excessive firmness, and yellowish-brown discoloration are all indications of abnormality. Adrenal tumors range in size from only slightly larger than the normal gland up to 3 cm in diameter.

Excision of the left adrenal gland is usually easier than that of the right, which is often adherent to the caudal vena cava. The glands lie craniomedial to the kidneys. The left adrenolumbar vein passes ventrally over the left gland.[10] The right gland lies along the vena cava under a tip of the right lobe of the liver.

Gently dissect the left adrenal gland free of the fat, ligating the adrenolumbar vein and other minor vasculature encountered. Dissection is aided by the use of sterile, cotton-tipped applicator swabs (Fig. 13–6*A*). Apply a gelatin sponge to control hemor-

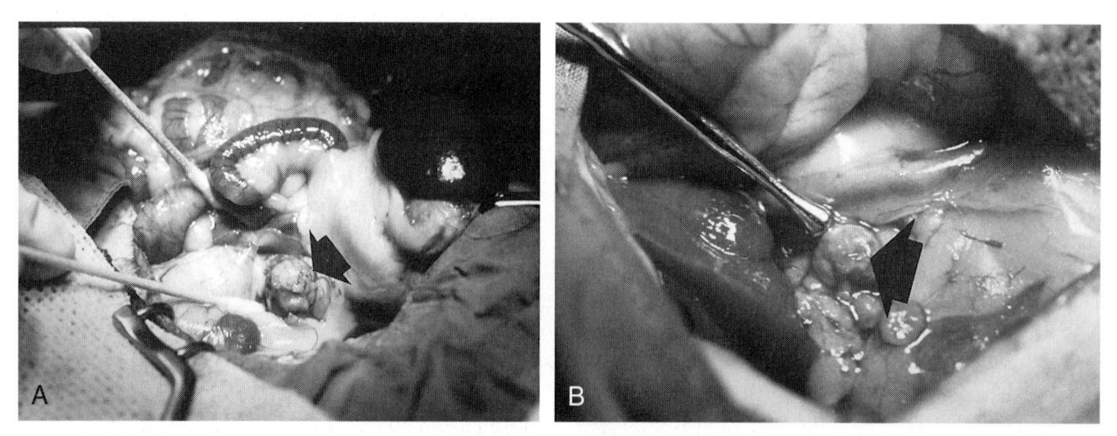

FIGURE 13–6

A, Dissection of a left adrenal tumor 2 cm in diameter in a 5-year-old ferret. The tumor *(arrow)* is craniomedial to the cranial pole of the left kidney. *B*, Dissection of a right adrenal tumor 1 cm in diameter *(arrow)*. The liver lobe is reflected cranially. Note proximity of the mass to the caudal vena cava.

rhage from small vessels in the fat. If the tumor is large enough that it approaches midline, be very careful not to disrupt the mesenteric blood supply, otherwise intestinal ischemia will result.

Expose the right adrenal gland by cranially reflecting the tip of liver lobe covering the vena cava (see Fig. 13–6*B*). The gland is usually adherent to the vena cava. In my experience, the vena cava usually tears if you try to peel off the adrenal gland. Two methods for successful removal of the gland are recommended. Incise the adrenal capsule and shell out the contents of the gland. Often, the enlarged tumor is well-circumscribed and shells out easily. Alternatively, free the gland as much as possible from its attachment to the vena cava. Using hemostatic clips, ligate the longitudinal border of the vena cava where it joins the gland (Fig. 13–7). One or two clips are all that are usually needed. Trim away the gland and border of the vessel. Control minor hemorrhage, if any, with gelatin sponge.

When bilateral tumors are present, I resect the left adrenal gland and debulk the right, using the capsular incision method. When this method has been used, no ferret has shown signs of hypoadrenalism and all have had regression of clinical signs. Successful medical management of a pet ferret with hypoadrenocorticism has not been reported.

Close the abdomen in a routine fashion after adrenalectomy. No special postoperative care is needed unless a true Cushing's syndrome was present, in which case glucocorticoid supplementation is required for several weeks until the contralateral gland begins functioning normally.

Within 24–48 hours of surgery, the swollen vulva will become less turgid. The vulva usually returns to its normal size within 1–2 weeks postoperatively. In males, strangury and dysuria from paraurethral cysts usually begin to subside within 48 hours. Regrowth of the pelage begins within 2 weeks and is usually complete by 2 months.

PARAURETHRAL OR PROSTATIC CYSTS

A small number of neutered male ferrets with adrenal neoplasia present with the complaint of strangury and dysuria and have a palpable caudal abdominal mass that is not the urinary bladder. Alopecia and pruritus consistent with hyperadrenocorticism may be incidentally noted by the owner.

At surgery, an adrenal tumor is present along with an enlarged, cystic structure encompassing the proximal urethra just caudal to the urinary bladder (Fig. 13–8). Typically, these masses are less than 4 cm in diameter and are partially fluid-filled and partially solid. Multiple cavitations may exist within the mass. Fluid aspirated from the mass is usually an acellular transudate or exudate. Cultures of this fluid have shown no bacterial growth. Occasionally, urine may be aspirated and, if the cyst is opened, direct communication with the urethra may be seen.

It is possible to debulk the cyst by opening the cyst wall and resecting some of the parenchyma. Be very careful not to damage the urethra and to close the cyst wall so that urine cannot leak into the abdomen.

Biopsy findings of the wall and parenchyma of these structures are consistent with the presence of inflammatory cysts—hence, the term *paraurethral cyst*. No prostatic tissue or urinary tract epithelial cells have been noted in these biopsy specimens at The Animal Medical Center in New York City; however, another pathologist believes that these cysts arise from prostatic tissue.* The cysts occur in the area of the prostate gland, which is a small, indistinct structure in ferrets. Because the cysts have only been found in ferrets with non-glucocorticoid-secreting adrenal tumors, and they regress in size after adrenalectomy, I suspect that they are glandular in origin.

Despite negative biopsy findings, the possibility of these cysts arising from prostatic tissue is likely. Cystic prostatic hypertrophy occurs in the presence of endogenous or exogenously administered estrogenic compounds in many species, including dogs and humans. These masses in ferrets regress in size, and clinical signs of partial urethral obstruction diminish rapidly after adrenalectomy. It is possible that the cystic prostatic hypertrophy is so marked that only the cyst wall and cystic tissue is available for biopsy without radical urethral resection. Without complete sectioning of the prostatic urethra, prostate tissue may not be identified.

It is not known why only some males with adrenal neoplasia have paraurethral cysts. Further experience is needed if the origin of these structures is to be determined. I have not seen a paraurethral cyst in a male ferret that did not have successful resolution of clinical signs (dysuria, strangury) following adrenalectomy. Based on this experience, I no

*Williams B: Personal communication, April 1995.

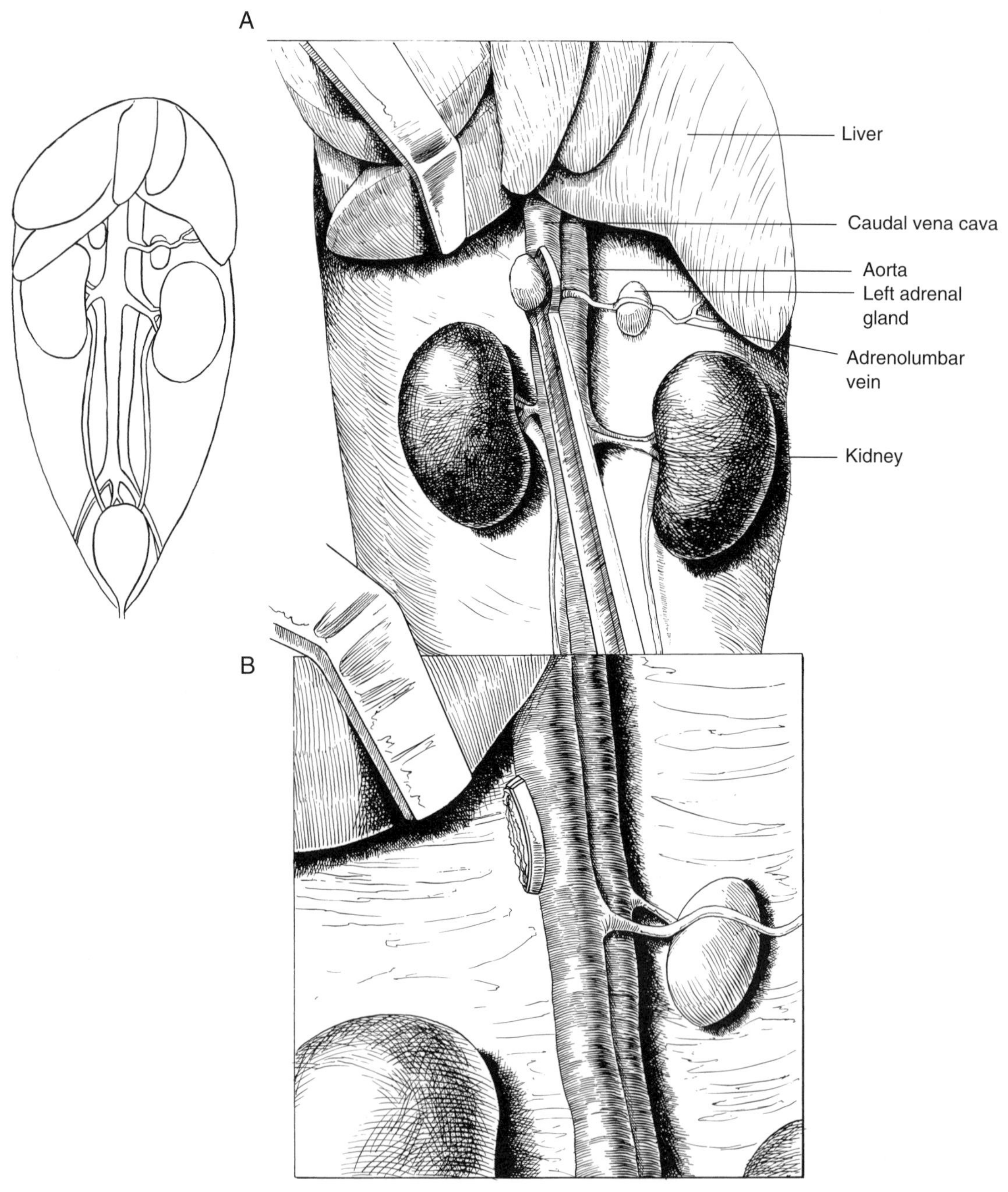

FIGURE 13–7

Hemostatic clip method for right adrenalectomy. *A,* Retract the adherent adrenal mass gently while placing a hemostatic clip between it and the vena cava. Take care not to occlude the caval lumen. *B,* Appearance of the vena cava after the right adrenal mass has been resected. Excise the mass 2–3 mm lateral to the clip to prevent retraction of the caval wall through the clip, which would result in rapid hemorrhage.

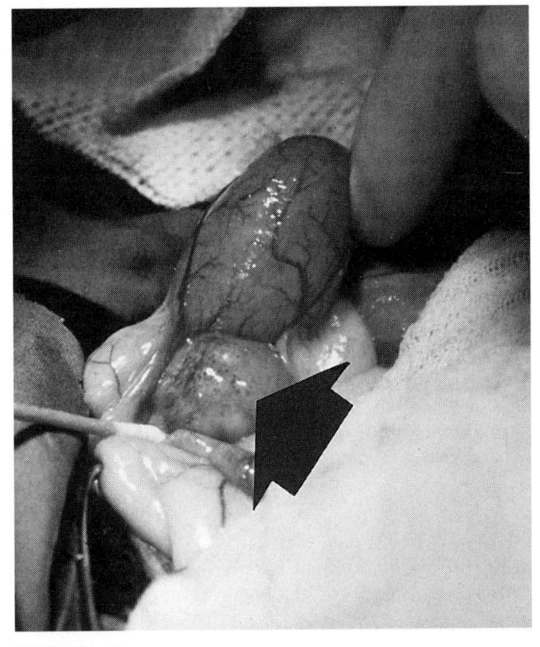

FIGURE 13–8
Paraurethral cyst *(arrow)* at the neck of the urinary bladder in a 6-year-old male ferret with strangury and a left adrenal mass.

longer attempt surgical debulking of the mass unless it is larger than 2 cm in diameter.

CYSTOTOMY

Like cats, ferrets can suffer from urolithiasis and cystic calculi (Chapter 5). Struvite (magnesium ammonium phosphate) calculi are the most commonly reported type in ferrets.[6] Jills may develop urolithiasis during pregnancy (see Chapter 6).

Presenting signs are identical to those in similarly affected dogs and cats and include strangury, hematuria, and urethral blockage. If calculi or crystals ("sand") are noted in the bladder, a cystotomy should be performed. Make a caudal, midline incision (parapreputial in the male) and expose the urinary bladder. The anatomy and procedure for cystotomy are the same as in the cat. Diverticula have been noted in the ferret bladder.

Submit the calculi for culture and stone analysis. In addition, I culture the bladder mucosa by submitting a small piece in the same culture tube as the calculus, which has been crushed (some calculi contain more bacteria than are found on their surface). Close the cystotomy incision with 4–0 or 5–0 absorbable suture (chromic gut is not recommended) in a two-layer, inverting pattern, if possible. Lavage the abdomen, and close in a routine fashion.

Postoperative care consists of 48 hours of IV fluid supplementation. Use appropriate antibiotics based on culture and sensitivity testing.

Rupture of the urinary bladder is rare in ferrets. Possible causes include external trauma and unrelieved urethral blockage. Signs are similar to those in cats and include depression, abdominal distention, uroabdomen, and azotemia. Treatment is aimed at correcting fluid and electrolyte imbalances. Perform emergency surgery to locate and repair the tear when the affected ferret is stable.

PERINEAL URETHROSTOMY

Persistant urolithiasis (crystals, not calculi) in male ferrets may cause repeated urinary obstruction. The penis does not easily extrude from the sheath, and the male's urethra is difficult to catheterize because of the hook-shaped os penis. Repeated urinary blockages in the face of appropriate medical management can be treated palliatively with a perineal urethrostomy.

The anatomy of the ferret's penis more closely resembles that of the dog than that of the cat. The penis exits the pelvic canal, runs subcutaneously along the ventral pelvis, and lies along the caudal, ventral abdominal body wall. The preputial opening is located about 1–2 cm caudal to the umbilicus. The os penis extends from near the tip of the penis caudad to the ventral brim of the pelvis.

The urethrostomy site should be between the os penis and the pelvic urethra. This is a relatively small area. The urethrostomy stoma will open in the perineal area rather than ventrally; this prevents continued trauma to the site during normal ferret ambulation.

Position the ferret in a perineal stand, place a pursestring suture in the anus, and aseptically prepare the perineum for surgery. Make a full-thickness skin incision approximately 1 cm long, starting about 1 cm below the anus. The base of the penis will be exposed. Make a 1-cm longitudinal incision in the penile urethra, taking care to avoid the cavernosus tissue on either side of the urethra. Sectioning of the cavernous tissue causes remarkable hemorrhage.

At this point, an indwelling urinary catheter is easily inserted in the proximal portion of the urethra in order to ascertain the diameter of the urethra and to

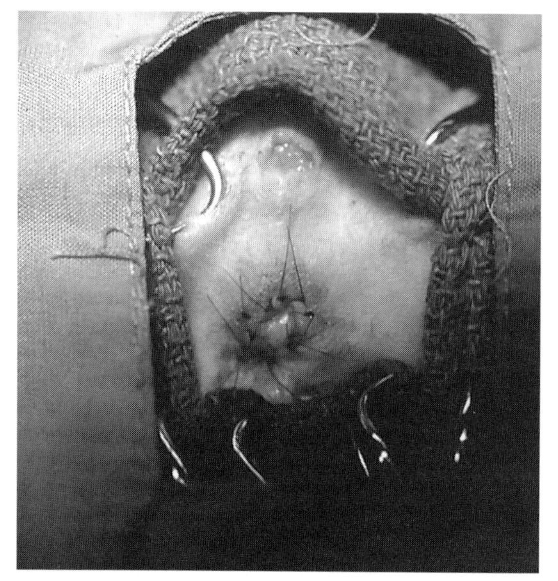

FIGURE 13–9
Immediate postoperative view of a perineal urethrostomy in a male ferret. Note the position of the mucosal drain site relative to the anus.

drain the urinary bladder if needed. Using nonabsorbable, monofilament, 5–0 or 6–0 suture material, appose the urethral mucosa to perineal skin with a simple, interrupted pattern. Make the urethral drain site at least 1 cm in length (Fig. 13–9).

Postoperative care includes the administration of antibiotics, the use of analgesics for 24 hours, and the application of an Elizabethan collar to prevent self-mutilation. The collar is usually unnecessary after the second day; this is good, because it is difficult to keep such a device on a ferret! I have performed perineal urethrostomy on two ferrets. Both had good clinical results, as characterized by the absence of recurrence of urethral obstruction, observation of a good urine stream, no urine scald, and no self-mutilation of the surgery site, which healed uneventfully.

PREPUTIAL MASSES

Tumors involving the preputial orifice are uncommonly seen in both neutered and intact ferrets.[8] These masses are located in the subcutis and may be either white to pink in color or darkly pigmented (Fig. 13–10). They may cause a partial functional obstruction to urination or may be an incidental finding.

Most of these masses are adenomas on biopsy, although an occasional adenocarcinoma is reported (see Chapter 10).[8, 15] Because of the possibility of malignancy and to prevent preputial obstruction, resect and biopsy all preputial masses. When resection of the mass involves the orifice, take care to recreate the opening by using 5–0 suture material for skin-to-preputial mucosa apposition. No special postoperative care is needed, and healing is uneventful.

MAMMARY GLAND NEOPLASIA

Mammary gland neoplasia is quite rare in ferrets. One case of malignant mammary tumor in a black-footed ferret has been reported.[8] I have not identified mammary neoplasia in a female ferret, but I have seen 11 cases in neutered male ferrets.

In ferrets, the typical presentation is one or more soft, subcutaneous, black-pigmented nodules lo-

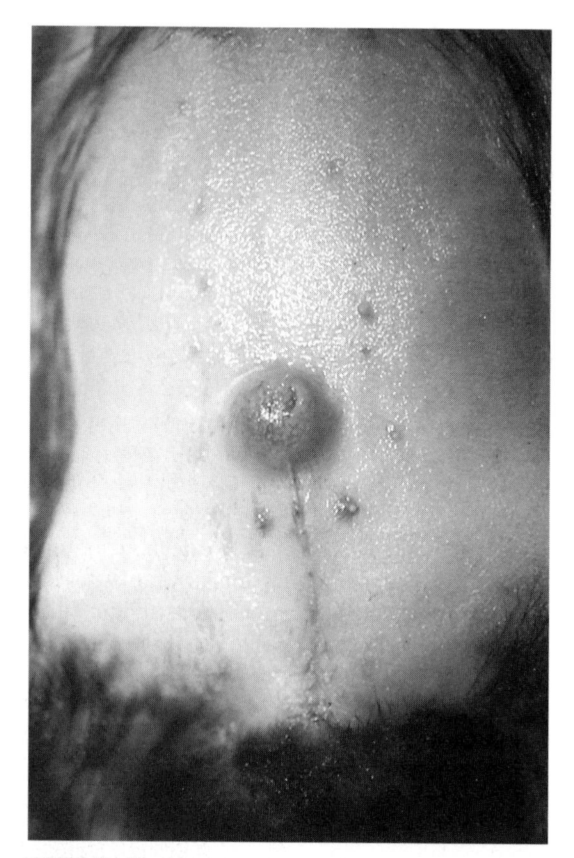

FIGURE 13–10
Preputial adenoma in a 2-year-old male ferret. Resection was uneventful. Note the two small darkly pigmented masses in the caudal mammary glands. These were identified as mammary adenomas on biopsy.

cated near a nipple in the mammary gland (Fig. 13–10). Mammectomy or lumpectomy was performed in all cases. All tumors were found to be benign mammary adenomas on biopsy, and there was no recurrence of tumor in any case.

DIAPHRAGMATIC HERNIA

Diaphragmatic hernia may occur in the traumatized ferret. I have seen three ferrets with diaphragmatic hernia. One was literally run over by the wheel of a car (and survived), and the other two had fallen from an open window ("high-rise syndrome"). Signs of diaphragmatic hernia include tachypnea, dyspnea, orthopnea, and muffled thoracic auscultation. Abdominal contents may be seen in the thorax on radiography (Fig. 13–11).

Treatment of diaphragmatic hernia includes treatment of shock and identification of other existing injuries. Pulmonary contusions, pneumothorax, ruptured bowel, and ruptured bladder may be seen in an animal that has sustained trauma with force sufficient to rupture the diaphragm.

An anesthetist is necessary for diaphragmatic hernia surgery in ferrets. Repair is the same as in dogs and cats. Identify the torn edges of the diaphragm, and débride and close the rent with nonabsorbable suture in a single, simple, interrupted pattern or in a continuous, double-layer pattern. Evacuate free air from the closed chest via thoracocentesis or an indwelling chest tube. If the ferret can survive complications of trauma in the immediate postoperative period, recovery of normal function is expected.

SALIVARY MUCOCELE

The five major pairs of salivary glands in ferrets include the parotid, mandibular, sublingual, buccal, and zygomatic glands.[1] Two reported cases of mucocele in ferrets appear to have involved the buccal glands.[2] Both were treated by marsupialization. One did not recur, and one recurred twice before finally resolving.

I have seen two cases of salivary mucocele in ferrets. Both presented with swelling over one side of the face and jaw. Neither ferret had swelling in the submandibular area, a common location for mucocele in the dog. On exploratory surgery, one ferret had a mucocele of the zygomatic gland. The gland and mucocele were resected. The zygomatic arch was removed to facilitate dissection of the gland. Recovery was uneventful, and the mucocele did not recur.

The second ferret also had an insulinoma and was euthanized. On necropsy, both the zygomatic and buccal glands appeared to be involved in the mucocele. Resection of both glands and the mucocele was not difficult once the zygomatic arch was removed.

Salivary mucocele may respond to marsupialization, but definitive treatment includes identification and surgical excision of the involved gland or glands. A thorough knowledge of anatomy is essen-

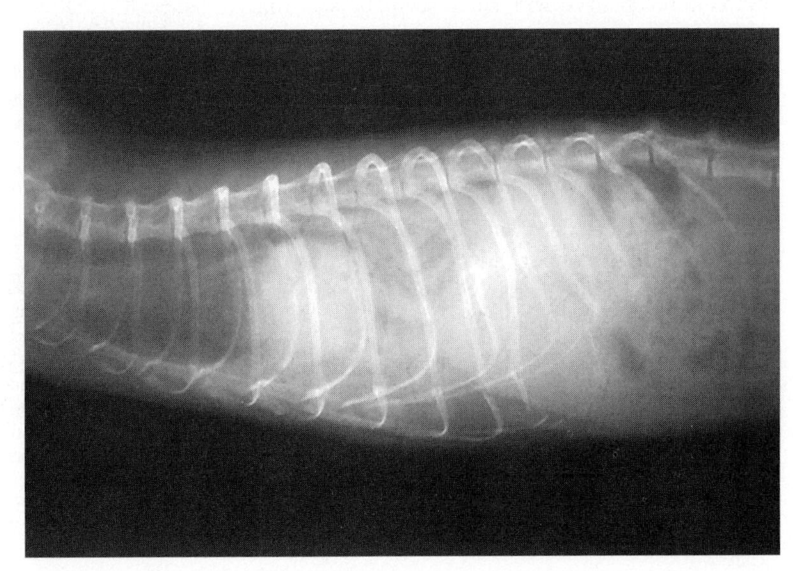

FIGURE 13–11
Lateral radiograph of a ferret with a diaphragmatic hernia and fractured ribs after being run over by a car. Linear intestinal gas patterns are seen in the thorax caudal to the heart.

tial for accurate identification and removal of the correct glands. It appears that salivary mucocele in ferrets may be found more frequently in the buccal and zygomatic glands than in the mandibular and sublingual glands, which are the most common locations in dogs and cats.

ONYCHECTOMY

Onychectomy (declawing) is rarely performed in ferrets. Ferrets have nails similar to those of dogs; they are not retractable claws like those of cats. A free-ranging ferret can do some damage to property by scratching and digging. Thus, ferrets should be confined when not directly observed. This prevents ingestion of foreign materials and allows any undesirable behavior to be monitored and eliminated early.

It is not accidental that onychectomy is addressed last in this chapter. I feel strongly that this procedure is rarely warranted and should never be offered as an elective surgery along with neutering and descenting. However, it is important to realize that declawing may be necessary in select circumstances—for example, if a ferret is predisposed toward psychogenic self-trauma, if it is owned by an immunosuppressed individual, or if the only alternative to the procedure is euthanasia.

Onychectomy in ferrets involves amputation of the distal phalanx of the toes. I have found that nail trimming instruments used with success to declaw the cat are not effective in ferrets. The best result seems to be obtained with sharp scalpel dissection.

Ferrets are fully anesthetized for onychectomy. Prepare the paw by trimming long hair from the toes and performing a surgical scrub on the feet. Have an assistant manually tourniquet one leg. Grasp the nail with a forceps and sharply incise the skin around the nailbed, sparing the digital pad. Sever the tendon attachments of the second and third phalanx and remove the third phalanx with its nail. Seal the wound with a drop of tissue glue or with a single, absorbable 5–0 suture. When all five toes are done, bandage the foot firmly. Analgesics should be used during the first 24 hours after surgery. Prophylactic antibiotics are not necessary.

The bandages are removed 24 hours after surgery. Ferrets should be restricted to cage rest for 7 days; thereafter, they can resume normal activity.

REFERENCES

1. An NQ, Evans HE: Anatomy of the ferret. *In* Fox JG, ed.: Biology and Diseases of the Ferret. Philadelphia, Lea & Febiger, 1988, pp 35–37.
2. Bauck LB: Salivary mucocele in two ferrets. Mod Vet Pract 1985; 66:337–339.
3. Caligiuri R, Bellah JR, Collins BR, et al: Medical and surgical management of esophageal foreign body in a ferret. J Am Vet Med Assoc 1989; 195:969–971.
4. Creed JE, Kainer RA: Surgical extirpation and related anatomy of the anal sacs of the ferret. J Am Vet Med Assoc 1981; 179:575–577.
5. Filion DL, Hoar RM: Adrenalectomy in the ferret. Lab Anim Sci 1985; 35:294–295.
6. Fox JG: Systemic diseases. *In* Fox JG, ed.: Biology and Diseases of the Ferret. Philadelphia, Lea & Febiger, 1988, pp 261–262.
7. Fox JG, Pearson RC, Gorham JR: Diseases associated with reproduction. *In* Fox JG, ed.: Biology and Diseases of the Ferret. Philadelphia, Lea & Febiger, 1988, p 192.
8. Goad MEP, Fox JG: Neoplasia in ferrets. *In* Fox JG, ed.: Biology and Diseases of the Ferret. Philadelphia, Lea & Febiger, 1988, pp 278–280.
9. Hillyer EV: Working up the ferret with a large spleen. Orlando, Proceedings of the North American Veterinary Conference, January 1994, pp 819–821.
10. Holmes RL: The adrenal glands of the ferret, *Mustela putorius*. J Anat 1961; 95:325–336.
11. Jergens AE, Shaw DP: Hyperinsulinism and hypoglycemia associated with pancreatic islet cell tumor in a ferret. J Am Vet Med Assoc 1989; 194:269–271.
12. Lawrence HJ, Gould WJ, Flanders JA, et al: Unilateral adrenalectomy as a treatment for adrenocortical tumors in ferrets: five cases (1990–1992). J Am Vet Med Assoc 1993; 203:267–270.
13. Lipman NS, Marini RP, Murphy JC, et al: Estradiol-17-beta–secreting adrenocortical tumor in a ferret. J Am Vet Med Assoc 1993; 203:1552–1555.
14. Marini RP, Ryden EB, Rosenblad WD, et al: Functional islet cell tumor in six ferrets. J Am Vet Med Assoc 1993; 202:430–433.
15. Miller TA, Denman DL, Lewis GC: Recurrent adenocarcinoma in a ferret. J Am Vet Med Assoc 1985; 187:839–841.
16. Mullen HS, Scavelli TD, Quesenberry KE, et al: Gastrointestinal foreign body in ferrets: 25 cases (1986 to 1990). J Am Anim Hosp Assoc 1992; 28:13–19.
17. Rosenthal K: How we treat an insulinoma in the ferret. Orlando, Proceedings of the North American Veterinary Conference, January 1994, p 822.
18. Rosenthal K: Adrenal disease in the ferret. Orlando, Proceedings of the North American Veterinary Conference, January 1994, pp 823–824.
19. Rosenthal KL, Peterson ME, Quesenberry KE, et al: Hyperadrenocorticism associated with adrenocortical tumor or nodular hyperplasia of the adrenal gland in ferrets: 50 cases (1987–1991). J Am Vet Med Assoc 1993; 203:271–275.
20. Ryland LM, Bernard SL: A clinical guide to the pet ferret. Compend Contin Educ Pract Vet 1983; 5:25–32.
21. Ryland LM, Lipinski E: A technique for vasectomizing male ferrets. Canine Pract 1994; 19:25–27.

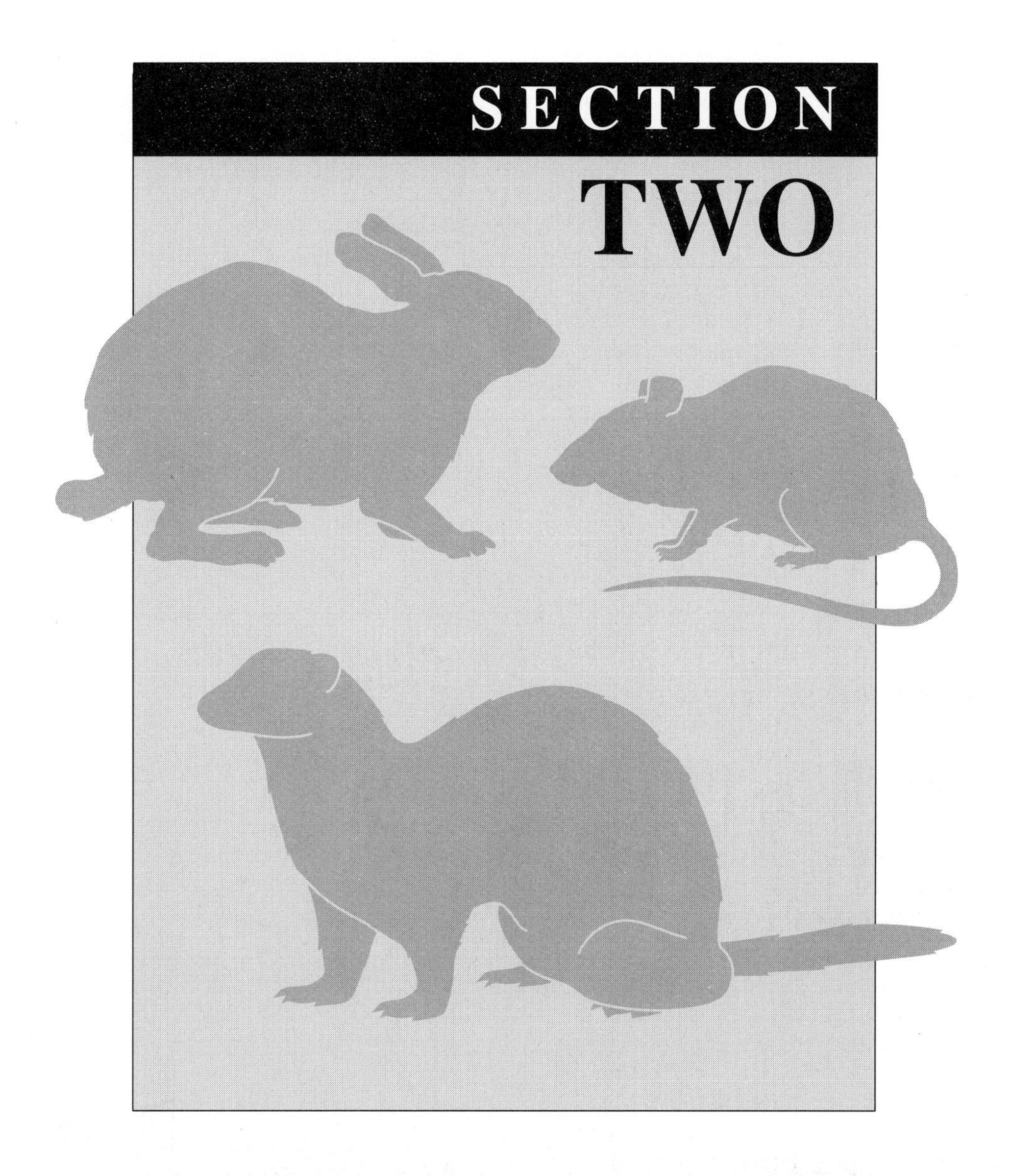

Rabbits

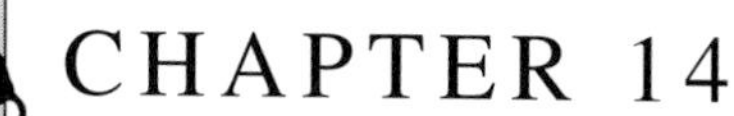

CHAPTER 14

Basic Anatomy, Physiology, and Husbandry

Thomas M. Donnelly, BVSc

TAXONOMY AND SIMILARITIES TO RODENTS

The Swedish naturalist Karl von Linne, who established the systematic classification of plants and animals, recognized the likeness of rabbits and rodents to each other and assigned them to a group called Glires. Later, naturalists designated Glires as the mammalian order Rodentia. Within this order, rabbits, hares, and pikas were grouped in the suborder Duplicidentata because they possessed a second pair of incisor teeth in the upper jaw. The majority of rodents that had only a single pair of upper incisors were grouped in the suborder Simplicidentata. Further classification in this century resulted in the redesignation of Duplicidentata as the mammalian order Lagomorpha. The order Rodentia is now restricted to the larger group of mammals with only one pair of upper incisors, such as squirrels, rats, mice, and guinea pigs. The discovery of a new fossil *(Tribosphenomys minutus)* in conjunction with recent morphologic and molecular evidence has suggested that rodents and lagomorphs are more closely related than had been suspected and that their similarities are not an example of convergent evolution.[16, 19] The term Glires is once again being used to describe the infraclass that encompasses these two orders.

Rabbits and rodents show a similarity to each other[23]: in both, the anterior incisors in the upper and lower jaws are modified to form chisel-like cutting organs. Their incisors remain in a permanently sharp condition from gnawing. Enamel is deposited on the front surface of these teeth only. The back surface is composed of dentin, and because enamel is harder than dentin, the front surface wears down more slowly. Also, teeth are absent between the last incisor and the first cheek tooth. This toothless interval is known as the *diastema*.

A range of normal physiologic values for healthy 2.5–3.0 kg New Zealand white rabbits, fed a standard pelleted diet, are presented in Table 14–1.

SKIN AND SCENT MARKING GLANDS

Female rabbits have a large fold of skin over the throat known as the *dewlap*. Breeding does pull fur from this area to line their nests before kindling. In older breeding does, the dewlap can be large and easily mistaken for an abscess. Moist dermatitis often develops in this area.

Rabbits do not have footpads; rather, the toes and metatarsal areas are covered with coarse fur. When a rabbit is sitting undisturbed, the plantar surface of the lower hindlimb, from the toes to the hock, is in contact with the ground. Heavy rabbits housed on wire floors often develop an ulcerative pododermatitis of this area referred to as *sore hocks*. The claws of rabbits are very sharp, and a rabbit that is picked up without appropriate support of its hindquarters can inflict painful scratches on the handler.

Rabbits are strongly territorial, and both sexes have three glands used in scent-marking behavior: the *chin glands,* which are specialized submandibular glands opening onto the underside of the chin; the *anal glands*; and a pair of pocket-like perineal glands referred to as the *inguinal glands*. The size of the glands and degree of marking are androgen-dependent and are related to the level of sexual activity. Males mark more frequently than do females, dominants of both sexes mark more frequently than subordinates, and dominants mark most in the presence of subordinate rivals. Rabbits leave behind messages expressing their dominance. Under natural conditions, both bucks and does on their own territory, surrounded by their own odor and that of their clan, win two thirds of all aggressive encounters.[18]

Does mark kits with chin and inguinal gland secretions, and they are openly hostile to young that are not their own. They harass young from their own colony but hotly pursue and kill young from other colonies. Kits smeared with odor from other rabbits are attacked and killed.[17]

TABLE 14–1

NORMAL PHYSIOLOGIC VALUES FOR RABBITS*

Body Weight	
Adult male (buck)	2–5 kg
Adult female (doe)	2–6 kg
Birthweight (kit)	30–80 g
***Clinical Examination*†**	
Rectal body temperature	38.5–40.0°C (101.3–104.0°F)
Normal heart rate	180–250 beats per min
Normal respiratory rate	30–60 breaths per min
Blood	
Whole blood volume	55–70 mL/kg
Plasma volume	28–51 mL/kg
Amounts of Food and Water	
Daily food consumption (rabbit pellets)‡	50 g/kg
Gastrointestinal transit time for hard feces	4–5 h after eating
Gastrointestinal transit time for cecotropes	8–9 h after eating
Daily hard feces excretion	5–18 g/kg
Daily water consumption§	50–150 mL/kg
Daily urine excretion	10–35 mL/kg
Age at Onset of Puberty and Breeding Life	
Sexual maturity, males	22–52 wk
Sexual maturity, females	22–52 wk
Breeding life, males	60–72 mo
Breeding life, females	24–36 mo
Female Reproductive Cycle	
Estrous cycle	Induced ovulators
Estrus duration	Prolonged
Ovulation rate	6–10 eggs
Pseudopregnancy	16–17 d
Gestation length	30–33 d
Litter size	4–12 kits
Male Copulatory Patterns	
Mounting time	2 seconds
Pre-ejaculatory intromissions	1
Ejaculations per mating	1–3

*The data listed are ranges for healthy 2.5- to 3.0-kg New Zealand white rabbits. Generally, New Zealand white rabbits reach this weight at about 18 wk of age. The data should be used as a guide only; these ranges are approximations, and actual values may vary, depending on the sex, age, and supplier of a rabbit.

†Lower values are expected in rabbits acclimatized to handling.

‡Food consumption is greater in growing, pregnant, and lactating animals.

§The amount of water required is influenced by food intake, feed composition, and environmental temperature. These values are for a normal rabbit fed standard rabbit pellets.

SENSE ORGANS AND NERVOUS SYSTEM

As is expected in animals subject to predation, the sense organs of rabbits are well developed. They are sensitive to catecholamines and have evolved for flight rather than fight. Temperature, heart rate, and respiratory rate significantly increase in a frightened animal.

Eyes*

Rabbits' eyes are directed more laterally than are those of most mammals; this provides them with a panoramic field of vision so that they are readily able to detect predators. Their eyes cannot, however, visualize the small area beneath the mouth, and rabbits depend on the sensitivity of the lips and vibrissae for food discrimination.[1]

The cornea is large, occupying 30% of the globe. The large spherical lens and poorly developed ciliary body confirm the limited need for accommodative vision in rabbits. The optic nerve is located above the horizontal midline of the eye, and retinal examination of this nerve involves looking upward into the eye. Retinal vessels spread out horizontally from the optic disc; also, rabbits have a depression or physiologic cup in their optic disc, as do dogs. Rabbits do not have a tapetum lucidum.

During anesthesia the third eyelid moves well across the cornea. Behind it and separated from the deep part of the cartilage is the harderian gland, which has a small, white upper lobe and a large, pink lower lobe. The excretory ducts from both lobes converge into a single duct that opens on the inner surface of the third eyelid. The harderian gland is larger in males than in females and is largest during breeding seasons. The lacrimal gland is small and light brown in color and is located behind the lower eyelid (location of the gland behind the upper eyelid is commonly seen in other species). However, the excretory duct opens into the conjunctiva of the upper lid.[26]

In rabbits, the primary channel for return of venous blood from the head, including that from the eye, is the external jugular vein.[25] In comparison, the primary drainage of the eye and head in humans occurs by the internal jugular vein. In other species, such as the dog, significant anastomoses exist between the branches of the internal and external jugular veins. In rabbits, such anastomoses are minor, and ligation or chronic catheterization of the external jugular vein results in swelling and protrusion of the eyeball for about 24 hours, after which its normal appearance returns.[11] The same pattern of vascularity also applies to the arterial blood supply of rabbit's eyes, but ligation of the external carotid artery results in ipsilateral ocular necrosis.

*Prince described the anatomy and physiology of the rabbit eye in great detail in the old but not outdated *The Rabbit Eye in Research*.[24]

Ears

The pinnae represent a large portion of the total body surface in rabbits—approximately 12%. They are highly vascular and have the largest arteriovenous shunts in the body when heated.[7] Noninvasive measurement of systemic arterial pressure in rabbits from the central ear artery has been described.[10] However, blood pressure in the central ear artery is about 10 mm Hg less than it is in the common carotid artery.

MUSCLES AND SKELETON

The skeleton of a rabbit is delicate and represents only 7–8% of its body weight; this is in contrast to the skeleton of the cat, which comprises 12–13% of body weight.[1, 7] Fractures, especially of the tibia, are always a potential problem. Rabbits have powerful hind legs that can kick violently. If rabbits are not securely held when picked up, their kicking can result in a vertebral fracture (nearly always at the seventh lumbar vertebra) and damage to the spinal cord. Proper handling of a rabbit is essential if injury to the rabbit and the handler is to be prevented.

In countries where rabbit meat is commonly eaten, clients may present a headless carcass that they suspect to be that of a cat. The color of the muscles distinguishes the two: rabbit muscles are pale pink, whereas those of cats are deep red. There are also skeletal differences, most noticeably between the scapula and pelvis. The infraspinous fossa of rabbits is sharply triangular, whereas that of cats is more rounded; also, the suprahamate process of the acromion is truly hook-shaped in rabbits (Fig. 14–1), whereas it is blunted in cats. The acetabulum of rabbits is formed by the ilium, the ischium, and a

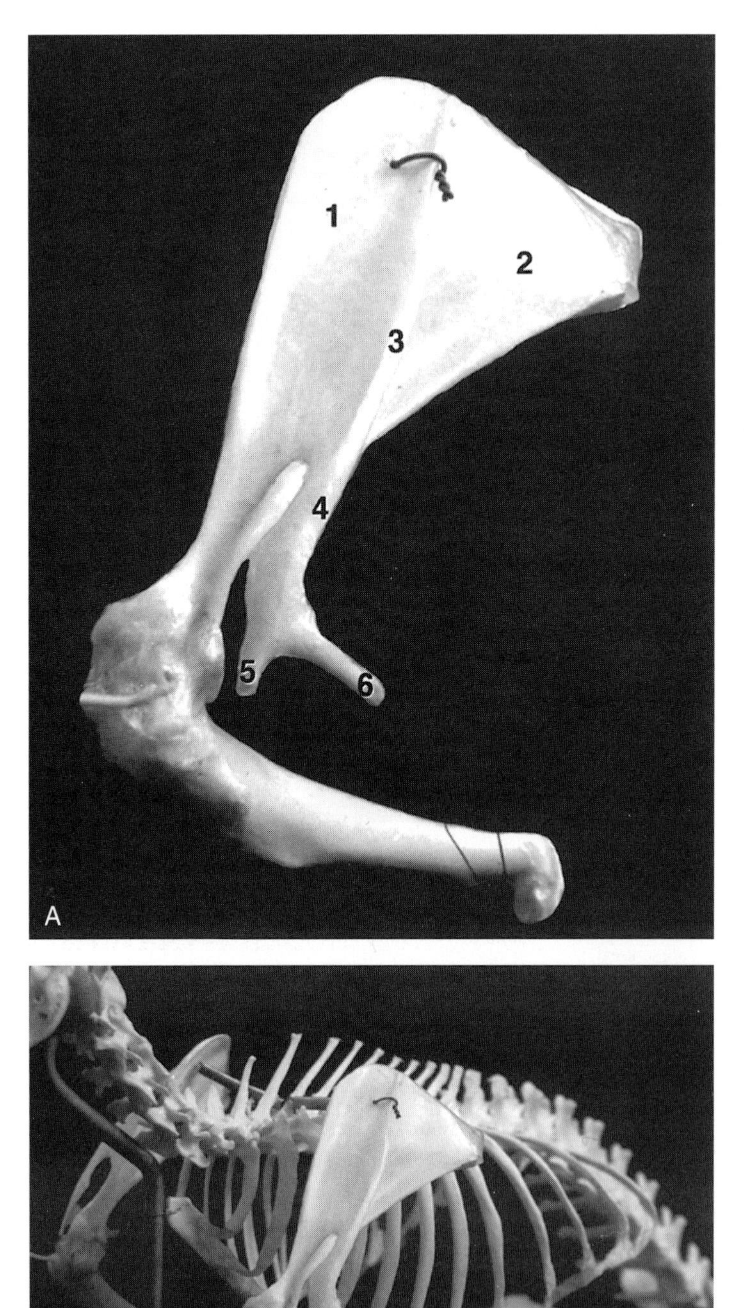

FIGURE 14–1

A, Lateral aspect of the left scapula of a rabbit. *B,* Skeleton of a rabbit showing the relationship of the left scapula to other bones.

Key to A: 1, supraspinous fossa; 2, infraspinous fossa; 3, spine of the scapula; 4, acromion; 5, hamate process; 6, suprahamate process.

small accessory bone, the os acetabuli, which excludes the pubis. In other animals, the acetabulum comprises the ilium, the ischium, and the pubis. Good drawings of these differences are found in Okerman's *Diseases of Domestic Rabbits.*[20]

The trochanteric fossa of the femur is a good site for intraosseous catheter placement and is easily located on palpation of the prominent greater trochanter.

Body conformation and ear size vary widely

among breeds of rabbits, and some unusual terms have been coined to describe types of lagomorph body shape and fall of ear. The small and chunky body of a dwarf rabbit, like a cobblestone, is referred to as "cobby"; the long and lean body of a Belgian hare is described as "racy"; and giant rabbits are often described as "mandolin-shaped" because of the high, curved topline over their hindquarters.[27] Most breeds of rabbits have upright ears, which can be long or short. However, some breeds have ears that hang downward; these are known as "lops."

DIGESTIVE SYSTEM

The definitive reference on the anatomy and physiology of the digestive tract of rabbits is Cheeke's *Rabbit Feeding and Nutrition.*[2] Most of the information described in this section is referenced from this book unless otherwise noted.

Oral Cavity

The mouth opening in rabbits is small, and the upper lip has a divided groove that continues by curving right and left to the nostrils—hence, the expression "harelip." Rabbits' teeth are curved, and the incisors and cheek teeth grow continuously. If the teeth are not aligned properly, they do not wear properly, and rabbits present with malocclusion problems, such as trouble with food prehension, or anorexia.

The muscles of the jaws extend both forward and backward. This confers a deceptively large appearance to the oral cavity, which is actually smaller than the size of the jaws suggests. The mandible is able to move forward, backward, and vertically but less so from side to side because the articular process forming the temporomandibular joint is longitudinally elongated.

Endotracheal intubation for anesthesia is not easily accomplished in rabbits because of their small mouth, large cheek teeth and tongue, and deep oral cavity. Relaxation of the jaw musculature signifies that the animal is sufficiently anesthetized for intubation. During intubation, it is easy to traumatize the oral and respiratory structures unless care is taken.[5]

Abdominal Cavity

The abdominal cavity of rabbits is large. The gastrointestinal tract is relatively long, and its contents can constitute 10–20% of the body weight. This is an important consideration when the appropriate dose of intravenous anesthetics is being determined. The two most striking organs in terms of their size are the stomach and cecum.

Stomach

The stomach serves as a reservoir for much of the ingested feed, and food and fecal pellets are almost always present in it. It is thin-walled and often appears ruptured at necropsy because of gas distention during autolysis. However, the cardia and pylorus are well developed. Rabbits are unable to vomit because of the anatomic arrangement of their cardia and stomach, and their pylorus is easily compressed by the duodenum, which exits at an acute angle. Gastric distention or compression caused by a furball, gas, or hepatomegaly contributes to pyloric compression and prevents emptying.

Small Intestine

The duodenum and jejunum have a relatively small lumen. The terminal portion of the ileum ends in the cecum and is expanded as the rounded sacculus rotundus. This structure has a minute honeycombed external appearance owing to the presence of a large number of lymph follicles and is sometimes referred to as the *ileocecal tonsil.* It is also a common site of foreign body impaction.[12]

Large Intestine

Rabbits have a large, thin-walled, coiled cecum (Fig. 14–2). It terminates in a thick-walled, pale vermiform appendix that is characterized, like the sacculus rotundus, by abundant lymphatic tissue. The cecum is the largest and most prominent organ in the abdominal cavity of rabbits. It folds onto itself three times as it coils around most of the inner surface of the abdominal cavity wall. The cecal contents are generally semifluid.

The colon is characterized by sacculations and the presence of bands. It starts from an area of cecum known as the *ampulla coli.* The proximal colon is separated from the distal colon by the *fusus coli,* a thickened section of colon heavily supplied with

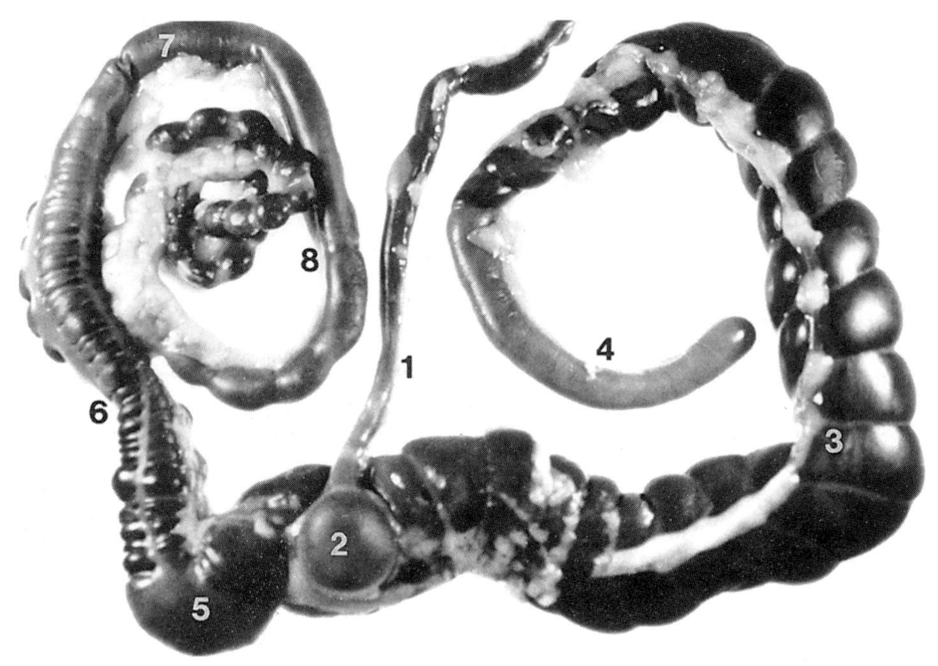

FIGURE 14–2
Dissected large intestine of a rabbit.

Key: 1, ileum; 2, sacculus rotundus; 3, body of cecum (note the long spiral fold along its length); 4, vermiform appendix; 5, ampulla coli; 6, proximal colon; 7, fusus coli; 8, distal colon.

ganglion cell aggregates that acts as a pacemaker for controlling the contractions for the excretion of the two types of feces.

Muscular contractions in the colon cause a separation of fiber particles from the nonfiber components of the feed. Peristaltic contractions rapidly move fiber through the colon for excretion in the hard feces. Antiperistaltic contractions move fluids and particles retrograde through the colon into the cecum, where they are retained for fermentation. At intervals, the cecum contracts and its fermentation contents are expelled through the colon and consumed directly from the anus by the rabbit. Thus, the products of bacterial growth are made available to the rabbit either by direct absorption or by consumption of the cecal contents. This latter process is known as *coprophagy* or *cecotrophy*. The consumed cecal contents are referred to as *soft feces, night feces,* or *cecotropes* and appear as a cluster rather than as the single pellets typical of hard feces. Cecotropes are surrounded by a mucilaginous membrane that acts as a barrier to the low pH of the stomach and that permits reabsorption in the small intestine.

Pancreas, Liver, and Gallbladder

Although closely associated with the duodenum, the pancreas of rabbits is diffuse and often difficult to differentiate from surrounding mesentery.

Rabbits have a small, circular hepatic lobe known as the *caudate lobe,* which has a narrow attachment or stalk to the dorsal, hilar region of the liver. This stalk is prone to displacement, and torsion of the caudate lobe has been infrequently reported.[9]

The gallbladder is located deceptively deep within the abdominal cavity from a midline approach. Like dogs, rabbits have separate openings for the bile duct and the pancreatic duct in the duodenum. They secrete mainly biliverdin in their bile, rather than bilirubin, as do most nonmammalian species.

RESPIRATORY SYSTEM AND THYMUS

Rabbits are obligate nose-breathers. This characteristic has important clinical and anesthetic consequences. Mouth-breathing is a poor prognostic sign, and inflammation of the upper respiratory tract enhances the risk of anesthetic mortality in nonintubated animals.

The thymus persists into adult life in rabbits. It retains considerable size, lies ventral to the heart, and extends forward to the thoracic inlet.

Rabbits have a relatively small thoracic cavity; in contrast, they have a large abdominal cavity and breathe primarily by contraction of the diaphragm. These characteristics allow for an efficient method of artificial respiration: suspend the rabbit horizontally in midair, holding the forelimbs in one hand and back legs in the other hand, and gently rock the rabbit from a head-up to a head-down position every 1–2 seconds.

CARDIOVASCULAR SYSTEM

As for many other organs of the body, the size of the heart is directly related to that of the body. Supplying the tissues with oxygen cannot be achieved with increases in the ventricular volume pumped out in one beat because this volume is limited by the heart's size. Instead, heart rate remains the major modifying variable, and as a consequence, small animals have higher heart rates than do larger ones. In rabbits, heart rate can vary from 180 to 250 beats per minute. Despite the small size and rapid contraction rate of rabbit hearts, quantitative Doppler echocardiographic methods have been validated for evaluation of their structural and functional abnormalities (Fig. 14–3).[15, 21, 28]

Rabbits have a relatively small heart, which comprises about 0.3% of body weight, and its right atrioventricular valve is unique because it is composed of two, rather than three, cusps. The rabbit aorta has a rhythmic contraction that is neurogenic in origin.

Muscle swellings in the pulmonary artery of rabbits make this vessel thicker and more muscular than it is in any other species. Death from anaphylaxis is caused by pulmonary hypertension, and at necropsy, severe constriction of the pulmonary arteries and dilation of the right side of the heart are observed.

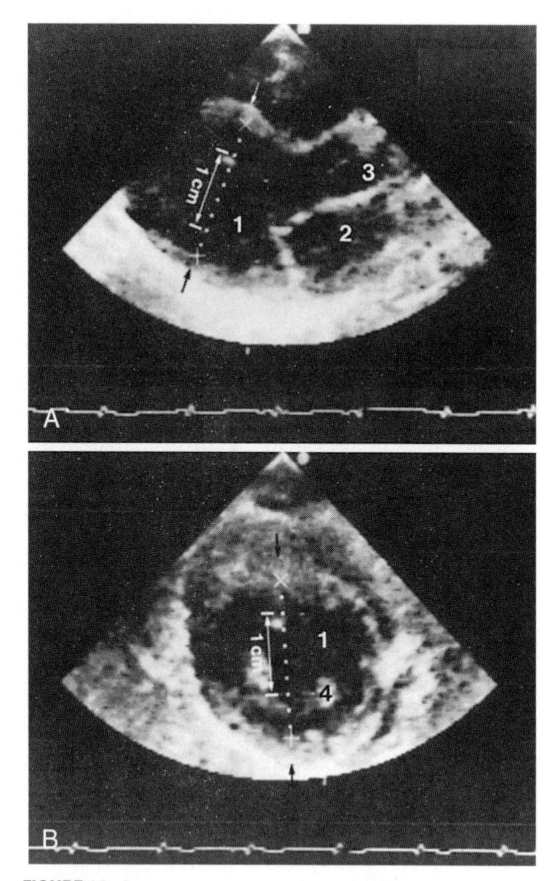

FIGURE 14–3

Two-dimensional echocardiographic long-axis *(A)* and short-axis *(B)* views of a rabbit with aortic regurgitation. Electrocardiographic signals were obtained simultaneously and are shown in the lower portions of the views. (Modified with permission from Young MS, Magid NM, Wallerson DC, et al: Echocardiographic left ventricular mass measurement in small animals: anatomic validation in normal and aortic regurgitant rabbits. Am J Noninvasive Cardiol 1990; 4:145–153.)

Key: 1, left ventricle; 2, left atrium; 3, aorta; 4, papillary muscle.

Rabbits' veins have thin walls and are susceptible to hematoma formation, which can be avoided through the judicious use of Teflon catheters and gentle pressure.

URINARY SYSTEM

Most mammalian kidneys are multipapillate, but those of rabbits and rodents are unipapillate. There is only one papilla and one calyx that enters the ureter directly.

The plasticity of the rabbit urinary system has not been fully recognized. Rabbits from Australian desert zones have large kidneys with powerful urine concentrating ability, small adrenal glands, and low levels of circulating aldosterone; rabbits from Australian alpine zones have small kidneys that are at least 25% less in weight, large adrenal glands, and high levels of circulating aldosterone.[17] At necropsy, the most striking difference is in the size of the renal medulla. In the desert-dwelling rabbits, which live on a high-fiber, high-salt, low-protein plant diet and which have limited access to water, the medulla is long. In contrast, in alpine rabbits, which enjoy a high-protein diet of lush grasses that are low in sodium, the renal medulla is short.

The capacity of the rabbit urinary system to vary its developmental pattern under different environmental conditions, combined with the various digestive strategies of rabbits, has probably accounted for these animals' successful colonization of diverse geographic regions.

Serum calcium levels of rabbits are unusual in that they are not regulated in a narrow range but rather reflect the level of dietary calcium. Urine is a major route of excretion for calcium and varies directly with serum calcium concentration. The consistency of the urine is often thick and creamy because of a white, calcium carbonate precipitate. Prolonged intake of diets high in calcium results in calcification of the aorta and kidney. Elevated vitamin D intake intensifies this effect.[13]

The color of normal rabbit urine varies from yellow to red because it contains pigments, which have not yet been identified. Certain types of feed such as alfalfa or a tropical legume in the genus *Leucaena* seem to increase the intensity of the pigmentation.[3] Rabbit owners often erroneously report the presence of blood in their pets' urine.

PUBERTY AND BREEDING LIFE

The age at which rabbits attain sexual maturity varies considerably, according to the breed. However, if the biologic pattern of growth is plotted graphically, puberty occurs just after maximal rate of growth. Sexual maturation occurs on the growth velocity curve where the rate of growth is decelerating rapidly. This means that body weight is more important than age in determining sexual maturity. Small breeds develop more rapidly and are mature at 4–5 months of age. Medium-sized breeds mature at 4–6 months, and large breeds reach maturity at 5–8 months of age.[22] Does mature earlier than do bucks, which do not achieve optimal sperm production and reserves until 40–70 days after puberty. Female New Zealand white rabbits reach maturity at approximately 5 months of age, and males at 6–7 months of age. The reproductive life of a rabbit again depends on its breed but is about 5–6 years for the buck and up to 3 years for the doe.

FEMALE REPRODUCTIVE SYSTEM AND BEHAVIOR

The reproductive tract of a doe lacks a uterine body; instead, each of two separate uterine horns has its own opening into the vagina (Fig. 14–4). If a cesarean section is performed, the fetuses must be removed through separate incisions in each horn. The mesometrium is a major fat storage site, and identification and ligation of the uterine vessels can be difficult.

Like cats and ferrets, rabbits are induced ovulators and do not have an estrous cycle. However, does vary in their sexual receptivity so that a certain rhythm can be ascertained; in domestic rabbits, this rhythm has been reported as intervals of 4–6 days. Ovulation occurs after coitus or after the injection of luteinizing hormone. The time of ovulation in induced ovulators varies among species. It is 10 hours after copulation in rabbits in contrast to 30 hours in cats and ferrets.

Sexual receptivity in a doe is characterized by lordosis, a reverse bending or flattening of the back, raising of the pelvis, or presentation of the perineum in response to attempts by a buck to mount. Similar behavior is seen in cats. Generally, female rabbits are hyperactive and brace themselves when touched. When not receptive, does do not allow males to mount. Depending on cage space, nonreceptive behavior often takes the form of running away, cornering, biting, and vocalizing.

In natural conditions, rabbits exhibit distinct breeding seasons that are influenced by both day length and temperature. In the northern hemisphere, rabbits in natural conditions exhibit their highest conception rate in spring and their lowest rate in autumn. When environmental conditions are controlled, male rabbits mate at any time. Maximal sexual receptivity in does is often accompanied by enlargement of the vulva, which also becomes reddish-purple and moist. Although females will al-

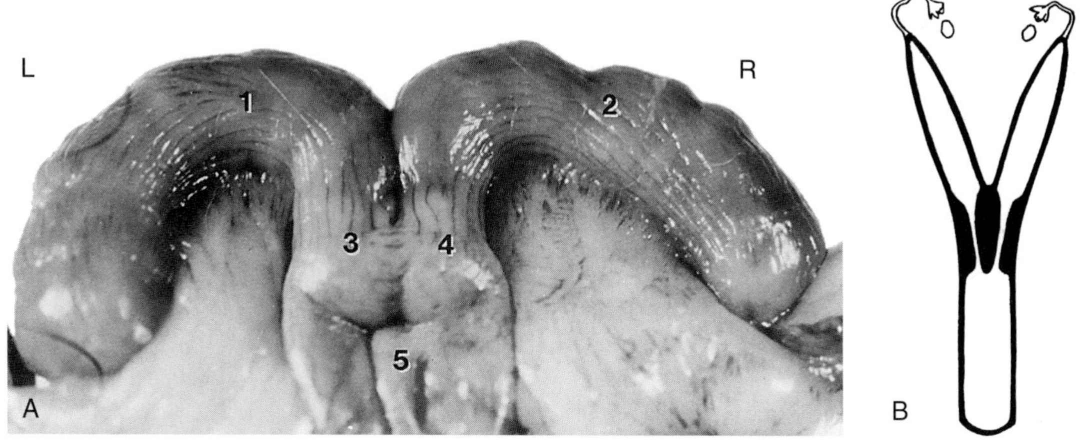

FIGURE 14–4

A, Dorsal surface of a dissected postparturient rabbit uterus. Note the abundant mesometrial fat, which makes identification and ligation of uterine vessels difficult. *B,* Diagrammatic representation of a doe's reproductive system showing two uterine horns and two cervices.

Key to A: 1, left uterine horn; 2, right uterine horn; 3, left cervix; 4, right cervix; 5, vagina.

most invariably mate in this condition, they also occasionally mate even when these changes have not occurred. Vaginal smears do not provide useful information. The most reliable indicator is lordosis that occurs when the female is firmly clasped in the lumbar region. Ovulation occurs between 10 and 13 hours after copulation. To ensure successful ovulation, many breeders give a single injection of 100 IU of human chorionic gonadotropin to does after mating to induce ovulation. Transportation of female rabbits may also result in spontaneous ovulation, with a resultant pseudopregnancy of approximately 18 days' duration.

The length of gestation in rabbits varies with the breed but is approximately 30–33 days. Litter size depends on the breed as well as on parity. Primiparous animals tend to produce smaller litters than they do in subsequent pregnancies. Small breeds such as the Dutch tend to produce small litters of 4–5 kits, whereas larger breeds such as the New Zealand white produce large litters of 8–12 kits.

Does usually give birth in the early morning. A few hours to days before kindling, rabbits pull fur from their abdomen, sides, and dewlap to make a nest. Although the underlying skin can look inflamed, this is normal behavior. The kits are born blind, helpless, and hairless and remain in the nest for about 3 weeks. Does nurse only once a day for 3–5 minutes. However, during this brief period, a young rabbit may drink 20% of its bodyweight. A healthy, well-fed litter bursts out of the fur covering like popcorn when the nest is examined. Olfactory cues are critical during the nursing period: a gland in the region of the nipple produces a pheromone that attracts kits; and does reject strange kits that do not smell the same as the rest of their litter. Successful cross-fostering requires healthy kits with the energy to suckle, and camouflaging of their scent by placement of the foster kits on the bottom of the litter and rubbing them in the nest bedding.[8]

MALE REPRODUCTIVE SYSTEM AND BEHAVIOR

The location of the two hairless scrotal sacs cranial to the penis is unlike that in most other placental mammals (in which scrotal sacs are caudal to the penis) but similar to that in marsupials. Rabbits do not have an os penis. The testes descend at about 12 weeks of age, and the inguinal canals do not close. The technique of choice for castration must take into account measures to prevent inguinal herniation.

Bucks show a constant libido after puberty. Initiation of copulation in rabbits is confined to basic patterns such as sniffing, licking, nuzzling, reciprocal grooming, and following of the doe. Bucks may also exhibit tail-flagging and enurination, the emission of a jet of urine at a partner during a display of courtship. Experienced males generally initiate copulation within minutes or even seconds after the introduction of a receptive female. Inexperienced males generally require a longer period of time.

The species-specific copulatory patterns of the male are related to ovulation and corpus luteum function in the female. Copulatory behavior of bucks may be understood by considering that the doe ovulates spontaneously after coitus. The stimulus of coitus is necessary only for ovulation and not the maintenance of corpus luteum function, which always follows ovulation. Bucks rapidly mount receptive females and accomplish intromission after a series of rapid copulatory movements. Reflex ejaculation follows immediately upon intromission. The copulatory thrust is generally so vigorous that the buck falls backward or sideways and may emit a characteristic cry. Vigorous bucks may attempt to copulate again within 2–3 minutes. A problem often encountered in male rabbits trained to use artificial vaginas is a reduced ability to induce lordosis during natural mating attempts. These conditioned bucks may become lazy. They fail to grasp and apply pressure to the flanks of the female when attempting to copulate and thus fail to induce lordosis.

Semen is deposited into the anterior vagina, and sperm passes as individual cells through the cervical mucus. This pattern also occurs in sheep, cattle, and humans. If a rabbit is inseminated during an active corpus luteal phase such as early pregnancy or pseudopregnancy, sperm transport does not take place. During this period, when blood progesterone levels are increasing in rabbits or in humans, the cervical secretions are thick and mucoid, and sperm transport is inhibited.

EATING AND DRINKING BEHAVIOR

Field studies on wild rabbits indicate that they are selective feeders with a wide food range. They prefer to eat tender, succulent plant parts as the major portion of their diet and consume small quantities of coarse roughage, which are believed to stimulate gastrointestinal motility. Rabbits chew their food thoroughly with highly organized tongue movements and up to 120 jaw movements per minute.[6] Nutritional studies in laboratory rabbits show that they are also adaptable to a high-roughage diet. Wild rabbits can consume a large volume of fiber without the need for a large gut because of the rapid digestive time. Furthermore, the relatively small gut does not interfere with the need for swift evasion of carnivorous predators.

The primary feeding times for rabbits are in the early morning and at night, with coprophagy commencing 3–8 hours after eating.[2] Rabbits like sweet materials and select diets containing molasses or sucrose over similar diets without added sugar.[2] This preference can be used to advantage when an anorectic rabbit is encouraged to eat, and medications are often given mixed with fruit jam.

Many pet owners feed their rabbits commercially available pelleted diets because they are convenient and balanced in their formulation. However, when pet rabbits are fed a diet of unlimited pellets, they become obese and develop chronically soft stools. Food restriction is practiced in some research laboratories in an effort to avoid these problems; 2- to 3-kg New Zealand white rabbits are fed 100–120 g of pelleted diet a day. Diet restriction in pet rabbits can lead to fur-pulling and gnawing of carpets, furniture, shoes, and sometimes fatally, electrical wires. Boredom and destructive behavior can be avoided through supplementation of the diet with fresh grass, hay, and a variety of vegetables, and by providing gnawing toys such as a small log from an untreated fruit tree or sturdy plastic animal toys.

Compared with other animals, rabbits have a high water intake. A rabbit's average daily water intake is 50–150 mL/kg of body weight, and a 2-kg rabbit drinks about as much water daily as does a 10-kg dog.[4] When food is withheld from rabbits, they develop polydipsia, and after 3 days of food deprivation they can increase their water intake by six and a half times.[1] With water deprivation, food consumption declines; after 3 days of deprivation, anorexia results.[4]

HUSBANDRY

Rabbits can be kept indoors or outdoors. An indoor pet rabbit can be either caged most of the time and let out for supervised exercise and play or can be given free range of a rabbit-proofed room. Because rabbits are quarry for carnivores, they seek hiding places when frightened; in the wild, the burrow is the primary haven, but other above ground hiding places are used in emergencies. If a pet rabbit is given free range in a house, it should still have a cage or box in which to escape.

Rabbits generally have clean habits, depositing their feces and urine in the same place each time. They can be trained to use a litter tray, if they are constantly placed in the litter tray every few minutes when first acquired. However, adult bucks deposit strong-smelling feces in scattered places to mark out their territory. Rabbits like to chew and scratch objects found in a home; two of the greatest hazards are electrical cords and poisonous plants. Electrical wires should be placed out of reach of rabbits. The decorative house plant dumbcane *(Dieffenbachia seguinae)* and the ornamental shrub oleander *(Nerium oleander)* are poisonous to rabbits.[2,3]

The area that a rabbit occupies in a cage can be divided into two functional spaces: a space for lying and sleeping, and a space for activities. An indoor rabbit that has free range requires a cage only large enough to stretch out in when lying on its side. A cage with a plastic bottom and a wire top is suitable because it can be easily cleaned and is well ventilated. The base of the cage can be covered with a layer of straw or shavings that should be changed daily. Glass terraria used for reptiles are not suitable for rabbits because they are poorly ventilated. If two or more pet rabbits are kept indoors, each animal should have its own separate cage because fighting can result when two rabbits are in the same cage.

Pet rabbits can be kept together in the same space with different pets as long as the other animals adapt to the rabbits. Pet birds such as parakeets cohabitate well with rabbits; well-behaved dogs also tolerate pet rabbits; cats are often unpredictable and generally should not be left alone with rabbits. Pet guinea pigs are often kept in the same household as rabbits, but this is not a good practice. Rabbits may carry *Bordetella bronchiseptica* without any ill effects; however, this organism is pathogenic for guinea pigs.

Outdoor rabbits should be housed in properly constructed hutches that provide shade and shelter from wind and cold below 4°C. Plans for the construction of hutches are available from libraries, feed manufacturers, or agricultural extension agents; assembled cages are available from farm supply stores or mail order houses that advertise in rabbit breeding journals. Professional and trade journals in laboratory animal science also advertise caging, but such caging is generally the most expensive. Space to move around in the hutch is important, and the space required for a rabbit to complete three hops is the minimum recommended length.[14] A fully grown New Zealand white rabbit moves forward 1.5–2.0 m in three hops. The hutch should also be tall enough for a rabbit to stand up on its hind legs. Laboratory rabbits have been observed to climb onto raised platforms and shelves placed 2 m above the cage floor; these have been used successfully for rabbit housing.[14]

Indoor and hutch rabbits can feed on lawn by means of a grazing ark. The ark can be a metal lid from an indoor rabbit's cage or a solid frame with wire mesh (Fig. 14–5). Move the grazing ark every day to a fresh area of grass. There should be a shaded area within the ark, and the ark should be pegged down so that the rabbit cannot tip it upward. Weedkillers used on lawn can be poisonous to rabbits.

Does primarily dig burrows, and only pregnant or pseudopregnant females attempt to dig very deep tunnels.[14,20] Appropriate bordering of gardens in which rabbits are kept with 30-cm concrete plates or wire mesh prevents unwanted escapes. Penned rabbits often dig shallow holes in which they lie or sleep; if fresh, green food is hidden in a heap of hay or a pile of soil, rabbits will root it out, and this redirects the digging behavior.

Rabbits tolerate cold better than heat. They shiver when exposed to cold because they do not possess brown fat. Shivering works well on a short-term basis, and rabbits are able to tolerate cold weather if properly acclimatized and sheltered. Rabbits are unusually sensitive to elevated temperatures greater than 28°C (82.4°F) and have little protection against high ambient temperatures. They cannot sweat, except through sweat glands confined to the lips; also, they pant ineffectively, and when sufficiently dehydrated, they stop panting. Rabbits do not increase water intake when the ambient temperature becomes high; heat actually seems to inhibit drinking. Although rabbits use their ears as organs to dissipate heat, they actively seek shade and burrow to achieve water conservation and relief from heat. Rabbits develop only a mild increase in pulse rate in response to an increase in body temperature. Shelter from direct sunlight is essential in the design of any rabbit housing.

The response of rabbits to high and low ambient temperatures is also important during transportation, and the risk of mortality is greater in hot

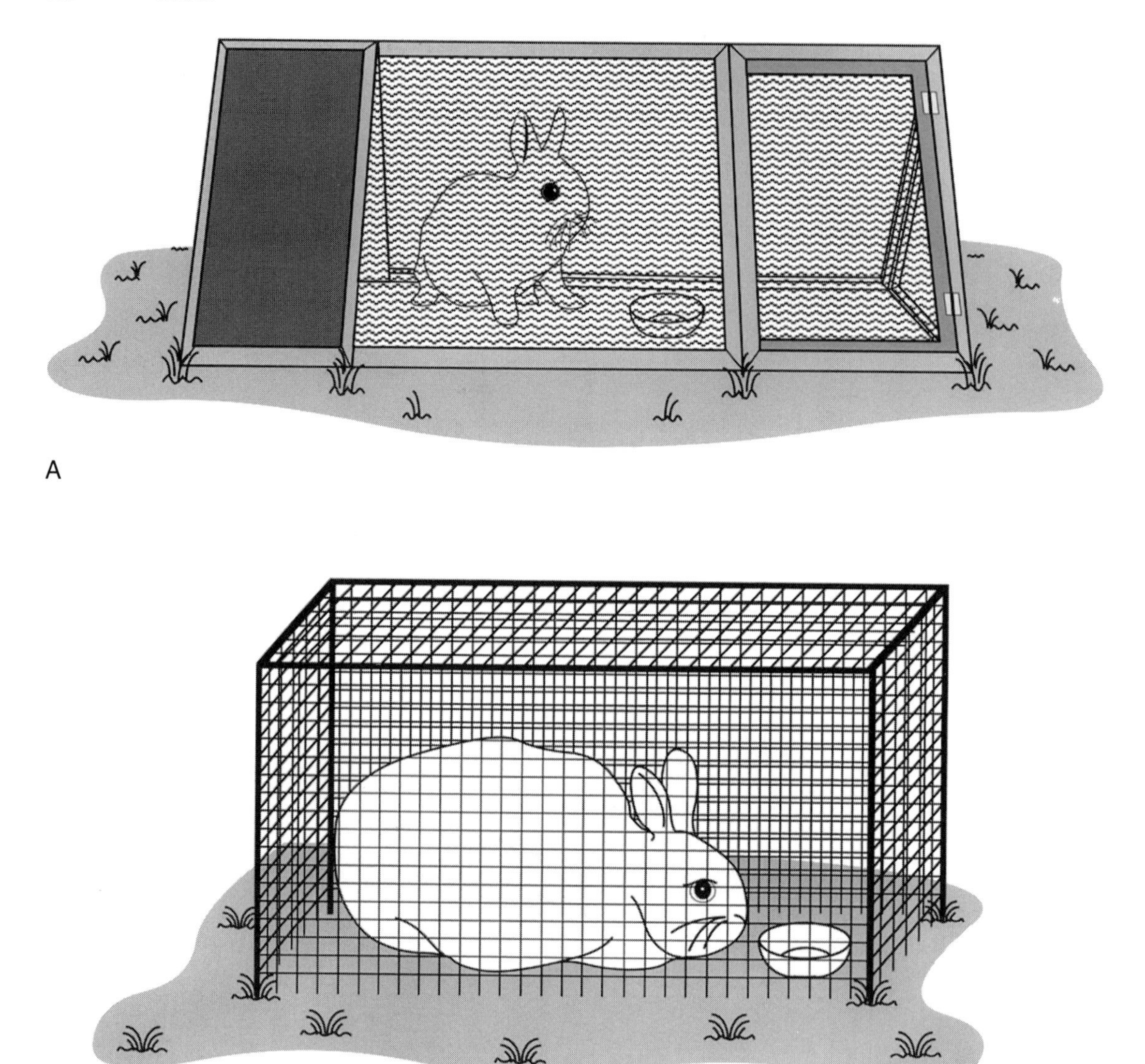

FIGURE 14–5

A grazing ark can be constructed from a solid frame and wire mesh *(A)*. Alternatively, the metal lid from an indoor rabbit's cage can be used as a small grazing ark *(B)*.

weather or in the presence of excessive indoor heating than in cold weather.

REFERENCES

1. Brewer NR, Cruise LJ: Physiology. *In* Manning PJ, Ringler DH, Newcomer CE, eds.: The Biology of the Laboratory Rabbit. 2nd ed. Orlando, FL, Academic Press, 1994, pp 63–70.
2. Cheeke PR: Rabbit Feeding and Nutrition. Orlando, FL, Academic Press, 1987, pp 15–33, and 160–175.
3. Cheeke PR, Patton NM, Lukefahr SD, et al: Rabbit Production. 6th ed. Danville, IL, The Interstate Printers and Publishers, 1987, pp 246–247.
4. Cizek LJ: Relationship between food and water ingestion in the rabbit. Am J Physiol 1961; 201:557–566.
5. Conlon KC, Corbally MT, Bading JA, et al: Atraumatic endotracheal intubation in small rabbits. Lab Anim Sci 1990; 40:221–222.
6. Cortopassi D, Muhl ZF: Videofluorographic analysis of tongue movement in the rabbit *(Oryctolagus cuniculus)*. J Morphol 1990; 240:139–146.
7. Cruise LJ, Brewer NR: Anatomy. *In* Manning PJ, Ringler DH, Newcomer CE, eds.: The Biology of the Laboratory Rabbit. 2nd ed. Orlando, FL, Academic Press, 1994, pp 47–61.
8. Donnelly TM, Kelsey SF, Levine DM, et al: Control of variance in experimental studies of hyperlipidemia using the WHHL rabbit. J Lipid Res 1991; 32:1089–1098.
9. Evering W, Edwards JF: Hepatic lobe deformity in a rabbit. Lab Anim 1992; 21:14–16.
10. Herrold EM, Goldweit RS, Carter JN, et al: Noninvasive laser-based blood pressure measurement in rabbits. Am J Hypertens 1992; 5:197–202.

11. Hoyt Jr RF, Powell DA, Feldman SH: Exophthalmia in the rabbit after chronic external jugular cathether placement. Contemp Top Lab Anim Sci 1994; 33:A19.
12. Jenkins JR: Rabbits. *In* Jenkins JR, Brown SA, A Practitioner's Guide to Rabbits and Ferrets. Lakewood, CO, American Animal Hospital Association, 1993, p 7.
13. Kamphues VJ, Carstensen P, Schroeder D, et al: Effect of increasing calcium and vitamin-D supply on calcium metabolism of rabbits. J Anim Physiol Anim Nutr 1986; 50:137–146.
14. Love JA: Group housing: meeting the physical and social needs of the laboratory rabbit. Lab Anim Sci 1994; 44: 5–11.
15. Magid NM, Opio G, Wallerson DC, et al: Heart failure due to chronic experimental aortic regurgitation. Am J Physiol 1994; 267:H556–H562.
16. Meng J, Wyss AR, Dawson MR, et al: Primitive fossil rodent from Inner Mongolia and its implications for mammalian phylogeny. Nature 1994; 370:134–136.
17. Myers K, Parer I, Richardson BJ: Leporidae. *In* Walton DW, Richardson BJ, eds.: Fauna of Australia: Mammalia. Vol. 1B. Canberra, Australia, Australian Government Publishing Service, 1989, pp 917–931.
18. Mykytowycz R: Territorial marking by rabbits. Sci Am 1968; 218:116–126.
19. Novacek MJ: Mammalian phylogeny: shaking the tree. Nature 1992; 356:121–125.
20. Okerman L: Diseases of Domestic Rabbits. 2nd ed. Oxford, Blackwell Scientific Publications, 1994, pp 10–13.
21. Okin PM, Donnelly TM, Parker TS, et al: High frequency analysis of signal-averaged ECG: correlation with left ventricular mass in rabbits. J Electrocardiol 1992; 25:111–118.
22. Patton NM: Colony husbandry. *In* Manning PJ, Ringler DH, Newcomer CE, eds.: The Biology of the Laboratory Rabbit. 2nd ed. Orlando, FL, Academic Press, 1994, pp 28–45.
23. Popesko P, Rajtova V, Horak J: A Color Atlas of the Anatomy of Small Laboratory Animals. London, Wolf Publishing, 1992.
24. Prince JH: The Rabbit Eye in Research. Springfield, IL, Charles C. Thomas, 1964.
25. Prince JH, Diesem CD, Eglitis I, et al: Anatomy and Histology of the Eye and Orbit in Domestic Animals. Springfield, IL, Charles C. Thomas, 1960, pp 260–297.
26. Render JA: Comparative ocular anatomy. Presented at a histopathology seminar on the eye and ear of laboratory animals sponsored by the International Life Sciences Institute, Washington, DC, San Diego, November 1992.
27. Williams CSF: Practical Guide to Laboratory Animals. St. Louis, CV Mosby, 1976.
28. Young MS, Magid NM, Wallerson DC, et al: Echocardiographic left ventricular mass measurement in small animals: anatomic validation in normal and aortic regurgitant rabbits. Am J Noninvasive Cardiol 1990; 4:145–153.

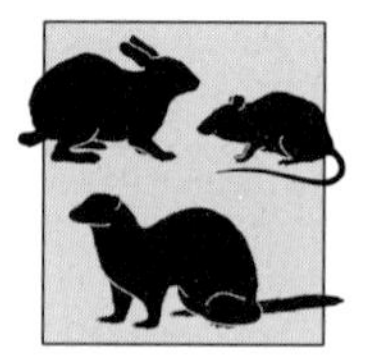

CHAPTER 15

Basic Approach To Veterinary Care

Douglas R. Mader, DVM

Few alterations need to be made to an existing veterinary practice for accommodating rabbits. Most of the challenges involve additional training for staff regarding husbandry, handling, and laboratory sample collection.

HOUSING

Housing requirements are readily met. Hospitalized rabbits can be kept in stainless steel cages designed for dogs and cats, or in hutch cages. The latter can be easily and inexpensively made or are readily available from pet or feed stores. Hutch cage units can also be adapted for use as tabletop cages with built-in catch pans or can be suspended with wire, as is commonly done in multianimal rabbitries. Cage floors should be constructed of 14-gauge wire mesh. The mesh openings should be rectangles no greater than 1 × 2.5 cm in size. This opening size facilitates cleaning, allows feces to drop through the cage floor, and is not so large that a rabbit might accidentally get its foot stuck. A portion of the floor should be solid so that there is a place for resting and to help prevent the rabbit's hocks from becoming sore.

If hospitalized rabbits are housed in standard stainless steel small animal cages, place a towel, a thick, roughly textured cage paper, or some other type of nonskid surface (not newspaper) on the bottom of the cage. A better alternative is providing the rabbit with a cage rack so that urine and feces can be separated from the patient. These racks also provide the appropriate nonslip surface.

Keep a supply of good-quality feed available for hospitalized rabbits. Rabbits can be finicky eaters, so check with the owner before hospitalizing a rabbit to find out what foods the rabbit prefers. If the diet is poor, it may be necessary to offer the rabbit some of the food to which it is accustomed while gradually introducing a more appropriate diet. A rapid change of diet, even a change from a poor diet to a proper one, may cause gastrointestinal upset and anorexia (see Chapter 16).

Fresh water should always be available. Consult with the owner to learn what type of watering system the rabbit is accustomed to. Rabbits easily learn to drink from sipper bottles. These should be cleaned daily. If water crocks are used, they should be of heavy ceramic so that they are not easily tipped over. Bowls with high sides are recommended because rabbits tend to hang their dewlap in the water when they drink. If the sides of the bowl are too low, this chronic wetting can lead to "wet dewlap" disease, which is an easily preventable moist dermatitis that is most often associated with colonization by *Pseudomonas* species.

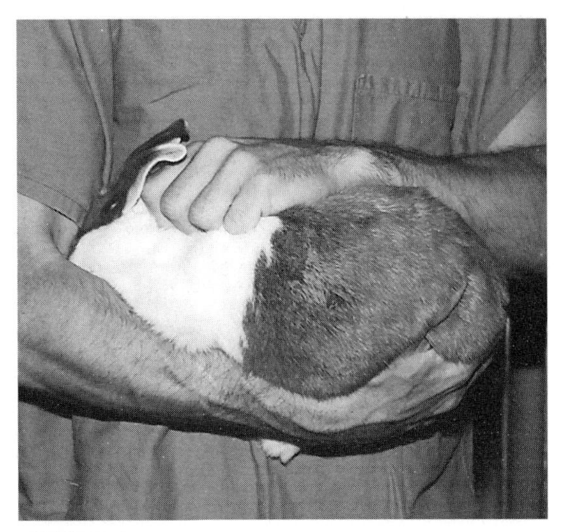

FIGURE 15–1
Proper technique for carrying a rabbit. Its head is tucked under one arm, and the back and feet are supported with the other.

HANDLING, RESTRAINT, AND PHYSICAL EXAMINATION

Rabbits have a relatively delicate skeleton that accounts for only 8% of their total bodyweight compared with 13% for cats of comparable size. In contrast, the muscles of rabbits are extremely strong and well developed for running. As a result, an improperly handled rabbit that kicks out or struggles is at risk of fracturing its long bones and spine.

Rabbits should never be picked up by their ears. Rather, they should be grasped by the scruff with one hand and have their hindquarters supported with the other. Never let a rabbit's rear legs dangle while carrying it.

When transporting a rabbit for any distance, tuck its head under your arm as if you were carrying a football (Fig. 15–1). With its head and eyes covered, the rabbit remains quiet and relaxed. This hold gives the handler extra security should the rabbit struggle or kick.

Cover the examination table with a nonslip surface such as a large heavy towel before placing the rabbit on the table. If a rabbit is placed on a Formica or stainless steel surface, it may slip and kick while trying to gain its footing and possibly break its back. Smaller hand towels are easily kicked off the table, making the examination even more difficult than if a bare table were used. An additional benefit to this technique is that it shows clients that you are taking special precautions with their pets.

During the examination, always maintain control of the rabbit. A rabbit often jumps off the table for no apparent reason. One method of restraint involves holding the rabbit with your forearm around it and tucking it into your abdomen as you stand against the table's edge. With this method, one hand is free to examine the patient, palpate the abdomen, and use any clinical instruments. When you are finished with one side, gently turn the patient end for end, using two hands, and examine the opposite side. If a two-handed palpation is required, tuck the rabbit's hindquarters into your abdomen and with its nose facing away from you, and hold on with both hands while palpating.

To examine the ventrum, gently roll the rabbit onto its back and cradle it like a baby in one arm, using the hand to support the rear legs (Fig. 15–2). The other hand is then free to do the examination. This position is also recommended for taking the rectal temperature. With your free hand, gently insert the lubricated probe into the rectum. Avoid using a glass thermometer as it can easily break if the rabbit should struggle. Electronic pediatric rectal thermometers are inexpensive, sturdy, and safe and record the patient's temperature more rapidly and accurately than their glass counterparts.

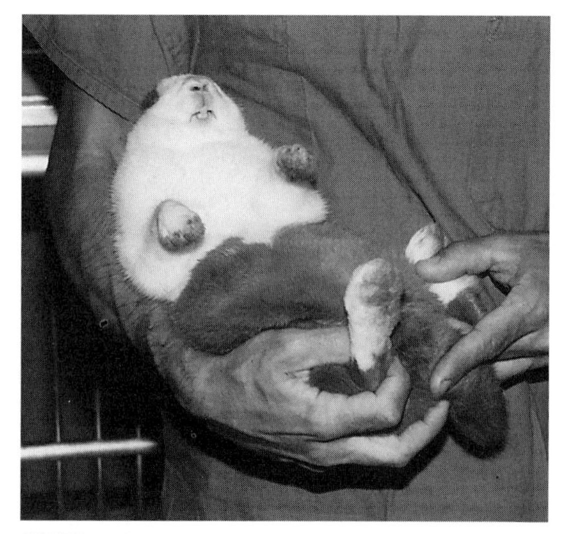

FIGURE 15–2
Cradling of a rabbit for examination of the ventral abdomen.

Perhaps the most difficult part of the physical examination is the evaluation of the rabbit's oral cavity. Rabbits do not like to have their mouths touched or manipulated. An assistant usually is needed to help with restraint, using the method described for a two-handed palpation. Have the assistant stand at the other side of the examination table so that the rabbit is facing you.

If an assistant is not available, roll the rabbit up in a soft towel, "burrito style," to facilitate examination and to provide the necessary restraint without using undue force. Commercial rabbit restraint devices are available and are used commonly in laboratory animal facilities (Fig. 15–3). These devices are made of stainless steel or plastic but tend to be very costly. An inexpensive alternative is a nylon cat bag, which is used in most small animal practices. A cat bag is especially useful when a rabbit must be restrained for the collection of laboratory samples or for doing minor procedures (Fig. 15–4).

A cursory oral examination is possible with your hands. Digitally palpate the jaws and lips. Gentle retraction of the lips allows access to the buccal area, the incisors, and the interdental region. Gently insert an otoscope cone through the interdental area to examine the tongue, hard palate, and molars. Use a dedicated ear cone, as the rabbit's sharp incisors will damage the outside of the cone, making it unusable for aural examinations.

Another method for oral examination is with a stainless steel oral speculum made for use in birds. Insert the narrow end of this instrument between the interdental region of the rabbit's mouth and gently turn it until the mouth gapes open. If a larger field of view is needed, the speculum can be slowly inserted to its next larger size. Examination can be enhanced with the use of a small light source, such as a transilluminator or penlight.

Be systematic and thorough when doing a physical examination and always follow the same procedure. Collect appropriate physical data such as body temperature, pulse rate, and respiratory rate. Start at the nose and work backward or follow any pattern to which you are accustomed. Special areas of concern in rabbits are the ears (mites are a common problem), the teeth (malocclusion and overgrown

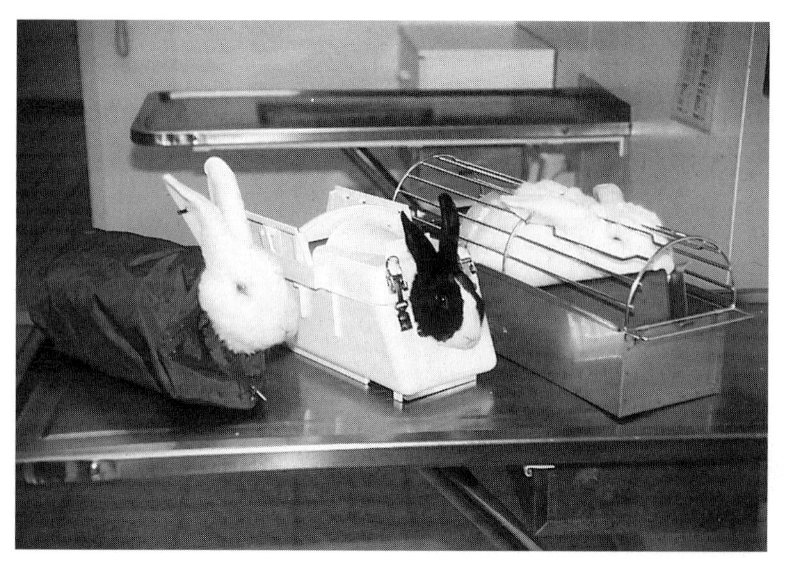

FIGURE 15–3
Rabbit restraint devices. The nylon bag is effective, inexpensive, and easy to store. Commercially available restrainers are very effective but are expensive and require a lot of storage space.

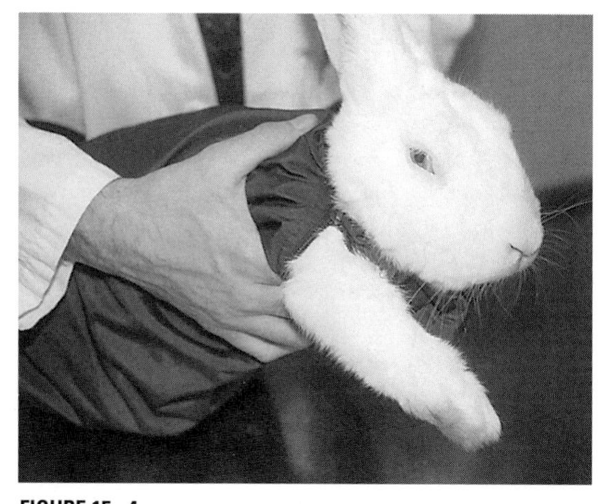

FIGURE 15–4
Nylon cat restraint bags have zippers that allow handlers to gain access to necessary veins for blood sampling or IV catheter placement.

molars), and the hocks (chronic abrasions from cage floors).

When placing a rabbit back into its cage, always return it caudal end first (i.e., with its head facing you when you release it; Fig. 15–5). This technique decreases the chance that the rabbit will kick when it is released. When a rabbit is released head first, its first reaction when its front feet are on the cage floor is to kick away. If the rabbit does not have its footing, it can easily slip.

Chemical restraint sometimes is needed for a thorough oral examination, positioning of the patient for radiography, or the collection of laboratory samples (see Chapter 32). Ketamine hydrochloride administered at 20 mg/kg IM produces adequate relaxation for most minor procedures. For longer procedures or when greater relaxation is needed, the dose is increased to 25–40 mg/kg IM and combined with acepromazine (1 mg/kg IM), diazepam (5–10 mg/kg IM, or 1–2 mg/kg IV) or xylazine (3–5 mg/kg IM; see also chapter 32).

For long procedures, give rabbits a volatile anesthetic such as isoflurane or halothane. Isoflurane is preferred and is the safest gas anesthetic in rabbits. Anesthesia can be administered by face mask; alternatively, and preferably, the patient can be intubated. Intubation is a difficult procedure in rabbits because of the deep, caudal placement of their glottis. However, with practice, the veterinarian can intubate most rabbits, with a blind technique or with the aid of either a curved neonatal laryngoscope or an otoscope cone and a stylet. Intubation is recommended for any involved or prolonged procedures. Premedication with ketamine and diazepam or acepromazine decreases the concentration of anesthetic gas needed and allows smoother induction.

CLINICAL TECHNIQUES

Venipuncture

Several different venipuncture sites can be used for blood collection in rabbits. These include the marginal ear vein, the central ear artery, the jugular vein, the cephalic vein, and the lateral saphenous vein. The marginal ear vein and the central ear artery are readily accessible even in the small Dutch breeds (Fig. 15–6). However, a possible sequela of ear

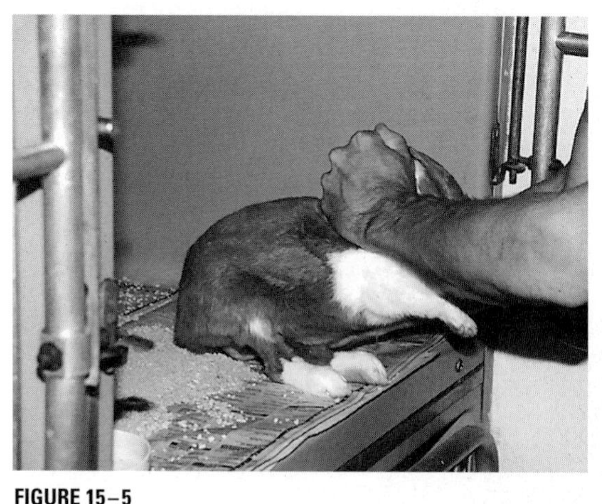

FIGURE 15–5
Proper placement of a rabbit back into its cage, rear end first.

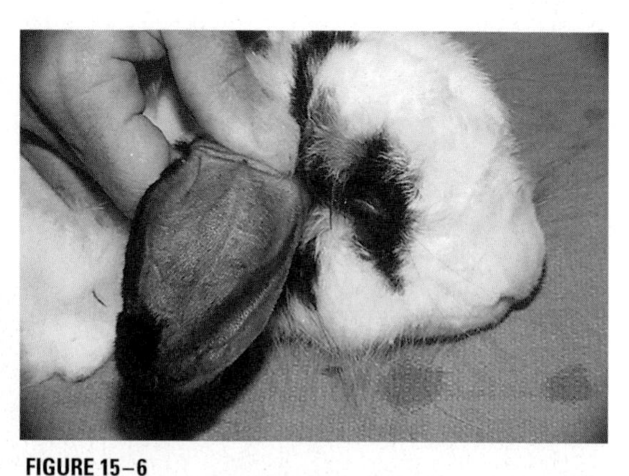

FIGURE 15–6
Ear vessels in a rabbit. The central ear artery or marginal ear veins can be used for collecting blood.

venipuncture is thrombosis of the vein, with subsequent sloughing of the skin. This is most common in breeds with small ears and very small veins.

For venipuncture, shave or gently pluck the fur over the vessel. Rub or tap the area with your finger to dilate the vein. Clean the skin with a mild soap or an alcohol wipe. If the vessel is not yet dilated, hold the ear in your hand for a few minutes, or wrap a warm cloth around the ear. Penetrate the vein with a small 25- or 27-gauge needle. Allow the blood to drip from the needle hub and free catch it in an appropriate collection tube (Fig. 15–7). Use of a syringe or Vacutainer tube generally collapses the vessel, but these instruments can be used on large-eared rabbits.

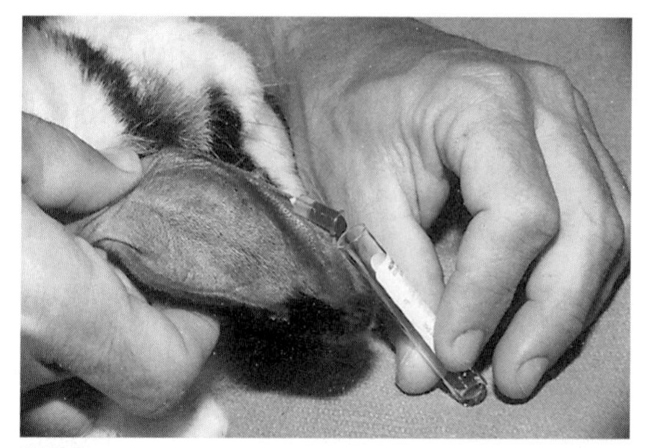

FIGURE 15–7
Collecting a small blood sample from the marginal ear vein.

Rabbits have accessible cephalic veins. However, small breeds have a short antebrachium, and the vessel can be difficult to locate and hold off. When easily visible, these veins are a good site for venipuncture.

Another vein that is commonly used for blood collection is the lateral saphenous vein (Fig. 15–8). This vein is readily accessible as it courses from medial to lateral diagonally across the lateral aspect of the tibia. Blood can be withdrawn quickly and easily from this vein, especially in large rabbits. For venipuncture, the rabbit is restrained on its side, with the assistant holding off the vein just above the hock joint.

Rabbits have large paired jugular veins. A number of methods are suggested for jugular blood collection, but I have found that the easiest technique includes some form of sedation, either with injectable tranquilizers or isoflurane administered by face mask.

Shave and prepare the neck area over the midtrachea cranial to the thoracic inlet. With the patient in dorsal recumbency, have your assistant hold the rabbit on the worktable with its head over the edge, grasping the rabbit's body with one hand and pulling the front feet back toward the rear with the other. Take the rabbit's head with your free hand and gently tip it back to expose the ventral neck region. In all but the most grossly obese rabbits, the jugular veins should be readily apparent (Fig. 15–9). Large amounts of blood can be readily collected from this position. Jugular venipuncture can be done without sedation in many rabbits. For this procedure, restrain the rabbit as you would a cat, with the rabbit held at the edge of a table, the front legs held down, and the head extended up. Pluck or shave the fur from the jugular furrow to enhance visibility of the vein. This technique may be difficult in does with large dewlaps. Use your thumb to push the dewlap ventrally and hold off the jugular vein at the same time. This technique should expose a short section of neck (and raised jugular vein) above the dewlap.

Cardiocentesis is commonly used in research for collection of large blood samples or for exsanguination under anesthesia. However, this method should

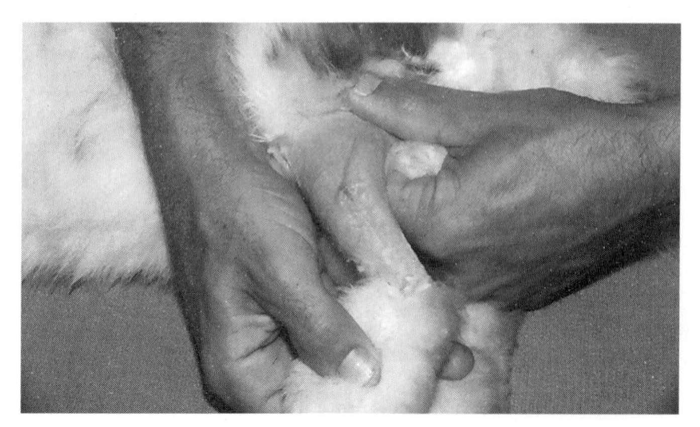

FIGURE 15–8
The lateral saphenous vein of a rabbit is easily accessible for venipuncture or catheter placement.

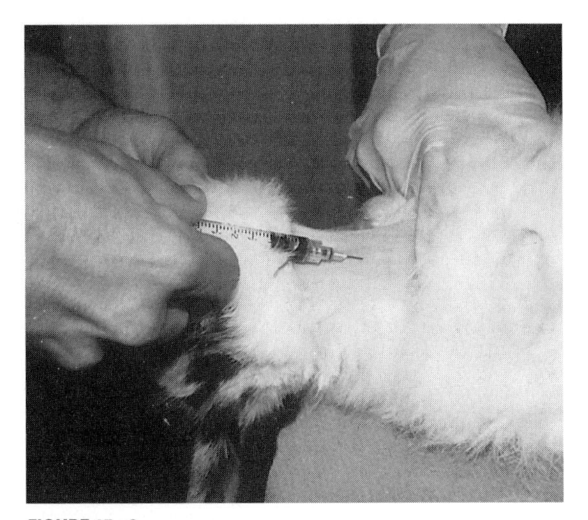

FIGURE 15-9
Two-person restraint for jugular venipuncture in a rabbit. The rabbit is restrained in a nylon cat bag.

not be used in clinical patients for blood collection because of the inherent risks of myocardial damage, cardiac tamponade, and death.

Reference ranges for hematologic and serum biochemistry values are presented in Tables 15-1 and 15-2.

TABLE 15-2
REFERENCE RANGES FOR SERUM BIOCHEMISTRY VALUES IN THE RABBIT

Serum protein	5.4-8.3 g/dL
Albumin	2.4-4.6 g/dL
Globulin	1.5-2.8 g/dL
Glucose	75-155 g/dL
Blood urea nitrogen	13-29 mg/dL
Creatinine	0.5-2.5 mg/dL
Total bilirubin	0.0-0.7 mg/dL
Cholesterol	10-80 mg/dL
Total lipids	243-390 mg/dL
Calcium	5.6-12.5 mg/dL
Phosphorus	4.0-6.9 mg/dL
Sodium	131-155 mEq/L
Potassium	3.6-6.9 mEq/L
Chloride	92-112 mEq/L
Bicarbonate	16-38 mEq/L
Amylase	166.5-314.5 U/L
Alkaline phosphatase	4-16 U/L
Alanine aminotransferase (ALT)	48-80 U/L
Aspartate aminotransferase (AST)	14-113 U/L
Lactic dehydrogenase	34-129 U/L

Adapted from Quesenberry KE: Rabbits. *In* Birchard SJ, Sherding RG, eds.: Saunders Manual of Small Animal Practice. Philadelphia, WB Saunders, 1994, p 1346.

Cystocentesis

Urinalysis is a useful diagnostic tool in rabbits. Interpreting samples is often difficult because of the sometimes heavy but normal mineral or pigment content of the urine. Samples can be collected by cystocentesis with a method similar to that used in cats. Cystocentesis can be done without tranquilization in most rabbits.

TABLE 15-1
REFERENCE RANGES FOR HEMATOLOGIC VALUES IN THE RABBIT

Erythrocytes	5.1-7.9 × $10^6/\mu L$
Hematocrit	33-50%
Hemoglobin	10.0-17.4 g/dl
Mean corpuscular volume	57.8-66.5 μm^3
Mean corpuscular hemoglobin	17.1-23.5 pg
Mean corpuscular hemoglobin concentration	29-37%
Platelets	250-650 × $10^3/\mu L$
Leukocytes	5.2-12.5 × $10^3/\mu L$
Neutrophils	20-75%
Lymphocytes	30-85%
Monocytes	1-4%
Eosinophils	1-4%
Basophils	1-7%

Adapted from Quesenberry KE: Rabbits. *In* Birchard SJ, Sherding RG, eds.: Saunders Manual of Small Animal Practice. Philadelphia, WB Saunders, 1994, p 1346.

Have an assistant stretch the patient by holding the scruff in one hand and the rear legs in the other. After appropriate preparation of the antepubic region, collect the urine with a small-diameter needle (23- to 25-gauge) attached to a sterile 6-mL syringe.

After collection, analyze the sample with standard laboratory techniques. Reference ranges for urinalysis values are presented in Table 15-3.

Cerebrospinal Fluid Tap

Occasionally, the collection of cerebrospinal fluid may be indicated. Perform the tap with the patient under anesthesia, using techniques similar to those employed in cats. The best site to collect spinal fluid is the cisterna magna.

Position the rabbit in lateral recumbency with the head flexed toward the chest. Shave the fur on the nape of the neck from the occipital protuberance to

TABLE 15–3

REFERENCE RANGES FOR URINALYSIS VALUES IN THE RABBIT

Urine volume	
Large	20–350 mL/kg per d
Average	130 mL/kg per d
Specific gravity	1.003–1.036
Average pH	8.2
Crystals present	Ammonium magnesium phosphate, calcium carbonate monohydrate, anhydrous calcium carbonate
Casts, epithelial cells, or bacteria present	Absent to rare
Leukocytes or erythrocytes present	Occasional
Albumin present	Occasional in young rabbits

From Quesenberry KE: Rabbits. *In* Birchard SJ, Sherding RG, eds.: Saunders Manual of Small Animal Practice. Philadelphia, WB Saunders, 1994, p 1346.

the level of the third cervical vertebra and laterally past the margins of the atlas.

The cranial margins of the wings of the atlas and the occipital protuberance are the landmarks for needle placement. The 22-gauge, 1.5- to 3.5-inch spinal needle should enter the skin midway between these points and be directed toward the patient's nose. A stylet is usually not necessary because of the relatively small size of most rabbits. After the needle has penetrated the dura and arachnoid membranes, watch carefully for the appearance of spinal fluid. After placement is confirmed, attach a manometer or syringe and proceed with diagnostic tests. Reference values for constituents of cerebrospinal fluid in rabbits are presented in Table 15–4.

TREATMENT TECHNIQUES

Intravenous Catheter Placement

Many hospitalized rabbits can be treated effectively with maintenance fluids administered SC. However, rabbits that are azotemic, in shock, or critically ill should be given fluids by the IV route. All of the vessels mentioned for venipuncture can also be used for venoclysis. Simple injections are easily administered into the cephalic or the saphenous vein. Prolonged infusions, such as those used with IV fluid therapy, should be given through indwelling catheters.

Although small-bore IV catheters can be used for the marginal ear veins, sloughing of the ear tips can occur even with the short-term placement of catheters. This may result from chemical phlebitis caused by solutions or medications infused into the delicate ear veins, mechanical irritation from the catheter itself, or aggressive taping of the catheter to the ear.

Larger veins, such as the cephalic, the saphenous, and the lateral thoracic veins in does (Fig. 15–10), are better suited for catheter placement. Large jugular catheters can be inserted, but the insertion procedure often requires sedation or anesthesia.

In an emergency or when a rabbit is severely dehydrated and its peripheral veins are collapsed, fluids can be administered intraosseously. Intraosseous catheters are best placed in the greater trochanter of the femur. With the rabbit sedated, clip the fur over the head of the femur and prepare the skin for surgery. Wearing a sterile glove, palpate the top of the greater trochanter with your finger. Pass the needle (the size of which depends on the size of the patient but can vary from 18 to 23 gauge and from 1 to 1.5 inch in length) directly through the top of the trochanter, parallel to the long axis of the

TABLE 15–4

VALUES FOR CONSTITUENTS OF RABBIT CEREBROSPINAL FLUID

Constituent	Concentration
Glucose	75 mg/dL
Urea nitrogen	20 mg/dL
Creatinine	17 mg/dL
Cholesterol	33 mg/dL
Total protein	59 mg/dL
Alkaline phosphatase	5.0 U/dL (Kings-Armstrong)
Carbon dioxide	41.2–48.5 mL%
Sodium	149 mEq/L
Potassium	3.0 mEq/L
Chloride	127 mEq/L
Calcium	5.4 mg/dL
Magnesium	2.2 mEq/L
Phosphate	2.3 mg/dL
Lactic acid	1.4–4.0 mg/dL
Nonprotein N	5.6–16.8 mg/dL

From Weisbroth SH, Flatt RE, Kraus AL: The Biology of the Laboratory Rabbit. New York, Academic Press, 1974, p 65.

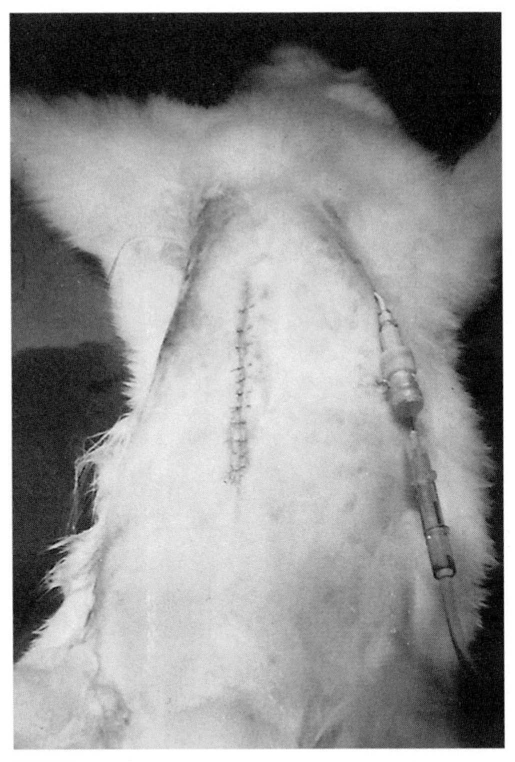

FIGURE 15–10
An IV catheter placed in the lateral thoracic vein. This large vein is easy to catheterize. The catheter port is sutured to the skin over the access area.

femur, and into the medullary cavity. Flush the needle gently with sterile saline and attach a male adapter. Apply an antimicrobial ointment to the insertion site and place a light dressing over the entire unit. Administer replacement fluids by slow drip into this needle. When the patient has been adequately rehydrated, the intraosseous catheter can either be replaced with an IV catheter or removed.

Most rabbits tolerate peripheral catheters well. Occasionally, an Elizabethan collar is needed to prevent a rabbit from chewing on or pulling out a catheter. Avoid using collars in very sick or stressed animals if possible.

Fluid selection and the principles of fluid therapy can be based on those used in other small mammals. However, the exact fluid requirements of rabbits are not well worked out, especially those in sick rabbits. The role of the cecum, the amount of ongoing fluid loss, and the disease process all may be factors in daily fluid maintenance requirements. Therefore, calculate the quantities of maintenance fluids on the basis of the normal water consumption of adult rabbits, which is 50–150 mL/kg per day (see Chapter 14 for discussion of water intake in rabbits), or use an average amount of 60–100 mL/kg per day. Divide the total calculated fluid volume into three equal treatments or give fluids by continuous infusion. Use an infusion pump or a Buretrol device for fluid administration in small rabbits.

Injection Techniques

Injection techniques in rabbits are similar to those used in cats. Administer SC injections over the scruff or laterally, just cranial to the hips. Give IM injections into the large lumbar muscles on either side of the spine, just cranial to the pelvis. One person can easily do this by tucking the rabbit under an arm as if carrying it. Before penetrating the skin with the needle, squeeze the rabbit gently with your arm to prevent it from jumping during injection.

Exercise caution when giving IM injections in the rear leg because of the risk of damaging the ischiatic nerve, especially when certain drugs such as ketamine are used. It is best to give all injections into the cranial aspect of the rear leg in the quadriceps muscle group.

Oral Medications

Administering pills to rabbits is difficult. One method involves the insertion of the pill into the oral cavity through the diastema. If the medication is relatively palatable, such as enrofloxacin (Baytril, Miles Inc., Shawnee, KS), a rabbit may chew and swallow it. Oral medications are best given in suspension form. Many drugs that are available only in tablet form can be made into suspensions by compounding pharmacists for use in rabbits. Alternatively, crush the pill and mix it with jam or a paste nutritional supplement. Place oral medication as far back in the oral cavity as possible to prevent the rabbit from spitting it out.

Nasogastric Tubes

Nasogastric tubes are sometimes indicated for management of anorectic rabbits. The technique used for placement is similar to that used in cats. Premeasure an infant nasogastric tube by placing it against the rabbit and estimating the position of the stomach.

Mark the end of the tube where it should exit the nasal opening. Place several drops of a topical ophthalmic anesthetic, such as proparacaine (Ophthaine, Solvay Animal Health, Inc., Mendota Heights, MN), into the nasal mucous membranes, or use xylocaine gel. After several minutes, introduce the nasogastric tube into the nasal meatus, directing it caudad and dorsally. If the rabbit objects, withdraw the tube and instill more anesthetic into the nasal opening. After passing the tube, secure the tube by applying a butterfly piece of tape and suturing it to the top of the rabbit's head, between the ears. Check the placement of the tube by taking a radiograph of the thorax in a lateral view. Once the tube has been inserted correctly, place an Elizabethan collar on the rabbit to prevent it from pulling the tube out with its feet. Nutritional supplements used must be in liquid form so that they can pass easily through the tube. Lactose-free soy-based supplements such as Deliver (Mead Johnson, Evansville, IN) work well.

VACCINATIONS

Currently, no vaccines are routinely given in pet rabbits.

GENERAL REFERENCES

Brown SA: Husbandry, restraint, diagnostic sampling and surgical techniques in the rabbit. Proceedings of the Atlantic Coast Veterinary Conference, October 1993.

Harkness JE, Wagner JE: The Biology and Medicine of Rabbits and Rodents. 4th ed. Baltimore, Williams & Wilkins, 1995, pp 13–30.

Krauss AL, Weisbroth AH, Flatt RE, et al: Biology and diseases of rabbits. *In* Fox JG, Cohen BJ, Loew FM, eds.: Laboratory Animal Medicine. Orlando, FL, Academic Press, 1984, pp 207–240.

Manning PJ, Ringler DH, Newcomer CE: The Biology of the Laboratory Rabbit. 2nd ed. San Diego, Academic Press, 1994.

Quesenberry KE: Rabbits. *In* Birchard SJ, Sherding RG, eds.: Saunders Manual of Small Animal Practice. Philadelphia, WB Saunders, 1994, pp 1345–1362.

Weisbroth SH, Flatt RE, Kraus AL: The Biology of the Laboratory Rabbit. New York, Academic Press, 1974.

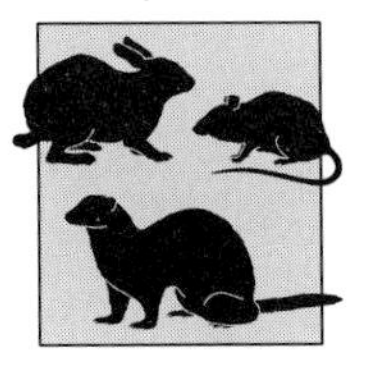

CHAPTER 16

Nutrition and Gastrointestinal Physiology

Dale Brooks, DVM, PhD

In natural habitats, rabbits are a frequent prey species for predators. Their primary and first survival reaction is to be very still in an effort to avoid detection. They have adapted to "fight or flight" by developing sensitive hearing and an acute sense of smell as well as a light skeleton, small forelimbs, and powerful, well-developed hindquarters, which make possible rapid bursts of speed and quick changes of direction for short distances. These survival reactions still exist in most domestic rabbits that appear stoic, but these rabbits respond poorly to disturbances and are easily stressed by change. Stressed animals are more susceptible to health, reproductive, and behavioral problems, which initially result in anorexia and changes in the frequency and consistency of their fecal pellets.

GASTROINTESTINAL PHYSIOLOGY

The Role of Fiber

Dietary fiber primarily stimulates gut motility rather than serving as a source of nutrition. Wild rabbits prefer to be browsers, eating the more succulent buds and young leaves of bushes, but they easily adapt to grazing on grasses, weeds, and the bark around bushes and trees in arid and wintery environments. It is interesting that anorectic and diarrheic rabbits often select foods such as hays, grasses, and straw before alfalfa pellets. These naturally chewed roughages result in a larger, coarser particle than do the commercially milled alfalfa meal–based pellets. Fiber or particle size, referred to as the "scratch factor" by French rabbiters, is important in normal digestion; coarse, nondigestible particles stimulate normal gastrointestinal processes of cell regeneration, secretion, digestion, absorption, peristalsis, and excretion.

Principles of Digestion

The teeth of rabbits are developed for a high-fiber, herbivorous diet. The dental formula is $2(I\frac{2}{1}\ C\frac{0}{0}\ P\frac{3}{2}\ M\frac{3}{3}) = 28$. A small second set of incisors sits just behind the larger upper incisors. Chewing is characterized by a lateral motion, which helps keep the constantly growing teeth worn down to their proper occlusal surfaces. Malocclusion secondary to mandibular prognathism, a recessive genetic trait, results in overgrown teeth.[10] Malocclusion occurs frequently with the incisors, but is also seen with the premolars and molars and is somewhat analogous to horses that need their teeth floated. Malocclusion of the premolars and molars is common in middle-aged to older animals and may result from many factors. It leads to overgrowth and sharpening of the lateral (upper arcade) and the medial (lower arcade) edges.

Rabbits have a simple stomach with a relatively small, nondistensible lumen and a well-developed muscular pyloric sphincter. These features along with their inability to vomit and their self-licking grooming behavior, increase the incidence of gastric trichobezoars, or "hairballs," especially when they are fed a diet low in fiber.[8] The hairballs may occlude the pyloric sphincter or the first few centimeters of the small intestine.[1]

Once ingesta enters the small intestine, the fiber moves rapidly through the intestine while the remaining digestible suspension of small particles and those of heavier specific gravity separates (as occurs from the rumen to the reticulum), passes from the ileum, and concentrates in the haustra of the proximal colon. By a reverse peristaltic action, the haustra's contents are returned to the cecum for a more efficient fermentation and concentration of proteins, amino acids, and volatile fatty acids (Fig. 16–1).[4] The digestive process in the rabbit differs from the usual cecal and colonic fermentation process in other animals in that fiber is eliminated as rapidly as possible. This rapid separation of fiber and concentration of energy for cecal fermentation more readily conforms to rabbits' small size and high metabolic rate; in comparison, the hindgut fiber fermentation process is more suited to horses' greater size.[3]

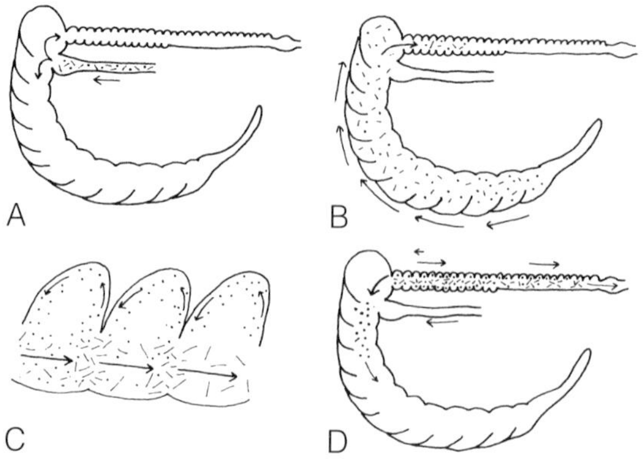

FIGURE 16–1
Mechanisms for the selective excretion of fiber and retention of small particles and solubles for fermentation in the cecum. *A*, Intestinal contents enter the hindgut at the ileocecal-colonic junction and uniformly disperse in the cecum and colon. *Dashes* represent large fiber particles, and *dots* represent nonfiber particles. *B*, Contraction of the cecum moves material into the proximal colon. *C*, Peristaltic action moves large fiber particles *(dashes)* down the colon for excretion as hard feces. Contractions of the haustrae of the colon move small particles *(dots)* and fluids backwards into the cecum. *D*, Small particles and fluids are thus separated from fiber. (From Cheeke PR, Grobner MA, Patton NM: Fiber digestion and utilization in rabbits. J Appl Rabbit Res 1986; 9:25–30.)

The well-developed large cecum of rabbits is adapted for microbial hindgut fermentation, which digests starches and fiber. The cecal production of carbohydrates and nitrogenous substances, along with cecal goblet cell mucin production, supports abundant microbial synthesis. Cyclic segmental contractions of the cecum carry the contents rapidly through the large bowel,[23] with the resultant production of cecotropes. This process is variously referred to as "hindgut fermentation," "pseudorumination," or "coprophagy," and the cecal output is referred to as "soft feces," "night feces," or "cecotropes."[21]

Coprophagy is practiced by rabbits, most rodents, and a variety of other animals.[22] It is part of rabbits' normal circadian behavior, beginning during the second and third week of age, when the kits start to consume solid food.[9] Hard, round fecal pellets are excreted during the day, and the seldom observed soft fecal pellets at night, most often during the early morning hours.[15] These night feces are small, soft, sweet-smelling cecotropes that are the size of a pea. The cecotropes have an outer greenish membrane of mucus that encloses semi-liquid cecal ingesta; they contain high levels of vitamins B and K with twice the protein and half the fiber of hard feces. The coprophagic rabbit eats these soft cecal droppings directly from its anus; they resemble a bunch of light green sheen-covered peas in the rabbit's stomach.[6,12] This "pseudorumination" process for redigestion helps in the absorption of previously undigested nutrients and reinoculates the gut with essential nutrients. In this way, portions of ingested food may pass through the gastrointestinal tract twice during a 24-hour period.

Once reingested into the stomach, the cecotropes remain intact up to 6 hours with continued bacterial synthesis. As the mucus layer dissolves, most of the cecal bacteria are lost to the low pH environment of the stomach. Occasionally, a cecotrope passes intact into the intestine. This circadian coprophagic behavior occurs only in healthy rabbits, and it helps them to survive periods during which no food is available as well as in different habitats—from snowy mountains to arid deserts, and over periods of droughts and severe storms.[13]

Microbial Flora

The rabbit possesses several interesting gastrointestinal characteristics. The suckling feeds for only 3–5 minutes once every 24 hours.[24] Suckling rabbits are unique among nursing neonates, having a stomach and intestine devoid of living microorganisms.[19] Normally, kits have a fully distended stomach filled with a firm milk curd. This milk curd and its relatively high pH (5.0–6.5), which in other species supports a luxuriant growth of gastrointestinal flora within the first days of life,[2] does not support such growth in rabbits.[18,20] Rabbits have so-called "milk oil," an antimicrobial fatty acid distinct from that of secreted gastric acids. This antimicrobial fatty acid is produced from an enzymatic reaction with a substrate in the doe's milk in a suckling rabbit's stomach. This special physiologic adaptation controls the gastrointestinal microbial contents of young rabbits. Rabbits fed milk from other species do not develop this antimicrobial factor and are more susceptible to infections.[2]

Up to 21 days of age, the neonates' diet is derived from nursing; after the first 21 days, they start coming out of the nest to explore and nibble. Over the next 4–6 weeks, young rabbits lose the guarding "milk oil" factors and gradually develop the mature antimicrobial stomach pH of 1–2. Depending on the type of diet, available microorganisms, and stress, the kits' sterile gut may not be colonized with a normal flora and instead may become overgrown by infective organisms that can cause enteroxemias.

The few microorganisms that pass through a young rabbit's stomach "milk oil" and the adult's low gastric pH gradually undergo a logarithmic increase in their growth rate as they pass through the small intestine. With normal peristalsis, the ingesta is quickly deposited in the cecum and colon, where the first significant flora growth and hindgut fermentation flora appear in the rabbit.

The ileum forms the transitional zone between the upper small intestine, where few bacteria are present, and the lower intestine, where there are large numbers of bacteria. The cecum and colon have well-established indigenous numbers of strict anaerobes (*Bacteroides* species) and fewer facultative anaerobes. The results of microbiologic analyses may be confusing; in many diarrheas, no pathogens are detectable (use anaerobic techniques and test for toxins), and so-called "enteric" pathogens often are cultured from asymptomatic rabbits. Many diarrheas are the result of microbial overgrowth, into the small intestine, of inhabitants of the lower intestine.[1,3,5,8]

The most important factor in the bacterial pathogenesis of rabbit diarrhea is the establishment of an infective dose of intestinal pathogens. The common rabbit enteropathogens *Escherichia coli* and *Clostridium spiroforme* are not infective as long as their numbers are small. With overgrowth, these organisms become invasive or produce toxins. Factors that further decrease immunity and the host's ability to respond are an inadequate amount of the "milk oil," a higher than normal pH, inadequate consumption of fiber, an unbalanced diet (especially one low in fiber, high in protein, and with excessive amounts of carbohydrates), poor sanitation, and stress, especially during the weaning age.[7] The delicate balance of intestinal transport of water is also altered by minor shifts in solute fluxes induced by microfloral changes.

Normally, consumed microorganisms never reach an infective dose in the small intestine because they succumb to the antimicrobial factors in the rabbit's stomach. Experimental data show that gastric pH is higher in diarrheic rabbits, with an average pH of 3–7, than in normal controls, with a pH of 1–2.[1]

Normal peristalsis is achieved with the ingestion of a high-fiber diet, which provides a large particle size and which results in a lattice-like food ball for effective gastric acid penetration. Incomplete penetration of gastric acid may occur with the use of alfalfa meal–based pellets, which have small particle sizes, resulting in the production of a more dense, hard-packed food ball, especially in rabbits with marginal water consumption. A large food ball, often found in the stomachs of the largest and greediest of rabbits, may not allow complete penetration of gastric acid, thus enabling an infective dose of microorganisms to enter the intestine. The normal peristalsis of the small intestine, aided by a high-fiber diet, quickly flushes ingesta into the cecum, reducing microbial colonization. Low-fiber diets decrease peristalsis; this increases passage time, and with the limited indigenous microflora of the small intestine, large numbers of potentially pathogenic bacteria can quickly proliferate. It is interesting that rabbits digest fiber poorly even though it is a critical dietary component essential to the stimulation of normal peristalsis and the control of gut transit time.

The use of therapeutic antibiotics, especially gram-positive and anaerobic spectrum drugs, may produce a dysbiosis (unbalanced flora). Experimental oral inocula of *E. coli* and *C. spiroforme* usually do not produce diarrhea unless the stomach pH is neutralized with 10 mL of 10% sodium bicarbonate solution (to raise the gastric pH), or unless antibiotics are administered before the inoculation, reducing the competitive protection of indigenous intestinal flora.[1]

NUTRITION

Pellets

Commercially milled alfalfa meal–based pellets are the predominant feed for rabbits. The pellets' fiber content ranges from a low of 10–12% to a high of 20–22%, with the average content being 15–16%. The protein content averages 16–18%, with a low of 12–14% to a high of 22–24%. The feed with higher protein levels, used for maximal growth and weight gains in meat production rabbits, often has a lower fiber content in order to increase its palatability. However, feeding high-protein and low-fiber feeds also causes increased morbidity and mortality from diarrhea. The most successful pellet rations for commercial rabbits have a fiber content of 16% and a reduced protein content of 16%. A fiber content below 15% may increase the potential for anorexia and diarrhea, and one over 16% reduces feed palatability. A higher fiber content (18–22%) helps to prevent obesity in pet rabbits and is useful for mature long-term–use laboratory animals. A protein content of up to 18% may be safely fed for achieving extra weight gain in meat production rabbits and for the conditioning of show rabbits.

The free-choice feeding of pellets often increases the incidence of overeating, obesity, and diarrhea. Providing a measured daily pellet intake is the preferred feeding practice for domestic rabbits. An adequate dietary intake for the average adult New Zealand white rabbit (8–10 lbs) should be 4–6 oz (approximately ½–1 cup) of pellets per day, or 120–180 g of pellets for a 3.6- to 4.5-kg rabbit. Sedentary pet rabbits should be fed less (⅛–½ cup/day, depending on size).

Lactating does and growing young should be fed as much as they will eat each day. A feeding routine is successful when no pellets are left in the food hopper at the next feeding. This can be accomplished by following the "5/5 feeding schedule": 5 days after birth, increase the amount of pellets given by 5 oz (150 g) and by an additional 5 oz each succeeding 5-day period thereafter. Cut back on the number of pellets provided only when excess pellets remain at the next feeding. Waiting 5 days after parturition prevents milk overproduction and reduces the incidence of mastitis ("caked breast"), milk fever, and ketosis. By the time they are 5 days of age, healthy kits have developed a full appetite and will depend on a milk diet up to 21 days of age. Increasing the amount of pellets in the doe's diet is continued in 5-oz increments each 5 days of the litter's age until the doe is receiving 25 oz (750 g) of pellets (when the kits are 3 weeks old). At the age of 3 weeks, the kits are starting to crawl and tumble out of their nesting box and begin to nibble at the pellets, decreasing their dependence on their dam's milk. This is a good time to record litter weights as a measure of the dam's milk production (for use in culling and selection breeders).

The rabbit owner must evaluate how much to continue increasing and decreasing the number of pellets by monitoring the amount left in the feeder until the average weaning age of 42 days is reached. At weaning, rabbit owners often move the weanlings to an unfamiliar new cage; this adds further stress to the weaning process. It is less stressful to remove the dam and leave the weanlings in a familiar cage until they are selected for future use, separated by sex, or butchered at about 60 days of age.

Hay

Most show and commercial as well as some pet rabbits do well on a diet of alfalfa meal–based pellets measured daily. However, many pet rabbits, especially older sedentary animals, do better on a limited pellet diet supplemented with hay and a few greens. Some rabbits, especially those of the Angora breeds, fare better on a free-choice hay diet supplemented with a few vegetables. The quality of hay varies tremendously with regions, seasons, and farming techniques, and it is difficult to generalize on what is the best type of hay and on differences in nutritional content. Overall, the most economical and readily available hay is alfalfa.

Some rabbitries claim that alfalfa hay is too high in calcium and should not be fed as a further supplement to an alfalfa meal–based pelleted diet. However, alfalfa is the major feed source for many rabbits, and there is little validity to the contention that alfalfa hay alone is harmful to a healthy rabbit. However, problems with excessive calcium in the urine are seen in some pet rabbits, especially those given excessive vitamin or mineral supplements (see later in this chapter) or sedentary obese animals.

Timothy hay is often suggested to be the best for rabbits. It can be expensive and frequently is not available in many regions of the United States. The grain hays, primarily oats and barley, may also be hard to find. The clover hays are frequently musty and dusty. When available, the local grass hays are the best buy for pet rabbits.

Remember that the dietary requirements vary, according to the age and use of a rabbit. A balance of timothy and grass hay and vegetables may be the best diet for some pet rabbits; in contrast, meat production and most show rabbits do well on a commercially produced alfalfa meal–based pellet (16–18% protein and 16% fiber) for reproduction, lactation, and growth. *Mature* laboratory rabbits as well as pet rabbits do better on a higher fiber (18%) and lower protein (14%) diet, which helps reduce obesity, diarrhea, and hairball problems.

In conclusion, the overall best pet rabbit diet is a measured daily alfalfa meal–based pellet with a hay supplement provided daily and a treat of "greens," or a free-choice hay diet with vegetable supplement.

Other Nutritional Considerations

Other components of rabbit nutrition need to be considered. A dietary fat component of up to 8% increases pellet palatability, especially that of the high fiber ones, and helps to decrease dustiness and crumbling of pellets.[3] Proper feed storage and quick use prevent rancidity. Synthetic antioxidants and vitamin E are often added to increase shelf life. Excess dietary fat, such as that provided by milk supplements, may increase the incidence of arteriosclerosis, which occurs as whitish-yellow arterial wall plaques especially noticeable in the aorta. Some strains of rabbits have a genetic predisposition to arteriosclerosis and may develop these plaques even on a fat-free diet.

Vitamin A deficiency may result in infertility, resorptions, abortions, stillbirths, neonatal mortality, and central nervous system defects such as hydrocephalus. Conversely, an excess of vitamin A can also cause hydrocephalus when fresh alfalfa pellets, already high in vitamin A, are further supplemented with a vitamin-mineral premix that is high in vitamin A.[3]

The vitamin B complex is adequately synthesized by the hindgut fermentation and the consumption of cecotropes.[14]

Pellets high in calcium or containing excessive vitamin D can occasionally produce gross signs of dystrophic calcification.[11] The normal color and consistency of a rabbit's urine can vary from a clear straw color to a cloudy-milky color to a reddish-brown color, depending on the animal's diet. Rabbits uniquely absorb all of the dietary calcium from their intestines and excrete the excess in the urine; this can result in a chalky-white, cream-colored urine. Excess calcium may cause urinary lithiasis or excessive excretion of calcium "sand," especially when rabbits are overly supplemented with some types of greens, weeds, and vitamin-mineral mixes. Urinary calculi can occur in the kidneys, ureters, and urinary bladder (see Chapter 19). Urolithiasis and excessive calciuria are seen most commonly in pet rabbits, probably because of dietary management and their more frequent presentation to veterinarians. Most alfalfa meal–based diets provide more than enough calcium, and further supplementation is not needed.

Vitamin E deficiencies can cause infertility, resorptions, abortions, stillbirths, neonatal mortality, and muscular dystrophies.[17] Selenium does not seem to be involved as it is in some other species with white muscle–type dystrophies.

Some rabbitries suggest providing dietary copper at a supplemented level of 400 ppm for increasing weight gains and reducing diarrhea in commercial fryer rabbits.[16]

All commercial feeds should have a mill location and date of manufacture clearly printed on the bag. Optimally, the feed sacks should be stored at 15.5°C (60°F) in a vermin-proof area and fed within 90 days of the milling date. Never purchase more feed than can be used in the shortest convenient period of time. Food over 6 months old has a compromised nutritional quality and reduced shelf-life, especially during the hot summer months. Refrigeration should be available for perishable vegetables, greens, and fruits. Grass clippings, weeds, and the outer leaves and tops of vegetables may be contaminated with fertilizers, insecticides, herbicides, feces, and urine that can result in intoxications, infections, and an unbalanced diet when present in excess. Available greens are often the outer leaves and therefore are more likely to be contaminated. A good rinse in fresh water before feeding is advised. Some greens are primarily water and have little nutrient value; thus, they should be fed only as a special treat or as an appetite stimulant.

Commercial animal feeds may become contaminated with antibiotics found as residue in milling apparatus that previously was used to mix a batch of medicated feed. A few approved commercial rabbit pellet formulations contain low levels of sulfaquinoxaline for coccidia control and low levels of tetracycline for growth stimulation. Remember the legal liabilities of drug administration because rabbits may be used for human consumption and presently there are no governmental approvals for residue withdrawal times. Also, some antibiotics may disrupt the balance of the intestinal flora, resulting in dysbiosis, anorexia, diarrhea, and death.

Water

Rabbits need access to water at all times. A rabbit can go for several days without feed, relying on coprophagy. However, it cannot endure a lack of water for longer than 24 hours, or less in hot weather. Potable water should be free of harmful contaminants and provided in a manner that minimizes contamination by urine and feces. Check watering devices such as water bottles with drinking tubes and automatic "lixits" each day to ensure proper operation and availability of water. It may be necessary to train some rabbits that are accustomed to a different watering system how to use automatic lixit-type devices. The application of a sweet sticky molasses or corn syrup to the surface of the water delivery system helps the animal to find and use automatic waterers. Water bowls are easily contaminated and spilled and need to be cleaned and filled at least daily. The use of heavy clay crocks and bowls containing a heavy round rock reduces tipping. A wet dewlap and resultant "green fur" *Pseudomonas*-related moist dermatitis may result in some rabbits that use water bowls.

This overview of the rabbit gastrointestinal system primarily relates to the domestic *Oryctolagus* rabbits and does not address the nutritional specifics for wild hares (*Lepus*), cottontails (*Sylvilagus*), and rock rabbits (*Pika*), all of which do poorly in captivity. If additional information is desired, *Rabbit Feeding and Nutrition* by Peter R. Cheeke is an excellent reference.[3] The dietary requirements for pet, show, meat production, and laboratory rabbits may vary somewhat.

REFERENCES

1. Brooks DL: Rabbit gastrointestinal disorders. *In* Kirk RW, ed.: Current Veterinary Therapy VIII. Philadelphia, WB Saunders, 1983, pp 654–657.
2. Canas-Rodriguez A, Smith HW: The identification of the antimicrobial factors of the stomach contents of suckling rabbits. Biochem J 1966; 100:79.
3. Cheeke PR: Rabbit Feeding and Nutrition. Orlando, FL, Academic Press, 1987.
4. Cheeke PR, Grobner MA, Patton NM: Fiber digestion and utilization in rabbits. J Appl Rabbit Res 1986; 9:25–30.
5. De SN, Bhattacharya K, Sarkar JK: Study of pathogenicity of strains of *Bacterium coli* from acute and chronic enteritis. J Pathol Bacteriol 1956; 71:201–209.
6. Eden A: Coprophagy in the rabbit: origin of 'night' faeces. Nature [Lond] 1940; 145:628–629.
7. Gorden RF: The problems of backyard poultry and rabbits. Vet Rec 1943; 55:83–85.
8. Harkness JE, Wagner JE: The Biology and Medicine of Rabbits and Rodents. 3rd ed. Philadelphia, Lea & Febiger, 1989.
9. Hornicke H, Batsch F: Coecotrophy in rabbits: a circadian function. J Mammal 1977; 58:240–242.
10. Huang CM, Mi MP, Vogt DW: Mandibular prognathism in the rabbit: discrimination between single and multifactorial models of inheritance. J Hered 1981; 72:296–298.
11. Kamphues VJ, Carstensen P, Schroeder D, et al: Effect

of increasing calcium and vitamin D supply in calcium metabolism of rabbits. J Anim Physiol Anim Nutr 1986; 56:191–208.
12. Kardatsu M, Yoshihara I, Yoshida T: Studies on cecal digestion: II. study on excretion of hard, soft feces and fecal composition in rabbits. Jpn J Zoo Tech Sci 1959; 29:365–371.
13. Krull WH: Coprophagy in the wild rabbit *Sylvilagus nutalli granger* (Allen). Vet Med 1954; 35:481–483.
14. Kulwich R, Struglia H, Pearson PB: The effect of coprophagy on the excretion of B vitamins by the rabbit. J Nutr 1953; 49:639–645.
15. Lockley RM: The Private Life of the Rabbit. New York, Avon Books, 1975.
16. Patton NM, Harris DJ, Grobner MA, et al: The effect of dietary copper sulfate on enteritis in fryer rabbits. J Appl Rabbit Res 1982; 5:78–82.
17. Ringler DH, Abrams GD: Nutritional muscular dystrophy and neonatal mortality in a rabbit breeding colony. J Am Vet Med Assoc 1970; 157:1928–1934.
18. Smith HW: The antimicrobial activity of the stomach contents of suckling rabbits. J Pathol Bacteriol 1966; 91:1–9.
19. Smith HW: The development of flora of the alimentary tract in young animals. J Pathol Bacteriol 1965; 90:495–513.
20. Smith HW: Observations on the flora of the alimentary tract in young animals. J Pathol Bacteriol 1965; 89:95–122.
21. Taylor EL: Pseudorumination. Vet Med 1940; 35:481–482.
22. Thacker EJ, Brandt CS: Coprophagy in the rabbit. J Nutr 1955; 55:375.
23. Yoshihara T, Kardatsu M: Studies in cecum digestion: IV. movement of cecal contents in rabbits. Bull Agric Chem Soc Jpn 1960; 24:543–546.
24. Zarrow MX, Denenberg VH, Anderson CO: Rabbit: frequency of suckling pup. Science 1965; 150:1835–1836.

CHAPTER 17

Gastrointestinal Diseases

Jeffrey R. Jenkins, DVM

The most common clinical problems seen in rabbits involve the gastrointestinal tract. This is true both for pet rabbits and for rabbits raised for meat and fur. To understand the pathogenesis of nutrition-related and gastrointestinal diseases of the rabbit, you must first be knowledgeable of normal anatomic and physiologic aspects of rabbit digestion (see Chapters 14 and 16).

The history and management are very important in the diagnosis of gastrointestinal diseases in rabbits. Question the owner in detail about the diet and environment of the pet rabbit. Most pet rabbits are caged when they are not supervised, but they are allowed to roam the house for part of the day. This allows them some exercise but exposes them to a variety of potentially noxious food items and dangerous materials, such as electrical cords, carpet fibers, and other foreign materials. Frequently, pet rabbits are fed foods inappropriate for herbivores, such as those high in simple sugars or those high in protein and fat (e.g., dog or cat food).

Disease processes that rarely occur in short-lived "working rabbits" are common in pet rabbits because of their longer life span. Complications of uterine disease (common in old rabbits) and adhesions resulting from ovariohysterectomy have both been associated with gastrointestinal problems.

CLINICAL ASPECTS OF DIGESTIVE PHYSIOLOGY

As was discussed in Chapter 16, rabbits are herbivores, but their digestive strategy differs from those of horses (colon fermenters) and large ruminants. Similar to horses, rabbits are hindgut fermenters; however, unlike horses, rabbits have adapted to a system that eliminates fiber from the gut as rapidly as possible. This allows efficient digestion of the nonfiber portion of forage. It is interesting, however, that this system is driven by the presence of fiber in the diet. The rapid digestive transit allows a high feed intake, increasing the total amount of energy extracted and minimizing the quantity of fiber stored.

Rabbit diets high in fiber have been shown to have a protective effect against enteritis. The beneficial effect is associated with the indigestible component *lignocellulose*. The digestible fiber sources do not afford the same protection. Fiber stimulates cecocolic motility, either directly or by a distention effect of the bulk. Conversely, diets low in fiber cause cecocolic hypomotility, which predisposes rabbits to abnormal cecal fermentation and prolonged retention of digesta in the cecum; they also stimulate volatile fatty acid production, alter pH and substrate concentrations, and ultimately produce changes in cecal microflora. Other effects of fiber consumption are indirect. High-fiber diets have a low level of available carbohydrate and thus decrease the risk of enterotoxemia caused by carbohydrate overload of the hindgut. Carbohydrate provides an environment in which pathogens such as *Escherichia coli* and *Clostridium* species proliferate. Glucose, a byproduct of carbohydrate digestion, is necessary for the production of iota toxin by *Clostridium* species.

The pelleted diets fed exclusively to feeder rabbits are high in calories (high in digestible carbohydrate), high in protein, and highly digestible, being designed to increase weight gain in growing rabbits raised for their meat. From the previous discussion, the potential for gastrointestinal complications in a rabbit given this diet is obvious.

Both energy and protein levels of a diet affect coprophagy. With energy deficiency, rabbits consume the total quantity of the produced cecotropes. During ad libitum feeding, cecotrope intake depends on the protein and fiber levels of the diet. Therefore, cecotrophy is greater if a ration is low in protein or high in fiber.[13] The relative composition of feces and cecotropes is listed in Table 17–1. Coprophagy is discussed in detail in Chapter 16.

Insulin appears to have a minor role in the energy metabolism of rabbits. Rabbits are reported to survive for long periods following pancreatectomy,[1, 23, 24] and diabetes mellitus is not reported as a clinical disease in rabbits.[15] Diabetes mellitus has been induced in rabbits by treatment with alloxan, a drug that selectively destroys beta cells, in experimental efforts to create a model of human diabetes.[12]

TABLE 17–1

COMPOSITION OF RABBIT FECES AND CECOTROPES

	Feces	Cecotropes
Dry matter (%)	52.7	38.6
Crude protein (%)	15.4	34.0
Ether extract (%)	3.0	5.3
Crude fiber (%)	30.0	17.8
Ash (%)	13.7	15.2
Nitrogen-free extract (%)	37.9	36.7
Gross energy (mJ)	18.2	19.0
Sodium:potassium	0.4	0.6

From Fekete S: Recent findings and future perspectives of digestive physiology in rabbits: a review. Acta Vet Hung 1989; 37:265–279.

Rabbits may have a higher total serum calcium (Ca) concentration than do other mammals. In a study in which rabbits were fed a diet comparable with commercially available diets containing between 0.9 and 1.6 g of Ca per 100 g of feed and between 220 and 560 IU of vitamin D, the mean fractional excretion of Ca was 44%. The fractional excretion of Ca in most mammals is less than 2%.[3] It is reported that in the rabbit, the absorption of Ca from the gut is *not* regulated by 1,25-dihydroxyvitamin D (vitamin D_3). Rather, it is believed that parathyroid hormone (PTH) and calcitonin protect the rabbit from dangerously high serum Ca concentrations, which vary directly with the level of Ca in the diet. Interestingly, the ionized fraction of Ca is comparable with that of other mammals.[2]

Physiologists and microbiologists generally agree that the most common cecal bacteria are nonsporulated gram-negative bacilli in the genus *Bacteroides,* at 10^2–10^9/g.[6, 13] Large anaerobic metachromatic staining bacteria (LAMB) were found to be the most abundant, at 10^8–10^{10}/mL of cecal contents, by one group of researchers.[20] Other bacteria normally present include gram-negative oval and fusiform rods. Coliform bacteria are not isolated from normobiotic animals; if they are present, they represent a very small percentage of the total bacterial population. Large ciliated protozoa, similar to those of the genus *Isotricha* found in ruminants, were present at 10^7/mL.[20] A rabbit-specific ascosporogenous yeast in the Saccharomyces family, *Cyniclomyces guttulatulus,* also has been found and identified at 10^6/g.[14] Veterinarians unfamiliar with rabbit fecal and cecal flora commonly mistake this yeast for coccidia on fecal examinations.

DIET-RELATED DISEASES OF THE RABBIT

Nearly all of the important disease problems that rabbits experience are directly or indirectly related to diet. Nearly every case of enteric disease is related to diet and feeding practices. Even respiratory diseases (e.g., pasteurellosis) are influenced by environmental conditions, particularly the concentration of ammonia in the air, which is associated with the feeding of a high protein diet. Fur chewing (barbering) and hair-related gastric motility problems ("hairballs," "wool block," or "trichobezoars") are largely a result of dietary inadequacies and may be prevented with proper dietary management. Other diseases, including pregnancy toxemia, are also associated with nutritional status. Abortions, fetal absorption, small litter size, and weak kits usually result from poor nutrition, and particularly from inadequate energy intake.

The bacterial flora of the hindgut of rabbits has been well studied. The problems induced by diet and nutrition often involve the disruption of this complex flora and the environment in which it grows. Populations of spore-forming anaerobes, consisting mostly of *Clostridium* species, and coliform species such as *E. coli,* increase as the populations of normal organisms decrease. Frequently, a reduction in the amount of fiber in the diet, an increase in carbohydrate consumption, and disruption of gastroenteric motility lead to alterations in the cecal pH or in the composition of the cecal chyme.

Subacute to Chronic Gastric Stasis (Trichobezoars)

Gastric stasis, also known as "wool block," is a common syndrome in rabbits and is characterized by anorexia, decreased or no stool production, and a large stomach filled with doughlike stomach contents and hair. It is classically associated with the ingestion and accumulation of excessive amounts of hair in a rabbit's stomach (Fig. 17–1). Rabbits that are on a high-carbohydrate, low-fiber diet; are caged; and are under some stress are affected most often. A trichobezoar may also occur in a rabbit receiving a high-carbohydrate, low-fiber diet that grooms excessively for any reason (e.g., because of a heavy molt, the prepartum state, or fleas).

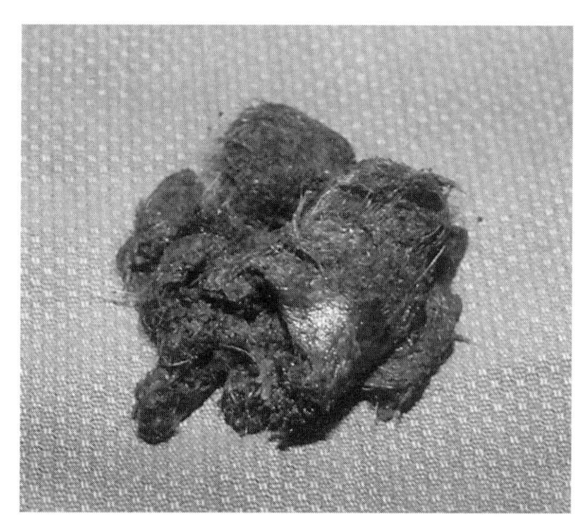

FIGURE 17–1
A trichobezoar that was surgically removed from the stomach of a rabbit with clinical signs of "wool block."

The history most often includes anorexia of 2–7 days' duration. Water consumption may be normal or decreased. Rabbits may be alert or depressed, depending on the chronicity of the problem and the hydration status. Weight loss may be noted in some rabbits. Occasionally, a firm, doughlike mass can be palpated in the cranial region of the abdomen. Gas may be palpable in the stomach or intestines, supporting the diagnosis of gastric stasis or hairball. Frequently, the number of fecal pellets is significantly reduced, and those that are passed are much smaller than normal or may contain hair.

Radiography may or may not be helpful in diagnosis because the mass of food and hair appears similar to normal ingesta, even with contrast radiography. However, visualization of a large, ingesta-filled stomach on a radiograph of a rabbit that has been anorectic for 4–7 days suggests the presence of a hairball (see Fig. 31–6). Furthermore, large amounts of gas in the stomach or intestine may indicate gastric stasis (Fig. 17–2). However, a definitive diagnosis often can be made only with exploratory laparotomy, which is a risky procedure to perform in these patients.

I believe that the pathophysiologic mechanism of this syndrome is often not gastric obstruction, but rather changes in gastric motility and normal gastric function that result in the loss of liquid from the material in the stomach. The resultant dehydrated mass

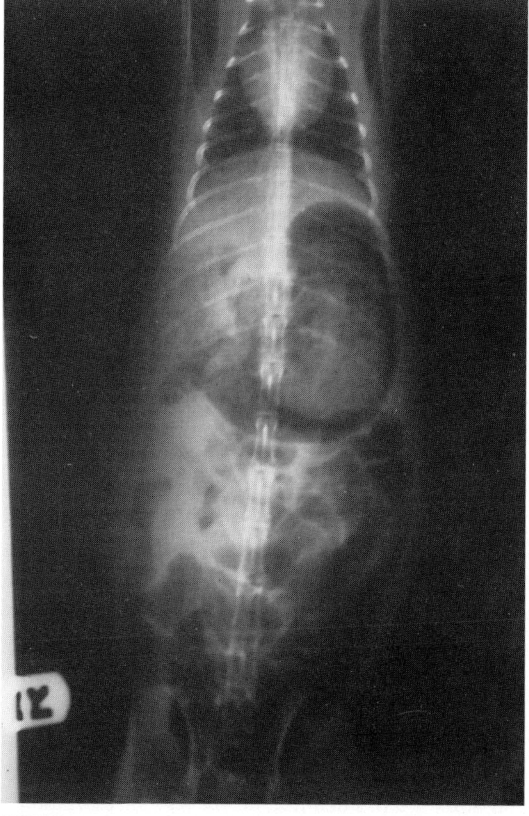
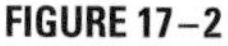

FIGURE 17–2
Survey radiograph of a rabbit suspected of having a hairball. Note the enlarged gas- and ingesta-filled stomach and the large amount of intestinal and cecal gas, which are suggestive of gastrointestinal stasis.

of gastric ingesta may not be passed by the rabbit, and its presence leads to clinical changes. The underlying cause of these changes may or may not involve the presence of hair in the rabbit's stomach. Certainly, this syndrome exists in rabbits that have not ingested large amounts of hair; the material in the stomach may consist primarily of ingested food. Providing rabbits a diet high in fiber has been shown to prevent this syndrome, possibly because the increased fiber component decreases hair accumulation; however, it is more likely that a high-fiber diet stimulates gastrointestinal motility and the creation of a more healthy digestive environment.

The use of a variety of lubricants (e.g., petroleum laxatives, paraffin oil) and protein-digesting enzymes or agents (e.g., pineapple for bromelain, papain) has been advocated for treating this syndrome. However, the response to such treatment often is equivocal.

Very good results have been obtained with a medical treatment based on rehydration of the patient, rehydration of the stomach contents, and stimulation of gastric motility. Force-feed fluids (e.g., water, electrolyte solutions, fruit juices) and fruit and vegetable purees (e.g., fruit or vegetable baby food) to rehydrate the rabbit. If indicated in hospitalized animals, administer SC fluids. Give systemic antibiotics, such as trimethoprim-sulfa (30 mg/kg PO q12h), to decrease bacterial overgrowth. Administer metoclopramide hydrochloride (0.5 mg/kg SC q4–8h) or cisapride (0.5 mg/kg SC q8–12h) to stimulate gastric motility. However, do not give motility stimulants if there are clinical signs of an acute abdomen (e.g., gastric dilatation, painful abdomen, signs of shock). Continue this treatment for 3–5 days; usually, the rabbit begins eating food by the third or fourth day of treatment.

Hepatic lipidosis can develop rapidly in rabbits with a negative energy balance. The hepatic changes occur almost immediately if ketosis develops. Use urine test strips to quickly screen for ketosis in anorectic rabbits. The return of a positive energy balance in the rabbit is the first priority of treatment. Place an IV or intraosseous catheter and administer IV fluids to correct dehydration. Once the rabbit is hydrated, continue administering glucose-containing IV fluids.

Occasionally, the mass of material in the stomach is so dehydrated that the rabbit fails to respond to medical treatment, and surgical intervention is necessary. However, the prognosis for a successful outcome is greatly reduced in rabbits that are treated surgically. Complications of hepatic lipidosis are a common cause of death in these patients.

Acute Gastric or Intestinal Obstruction

Rarely, a rabbit is presented with an acute onset of abdominal pain and gastric dilatation that is the result of gastric (most often pyloric) or duodenal obstruction. The most commonly implicated object is a mat of hair. In contrast to the trichobezoars found in the pet cat or ferret, hair found in a rabbit appears to have become matted while still on the coat of the animal rather than in its stomach. Obstruction from carpet fiber or plastic foreign bodies may present similarly. Gastric and intestinal obstructions are life-threatening, and affected rabbits must be treated rapidly and aggressively if they are to survive. Treatment protocol consists of the administration of analgesics, such as buprenorphine (0.01–0.05 mg/kg IM or SC q12h); a shock dose of IV or intraosseous crystalloid solution;

and short-acting corticosteroids, such as hydrocortisone sodium succinate, 10 mg/kg IV (Solu-Cortef, The Upjohn Company, Kalamazoo, MI) or prednisolone sodium succinate, 11–25 mg/kg IV (Solu-Delta-Cortef, The Upjohn Company, Kalamazoo, MI). Take radiographs to confirm the location of gas. In some rabbits, a tube can be passed into the stomach for decompression. Most often, this is done with the patient under isoflurane anesthesia, either while radiographs are being taken or while the rabbit is being prepared for surgery. If obstruction is confirmed, immediate surgery is indicated. Very often, a section of the duodenum is necrotic and thus must be resected. The prognosis in these animals is guarded to poor.

Other Gastrointestinal Foreign Bodies and Cecoliths

A variety of foreign materials can be ingested by rabbits. In addition to those locations already mentioned, foreign bodies may be found at the ileocecal-colonic junction, in the cecum, or in the colon. Rabbits with gastrointestinal foreign bodies most often are presented with intermittent abdominal pain, gas, or diarrhea. Much less common in rabbits are cecoliths and cecal phytobezoars. Some foreign bodies can be identified on radiographic survey films. Contrast studies may be helpful, but their interpretation may be complicated by the presence of intestinal, cecal, and colonic gas and by the recirculation of barium through the ingestion of cecotropes. Exploratory surgery is required for both diagnosis and correction in most cases (see Chapter 22).

ENTERITIS COMPLEX AND ENTEROTOXEMIA

Enteritis complex, with signs ranging from soft stool and diarrhea to enterotoxemia, sepsis, and death, is one of the most common diseases of rabbits in clinical practice. Pathogenic bacteria and the factors that allow them to proliferate are the usual causes. These factors involve changes in diet, the effects of antibiotics, stress, and genetic predisposition to gut dysfunction. Simple cases of enteritis, resulting in soft or pasty stool, may be caused by minor disruption of cecal flora, pH, or motility. Simple correction of the diet, the addition of fiber in the form of hay to the diet, and removal of stress often correct the problem.

Enterotoxemia in rabbits, which is characterized by more significant dysbiosis than is enteritis, is caused by the iota-like toxin from *Clostridium spiroforme*. Other *Clostridium* species, especially *C. difficile* and *C. perfringens,* also have been reported but are now not thought to be the cause of the disease.[8, 24] Newly weaned animals (3–6 weeks of age) are most often affected, and they have the greatest mortality. This group of rabbits may develop enterotoxemia from simple exposure to *C. spiroforme*. This is likely because these young rabbits have an undeveloped population of normal gastrointestinal flora and a high gastric pH, which allows the proliferation of *C. spiroforme*. Adult rabbits are more resistant and generally require some dietary, environmental, or other stress for the dysbiotic state to be induced and growth of the bacteria allowed. Rapid multiplication of *C. spiroforme* results in significant alteration of the rabbit's normal cecal flora. Nursing does with enterotoxemia can develop a so-called "milk enterotoxemia" that is thought to be caused by *Clostridium* endotoxin produced in the does' cecum and passed to the kits in their milk.

In acute disease, rabbits become anorectic and markedly depressed. Diarrhea is brown and watery and soils the perineum and rear legs of the rabbits. It may contain blood or mucus. As the disease process progresses, affected rabbits become hypothermic and moribund, and they die after 24–48 hours. Occasionally, a chronic form of the disease characterized by intermittent diarrhea, anorexia, and weight loss is seen. Postmortem findings in these rabbits include petechial and ecchymotic hemorrhages on the serosal surface of the cecum. The appendix and proximal colon also may be involved. Various amounts of gas throughout the intestinal tract, cecum, and colon result from ileus. Hemorrhages, pseudomembranes, or mucus may be present on the mucosa of the cecum and proximal colon.

Mucoid Enteritis

Mucoid enteritis is one of the major causes of morbidity and mortality in young rabbits 7–14 weeks of age. It is characterized by anorexia, lethargy, weight loss, diarrhea, cecal impaction, and excessive production of mucus by the cecum. Its cause is unknown; however, studies have convincingly established the relationship between bacterial dysbiosis and hyperacidity of the cecum and the symptoms of mucoid enteritis.[20] Alterations in cecal pH resulting from changes in the production or absorption of volatile fatty acids or from vigorous fermentation of carbohydrates can destabilize the cecal microbial population and stimulate mucus production within the cecum and colon. Feeding a diet high in fiber and low in simple carbohydrates is preventative.

Dysbiosis Secondary to Treatment with Antibiotics

Other factors involved in the development of enteritis include antibiotic administration and stress. Some antibiotics suppress normal flora, allowing pathogens to proliferate. Clindamycin, lincomycin, penicillin, ampicillin, amoxicillin, amoxicillin-clavulanic acid, cephalosporins, and erythromycin can induce enteritis in rabbits. Epinephrine-mediated inhibition of gut motility is believed to be the cause of stress-induced enteritis.

Treatment of Enteritis

Treatment of rabbits with severe enteritis, enterotoxemia, and mucoid enteritis consists of aggressive supportive care and efforts aimed at increasing cecal and colonic motility, discouraging the growth of pathogenic bacteria and the production of toxins, and supporting the growth of normal flora. Antimicrobial drugs have limited value in treatment of the disease and are used primarily as "supportive" therapy. *C. spiroforme* has been shown to be sensitive to chloramphenicol, sulfaquinoxaline, and other antibiotics (erythromycin and ampicillin) that may contribute to the state of dysbiosis. These have not been proved effective in the treatment of the disease. The use of metronidazole has been reported to reduce the number of deaths from enterotoxemia.[4] I suggest a metronidazole dosage of 20 mg/kg q12h. Correction of dehydration and maintenance of normal hydration is of paramount importance, and administration of IV or intraosseous fluids often is indicated. In my experience, use of motility-stimulating drugs (e.g., cisapride or metoclopramide) and giving a diet high in fiber (force-fed, if necessary) yield the most favorable results. Administration of cholestyramine, an ion exchange resin capable of binding bacterial toxins, has been suggested at a dose of 2 g per 20 mL water q24h by gavage. Cholestyrine has prevented death in rabbits with clindamycin-induced enterotoxemia.[21]

To prevent enterotoxemia, maintain optimal husbandry and minimize stress. Feed a pelleted diet containing no less than 18–20% fiber supplemented with a good-quality grass hay. Avoid sudden changes in the diet. Make feed and hay available to weanling rabbits from 3 weeks of age; avoid early or forced weaning.

Bacterial Enteritis

Colibacillosis

Enteritis caused by exposure to or overgrowth of gram-negative enteric bacteria is less common than enterotoxemia. Serotypes of *E. coli* have been divided into four major groups on the basis of virulence and pathogenesis in humans: enterotoxigenic, enteroinvasive, enteropathogenic, and enterohemorrhagic. Diarrhea in the rabbit is most often caused by a strain similar to enteropathogenic *E. coli*, which causes chronic diarrhea in human infants. This strain, called "rabbit enteropathogenic *E. coli*," has also been referred to as "attaching and effacing *E. coli*" because of how the bacteria attach and efface the intestinal microvillous border with adhesin or adhesion factor.[24] Serotyping of *E. coli* isolated from rabbits is not available to clinical veterinarians and remains a tool of research only. Biotyping may be available from some laboratories.

E. coli–related diarrhea is common in neonatal rabbits between 1 and 14 days of age. The diarrhea is typically watery and stains the abdomen and perineum yellow. The morbidity and mortality within a litter approaches 100%. Subsequent litters of the doe may have passive immunity. The serotype most often isolated from these neonates, O109, does not form an enterotoxin as do the strains that cause similar diarrhea in calves or piglets. These bacteria are not invasive but attach to the brush border of the cells of the intestinal wall. Treatment consists of appropriate antibiotic therapy. Positive results may be obtained with early treatment.

E. coli–related diarrhea in postweaning rabbits may be caused by a variety of different serotypes. All are noninvasive strains and do not form enterotoxin. They do attach to the brush border of intestinal cells and belong to the rabbit enteropathogenic *E. coli* group. Morbidity and mortality vary with the serotype; signs range from mild diarrhea and weight loss to death, and the mortality rate can be 50% or greater. Those animals that recover may have retarded growth. The disease process is limited to the cecum and colon. The cecal wall may be inflamed with longitudinal "paintbrush" hemorrhages. In severe cases, intussusception and rectal prolapse may be present. Presumptive diagnosis may be based on isolation of *E. coli* from stool or tissue samples from affected animals; however, nonpathogenic *E. coli* routinely proliferates in any rabbit with dysbiosis. Confirmation of the diagnosis requires histologic examination of tissues and observation of *E. coli* attachment to the intestinal cells. Treat individual rabbits with appropriate antibiotics, guided by the results of culture and sensitivity testing. Use trimethoprim-sulfa combination antibiotics (30 mg/kg PO q12h) or enrofloxacin (10 mg/kg q12h) until culture and sensitivity test results are obtained.

Tyzzer's Disease

Tyzzer's disease is caused by *Clostridium piliforme* (formerly *Bacillus piliformis*), a motile, gram-variable, spore-forming, obligate intracellular bacterium. The disease occurs in many rodents and other mammalian species in addition to rabbits. Stress (i.e., that produced by overcrowding, unsanitary conditions, high temperatures, or breeding) may be an important component of this disease. Clinical signs of Tyzzer's disease include watery diarrhea, depression, and death. Morbidity and mortality may be especially high in weanling rabbits. Older rabbits can develop a more chronic form of the disease that results in chronic weight loss. Postmortem examination of rabbits with Tyzzer's disease may show the characteristic foci of necrosis in the liver and degenerative lesions of the myocardium. More often, the intestinal wall is edematous, with areas of necrosis in the mucosa of the proximal colon. Treatment is palliative once clinical signs have been observed. The intracellular location of the bacteria may contribute to the difficulty in treating affected animals. If exposed animals are treated early (i.e., they are isolated from affected animals, good hygiene is promoted, and supportive care and a high fiber diet are provided), they may not develop the disease. Prevention of the disease depends on good husbandry. Bacterial spores are killed with a 0.3% sodium hypochlorite solution or with heating to 80°C (173°F) for 30 minutes. There is no vaccine available for Tyzzer's disease.

Other Bacterial Enteritides

Other causes of enteritis include *Salmonella, Pseudomonas,* and *Campylobacter*-like species. Salmonellosis is not common but can cause disease with both high morbidity and mortality. The species and serovar most often associated with salmonellosis in rabbits are *S. typhimurium*; however, other species and serovars have been reported. Transmission of the disease most often is associated with contaminated food or water. Usually, affected rabbits develop sepsis, which quickly leads to death; however, diarrhea may occur as well. Postmortem findings are consistent with septicemia and include vascular congestion of organs and diffusely distributed petechial hemorrhages. Lymph nodes and gut-associated lymphoid tissue may be edematous and contain similar foci of necrosis. I have seen an epidemic of lethal diarrhea in rabbits associated with *P. aeruginosa,* which was isolated from the watering system. The morbidity associated with this outbreak was low to moderate, but mortality was high. *Campylobacter*-like species–related diarrhea is characterized by not only the presence of the bacteria but also the disruption of normal flora. These organisms appear to be similar to organisms identified in pigs, hamsters, and ferrets with proliferative enteritis (*Lawsonia intracellularis*; see Chapters 4 and 27); organisms from rabbits react to monoclonal antibodies prepared to organisms isolated from these species but are thought to be a different bacterial species.[27]

VIRAL DISEASES OF THE DIGESTIVE TRACT

Papillomatosis

Rabbit oral papillomatosis is a benign, rare disease caused by a papillomavirus. Lesions consist of small white growths on the ventral surface of the tongue but only rarely elsewhere in the mouth. Early lesions are sessile, later becoming rugose or pedunculated and, ultimately, ulcerated. The lesions can exceed 4–5 mm at their greatest dimension but are typically smaller (1–3 mm). Lesions may persist as long as 145 days, but they usually disappear within weeks.[9]

Rabbit Enteric Coronavirus

In 1980, a coronavirus was found to be the cause of diarrhea in rabbits.[19] Further research has shown that this virus affects rabbits 3–10 weeks of age. This coronavirus also has been found in clinically normal adult rabbits. Clinical signs in naturally occurring outbreaks include lethargy, diarrhea, abdominal swelling, and death. The disease is associated with high morbidity and mortality; in one described outbreak, 40–60% of rabbits were affected; death occurred in almost 100% of these animals within 24 hours of the onset of clinical signs.[9] Necropsy findings include fluid cecal contents, and histopathologic examination reveals atrophy of intestinal villi. Tentative diagnosis of this disease is based on clinical history, clinical signs, necropsy findings, and results of histopathologic analysis. The virus agglutinates red blood cells; therefore, evidence of hemagglutination activity in the feces supports a tentative diagnosis. The diagnosis is confirmed by demonstration of the virus in feces or cecal contents.

Pleural effusion and cardiomyopathy in rabbits have also been associated with coronavirus-like particles.[25]

Rotavirus

Infections caused by rotavirus alone may be only mildly pathogenic; in rabbits, however, the virus is associated with very high morbidity but variable mortality. Although poorly studied in pet rabbits, antibodies to rotavirus as well as the virus itself have been found in the feces of rabbits from commercial rabbitries throughout the world. A wide range of severity of diarrhea is associated with rotavirus infection and is likely influenced by synergy with various microorganisms associated with the infection. Severe anorexia, dehydration, and mucoid or greenish-yellow watery diarrhea have been reported. Rabbits between 30 and 80 days of age are those most often affected. Mortality in young rabbits with naturally occurring infections may be as high as 80%. In experimental studies, rotavirus caused soft or fluid feces in some rabbits, but in the majority diarrhea did not develop at all.[5] One study showed that a strain of rotavirus induced diarrhea, depression, anorexia, and death; however, the experiment was not reproducible.[10, 11] The clinical signs of naturally occurring infections involving rotavirus and other agents include marked congestion and distention of the intestines and cecum and petechial hemorrhages in the small intestine and colon. Histologic lesions include moderate to severe villous atrophy, with the most severe lesions found in the ileum. Apical enterocytes on the tips of villi are swollen, rounded, and desquamating, and the tips may be denuded. The lamina propria is usually infiltrated with lymphocytes and, occasionally, with neutrophils. Diagnosis is established on the basis of the results of histopathologic examination of the intestine, isolation of the virus, or demonstration of antibodies. Clinical signs and gross pathologic findings alone are not diagnostic.[9] The prevention and control of rotavirus infection is complicated by its highly infectious nature. Reduction of stress (e.g., by cessation of breeding, reducing crowding, removal of socially dominant animals, and addition of fiber to the diet) along with appropriate treatment of concurrent disease and improved hygiene should reduce mortality.

Rabbit Viral Hemorrhagic Disease

Hemorrhagic diseases have been recognized in rabbits in Europe (European brown hare syndrome) and in those in China imported from Europe in the late 1970s and early 1980s (rabbit viral hemorrhagic disease). The disease found in China has now spread to many other countries. It has not been found to occur in the United States; however, it is reasonable to expect that it will occur here in the future. It has been diagnosed in rabbits in many areas of Mexico.[16, 17] Although these two syndromes are very similar, only viral hemorrhagic disease is associated with diarrhea. The disease, which is thought to be caused by a calicivirus,[9] targets rabbits older than 2 months of age; younger rabbits are clinically unaffected. Transmission is horizontal, with fecal-oral spread being the major route; however, fomites such as water sipper tubes, feed, and utensils can transmit the virus. The virus enters the rabbit through the conjunctiva, nasal passages, or traumatized tissue. The disease course is acute, the duration of incubation being only 1–2 days. The virus is highly infectious and is associated with both high morbidity (70–80%) and high mortality (100%). The number of rabbits affected during outbreaks peaks in 2–3 days, and the disease course may last only 7–13 days. Initially, affected rabbits are febrile and show signs of depression, lethargy, and anorexia. Some may show signs of tachypnea, cyanosis, abdominal distention, and constipation or diarrhea. At the end-stage of the disease, the rabbit becomes hypothermic and recumbent and may have convulsions or epistaxis. Because of the rapid course of the disease, signs may not be noticed, and the affected rabbit is found dead. Surviving rabbits exhibit depression, anorexia, and fever that may last for 2–3 days. Hematologic testing often shows a lymphopenia and a gradual decline in the number of thrombocytes. In most moribund rabbits, prothrombin and thrombin times are prolonged; paracoagulation tests with protamine sulfate give a strong positive reaction; and fibrin degradation products can be detected. Gross pathologic changes are associated with viremia, and acute disseminated coagulopathy is associated with deep venous thrombosis. Congestion and hemorrhage may be seen in most organs but is most pronounced in the lungs. The liver is pale, and periportal necrosis with a fine reticular pattern is observed; often, a segmental catarrhal enteritis is identified.[9] A presumptive diagnosis may be made on the basis of data in the history, clinical signs, and pathologic findings. Definitive diagnosis requires demonstration of the virus by electron microscopic examination of tissues or with hemagglutination, immunoenzyme, or immunofluorescence tests. The virus is inactivated by 0.5% sodium hypochlorite or 1% formalin. A tissue-derived vaccine inactivated with formaldehyde has been shown to be safe and efficacious in preventing rabbit viral hemorrhagic disease.[9] Antisera also have been shown to be protective against the disease. Suspected cases of viral hemorrhagic disease or European brown hare virus should be reported to local agricultural authorities.

PARASITIC DISORDERS OF THE GASTROINTESTINAL TRACT

Coccidia

Coccidia are the most common parasites of the rabbit's gastrointestinal tract and are a common cause of illness. All rabbit coccidia are members of the genus *Eimeria*. Twelve species are reported to infect rabbits (Table 17–2). Only one species, *E. stiedae,* which parasitizes the liver, is found outside the intestinal tract. Very often, two or more species of coccidia are present in diseased rabbits; therefore, the precise role of the different species as pathogens is not clearly defined. The presence of only a few coccidial oocysts does not rule out coccidiosis nor does it confirm the diagnosis, as many rabbits are subclinically infected with coccidia.

Hepatic Coccidia

E. stiedae, the coccidium responsible for hepatic coccidiosis, is ubiquitous in open rabbitries in which rabbits are not treated preventatively with a coccidiostat or trimethoprim-sulfa drugs. In mild infections, the symptoms are inapparent retardation of growth; however, the disease may be fatal, especially in young rabbits. Heavily infected rabbits show signs related to the interference of hepatic function and the blockage of bile ducts. Infected rabbits become anorectic and debilitated; diarrhea or constipation may be noted in the terminal stages of the disease. Occasionally, the abdomen is enlarged and icterus is noted. On radiographs, the liver may appear enlarged and ascites may be present. On postmortem examination, the liver is enlarged and has yellowish-white, nodular, abscess-like lesions of varying size, some of which are within a fibrous capsule. Often, the gallbladder is enlarged by exudate. Diagnosis is based on the identification of oocysts in a sample of bile or on histologic examination.

Numerous agents have been used for preventing and treating *E. stiedae* hepatic coccidiosis. Sulfa drugs appear to be the most effective. The addition of sulfadimethoxine to the diet in an amount to ensure intake of 75 mg/kg for 7 days or 0.02% sulfamerazine sodium to the drinking water is safe and efficacious.[26] In my experience, sulfadimethoxine (15 mg/kg PO q12h for 10 days) and trimethoprim-sulfa combinations (30 mg/kg q12h PO for 10 days) have similarly proved effective. Amprolium 9.6% in drinking water (0.5 mL per 500 mL) also is effective. The major role of chemotherapeutic agents may be the limitation of multiplication until immunity develops. Once a rabbit is infected, it is rare for it to show clinical signs of coccidiosis, and immunity resulting from mild infections may be lifelong.[26] Currently, no effective vaccines against coccidiosis are available. Prevention depends on keeping rabbits in hygienic conditions and on avoidance of infected feces or feces-contaminated food and water.

Intestinal Coccidia

The most important species of intestinal coccidia are *E. perforans, E. magna, E. media,* and *E. irresidua,* with *E. perforans* being the most common. Infection is by ingestion of sporulated oocysts. Although rabbits are coprophagic, it is generally accepted that cecotropes eaten from the anus do not contain infectious oocysts. Clinical signs vary widely depending on the age of the rabbit, the organism involved, the degree of infection (i.e., the number of oocysts ingested), and the relative susceptibility of the animal (which is determined by factors such as age, stress, and diet). Most often, infections are not apparent. Clinical signs are most often seen in young rabbits. Weight loss, mild intermittent to severe diarrhea that may contain mucus or blood,

TABLE 17–2

COMPARISON OF *EIMERIA* SPECIES INFECTING RABBITS

Species	Mean Size of Oocyst (μm)	Shape	Distinguishing Characteristics	Part of Digestive Tract Affected	Pre-Patent Period (d)	Pathogenicity
E. stiedae	37 × 20	Ellipsoid	Smooth, light yellow wall; wide, thin micropyle; no residual body in oocyst; sporocyst with terminal knob (stiedae body)	Bile duct, epithelium	15–18	Variable
E. irresidua	38 × 26	Ovoid	Smooth, light yellow wall; prominent micropyle; small residual body variable	Small intestine	7–8	Significant
E. magna	35 × 24	Ovoid to ellipsoid	Dark yellow-brown wall; prominent micropyle with lipping; large residual body	Jejunum	6–7	Significant (serious diarrhea)*
E. media	31 × 18	Ellipsoid	Smooth, thick, light pink wall; micropyle; large residual body	Small, large intestines	6–7	Moderate
E. perforans	21 × 15	Ellipsoid	Smooth, colorless wall; indistinguishable micropyle; small residual body	Small intestine	5	Slight (nonpathogenic)*
E. exigua	15 × 13	Ovoid	Smooth wall; indistinguishable micropyle; no residual body	—	—	—
E. intestinalis	27 × 18	Ellipsoid	Smooth, yellow wall; micropyle; large granular residual body	Ileum	10	Significant (very pathogenic)*
E. matsubayashii	25 × 18	Ovoid	Smooth, light-colored wall; no residual body	Small intestine, cecum	7	Slight
E. nagpurensis	23 × 13	Barrel-shaped	Smooth, colorless wall; no micropyle; no residual body	—	—	—
E. neoleporis	39 × 20	Elongated and ellipsoid	Smooth, yellow wall; distinct micropyle; no residual body; sporocysts	Small intestine, cecum	12	Significant
E. coecicola	29 × 18	Ellipsoid	Smooth, light yellow-brown wall; prominent micropyle; no residual body	Jejunum, ileum	9–10	Significant (nonpathogenic)*
E. flavesceus	32 × 21	Broadly ellipsoid	Smooth, light yellow wall; prominent micropyle; no residual body	Lower small intestine, cecum, colon	9	Significant (very pathogenic)*

*Comments from Økerman L. Diseases of Domestic Rabbits. 2nd ed. Oxford, Blackwell Scientific Publications, 1994.

Modified from Pakes SP, Gerrity LW. Protozoal diseases. *In* Manning PJ, Ringler DH, Newcomer CE, eds. The Biology of the Laboratory Rabbit. 2nd ed. San Diego, Academic Press, 1994, p 206.

and dehydration may be observed. Animals with severe diarrhea may develop intussusception. Death most often is attributed to dehydration and secondary bacterial infections. Postmortem examination reveals lesions in the small or large intestine, depending on the agent involved. The epithelium of the intestine may be ulcerated. The presence of the organism (or organisms) in fecal samples or scrapings of the intestine supports a presumptive diagnosis. Definitive diagnosis is based on histologic findings. Treatment and prevention are similar to those for hepatic coccidiosis.

Cryptosporidia

Cryptosporidium parvum may cause a discrete and transitory diarrhea in infant rabbits that may lead to growth retardation. *C. parvum* infects the intestinal tract, especially the ileum and the jejunum. The organism apparently does not cause disease in adults. Currently, no effective treatment for cryptosporidiosis is recognized; however, in my experience, the use of potentiated trimethoprim-sulfa drugs has shown some promise.

Other Protozoa Found in Rabbits

Several nonpathogenic flagellates may be found in the feces of rabbits. They are more commonly found if the animal has diarrhea. *Giardia duodenalis* occurs rarely in the anterior region of the small intestine of rabbits and is not considered pathogenic. Other nonpathogenic protozoa found in the cecum and colon include *Monocercomonas cuniculi* and *Retortamonas cuniculi*, which are flagellates from the cecum; large ciliated protozoa found in the cecum that are similar to those of the genus *Isotricha* in ruminants; and *Entamoeba cuniculi,* which is commonly found in the cecum and colon of rabbits.

Helminthic Parasites

Passalurus ambiguus is the common pinworm of domestic rabbits, although *P. nonanulatus* also is reported. Occurrence is widespread in both wild and domestic rabbits; however, the presence of even relatively large numbers of pinworms is nonpathogenic. The adult parasite is found in the anterior portion of the cecum and colon. Adult worms are grossly visible in the lumen of the cecum and large intestine and when they are passed with fresh feces. Infection is through the ingestion of infected eggs. Juvenile stages are found in the mucosa of the small intestine and cecum. Pinworms are commonly seen during routine surgical procedures such as ovariohysterectomy. Diagnosis is made by identification of adult worms or by demonstration of the parasite's eggs in the feces or on tape preparations of the affected rabbit's perineum.

Obeliscoides cuniculi, a member of the family Trichostrongylidae, is found in the stomach of North American rabbits that have the opportunity to graze on grass or where fresh grass is used as a feed. Eggs of the parasite are passed in feces, and larvae hatch in 30 hours. Infectious, third-stage larvae develop in about 6 days. The larvae penetrate the gastric mucosa, where they develop into adults. Eggs may be found in feces as soon as 16–20 days after infection, and shedding continues for 61–118 days. Rabbits do not typically show signs of the infestation. Large numbers of the parasite may cause general malaise, anorexia, and a decrease in weight gain. Pathologic changes are limited to the stomach. On gross examination, the mucosa is thickened and has an irregular "cobblestone" appearance, with excess mucus on the surface. Adult worms are pink and may be seen in the gastric mucus. Eggs of *O. cuniculi* are thin shelled and oval.[18]

Treatment of helminthic infestation with a variety of drugs has been successful. The benzimidazoles are effective in greatly reducing if not eliminating pinworms. Thiabendazole (110 mg/kg for one treatment, followed by 70 mg/kg q4h for eight doses) showed 99% efficacy in the treatment of *O. cuniculi,* with no ill effects.[18] I have obtained good results with thiabendazole, 50 mg/kg PO repeated in 10–14 days, and fenbendazole (Panacur, Hoechst-Roussel Agri-Vet Co., Somerville, NJ), 10–20 mg/kg PO repeated in 10–14 days. I have used ivermectin (Ivomec 1%, Merck AgVet, Iselin, NJ), 0.4 mg/kg repeated in 10–14 days, to treat rabbits with *O. cuniculi* infestation, with no side effects and apparent good success. However, I have not observed the same in the treatment of *P. ambiguus* infection. My experience mimics that of studies showing the administration of ivermectin at doses of 0.4, 1.0 and 2.0 mg/kg to be ineffective against *P. ambiguus*.[29] Piperazine (200 mg/kg PO repeated in 14 days) can be used to treat individual rabbits, or it can be given in drinking water (100 mg per 100 mL of water for 1 day repeated in 10 days) to treat large numbers of animals.

Cestode and Trematode Parasites

The rabbit's gastrointestinal tract is host to five species of cestodes: *Cittotaenia variabilis, Mosgovoyia pectinata americana, M. perplexa, Monoecocestus americana,* and *Ctenotaenia ctenoides. C. variabilis* is found in domestic rabbits, whereas the other species are most often found in wild rabbits in North America and Europe. Adult parasites are found in the small intestine. The life cycles for some species are not well known; however, oribatid mites or ants are thought to act as intermediary hosts.

Trematode parasites of the rabbit gastrointestinal tract include *Hasstilesia tricolor* and *Fasciola hepatica. H. tricolor* is not associated with disease but most often is found incidentally at necropsy, or the ova are found on fecal examination. Adult *H. tricolor* are found in the small intestine of wild rabbits; the intermediary hosts are small terrestrial snails. *F. hepatica* occurs in rabbits that graze in wet pasture or along the banks of streams in endemic areas. These rabbits also may act as a reservoir for the parasite. Adults are found in the gallbladder and bile ducts. Signs of infestation include cachexia, poor coat, lethargy, and death. Eggs of the fluke may be found on examination of feces, or the adult may be found at necropsy. Treatment of cestode and trematode parasites consists of the administration of a single dose of praziquantel (Droncit, Miles Animal Health, Shawnee Mission, KS), 5–10 mg/kg PO. Prevent these parasites by not feeding rabbits grass from wet meadows.

NEOPLASIA

Neoplasms of the gastrointestinal tract include adenocarcinoma and leiomyosarcoma of the stomach, leiomyoma and leiomyosarcoma of the intestine, papilloma of the sacculus rotundus, papilloma of the rectal squamous columnar junction, and bile duct adenoma and carcinoma. Metastatic neoplasia, most commonly uterine adenocarcinoma, often involves the gastrointestinal tract. Surgical resection is the treatment of choice for many of these tumors. If diagnosed early, intestinal masses can be resected with good success.

Rectal papillomas (cauliflower-like, fungating masses arising from the anorectal junction) appear to be benign and are not related to the papillomas of skin or the oral cavity. Removal of these lesions often is curative.

Bile duct adenoma and adenocarcinoma occasionally occur in pet rabbits. These tumors often are multiple and consist of interlocking cysts filled with thick, viscous, myxoid fluid. A variety of noxious stimuli, particularly infection with *E. stiedae,* may be causative factors. Antemortem diagnosis in some rabbits is based on the results of radiography and ultrasound. Surgical removal often is not practical. Metastatic disease is most often miliary and carries a grave prognosis.[31]

AFLATOXICOSIS

Aflatoxins are secondary metabolites of fungi, produced primarily by *Aspergillus flavus* and *A. parasiticus*. Four major fractions—B_1, B_2, G_1, and G_2—are the major components of aflatoxins. Aflatoxin B_1 is the most toxic. The LD_{50} for aflatoxins in rabbits is among the lowest for any species studied.[7] Levels of aflatoxin B_1 greater than 100 ppm in the diet of rabbits have been shown to be associated with morbidity and mortality.[22]

REFERENCES

1. Brewer NR: Biology of the rabbit—X. Synapse 1991; 24:9.
2. Brewer NR: Biology of the rabbit—XVI. Synapse 1991; 24:27–29.
3. Buss SL, Bourdeau JE: Calcium balance in laboratory rabbits. Miner Electrolyte Metab 1984; 10:127–132.
4. Carman RJ, Evans RH: Experimental and spontaneous clostridial enteropathies of laboratory and free living lagomorphs. Lab Anim Sci 1984; 34:443–452.
5. Castrucci G, Frigeri F, Ferrari M, et al: Comparative study of rotavirus strains of bovine and rabbit origin. Comp Immunol Microbiol Infect Dis 1984; 7:171–178.
6. Cheeke PR, Patton NM, Lukefuhr SD, et al.: Rabbit Production. 6th ed. Danville, IL, The Interstate Printers and Publishers, 1987.
7. Clard JD, Jain AV, Hatch RC: Experimentally induced chronic aflatoxicosis in rabbits. Am J Vet Res 1980; 41:1841–1845.
8. Delong D, Manning PJ: Bacterial diseases. *In* Manning PJ, Ringler DH, Newcomer CE, eds.: The Biology of the Laboratory Rabbit. 2nd ed. San Diego, Academic Press, 1994, pp 129–170.
9. DiGiacomo RF, Maré CJ: Viral diseases. *In* Manning PJ, Ringler DH, Newcomer CE, eds.: The Biology of the Laboratory Rabbit. 2nd ed. San Diego, Academic Press, 1994, pp 171–204.
10. DiGiacomo RF, Thouless ME: Age-related antibodies to rotavirus in New Zealand rabbits. J Clin Microbiol 1984; 19:710–711.
11. DiGiacomo RF, Thouless ME. Epidemiology of naturally occurring rotavirus infections in rabbits. Lab Anim Sci 1986; 36:153–156.
12. Duff GL, McMillan GC: The effect of alloxan diabetes on experimental cholesterol atherosclerosis in the rabbit: I. The inhibition of experimental cholesterol atherosclerosis in al-

loxan diabetes. II. The effect of alloxan diabetes on the retrogression of experimental cholesterol atherosclerosis. J Exp Med 1994; 89:611–630.
13. Fekete S: Recent findings and future perspectives of digestive physiology in rabbits: a review. Acta Vet Hung 1989; 37:265–279.
14. Forsyth SJ, Parker DS: Nitrogen metabolism by the microbial flora of the rabbit caecum. J Appl Bacteriol 1985; 58:363–369.
15. Fox JG, Cohen BJ, Loew FM: Laboratory Animal Medicine. Orlando, FL, Academic Press, 1984.
16. Gregg DA, House C, Meyer R, Berninger M: Viral haemorrhagic disease of rabbits in Mexico: epidemiology and viral characterization. Rev Sci Tech 1991; 10:435–451.
17. Gutierrez JG: The outbreak of viral hemorrhagic disease of rabbits in Mexico and operation of the national animal emergency system. J Appl Rabbit Res 1990; 13:130–132.
18. Hofing GL, Kraus AL: Arthropod and helminth parasites. *In* Manning PJ, Ringler DH, Newcomer CE, eds.: The Biology of the Laboratory Rabbit. 2nd ed. San Diego, Academic Press, 1994, pp 231–257.
19. LaPierre J, Marsolais G, Pilon P, et al: Preliminary report on the observation of a coronavirus in the intestine of the laboratory rabbit. Can J Microbiol 1980; 26:1204–1208.
20. Lelkes L, Chang CL: Microbial dysbiosis in rabbit mucoid enteropathy. Lab Anim Sci 1987; 37:757–764.
21. Lipman NS, Weischedel AK, Conners MJ, et al: Utilization of cholestyramine resin as a preventative treatment for antibiotic (clindamycin)–induced enterotoxemia in the rabbit. Lab Anim 1992; 26:1–8.
22. Makkar HPS, Singh B: Aflatoxicosis in rabbits. J Appl Rabbit Res 1991; 14:218–222.
23. Manning PJ, Ringler DH, Newcomer CE, eds.: The Biology of the Laboratory Rabbit. 2nd ed. San Diego, Academic Press, 1994.
24. Økerman L: Diseases of Domestic Rabbits. 2nd ed. Oxford, Blackwell Scientific Publications, 1994.
25. Osterhaus AD, Teppema JS, Van Steenis G: Coronavirus-like particles in laboratory rabbits with different syndromes in the Netherlands. Lab Anim Sci 1982; 32:663–665.
26. Pakes SP, Gerrity LW: Protozoal diseases. *In* Manning PJ, Ringler DH, Newcomer CE, eds.: The Biology of the Laboratory Rabbit. 2nd ed. San Diego, Academic Press, 1994, pp 205–229.
27. Schoeb TR, Fox JG: Enterocecocolitis associated with intraepithelial *Campylobacter*-like bacteria in rabbits *(Oryctolagus cuniculus)*. Vet Pathol 1990; 27:73–80.
28. Smith HW: Observations on the flora of the alimentary tract of animals and factors affecting its composition. J Pathol Bacteriol 1965; 89:52–66.
29. Tsui TLH, Patton NM: Comparative efficacy of subcutaneous injection doses of ivermectin against *P. ambiguus* in rabbits. J Appl Rabbit Res 1991; 14:266–269.
30. Weisbroth SH, Flatt RE, Kraus AL: The Biology of the Laboratory Rabbit. San Diego, Academic Press, 1975.
31. Weisbroth SH: Neoplastic diseases. *In* Manning PJ, Ringler DH, Newcomer CE, eds.: The Biology of the Laboratory Rabbit. 2nd ed. San Diego, Academic Press, 1994, pp 205–229.

CHAPTER 18

Respiratory Disease and the Pasteurella Complex

Barbara J. Deeb, DVM

HISTORICAL INVESTIGATIONS

Respiratory disease is a major cause of morbidity and mortality in rabbits. Pasteurellosis is the primary respiratory disease entity affecting domestic rabbits. During the early 1920s, Webster and Smith studied the "epidemiology of a rabbit respiratory infection" and published a series of 11 reports on the subject in the *Journal of Experimental Medicine*. The findings from these classical studies, which established *Pasteurella multocida* as the causative agent, are still applicable today and deserve review.

Webster and Smith used the term "snuffles" to refer to upper respiratory disease (URD) in rabbits, which was common in the colony of rabbits at the Laboratories of the Rockefeller Institute for Medical Research. About 60% of the rabbits in the colony were found to be carriers of *P. multocida*. Following experimental procedures, 40% of the carriers developed URD, but spontaneous recovery from disease and infection occurred in about 8%. Postmortem examination of 100 rabbits from the colony revealed that 58% had URD. *P. multocida* was isolated from the nares of 55 of the rabbits with URD and from 8 rabbits with normal nares; 2% of the rabbits also had pneumonia, and 4% had bacteremia.

Histopathologic examination of the nares of 40 rabbits with rhinitis showed that 35 had erosion of the nasal turbinates. Fibrinous pleuritis, pericarditis, abscesses, and lung consolidation were also found. Otitis media was often, but not always, associated with torticollis or purulent exudate deep in the ear canal and with rhinitis in about half of the cases.

Only *P. multocida* was consistently associated with disease.

Webster and Smith studied the aerobic nasal flora of rabbits by culturing nasal swabs from 77 rabbits, selected at random, and identified the following (in order of frequency): *Moraxella catarrhalis*, *P. multocida*, *Bordetella bronchiseptica*, other gram-negative cocci or bacilli, and gram-positive cocci. Use of fresh blood agar plates with 5% rabbit blood was critical to successful isolation of *P. multocida.*

Webster and Smith performed experimental studies with various strains of *P. multocida* and *B. bronchiseptica* given at the same dose but by various routes. *B. bronchiseptica*, inoculated intranasally, caused a transient mucoid nasal discharge, followed by an asymptomatic carrier state. The more virulent type D nonmucoid strains of *P. multocida* were more likely to cause acute severe disease or to be cleared, whereas the mucoid strains were more likely to cause chronic infection. One virulent strain, inoculated intranasally, IV, SC, or intratesticularly, consistently induced pleuropneumonia. Webster and Smith concluded that rabbits may (1) resist infection, as did the controls housed with infected rabbits; (2) spontaneously eliminate infection; (3) become chronic carriers; (4) develop acute disease; (5) develop bacteremia and pneumonia; or (6) develop chronic disease. Pathogenesis depends on host resistance and on the virulence of the *P. multocida* strain.

Epidemiologic studies revealed factors that influenced respiratory disease in rabbits. Differences in susceptibility by breed were observed, and there was a high incidence of snuffles in spring and autumn. The prevalence of infection and incidence of disease increased in rabbits experimentally exposed to temperature fluctuations. Addition of fresh vegetables to a basic diet of hay and oats resulted in reduced prevalence of infection among the rabbits receiving the vegetables.

To have uninfected rabbits for experimental use, Webster and Smith established and maintained a *P. multocida*–free colony. Breeders were chosen on the basis of freedom from signs of snuffles and negative results for *P. multocida* on three nasal cultures. Human entry to the colony was restricted to attendants with clean hands and those wearing clean clothing. The room temperature was regulated at 68°F, and the cages were cleaned every other day. The food was always fresh, and the rabbits were given a "considerable amount of personal attention."

Before the studies of Webster and Smith, *B. bronchiseptica* and *Staphylococcus aureus* were thought responsible for URD in rabbits, but snuffles has not been experimentally reproduced by inoculation with either agent. However, a transient nasal discharge and a chronic subclinical infection of the nares, sinuses, and bronchi results after both experimental and naturally occurring exposure to *B. bronchiseptica.*[9, 38] Many rabbits carry both *B. bronchiseptica* and *Neisseria (Moraxella)* species in the nares (Table 18–1). The prevalence of infection varies from one rabbitry to another but increases with the age of rabbits in rabbitries where pasteurellosis is endemic.[12, 24, 31] There is an inverse relationship between *B. bronchiseptica* and *P. multocida* infections in rabbits: weanlings have higher rates of infection with *B. bronchiseptica*, whereas in adults *P. multocida* usually predominates.[9]

PASTEURELLOSIS

Features of *Pasteurella multocida*

Bacterial and Cultural Characteristics

P. multocida is a gram-negative, bipolar, nonmotile, asporogenous coccobacillus of the family Pasteur-

TABLE 18–1

NASAL FLORA OF RABBITS IN CONVENTIONAL RABBITRIES

	Prevalence of Infection (%)	
Bacteria	*Rabbitries A and B*[27] *(n = 135)*	*Rabbitry C*[*17] *(n = 60)*
Neisseria species†	70	—
Moraxella catarrhalis	—	13
Bordetella bronchiseptica	69	47
Pasteurella multocida	31	28
Staphylococcus epidermidis	3	35
Staphylococcus aureus	—	28
Streptococcus faecalis	—	30
Bacillus species	3	13
Other	—	52

*Study included does and weanlings.

†*Neisseria catarrhalis* has been reclassified as *Moraxella catarrhalis.*

ellaceae, or the HAP group, which includes *Hemophilus, Actinobacillus,* and *Pasteurella* species. *P. multocida* grows on blood agar and dextrose starch agar but not on MacConkey's agar. Some strains may require fresh blood for growth on nutrient agar, with cultural characteristics influenced by the type of blood used. Colonies grow larger and produce greenish discoloration on media with horse blood. *P. multocida* produces a distinctive odor, which bacteriologists liken to that of indole. Growth occurs under aerobic conditions or in 5% carbon dioxide. Temperature-sensitive and carbon dioxide–sensitive strains may exist. Most isolates require 24–48 hours' incubation to become apparent on blood agar, especially if mixed with other bacteria. Blood agar with 2 μg/mL of clindamycin can be used to inhibit other bacteria in mixed cultures. Colonies are convex and smooth but vary in coloration from bluish to greenish iridescence when observed in obliquely transmitted light, and they may vary in mucoid appearance. Colonies of the mucoid strains appear to run together, if their numbers permit. Capsular type A strains have large capsules and produce mucoid colonies, whereas colonies of the type D strains may appear iridescent.

P. multocida strains isolated from rabbits usually have the following biochemical characteristics: oxidase +, catalase +, indole +/−, hydrogen sulfide −, urease −, ornithine decarboxylase +, hexose +, and carbohydrate fermentation + for most sugars. These characteristics are useful in distinguishing *P. multocida* from other *Pasteurella* species that may be part of the normal flora.[36]

Serotypes

Serologic typing is done with the use of indirect hemagglutination to identify capsular types A, B, D, E, or F, and the gel diffusion precipitin test, which has been used to describe 16 somatic antigen determinants of lipopolysaccharide. The acriflavine flocculation test is specific for capsular type D strains, whereas a staphylococcal hyaluronidase inhibition test specifically inhibits type A strains. With these tests, the majority of isolates from rabbits were shown to be of type A. Serotypes vary by region, but in the United States, A:12 and A:3 are the most prevalent.[30]

Okerman and coworkers[32] substantiated the conclusion of Webster and Smith that some strains of *P. multocida* are more pathogenic than others. Capsular type D isolates from rabbits with bacteremia are significantly more pathogenic for mice than type A isolates from rabbits with rhinitis only. Somatic type 3 isolates are more pathogenic than type 12 ones.[35]

Virulence Factors

Virulence factors of *P. multocida* include adhesions, phagocyte resistance, endotoxin (lipopolysaccharide), exotoxin, and iron regulation. Pili or other adhesion proteins on the outer membrane of some strains of *P. multocida* enhance colonization. Type A strains are more adhesive to respiratory mucosa than type D strains.[22] Invasion and multiplication of the organism occurs because the capsule, largely consisting of hyaluronic acid and also present in host tissues, inhibits phagocytosis and complement-activated bactericidal activity of serum (opsonization). Some type D strains, although ingested by phagocytes, resist bactericidal activity.[2] Leukotoxic enzymes also are produced. Growth of some strains of *P. multocida* is regulated by the availability of iron, and most strains produce iron-binding outer membrane proteins, which enhance their survival in iron-poor cavities of the hosts.[5, 10, 25]

Endotoxin enhances resistance to bactericidal activity of serum and stimulates the release of inflammatory mediators, such as interleukin-1. In cases of bacteremia, free endotoxin in plasma causes fever and depression and may induce shock. A toxin with characteristics of an exotoxin is produced by some strains of *P. multocida*. Dermonecrotic toxin (now termed "*P. multocida* toxin") of some type D strains enhances attachment and colonization of mucosa. This protein toxin, which is similar to that causing atrophic rhinitis in pigs, also is associated with nasal turbinate atrophy in rabbits. Toxin has been demonstrated for type D[36] and for type A isolates,[15] but it is not clear whether it is the same toxin. Purified *P. multocida* toxin induces pneumonia, pleuritis, lymphoid atrophy, and possibly osteoclastic bone resorption in rabbits.[4]

Antibiotic resistance plasmids have been found in *P. multocida* from animals other than rabbits.[36] However, plasmid characterization of 14 isolates of *P. multocida* from rabbits showed no correlation with somatic serotype, toxigenicity, presence of pili, antimicrobial resistance, biochemical characteristics, or disease.[23]

Antibiotic Sensitivities

Antibiotic sensitivities for 42 isolates of *P. multocida* from rabbits are as follows[27]: 100% were sensitive to chloramphenicol, erythromycin, novobiocin, oxytetracycline, penicillin G, nitrofurazone, and nitrofurantoin; most were resistant to sulfonamides and streptomycin; and all were resistant to lincomycin and clindamycin. In my laboratory, four strains of *P. multocida* from rabbits were resistant to erythromycin and had moderate or intermediate sensitivity to penicillin G but otherwise were sensitive to 16 antibiotics, including several fluoroquinolones and cephalosporins. In my practice, most isolates of *P. multocida* tested on Mueller-Hinton agar with 5% sheep blood have been sensitive to chloramphenicol, ciprofloxacin, enrofloxacin, gentamicin, penicillin G, tetracycline, and trimethoprim-sulfa.

Clinical and Pathologic Manifestations

The clinical presentation of pasteurellosis in rabbits includes URD (rhinitis, sinusitis, conjunctivitis, lacrimal duct infection), otitis, pleuropneumonia, bacteremia, and abscesses of the subcutaneous tissues or internal organs, bones, joints, and genitalia.[19, 30]

Upper Respiratory Disease

URD (snuffles) in rabbits is caused primarily by *P. multocida*; however, predisposing factors influence pathogenicity. Rhinitis and sinusitis are the most common forms of pasteurellosis. A serous nasal discharge precedes the typical white or yellowish mucopurulent discharge associated with *P. multocida*. Exudate adheres to the fur around the nares and, because rabbits groom the face with their forepaws, to the medial aspects of the forepaws, where it mats and becomes yellowish-gray on drying. Affected rabbits often make audible sonorous noises and have bouts of sneezing with exudate forcibly expelled from the nares. Conjunctivitis is often a manifestation of URD. Infection of the nasal lacrimal duct may extend to the conjunctiva. Exudate occluding the duct causes excessive tearing and scalding of the face, alopecia, and pyoderma.

Auscultation of the trachea and nares reveals rales and rattles caused by exudate in the upper respiratory tract. The origin of these respiratory sounds must be determined so that rales from the lungs are not misinterpreted. Signs of rhinitis may subside or even disappear, with affected rabbits harboring infection in the paranasal sinuses or middle ears. Recovery from acute disease and elimination of infection may occur, but spontaneous recovery from chronic infection is unlikely.

Acute infection of the nares is accompanied by edema and hyperemia of the mucosa. Chronic infection may be accompanied by mucosal erosion and atrophy of the turbinates[13] (Fig. 18–1).

Otitis

Extension of infection from the nares to the middle ears probably occurs through the eustachian tube. Most rabbits with otitis media also have rhinitis, but some clear the infection from the nares while the middle ears remain infected.[9] Otitis media may be asymptomatic or, if infection spreads to the inner ear, torticollis, nystagmus, and ataxia can occur. Infection extends to the external ear if the tympanic membrane ruptures. What appears to be accumulation of wax deep in the ear canal may be dried exudate, which, if removed, reveals the typical white purulent exudate underneath. Exudate may be physically expressed by gentle pressure at the base of the ear, and its origin can be determined by otoscopic examination. Consider otitis media in a rabbit that scratches excessively at the base of the ear and in which external parasites are not present. A dorsoventral radiograph of the skull aids in diagnosis of otitis media; increased soft tissue opacity caused by the exudate can be visualized within the bulla, and the bone shows thickening (Fig. 18–2). The tympanic bullae are normally thin walled and hollow.

Bacteremia

The more pathogenic strains of *P. multocida* are likely to spread hematogenously, causing acute generalized disease, fever, and sudden death. Pathologic examination may reveal congestion, petechiation, and microscopic abscesses throughout the viscera. Pleuropneumonia is another sequela of hematogenous spread.

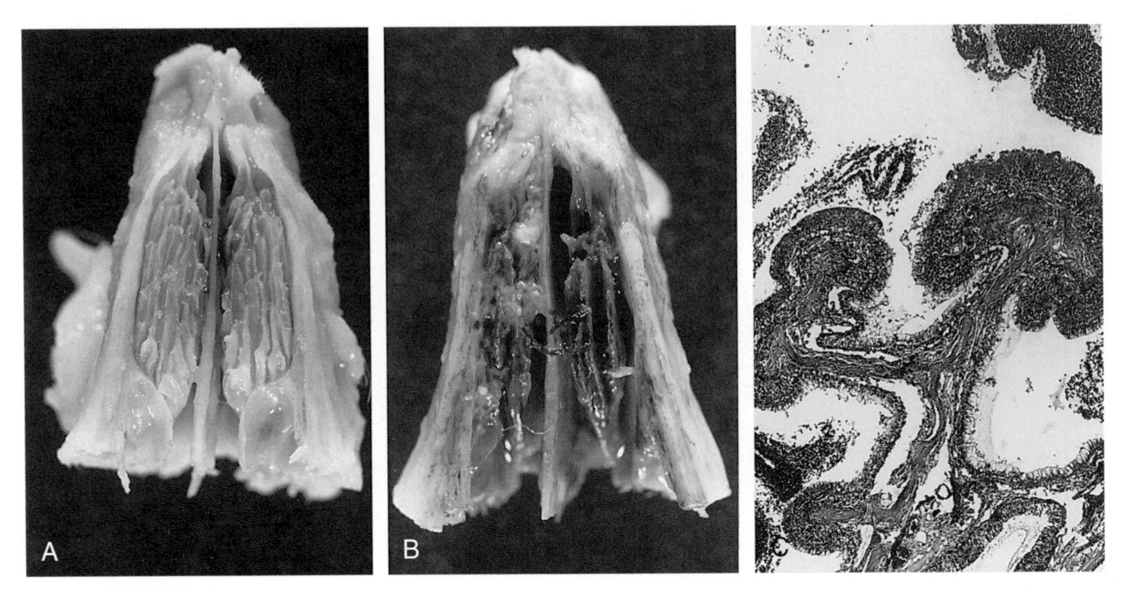

FIGURE 18–1

A, Frontal section of normal maxilloturbinates of a New Zealand white rabbit after removal of the nasal bones. The tissue was fixed in neutral buffered 10% formalin. *B,* Frontal section of maxilloturbinates of a New Zealand white rabbit with *P. multocida* infection of the nares. Hyperemia, mucopurulent exudate, and turbinate atrophy are apparent. *C,* Photomicrograph of a turbinate from a rabbit with *P. multocida* infection of the nares. Marked inflammatory infiltration, blunting, and erosion of bone characterize midstage turbinate atrophy (hematoxylin & eosin stain × 375).

Pneumonia, Pleuritis, Pericarditis

Chronic infection within the thoracic cavity may go undetected until long after the acute phase of infection, and it is likely to take the form of pleuropneumonia or pericarditis, with abscesses developing in or around the lungs or heart (Fig. 18–3). Anorexia, weight loss, depression, and rapid fatigue are nonspecific signs, but in rabbits they should arouse suspicion of lower respiratory disease caused by *P. multocida* infection. Dyspnea occurs on exertion. Auscultation may reveal areas in the thorax where

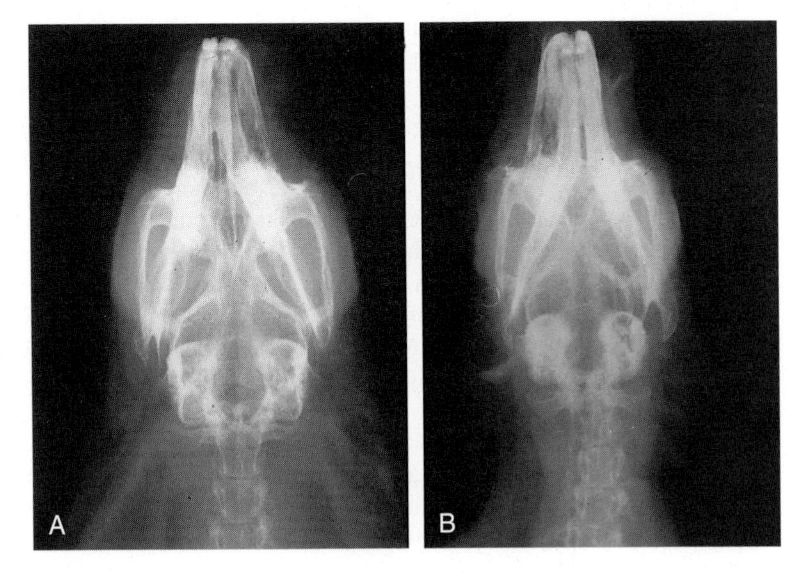

FIGURE 18–2

A, Radiograph of the skull of a Dutch rabbit showing normal tympanic bullae. *B,* Radiograph of the skull of a New Zealand black rabbit with otitis media showing thickened bone of the tympanic bullae and increased opacity resulting from exudate in the middle and external ear. (Courtesy of Mark Mitchell, Northwest Veterinary Hospital, Seattle, WA.)

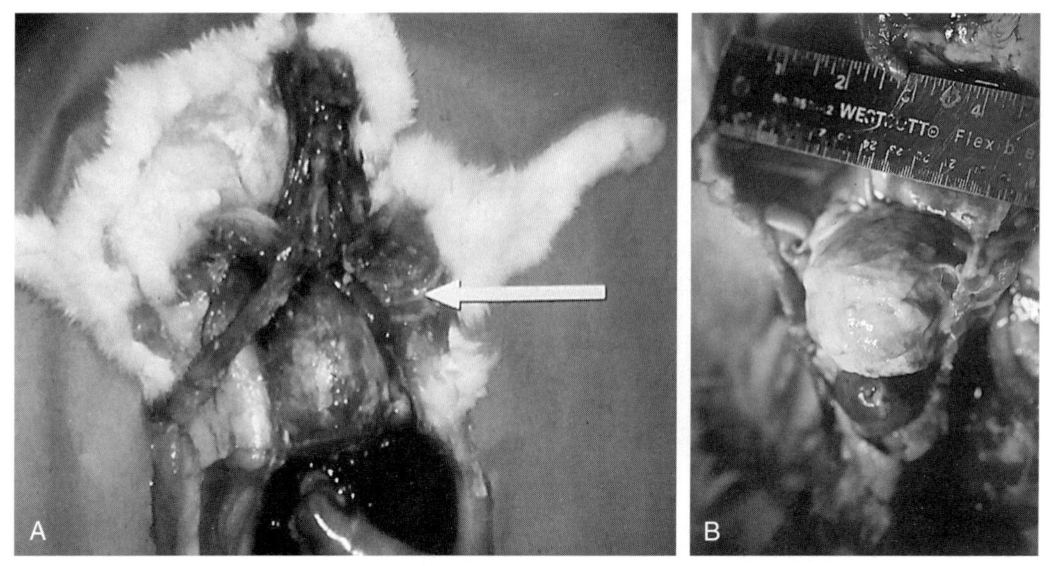

FIGURE 18–3

A, Necropsy of a New Zealand white rabbit with fibrinous pleuritis *(arrow). P. multocida* was isolated. *B,* A massive abscess filling the thoracic cavity of a New Zealand white rabbit. *P. multocida* was isolated.

lung sounds are absent because of consolidation or abscessation. Pulmonary rales must be differentiated from those referred from the upper respiratory tract. Radiographs help to determine the extent of involvement. Rabbits often appear relatively normal even with surprisingly minimal functional lung.

Pathologically, pasteurellosis in the thorax is characterized by the presence of fibrinopurulent exudate in the airways and on serosal surfaces. Neutrophils (also called *heterophils*) are the principal inflammatory cells, but macrophages and erythrocytes may be present. Lymphocytic peribronchial and perivascular cuffing also occur.

Abscesses and Genital Infections

Abscesses in subcutaneous tissues, retrobulbar tissues, or the internal organs of rabbits frequently are caused by *P. multocida.* These abscesses are well encapsulated, contain thick white exudate that does not drain, and enlarge slowly. Mandibular abscesses and infections of the hock joints are common. Genital tract infections occur in both males and females; pyometra is common. A note of caution: abscesses in rabbits tend to appear similar regardless of cause, and not all are caused by *P. multocida.* For example, I have cultured the following organisms in pure culture from abscesses that appeared as described: *Pseudomonas aeruginosa* from mandibular abscesses, *S. aureus* from a pericardial abscess, and *Enterococcus* species from a joint abscess. It is important to document the cause and antibiotic sensitivity and not assume that the cause is *P. multocida.*

Transmission and Pathogenesis

Spread of Infection

Transmission of *P. multocida* is by aerosol from acutely affected rabbits, direct contact, or fomites.[30] Venereal transmission also occurs with genital infections, and kits may be infected at birth if the doe has genital infection. However, kits generally remain uninfected for several weeks, and prevalence of infection increases with age and exposure.

P. multocida gains entry to the host primarily through the nares or wounds. If the host does not resist infection, the bacteria colonize the nares or cause production of nasal exudate. The incubation period is difficult to define because many rabbits are subclinical carriers of infection; however, in experimental studies, rhinitis occurred 1–2 weeks after intranasal inoculation of *P. multocida.* Once established in the nasal passages, infection spreads to contiguous tissues (paranasal sinuses, nasolacrimal duct and conjunctiva, eustachian tube and middle ears, trachea, bronchi, and lungs). Hematogenous spread also accounts for infection reaching the middle ears, lungs, and internal organs.

Host Response

Most of the Pasteurellaceae are commensal organisms on mucous membranes but exhibit pathogenicity under conditions of immunodeficiency and stress in the host. Thus, nutritional, climatic, managerial, or social changes may predispose to disease, as may concomitant infection and physical or chemical injury to the mucosa. Exposure of mucous membranes to ammonia or dilute acetic acid increased susceptibility of rabbits to *P. multocida* infection, and stress or hydrocortisone treatment increased pathogenicity.[7, 28, 34] With disseminated pasteurellosis, fever enhances neutrophil response and increases survival.

The protective role of the humoral immune response to *P. multocida* is unclear. Immunization partially protects against severe disease but does not prevent infection.[30] Antibodies to antigens of *P. multocida* or to cross-reacting antigens of other bacteria may enhance opsonization and phagocytosis. Common epitopes do occur between *P. multocida* and other gram-negative bacteria, notably *Pasteurella, Yersinia,* and *Moraxella* species.

Serum with immunoglobulin G to *P. multocida* is not bactericidal in vitro or in vivo.[30] Rabbits with chronic and severe infections usually have high immunoglobulin G titers to *P. multocida*. Also, the secretory immune response (immunoglobulin A) does not protect against nasal infection,[9] although it may play a role in limiting spread. The protective role of cell-mediated immunity in *P. multocida* infection has not been well studied, but depressed T lymphocyte function resulted in severe disease in infected rabbits.[7]

Characterization of the protein patterns and immunogenic epitopes of *P. multocida* by electrophoresis and immunoblotting indicates that several proteins are consistently recognized by infected rabbits.[11, 41] Several antigens associated with virulence have been identified.[5, 10, 20, 25, 29] Their identification offers promise for their use in subunit vaccines.

Diagnosis

Isolation of Bacteria

Although rhinitis, conjunctivitis, respiratory distress, torticollis, and abscesses in rabbits are suggestive of pasteurellosis, a causative diagnosis cannot be made on the basis of clinical signs alone. Hematologic evaluation is recommended, but even in severe pasteurellosis, hematologic values are not always indicative of infection. Isolation of the causative agent from affected tissues requires culture before the use of antibiotics. Once antimicrobial therapy has been initiated, bacteria may be attenuated, even if not eliminated, and difficult to grow in vitro. To determine whether a bacterial pathogen is present in the nares, in the case of rhinitis or in screening for *P. multocida*, insert a No. 4 calcium alginate swab 1–4 cm into the nares along the nasal septum on both sides (nasal infection may be unilateral). The nasopharynx may be a better site to recover *P. multocida* but is less accessible. A bacterial agent causing rhinitis is likely to be present in nearly pure culture from the nares, but there is no need to do multiple sensitivity tests on normal nasal flora in a mixed culture (see Table 18–1).

For various reasons, *P. multocida* is sometimes difficult to recover, and more than one attempt should be made before ruling it out. To maximize success, the swab of the affected tissue should be inoculated directly or within a short time onto a blood agar plate. Incubate the culture for at least 48 hours for the best visualization of the slowly growing *P. multocida* colonies. Some strains grow better in 5% carbon dioxide, and some at 34–35°C (93.2–95.0°F), a temperature range that approximates that in rabbit nares. When collecting a swab sample from an abscess for culture, insert the swab against the inner wall of the capsule because the centers of abscesses are often sterile.

Serodiagnosis

Because rabbits infected with *P. multocida* develop antibodies but usually remain infected, serologic testing is helpful in detecting internal infections or subclinical carriers. Enzyme-linked immunosorbent assays (ELISAs) have been developed to detect immunoglobulins against *P. multocida*.[30] ELISAs are reliable in screening for *P. multocida* infection in rabbit colonies.[39] The practitioner must understand the limitations of these tests and not misinterpret results. High levels of antibody to *P. multocida* correlate well with chronic infection. The test does not detect antibody very early in infection, as it takes 2–3 weeks for the titer to rise substantially. Antibody in a rabbit younger than 8 weeks of age is likely maternally acquired. Sera with antibodies to related bacteria, possibly normal flora, react at low levels in the test, giving false-positive results. Immunosuppression results in decreased antibody and possibly false-negative results. If a serum sample is reactive at a low level, testing a second sample about 3 weeks later helps in determining whether the antibody level is increasing (an early infection), decreasing (maternal antibody or infection eliminated), or remaining about the same (probably because of infection with related bacteria that are not necessarily pathogenic). Of course, the ideal test would be one that detects antibody to an antigenic epitope unique to *P. multocida* and present in all strains.

The relationship of serum antibodies against *P. multocida* to signs of URD in 100 pet rabbits is shown in Table 18–2. Interpretation was based on epidemiologic and experimental studies.[9, 14] Optical density readings greater than 0.6 were recorded as positive, and those less than 0.3 as negative. When values were between 0.3 and 0.6, a second serum sample, taken 3 weeks after the first, was requested, and the two samples were compared in tests done at the same time. Data from bacterial culture were unavailable. Among the 100 rabbits, 35 had second serum samples submitted. Optical density values of 22 of the 35 samples were within 0.1 of the first sample (unchanged); 5 increased more than 0.1 (changed to positive); and 8 decreased more than 0.1 (these rabbits had been treated with antibiotics). Thus, not all pet rabbits have antibodies to or are carriers of *P. multocida* infection; those rabbits with serum samples showing high optical density values are likely to have signs of URD; and some rabbits with signs of URD but with low optical density values or no increase in optical density values may have infections with bacteria other than *P. multocida.*

Regardless of bacteriologic or serologic findings, if a rabbit has respiratory distress or if a middle ear infection is suspected, radiography is indicated as an aid in diagnosis and prognosis (Table 18–3).

Treatment and Control

Antibiotics

Studies for determining the effectiveness of various antibiotics in treating *P. multocida* infection generally have involved rabbits with chronic disease. They have shown diminishment or cessation of clinical signs during treatment for 7–14 days but recurrence when treatment was discontinued as well as a failure to eliminate infection. Infection was eliminated in seven of eight rabbits treated with enrofloxacin (5 mg/kg SC q12h) for 14 days.[3] Enrofloxacin given in the drinking water (50–100 mg/L) before and continuing for 48 hours after inoculation with a virulent strain of *P. multocida* protected rabbits against bacteremia, provided that daily intake of the drug was greater than 5 mg/kg.[33] I have had success with some chronic severe cases of pasteurellosis when enrofloxacin (5–10 mg/kg

TABLE 18–2
ANTIBODIES AGAINST *PASTEURELLA MULTOCIDA* IN PET RABBITS

	Optical Density (sera diluted 1:100)*									
	<0.3†		*0.3–0.5*		*0.6‡–1.0*		*>1.0*		*Total*	
Age (y)	*n*§	*URD*‖	*n*	*URD*	*n*	*URD*	*n*	*URD*	*n*	*URD*
<1	21	2	7	3	4	0	3	3	35	5
>1	20	5	23	7	13	6	9	8	65	26
Total	41	7	30	10	17	6	12	11	100	31
% with URD	17		33		35		92		31	

*Positive control serum reads about 1.5; negative control about 0.03.
†Optical density <0.3 considered negative.
‡Optical density >0.6 considered positive.
§*n* = number tested.
‖Number with nasal and/or ocular discharge (upper respiratory tract disease).

TABLE 18–3
DIFFERENTIATION OF RESPIRATORY DISEASE IN RABBITS

Signs	*Upper:* Nasal/ocular discharge; matted fur on face, forepaws; sneezing, snoring	*Lower:* Anorexia, depression, fever, fatigue, dyspnea, cyanosis		
Auscultation	*Rhinitis/Sinusitis:* Nasopharyngeal rales	*Bronchopneumonia:* Pulmonary rales; patchy absence of respiratory sounds	*Pleuritis:* Friction sounds; exaggerated heart sounds	*Pulmonary edema:* Wheezing and fluid sounds
Radiographic Findings	*Nasal turbinates/sinuses:* ↑ Opacity—exudate ↓ Opacity—atrophy	↑ Peribronchial opacity; pulmonary consolidation	Effusion line; thoracic masses	Generalized ↑ in pulmonary opacity

PO q12h) or chloramphenicol (50 mg/kg PO q12h) was given for extended periods (2–3 months); signs of disease were eliminated and antibody titers diminished. Some owners are willing to use antibiotics in the long-term to improve the health and extend the lives of their pets. Adjunct therapy includes instillation of antibiotic drops such as ciprofloxacin ophthalmic drops (Ciloxan, Alcon Laboratories, Inc., Fort Worth, TX) or gentamicin ophthalmic drops into nares, ear canals, or conjunctival sacs, or nebulization with antibiotics. When indicated, lacrimal ducts should be flushed and abscesses surgically removed or lanced and débrided.

Choose an antibiotic based not only on in vitro sensitivities but also on the sensitivity of the rabbit's intestinal flora. Enteric dysbiosis can result in fatal enterocolitis or enterotoxemia. Antimicrobials less likely to cause this side effect are trimethoprim-sulfa, the fluoroquinolones, chloramphenicol, and tetracyclines. The use of any antimicrobial agent in rabbits warrants monitoring. In the event of anorexia, diarrhea, or excretion of abnormal feces, discontinue use of the antibiotic and select a different drug.

Control

Pasteurella-free rabbit colonies were first established by Webster. Webster's methods are still used today and are referred to as "barrier housing."[30] *Pasteurella*-free rabbits are selected by bacteriologic and serologic screening and housed away from rabbits of unknown or infected status. Traffic of materials and caretakers from infected to uninfected rabbits is prevented. Cesarean derivation and fostering of kits onto *Pasteurella*-free does is another method of establishing a *Pasteurella*-free colony. Early weaning, with or without the use of antimicrobials for infected does, can give *Pasteurella*-free weanlings.

Rabbits available at pet stores are not likely to be from *Pasteurella*-free colonies. Thus, a rabbit recently acquired from a pet store should be examined, tested for *P. multocida* infection, and if infected, treated with antibiotics. Elimination of infection may be easier in young rabbits before disease becomes chronic. If rhinitis is severe and exudate is being expelled by sneezing, isolate the affected rabbit from other rabbits and ensure that infectious exudate is not spread by fomites. Transmission from rabbits with chronic pasteurellosis is less common than from those acutely affected. Sometimes, infected rabbits have lived in relatively close contact with uninfected rabbits and have not transmitted the organism. Germicidals effective against *P. multocida* include a 10% solution of sodium hypochlorite 5.25%, 1 oz/gal of 2% chlorhexidine diacetate, and 2 mL/gal of 20% benzalkonium chloride, but not 70% alcohol. Controlling spread of infection in the host generally depends on proper diet, avoidance of stress or changes in ambient temperature, and good husbandry practices, including good ventilation, as well as treatment with antibiotics.

Vaccines

No vaccine is currently available for the prevention of pasteurellosis in rabbits. The following vaccine preparations have been evaluated and have *not* prevented nasal infection on challenge: bacteria killed with heat or formalin; potassium thiocyanate extracts; and live but avirulent strains, such as a streptomycin-dependent strain.[30] New strategies based on virulence factors of *P. multocida* and host response to antigenic epitopes are under consideration.

OTHER INFECTIOUS CAUSES OF RESPIRATORY DISEASE

Bacteria

Bordetella bronchiseptica

B. bronchiseptica is a common inhabitant of the respiratory tract of rabbits. The prevalence of infection increases with age, and both the nares and the bronchi become colonized. Respiratory disease usually is not associated with *B. bronchiseptica* infection.[9] Experimentally, intranasal inoculation of *B. bronchiseptica* caused serous nasal discharge and bronchopneumonia and pleuritis in suckling or weanling rabbits.[21, 38]

B. bronchiseptica is pathogenic in guinea pigs, dogs, cats, and pigs. It adheres to ciliated mucosa, resists respiratory clearance, and induces ciliostasis and reduced macrophage adherence and phagocytosis.[40] Cytotoxic *B. bronchiseptica* enhances colonization by toxigenic *P. multocida*.[18] Therefore, *B. bronchiseptica* is suspected as a copathogen or predisposing factor in *P. multocida* infections. More pathogenic strains of *B. bronchiseptica* may exist. For example, an investigation of URD in rabbits from a colony of inbred rabbits showed them free of *P. multocida*; however, the nares were colonized by *B. bronchiseptica,* which was resistant to several commonly used antibiotics. In such a case, selective antibiotic therapy for *B. bronchiseptica* is indicated.

Staphylococcus aureus

S. aureus is often isolated from the nares of both healthy and diseased rabbits. It is probably a secondary agent that increases suppurative inflammation of compromised mucosa. As with *P. multocida* infection, pathogenicity depends on host susceptibility and bacterial virulence. *S. aureus* produces toxins lethal for rabbit neutrophils as well as protein A, which binds the Fc portion of immunoglobulin G. Thus, bactericidal mechanisms of the host are blocked.[6]

Disseminated staphylococcosis results in fibrinous pneumonia or abscesses in the lungs or heart. Abscesses caused by *S. aureus* appear similar to those caused by *P. multocida. S. aureus* more often shows in vitro resistance to a variety of antibiotics than does *P. multocida*. Thus, a culture and sensitivity test is advisable, but the abscess may be in an area that is inaccessible. Chloramphenicol, enrofloxacin, or trimethoprim-sulfa combinations are antibiotics of choice for rabbits when a culture specimen cannot be obtained.

Pasteurella Species

Pasteurella species other than *P. multocida* are often reported by bacteriology laboratories from nasal cultures of rabbits. Unless the organism is present in pure culture and is associated with clinical disease, it is likely a commensal rather than a pathogen.

Moraxella catarrhalis

This organism, previously known as *Micrococcus, Neisseria,* or *Branhamella catarrhalis*, is a well represented member of the nasal flora of rabbits. Like *B. bronchiseptica*, it is sometimes isolated from clinical cases of rhinitis or conjunctivitis. If isolated in pure culture, one suspects that the organism may have a role in the disease, probably as an opportunist on unhealthy mucosa. However, unless clinical disease is present, there is no justification for antibiotic therapy to eliminate *M. catarrhalis* from the nares.

Other Bacterial Agents

Other bacterial agents that have caused pneumonia in rabbits are *Mycobacterium bovis, M. avium, and M. tuberculosis, Francisella tularensis, Moraxella bovis,* and *Pseudomonas aeruginosa*.[19] Tularemia is rare in domestic rabbits. *P. aeruginosa* can cause abscesses similar to those of *P. multocida* as well as septicemia and pneumonia.

Cilia-associated respiratory bacillus colonizes ciliated epithelial cells of the respiratory tract and causes chronic respiratory disease in rodents. Although it occurs in rabbits, cilia-associated respiratory bacillus induces only mild hyperplasia of ciliated epithelium and inflammatory infiltration.[26]

Mycoplasma/Chlamydia

Mycoplasma pulmonis was isolated from the nasopharynx of rabbits with signs of URD.[8] Specimens from the rabbits were not cultured for *P. multocida*. The rabbits were housed in close proximity to rats, which may have been the source of the infection. *M. pulmonis* causes chronic respiratory disease in rats, but the pathogenicity of *M. pulmonis* in rabbits has not been investigated. Isolation of *Mycoplasma* species requires special media and methods and precludes routine examination for these organisms. In 1986, I attempted to isolate *Mycoplasma* species from the nasopharynx and lungs of 52 rabbits from 4 commercial rabbitries where respiratory disease was endemic. *Mycoplasma* species were not recovered (unpublished study).

Chlamydia species have been isolated from the lungs of domestic rabbits with pneumonia. A mild interstitial pneumonia occurred when the agent was inoculated into the trachea of laboratory rabbits.[19]

Viruses

Viral agents of respiratory disease in rabbits are not well studied; they may be insignificant as pathogens in the respiratory tract, or they may be underreported.[16]

Myxoma virus causes nasal and ocular discharge and dyspnea in protracted cases. However, respiratory disease is not a hallmark of myxomatosis and is not likely to occur in the absence of generalized disease, edema, and tumors.

A herpesvirus has been recovered from the nares of European rabbits with respiratory disease. Rabbits develop antibodies to Sendai virus, a paramyxovirus that causes respiratory disease in rodents. However, experimental inoculation did not induce disease in rabbits.

A coronavirus has been implicated in association with pleural effusion disease/infectious cardiomyopathy. The disease occurred in the 1960s in Scandinavia in rabbits used to propagate *Treponema pallidum*. As yet, no cases of the disease outside the laboratory environment have been reported; thus, the agent may have been a contaminant of suspensions of testicular cells infected with *T. pallidum*. The target organ of the viral agent was the heart. Clinical signs were typical of acute viremia and, in survivors, of myocarditis and congestive heart failure.

NONINFECTIOUS RESPIRATORY DISEASE

Immunologic Causes

Rhinitis and chronic bronchitis resulting from exposure to allergens occurs in rabbits. If the allergen cannot be identified and eliminated from the rabbit's environment, corticosteroids or antihistamines are used to reduce and control inflammation. Pasteurellosis or infections with other pathogenic agents must be ruled out. Prolonged use of corticosteroids in rabbits with chronic *P. multocida* infection is contraindicated.

Neoplastic Disease

Thymomas are occasionally seen in both young and adult rabbits. These tumors can be of either lymphoid or epithelial origin. Clinical signs include tachypnea and moderate to severe dyspnea. Bilateral exophthalmos is occasionally observed[37] and may be related to interference of vascular return to the heart caused by the mass (see Chapter 14). Radiographs reveal a rounded, soft tissue opacity cranial to the heart. There is no treatment for thymoma.

Cardiovascular Disease

Pulmonary edema, the accumulation of fluid in the interstitial tissue, alveoli, and bronchi, occurs in conjunction with circulatory disorders. How often pulmonary edema occurs in rabbits is unknown, but it may be fairly common. Heart failure and arteriosclerosis are likely in pet rabbits because their life span is extended (more than 10 years is common). Differentiation from infectious processes involves auscultation of the lungs for typical wheezing sounds, radiographic evaluation, and hematologic testing. If pulmonary edema is confirmed, treat with diuretics and bronchodilators.

Traumatic Causes

Traumatic tracheitis may result from endotracheal intubation for inhalant anesthesia. Rabbits maintained for 3–4 hours on halothane developed severe necrotizing tracheitis, submucosal edema, and mucosal erosion where the tip of a Sheridan cuffed endotracheal tube touched the trachea.[1] Use a soft pliable silicone endotracheal tube or face mask when administering gas anesthesia in rabbits.

Irritation to the respiratory tract occurs with aerogenous exposure to chemicals, such as excessive ammonia from urine build-up or possibly cigarette smoke. Such exposure may predispose the mucosa to infection.

REFERENCES

1. Abbott LJ, Deeb BJ, Dickinson EO, et al: Use of an atraumatic endo-tracheal tube in rabbits. Lab Anim Sci 1989; 39:493.
2. Anderson LC, Rush HG, Glorioso JC: Strain differences in the susceptibility and resistance of *Pasteurella multocida* to phagocytosis and killing by rabbit polymorphonuclear neutrophils. Am J Vet Res 1984; 45:1193–1198.
3. Broome RL, Brooks DL: Efficacy of enrofloxacin in the treatment of respiratory pasteurellosis in rabbits. Lab Anim Sci 1991; 41:572–576.
4. Chrisp CE, Foged NT: Induction of pneumonia in rabbits by use of a purified protein toxin from *Pasteurella multocida*. Am J Vet Res 1991; 52:56–61.
5. Choi-Kim K, Meheswaran SK, Felice LJ, et al: Relationship between the iron regulated outer membrane proteins and the outer membrane proteins of *in vivo* grown *Pasteurella multocida*. Vet Microbiol 1991; 28:75–92.
6. Cohen JO: Staphylococcus. *In* Baron S, ed.: Medical Microbiology. New York, Churchill Livingstone, 1991, pp 203–214.
7. Corbeil LB, Strayer DS, Skaletsky E, et al: Immunity to pasteurellosis in compromised rabbits. Am J Vet Res 1983; 44:845–850.
8. Deeb BJ, Kenny GE: Characterization of *Mycoplasma pulmonis* variants isolated from rabbits: I. identification and properties of isolates. J Bacteriol 1967; 93:1416–1424.
9. Deeb BJ, DiGiacomo RF, Bernard BL, et al: *Pasteurella multocida* and *Bordetella bronchiseptica* infections in rabbits. J Clin Microbiol 1990; 28:70–75.
10. Deeb BJ, DiGiacomo RF, Stewart JS: Iron-regulated growth and expression of proteins in rabbit strains of *Pasteurella multocida*. Microbiol Pathog (in press).
11. DeLong D, Manning PJ, Gunther R, et al: Colonization of rabbits by *Pasteurella multocida*: serum IgG responses following intranasal challenge with serologically distinct isolates. Lab Anim Sci 1992; 42:13–19.
12. DiGiacomo RF, Garlinghouse LE, Van Hoosier GL: Natural history of infection with *Pasteurella multocida* in rabbits. J Am Vet Med Assoc 1983; 183:1172–1175.
13. DiGiacomo RF, Deeb BJ, Giddens WE, et al: Atrophic rhinitis in New Zealand White rabbits infected with *Pasteurella multocida*. Am J Vet Res 1989; 50:1460–1465.
14. DiGiacomo RF, Taylor FGR, Allen V, et al: Naturally acquired *Pasteurella multocida* infection in rabbits: immunologic aspects. Lab Anim Sci 1990; 40:289–292.
15. DiGiacomo RF, Deeb BJ, Brodie SJ, et al: Toxin production by *Pasteurella multocida* isolated from rabbits with atrophic rhinitis. Am J Vet Res 1993; 54:1280–1286.
16. DiGiacomo RF, Maré CJ: Viral Diseases. *In* Manning P, Ringler DH, Newcomer CE, eds.: Biology of the Laboratory Rabbit. Orlando, FL, Academic Press, 1994, pp 171–204.
17. Duclos P, Caillet J, Javelot P: Flore bacteriènne aerobie des cavités nasales du lapin d'élévage. Ann Rech Vet 1986; 17:185–190.
18. Dugal F, Bélanger M, Jacques M: Enhanced adherence of *Pasteurella multocida* to porcine tracheal rings preinfected with *Bordetella bronchiseptica*. Can J Vet Res 1992; 56:260–264.
19. Flatt RE: Bacterial diseases. *In* Weisbroth SH, Flatt RE, Kraus AK, eds.: The Biology of the Laboratory Rabbit. New York, Academic Press, 1974, pp 193–236.
20. Foged NT, Nielsen JP, Jorsal SE: Protection against progressive atrophic rhinitis by vaccination with *Pasteurella* toxin purified by monoclonal antibodies. Vet Rec 1989; 125: 7–11.
21. Glavits R, Magyar T: The pathology of experimental respiratory infection with *Pasteurella multocida* and *Bordetella bronchiseptica* in rabbits. Acta Vet Hung 1990; 38: 211–215.
22. Glorioso JC, Jones GW, Rush HG, et al: Adhesion of type A *Pasteurella multocida* to rabbit pharyngeal cells and its possible role in rabbit respiratory tract infections. Infect Immunol 1982; 35:1103–1109.
23. Gunther R, Manning PJ, Bouma JE, et al: Partial characterization of plasmids from rabbit isolates of *Pasteurella multocida*. Lab Anim Sci 1991; 41:423–426.
24. Hagen KW: Enzootic pasteurellosis in domestic rabbits: I. pathology and bacteriology. J Am Vet Med Assoc 1958; 133:77–80.
25. Ikeda JS, Hirsh DC: Antigenically related iron-regulated outer membrane proteins produced by different somatic serotypes of *Pasteurella multocida*. Am J Vet Res 1988; 56:2499–2502.
26. Kurisu K, Kyo S, Shiomoto Y, et al: Cilia-associated respiratory bacillus infection in rabbits. Lab Anim Sci 1990; 40:413–415.
27. Lu YS, Ringler DH, Park JS: Characterization of *Pasteurella multocida* isolates from the nares of healthy rabbits and rabbits with pneumonia. Lab Anim Sci 1978; 28:691–697.
28. Lu YS, Pakes SP, Rehg JE, et al: Pathogenicity of serotype 12:A *Pasteurella multocida* in hydrocortisone treated and nontreated rabbits. Lab Anim Sci 1982; 32:258–262.
29. Lu YS, Lai WC, Pakes SP, et al: A monoclonal antibody against a *Pasteurella multocida* outer membrane protein protects rabbits and mice against pasteurellosis. Infect Immunol 1991; 59:172–180.
30. Manning PJ, DiGiacomo RF, DeLong D: Pasteurellosis in laboratory animals. *In* Adlam C, Rutter JM, eds.: *Pasteurella* and Pasteurellosis. London, Academic Press, 1989, pp 263–302.
31. Nakagawa M, Nakayama K, Saito M, et al: Bacteriological and serological studies on *Pasteurella multocida* infection in rabbits. Jikken Dobutsu 1986; 35:463–469.
32. Okerman L, Spanoghe L, DeBruycker RM: Experimental infections of mice with *Pasteurella multocida* strains isolated from rabbits. J Comp Pathol 1979; 89:51–55.
33. Okerman L, DeVriese LA, Maerten L, et al: In vivo activity of orally administered antibiotics and chemotherapeutics against acute septicaemic pasteurellosis in rabbits. Lab Anim 1990; 24:341–344.

34. Patton NM, Holmes HT, Caveny DD, et al: Experimental inducement of snuffles in rabbits. J Appl Rabbit Res 1980; 3:8–12.
35. Percy DH, Prescott JF, Bhasin JL: Characterization of *Pasteurella multocida* isolated from rabbits in Canada. Can J Comp Med 1984; 48:162–165.
36. Rimler RB, Rhoades KR: *Pasteurella multocida*. *In* Adlam C, Rutter JM, eds.: *Pasteurella* and Pasteurellosis. London, Academic Press, 1989, pp 37–73.
37. Vernau KM, Grahn BH, Clarke-Scott HA, Sullivan N: Thymoma in a geriatric rabbit with hypercalcemia and periodic exophthalmos. J Am Vet Med Assoc 1995; 206:820–822.
38. Watson WT, Goldsboro JA, Williams FP, et al: Experimental respiratory infection with *Pasteurella multocida* and *Bordetella bronchiseptica* in rabbits. Lab Anim Sci 1975; 25:459–464.
39. Zaoutis TE, Reinhard GR, Cioffe CJ, et al: Screening rabbit colonies for antibodies to *Pasteurella multocida* by an ELISA. Lab Anim Sci 1991; 41:419–422.
40. Zeligs BJ, Zeligs JD, Bellanti JA: Functional and ultrastructural changes in alveolar macrophages from rabbits colonized with *Bordetella bronchiseptica*. Infect Immunol 1986; 53:702–706.
41. Zimmerman TE, Deeb BJ, DiGiacomo RF: Polypeptides associated with *Pasteurella multocida* infection in rabbits. Am J Vet Res 1992; 53:1108–1112.

ACKNOWLEDGMENTS

The author thanks Ronald DiGiacomo and Lillian Price for reviewing the manuscript, Alice Ruff for editorial assistance, and Sandi Ackerman of the House Rabbit Society for encouragement.

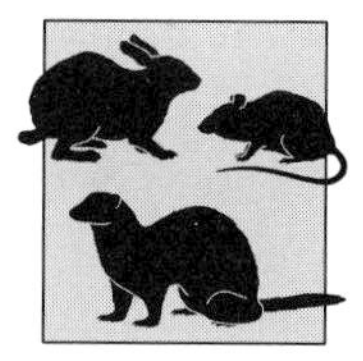

CHAPTER 19

Reproductive and Urogenital Disorders

Joanne Paul-Murphy, DVM

DISORDERS OF THE REPRODUCTIVE SYSTEM

Adenocarcinoma

Uterine adenocarcinoma is the most common neoplasia of female rabbits. Age is the most important factor in the development of adenocarcinoma, and occurrence is independent of breeding history. When older than 4 years of age, rabbits of certain breeds (tan, French silver, Havana, and Dutch) have an incidence of 50–80%.[1, 20] With age, the endometrium undergoes progressive aging changes, a decrease in cellularity, and an increase in collagen content. These changes are associated with the development of uterine cancer.[1] Adenocarcinoma of the uterus is a slowly developing tumor. Local invasion of the myometrium and peritoneal cavity occurs early; hematogenous metastasis to the lungs, liver, and bones may occur within 1–2 years.

Early clinical signs such as decreased fertility, small litter size, and increased occurrence of fetus retention or resorption and of stillbirths may be recognized in a breeding doe. The first sign observed in many pet rabbits is hematuria or a serosanguineous vaginal discharge. Commonly, frank blood in the urine is most pronounced at the end of urination. Cystic mammary glands can occur concurrently with uterine hyperplasia or adenocarcinoma.[17, 26] Clinical signs of late stage adenocarcinoma may include depression, anorexia, and

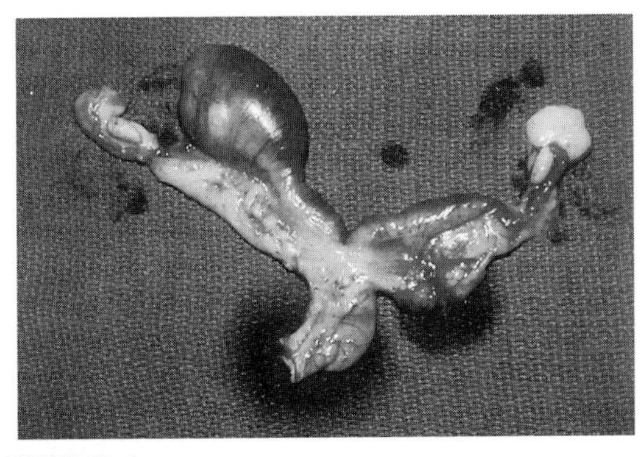

FIGURE 19–1
Uterine adenocarcinoma often is multicentric and involves both uterine horns.

dyspnea if pulmonary metastasis has occurred. The diagnosis relies on palpation of an enlarged uterus or of uterine masses or nodules, 1–5 cm in diameter, in the caudal abdomen. Adenocarcinomas are often multicentric, involving both horns[1] (Fig. 19–1). Other causes of uterine enlargement include pregnancy, pyometra, metritis, venous aneurysms, endometrial hyperplasia, and other tumors such as leiomyosarcoma.

Radiographs and ultrasound imaging assist in establishing the diagnosis when a caudal abdominal soft tissue mass or uterine enlargement can be identified. Ultrasound imaging can help you differentiate the cause of uterine enlargement, measure masses, and scan for multiple nodules. Evaluate thoracic radiographs for the presence of pulmonary metastasis. Pulmonary involvement carries a grave prognosis.

If you identify abdominal masses in the early stages of disease, prior to metastasis, surgical excision and ovariohysterectomy is the treatment of choice. The prognosis is good with ovariohysterectomy if the tumor is contained within the uterus. If local invasion is observed at the time of surgery, reexamine the rabbit every 6 months for a 1–2-year period after surgery for evidence of pulmonary metastasis. Successful chemotherapy for this tumor has not been reported.

Prevention is the key to the management of this disease. Ovariohysterectomy is recommended for pet rabbits before they reach 2 years of age. I prefer to spay rabbits between the ages of 6 and 12 months, because the amount of abdominal fat is less than that in older rabbits. Twice yearly, schedule preventative health checks for intact females 3 years of age and older to monitor for early signs of disease.

Endometrial Hyperplasia or Uterine Polyps

Endometrial changes may occur along a continuum, from polyp formation to cystic hyperplasia to adenomatous hyperplasia to adenocarcinoma, as it does in humans.[11, 20, 26] Some reports have found no association between cystic hyperplasia and adenocarcinoma in rabbits because adenocarcinoma is associated with senile atrophy of the endometrium.[1] Uterine hyperplasia is associated with aging, but with aging the endometrial glands become cystic and hyperplastic.

Clinical signs can include intermittent hematuria, anemia, and a decrease in activity. A firm, irregular uterus sometimes can be detected on palpation. Cystic mammary glands can occur with this condition.[26] Radiography and ultrasound can help in diagnosis of the uterine changes; cystic ovaries can be identified concurrently.[17] Ovariohysterectomy is the recommended treatment, and exploration of the abdomen is warranted.

Pyometra and Endometritis

Vaginal discharge, anorexia, lethargy, weakness, and an enlarged abdomen are frequent clinical signs that accompany endometritis or pyometra. Clinical signs of mild endometritis can be subtle, making the condition difficult to diagnose. Rabbits with chronic disease may have no overt clinical signs. The history of a breeding doe often includes a recent parturition, pseudocyesis, or an inability to rebreed. Rabbits with mild endometritis may kindle successfully or have fetal resorptions and stillbirths. Pyometra and endometritis can also develop in virgin does. Diagnosis relies on palpation of a doughy uterus and on enlargement of the uterus, as identified on abdominal radiographs. Use caution when palpating the abdomen if the uterus is greatly enlarged because the uterine wall becomes very thin. Results of ultrasound imaging can rule out other uterine conditions such as polyps, masses, or cystic changes. The results of a complete blood count (CBC) may be normal or show a slight leukocytosis with neutrophilia. Evaluate serum biochemistry values because chronic inflammation of the uterus has been reported to induce amyloid deposition in the kidneys.[19] Cytologic assessment and a Gram's stain of the cervical mucus or drainage can assist diagnosis.

Exploratory laparotomy and ovariohysterectomy may be the procedures of choice for confirming a diagnosis. Multiple adhesions to adjacent viscera often complicate the procedure. Before surgery, obtain a guarded deep vaginal or cervical swab for bacterial culture and sensitivity testing, or take an intraoperative culture. IV or intraosseous fluids are an important component of therapy. Begin broad-spectrum antibiotic therapy as soon as a sample for culture has been collected.

Pasteurella multocida and *Staphylococcus aureus* are frequently isolated from rabbits with pyometra or metritis. Venereal transmission occurs when infected does breed with uninfected bucks, or vice versa. *P. multocida* can localize in the genital tract from hematogenous spread from another location, or retrograde infection can occur from a vaginitis.[13] Ovarian abscesses can occur in conjunction with *P. multocida* pyometra.[21] Rare cases of naturally occurring metritis or pyometra have been associated with *Chlamydia, Listeria monocytogenes, S. aureus, Moraxella bovis, Actinomyces pyogenes, Brucella melitensis,* and *Salmonella* species.[18, 32, 37, 41] Postpartum metritis can occur in conjunction with hypervitaminosis A, and the delivery of stillborn young and metritis have been associated with uterine torsion.[18]

For a breeding rabbit with mild endometritis, appropriate antibiotic and fluid therapy may be sufficient, but the tenacious nature of inflammatory exudates in rabbits makes it extremely difficult for the uterus to drain adequately. The use of prostaglandins to assist uterine contraction and drainage has not been reported. Ovariohysterectomy is the best choice for treatment of pyometra because of the high incidence of *P. multocida* infections.

Orchitis/Epididymitis

Clinical signs of orchitis include fever, an intermittent appetite, and weight loss. The testicles may be enlarged with obvious abscesses, or abscesses may be small and internal, with minimal swelling of the testicles. The epididymis rather than the testis may be infected. An affected breeding buck has low conception rates. Treatment is castration and antibiotic therapy. *P. multocida* is often isolated from exudate or abscessed tissue on bacterial culture; specific culture for *Treponema* should also be requested. House male rabbits separately to prevent fighting injuries that lead to abscesses.

Venereal Spirochetosis: *Treponema paraluis-cuniculi*

Treponema paraluis-cuniculi is the spirochete responsible for rabbit syphilis or vent disease. This is not a zoonotic disease. Transmission between rabbits is by direct and venereal contact. Bucks can spread the disease to several does, and young rabbits can be infected. It is a self-limiting disease, but asymptomatic carriers can remain. Infection may be subclinical until stress occurs. Lesions first appear on the skin of the perineum and genitalia and begin as areas of redness that progress to edema, vesicle formation, ulcerations, and scabs. The lesions can be painful and impair breeding activity. Autoinfection can lead to facial lesions around the chin, lips, nostrils, and eyelids. Inguinal lymph nodes may be enlarged. Colony epidemics result in a decrease in the rate of conception, metritis, placenta retention, and neonatal deaths.

Clinical signs are often diagnostic. Few other skin problems resemble those of rabbit syphilis, but dermatitis, dermatophytosis, acariasis, and myxomatosis are possibilities. Lesions on the nose and lips are often proliferative and scaly and are commonly mistaken as dermatophyte lesions. For a definitive diagnosis, submit a skin biopsy sample and request silver staining. Examine skin scrapes of the lesions by darkfield microscopy to identify the organism. Large rabbitries can benefit from a serologic survey with the microhemagglutination test to screen and verify affected animals. Other serologic tests are available, such as the rapid plasma reagin card test, which is very specific.[10] In rabbitries, the prevalence of *T. paraluis-cuniculi* infection increases with parity: females that have had six or more litters will be seropositive; bucks in a breeding program 6–12 months will also be seropositive.[10] Bucks are often asymptomatic carriers and may have small star-shaped scars on their scrotum.

Treponema is effectively treated with penicillin. Administer either penicillin G benzathine and penicillin G procaine (42,000–84,000 IU/kg SC at 7-day intervals for 3 injections),[8] or penicillin G procaine (40,000–60,000 IU/kg IM q24h for 5–7 days). Tetracyclines and chloramphenicol can also be effective. Treat all exposed rabbits.

Pregnancy Toxemia

Pregnancy toxemia usually occurs during the last week of gestation, when nest building behavior begins. It is common in obese rabbits. Inadequate caloric intake predisposes pregnant rabbits to toxemia, and environmental change or stress can precipitate the disease. Weakness, depression, incoordination, anorexia, abortion, convulsions, and coma are common clinical signs. Signs can progress over 1–5 days, or acute death may occur. Some rabbits may be dyspneic, and their breath may have an acetone-like odor. The urine becomes acidic and clear because the lower pH decreases the concentration of calcium carbonate crystals. Rabbits should be evaluated for trichobezoars because hair pulling for nesting can contribute to hairball formation and inappetence.[33] Clinical findings that support the diagnosis include acidic urine (pH 5–6), proteinuria, ketonuria, hyperkalemia, ketonemia, hyperphosphatemia, and hypocalcemia. Hepatic lipidosis is a common finding at necropsy.

There are no consistently effective treatments for pregnancy toxemia. Keep rabbits warm and provide intravenous or intraosseous fluids. Calcium gluconate and corticosteroids may be helpful if the animal is in shock. In rabbits with trichobezoars, administer metoclopramide or cisapride and oral fluids. Pregnancy toxemia has a very grave prognosis, and treatment is usually unrewarding. The best approach is prevention. Avoid fasting or undernutrition in late pregnancy, and prevent obesity and sudden stress at all times.

Dystocia or Retained Fetuses

Dystocia is unusual in rabbits, and normal delivery is usually complete within 30 minutes of onset. Rarely, the young are delivered several hours apart. Anterior and breech positions are normal for rabbits. Palpate does 24 hours after delivery to determine whether any fetuses have been retained. A rabbit may be predisposed to dystocia by obesity, large fetuses, a small pelvic canal, or uterine inertia. Signs of dystocia include contractions, straining, and bloody or greenish-brown vaginal discharge. Assistance usually requires gentle manual removal of the fetuses and rapid removal of fetal membranes from the fetuses. Oxytocin (1–2 units IM, SC) can assist uterine contraction. If uterine inertia is suspected, give 5–10 mL of 10% calcium gluconate PO 30 minutes before injection of the oxytocin. Place the doe in a quiet dark room for 30–60 minutes after administration. Cesarean section is indicated if there is no result from this treatment, and the prognosis is guarded.

Abortion/Resorption

The owner of a single rabbit or a rabbitry may seek veterinary advice when abortions or fetal resorptions are suspected. A thorough history-taking is extremely important. Ask questions such as, Is this the first litter? Is there a prior history of abortion? Have any drugs been administered recently? Has there been a recent change in environment? and, Are other rabbits aborting? Always check the doe for remaining fetuses. Submit the fetuses for bacterial culture and histopathologic examination. Possible causes of fetal resorptions or abortions can be numerous and include infection, stress, genetic predisposition, trauma, drug use, or dietary imbalances (e.g., vitamin E, vitamin A, and protein deficiencies). There is a critical period at 3 weeks of gestation in rabbits because of a temporary reduction in blood flow to the uterus and the changing size and shape of the fetuses. Fetal death before 3 weeks resolves as resorption, whereas fetal death after 3 weeks results in abortion. Listeriosis has a predilection for the gravid uterus and should be considered in rabbits with late-term abortion.[41]

Reduced Fertility

One or more factors can contribute to reduction in fertility, including malnutrition (e.g., deficiencies of vitamins A, D, or E, or excess vitamin A), heat stress, systemic illness, nitrate contamination of food or water, environmental disturbances, a decrease in daylight, endometrial carcinoma, metritis, or pyometra. Old age, sexual exhaustion, or breeding of rabbits that are too young may be causes of infertility. Vitamin E deficiency causes myodystrophy, which can lead to abortions, stillbirths, and neonatal deaths. A high concentration of serum creatine phosphokinase supports a diagnosis of hypovitaminosis E and indicates a need for dietary supplementation.[32] Hypervitaminosis A can cause fetal resorptions, abortions, and stillbirths. A suppurative metritis may follow the delivery of dead fetuses.[9] Hypovitaminosis A can cause similar reproductive disorders, resulting in poor fertility and weak, hydrocephalic young. The National Research Council recommends vitamin A levels of 1160 IU/kg of diet for gestation, or approximately 20 μg/kg of body weight per day.[39]

Prolapsed Vagina

A prolapsed vagina is easily recognized as a blood-covered mass of swollen and fragile tissue protruding from the vulva. The prolapse may be full of clotted blood. Affected rabbits are depressed or recumbent with an increased respiratory rate or are in shock with cold extremities. Pale mucous membranes or cyanotic ears and mucous membranes indicate severe shock. The hematocrit in such rabbits has been reported as low as 9%.[40] Treatment is directed at correcting hypovolemic shock and blood loss. Reduce the prolapse with the doe under anesthesia, or surgically amputate the tissue if it is necrotic. Prolapses start from the proximal circular part of the vaginal vault just distal to the urethral opening.[40]

Eight cases of vaginal prolapse were described in closely related rabbits during periods of increased sexual activity or receptivity; this finding suggests a genetic susceptibility.[40]

Endometrial Venous Aneurysms

Multiple endometrial venous aneurysms can cause hematuria because of episodic bleeding. This diagnosis was reported in only three New Zealand white rabbits and was confirmed on exploratory laparotomy and histopathologic examination of the uterus.[3] In rabbits with this condition, the uterine horns have multiple, blood-filled endometrial varices (veins) that periodically rupture into the uterine lumen, causing the clinical hematuria. Venous aneurysms in other species are caused by congenital defects of the adventitia, increased intraluminal pressure, or trauma.[3]

Hydrometra

Hydrometra is the accumulation of watery fluid in the uterus. It has been described in four unbred sandy half-lop rabbits from the same research colony[31] as well as in a New Zealand white rabbit.[18] Clinical signs include an enlarged, fluid-filled abdomen, increased respiratory rate, anorexia, and weight loss. Abdominal paracentesis yields clear fluid with a low specific gravity, a low cell count, and a moderate amount of protein.[18] Diagnosis can be supported by radiography and ultrasound. The rabbits in the reports were all euthanized or found dead, and no anatomic abnormalities could be correlated with this condition.[31] Ovariohysterectomy and supportive care are indicated if hydrometra is diagnosed in a pet rabbit.

Uterine Torsion

Torsion of the uterus is a rare occurrence in rabbits. It has been reported in association with pregnancy, hydrometra, or endometritis.[18] Clinical signs include cachexia and abdominal distention with hydrometra, or a bloody vaginal discharge with endometritis and torsion.[18] The cause of uterine torsion is difficult to identify, and the prognosis is grave.

DISORDERS OF THE MAMMARY GLAND

Septic Mastitis

Mastitis can occur in a lactating doe or a rabbit in pseudocyesis. Abscesses can develop in the mammary gland independent of lactation. Heavy lactation, poor sanitation, abrasive bedding or caging, or injury to the gland or teat predisposes the doe to mammary infection. Mastitis may occur in conjunction with metritis. Clinical signs include depression, fever, anorexia, polydipsia, septicemia, or death of the doe or the young. The mammary glands are firm, hot, and swollen, and the skin is discolored red to dark blue. Infection can begin in one gland and spread to other glands. The initial discharge may not be purulent. *S. aureus, Streptococcus* species, and *Pasteurella* species are most frequently isolated.

Submit samples of exudate or express the gland to obtain samples for bacterial culture. Choose systemic antibiotic therapy on the basis of the culture and sensitivity test results. Common antibiotic choices include enrofloxacin, a trimethoprim-sulfa combination, or penicillin. Supportive care includes fluid therapy, application of hot packs, and drainage of abscesses. Surgical excision may be necessary for severe infections. Consider analgesia with buprenorphine if the animal experiences pain. Force-feeding may be necessary if the doe is anorectic. Remove bunnies but do not foster them onto another doe because this is known to transmit infection. Disinfect the environment.

Cystic Mastitis

Noninfectious cystic mastitis occurs in breeding and nonbreeding does. The affected glands are swollen and firm, and a clear to serosanguineous discharge is expressible from the distended nipples. The glands do not seem painful, and the doe is not depressed. Epithelial hyperplasia, adenosis, and cystic mammary glands have been associated with uterine hyperplasia and adenocarcinoma.[17, 42] Cystic mammary glands may continue to progress and coalesce, with a fibrous connective tissue accumulating around the cysts.[42] Eventually, malignant cellular changes may occur, leading to invasive mammary adenocarcinoma. Metastasis to the regional lymph nodes, lungs, or other organs can occur with adenocarcinoma.

Evaluate rabbits with clinical signs of cystic mastitis for infectious mastitis and uterine tumors. The treatment for noninfectious cystic mastitis is ovariohysterectomy; clinical signs usually resolve within 3–4 weeks after surgery.

DISORDERS OF THE URINARY SYSTEM

Urolithiasis/Hypercalciuria

Urolithiasis refers to the presence of calculi in the urinary system. Rabbits can have any combination of cystic calculi, urethral calculi, renal calculi, and ureteral calculi. The cause of urolithiasis in rabbits is not well described, but several factors are involved, including nutrition, anatomy, physiology, and rarely, infection. Hypercalciuria is a similar clinical condition seen frequently in pet rabbits. Affected rabbits have a large amount of calcium "sand" in their bladder. Rabbits have an unusual calcium metabolism in that intestinal absorption of calcium is not directly dependent on vitamin D. The fractional urinary excretion of calcium is less than 2% in most mammals, whereas the range for rabbits is 45–60%. Increases in dietary calcium directly increase urinary excretion of calcium.[4, 7]

Rabbits with either urolithiasis or hypercalciuria tend to be obese, are fed a free-choice pellet and alfalfa hay diet, and have limited exercise. Often, the rabbits have a history of vitamin or mineral dietary supplementation. Clinical signs of urolithiasis include depression, anorexia, weight loss, lethargy, hematuria, anuria, straining to urinate, a hunched posture, grinding of teeth, and urine scald of the perineum. Rabbits with hypercalciuria usually have a thick, creamy urine. Often, voided urine appears only slightly turbid; however, with manual bladder expression, copious amounts of pasty urine are passed. Frequently, a doughlike mass is palpated in the caudal abdomen, or a turgid bladder is evident if urethral obstruction is present. An enlarged kidney or ureter may be palpated if hydroureter or hydronephrosis has occurred.[27] There is a single report of a large cystic calculus indirectly obstructing the bowel in a female rabbit by becoming wedged in the pelvic inlet.[38]

Confirm the diagnosis radiographically. A discrete calculus (see Fig. 31–7*A* and *B*) or the presence of homogenous dense material can be seen in the dependent portion of the bladder or completely filling a distended bladder (see Fig. 31–6*A* and *B*). A small amount of sand in the bladder is a common incidental radiographic finding because the presence of amorphous calcium carbonate crystals is normal in rabbits. Close inspection may be needed for identification of stones in the kidneys, ureters, or uretha. Perform ultrasound examination to detect the presence of discrete calculi in a bladder that is distended and diffusely opaque radiographically. Multiple renal cysts may be confused with hydronephrosis; use ultrasound examination to differentiate the two. If renal calculi are present, perform intravenous pyelography to evaluate renal function.

Obtain urine for analysis by cystocentesis or free catch. Analysis yields crystalluria; numerous calcium oxalate crystals are common, but ammonium phosphate, calcium carbonate, and monohydrate crystals are also frequently observed. Proteinuria and hematuria are common additional findings. If bacteria are found on cytologic examination, submit urine obtained on cystocentesis for culture. *Escherichia coli* and *Pseudomonas* species are bacteria known to cause cystitis. Results of a CBC and serum biochemistry testing assist in assessing renal function and in developing a prognosis.

Treatment of urolithiasis depends on the location and severity of the lesion. Cystotomy is the treatment of choice for cystic calculi. The procedure may be difficult because the neck of the bladder is flaccid and extends into the pelvic canal. Attempts to force small stones out of the urethra may result in their becoming lodged within the neck or proximal urethra. Use a surgical spoon to retrieve small stones from this region. Flushing and gentle surgical suction can aid removal of fine granular material. Submit the calculus for analysis, and obtain a swabbed sample of the bladder wall for bacterial culture. Preoperative and postoperative support includes IV fluid diuresis and systemic antibiotics. Subsequent radiographic monitoring is helpful because this condition can recur. Nephrectomy may be indicated if a calculus in the renal pelvis is causing obstruction and hydronephrosis. Extracorporeal shock wave lithotripsy has been experimentally applied to rabbit kidneys, but no information is available on a clinical application.[24] Prognosis is guarded for rabbits with either unilateral or bilateral renal calculi.

When hypercalciuria or nonobstructive calculi in the kidney or ureter is identified, consider a nonsurgical approach. Fluids, administered either IV or SC are necessary for increasing the flushing action of the urinary tract. Manually express the bladder daily for 2–4 days to encourage passage of crystals or calcium "sand" that may not be voided during normal micturition. A technique similar to voiding, urohydropropulsion, which is used in dogs and cats,[30] can be used in rabbits for the nonsurgical removal of fine granular or small, smooth cystic calculi. Rabbits must be anesthetized for this procedure. Hold the rabbit in an upright position so that the vertebral column is vertical, and apply steady pressure to the bladder. Administer preanesthetic diazepam to help relax the urethralis muscle; I recommend administering intraoperative butorphanol or buprenorphine because bladder expression is painful. Hematuria is expected to occur for 1–2 days after urohydropropulsion.[30]

Dietary changes are an important part of treatment and prevention. The alkaline pH of rabbit urine and high concentrations of calcium in the urine increase the risk of precipitation of solutes.[22] Decreasing dietary calcium directly lowers serum calcium levels and the amount of calcium excreted in the urine.[7, 23] To reduce calcium intake, give grass hay and green vegetables as the primary diet, and reduce the amount of pellets given daily to 1–2 oz or eliminate them altogether. Discontinue any vitamin or mineral supplementation. One report determined that a level of 0.22 g of calcium per 100 g of food is necessary for maximal growth[6]; most commercial rabbit pellets contain 0.90–1.60 g of calcium per 100 g of food.[4] Because many rabbits that develop urolithiasis are overweight, I recommend a decrease in total caloric intake and an increase in exercise. Acidifiers are not effective because rabbits are herbivores with naturally alkaline urine. Potassium citrate may be useful in the treatment of calcium oxalate crystals because it reduces urinary calcium ion concentrations.

Renal Failure

Both acute and chronic renal failure can occur in older rabbits. Clinical signs include lethargy, depression, anorexia, polyuria, polydipsia, and perineal urine scald. Serum creatinine and blood urea nitrogen levels are elevated, as are serum concentrations of calcium, phosphorus, and potassium. Urine specific gravity is isosthenuric. Other findings from urinalysis may include proteinuria, hematuria, pyuria, and cast formation. Submit a urine sample for bacterial culture to screen for infectious causes; blood cultures are indicated if clinical signs of septicemia are concurrent. Indicators of inflammation in the urine (pyuria, proteinuria, hematuria) occur more frequently with acute renal failure and nephritis than with chronic renal failure. Acute renal failure has a better potential response to treatment, but the prognosis remains guarded. Pyelonephritis in rabbits is often caused by *P. multocida* or *Staphylococcus* species. Noninfectious causes of chronic renal disease include hypercalcemia,[16] renal calcinosis resulting from hypervitaminosis D and hypercalcemia,[35] mineralization of the kidneys with interstitial fibrosis caused by excessive vitamin D in the diet,[43] and fatty degeneration in overweight animals.

Treatment should attempt to promote diuresis and diminish the consequences of uremia. Treatment is supportive in cases of chronic renal failure. Achieve diuresis with initial IV fluid administration in both acute and chronic renal failure; follow this with long-term SC fluid support in chronic renal failure. Antibiotics are indicated if infectious disease is suspected. The dietary changes discussed in the section on urolithiasis are indicated.

Nephrotoxicity

Several compounds are nephrotoxic in rabbits. Therapeutic use of gentamicin can result in acute tubular necrosis.[12, 25] Supplemental doses (10 mg) of vitamin B_6 given during gentamicin therapy may help protect the kidney.[12] Zolazepam (Telazol) is documented to cause nephrotoxicity in rabbits, inducing nephrosis at low doses and severe nonreversible nephrosis at high doses.[2]

Renal Cysts

The occurrence of multiple small subcapsular cysts in the kidneys is an inherited condition of rabbits. The cysts are either of tubular origin or primitive ductules, and the condition is similar to renal cortical dysplasia in humans.[28] The cysts do not create any clinical signs or change results of renal function tests but are detectable at ultrasound examination or necropsy.

Encephalitozoon: Nosematosis

Encephalitozoonosis or nosematosis is a common disease in rabbits caused by *Encephalitozoon cuniculi*, a microsporidian, obligate, intracellular protozoan. Transmission is by urine-oral passage, usually from doe to young. The organism is absorbed from the intestines into mononuclear cells and then is distributed to other organs. Spores have a predilection for kidney and brain tissue, where the most common lesions are found (see Chapter 21). Spores appear in the kidney 31 days after inoculation and are excreted in the urine up to 3 months after inoculation.[34] Spores can remain in the environment for longer than 1 month.

Signs are usually subclinical and chronic. No clinical signs of renal impairment occur, although early infections may have histologic foci of granulomatous nephritis if the organism is still present.[14] At necropsy, numerous small pits and stellate scars may be found on the cortical surface of the kidney caused by chronic interstitial nephritis from previous infection with *E. cuniculi*. Clinical signs and incontinence result from the central nervous system infection, not the renal lesions.

Several diagnostic tests are available, but the two most frequently used serologic tests are indirect fluorescence and ELISA (enzyme-linked immunosorbent assay). A positive titer indicates previous exposure to the parasite, but the assay cannot distinguish early infection, active infection, chronic asymptomatic infection, or previous exposure and recovery. Obtaining a negative titer for *E. cuniculi* is helpful for ruling out a diagnosis, indicating that another disease process may be responsible for clinical signs.

There is no treatment for nosematosis, but the use of sipper tubes and placing rabbit food off the ground helps to decrease urine contamination of food and water.

Urinary Incontinence

Urinary incontinence can be caused by lumbosacral vertebral fractures or dislocations or by central nervous system lesions of *E. cuniculi*. Ovariohysterectomized rabbits can develop urinary incontinence that is responsive to diethylstilbestrol.[5] Rabbits with urinary calculi or hypercalciuria often exhibit urinary incontinence and urine scald. Clinical signs include a urine-soiled perineum and ulcerations of the vaginal mucosa and intertrigonal pouches as well as sticky, strong smelling urine. Vertebral fractures can be ruled out by thorough neurologic examination and radiography. A positive titer to *E. cuniculi* and additional central nervous system signs support a diagnosis of protozoal infection. Urolithiasis or hypercalciuria can be identified on radiographs. A positive response to 0.5 mg of diethylstilbestrol given PO 1–2 times weekly in spayed females suggests a hormone-responsive urinary incontinence similar to that seen in dogs. Additional differentials include ectopic ureter, urinary tract infection, neoplasia, or pyoderma. Initial supportive care includes daily cleaning of the perineum and topical treatment for dermatitis with a drying agent such as Domeboro astringent solution (Miles Inc., West Haven, CT) in addition to treatment of the primary problem.

Tumors of the Urinary Tract

Benign embryonal nephromas are common in rabbits of all ages and are usually incidental findings at necropsy. In one report, an extremely large, palpable embryonal nephroma caused obliteration of the kidney and polycythemia.[29] Renal carcinoma and leiomyoma have also been reported in rabbits.

Red Urine

Rabbits can excrete a porphyrin-pigmented urine that often incorrectly suggests hematuria. It is probably caused by a plant pigment and does not affect the rabbits health. Pigmented urine tends to be intermittent and lasts only 3–4 days. It is speculated that dietary compounds, ingestion of pine needles, or antibiotic administration may be causes of increased pigment levels in rabbit urine (see Chapter 14).

True hematuria is determined on examination of a urine sediment and the finding of more than five red blood cells per high-power field; a positive reaction for blood with the use of a urine dipstick also indicates this condition. Hematuria can originate from the genital tract or the urinary tract. Blood from the reproductive tract can be associated with adenocarcinoma, polyps, abortion, or endometrial venous aneurysms. Blood originating from the urinary tract can be the result of cystitis, bladder polyps, pyelonephritis, renal infarcts, urolithiasis, or disseminated intravascular coagulation.[15] History, signalment, physical examination, laboratory tests, radiography, and ultrasound examination are helpful in determining the cause.

Hyperpigmented urine has also been associated with urobilinuria, which may appear similar to hematuria; however, test results are negative for blood and positive for urobilinogen.[15] There is one documented report of a New Zealand white rabbit with porphyria.[36] Porphyrias are diseases caused by impaired enzyme function in the heme biosynthesis pathway. No clinical signs were noted in the case reported, but necropsy findings included a pink tinge to the teeth, ultraviolet fluorescence of teeth and femur, and elevation of uroporphyrin levels in the urine.[36]

REFERENCES

1. Baba N, von Haam E: Animal model for human disease: spontaneous adenocarcinoma in aged rabbits. Am J Path 1972; 68:653–656.
2. Brammer DW, Doerning BJ, Chrisp CF, et al: Anesthetic and nephrotoxic effects of Telazol in New Zealand white rabbits. Lab Anim Sci 1991; 41:432–435.
3. Bray MV, Weir EC, Brownstein DG, et al: Endometrial venous aneurysms in three New Zealand white rabbits. Lab Anim Sci 1992; 42:360–362.
4. Buss SL, Bourdeau JE: Calcium balance in laboratory rabbits. Miner Electrolyte Metab 1984; 10:127–132.
5. Caslow D: Hormone responsive perineal urine soiling in two female ovariohysterectomized rabbits. Comp Anim Prac 1989; 19:32–33.
6. Chapin RE, Smith SE: Calcium requirement of growing rabbits. J Anim Sci 1967; 26:67–71.
7. Cheeke PR, Amberg JW: Comparative calcium excretion by rats and rabbits. J Anim Sci 1973; 37:450–454.
8. Cunliffe-Beamer TL, Fox RR: Veneral sporotrichosis of rabbits: eradication. Lab Anim Sci 1981; 31:379–381.
9. DiGiacomo RF, Deeb BJ, Anderson RJ: Hypervitaminosis A and reproductive disorders in rabbits. Lab Anim Sci 1992; 42:250–254.
10. DiGiacomo RF, Talburt CD, Lukehart SA, et al: *Treponema paraluis-cuniculi* infection in a commercial rabbitry: epidemiology and serodiagnosis. Lab Anim Sci 1983; 33:562–566.
11. Elsinghorst TA, Timmermans HJF, Hendriks HG: Comparative pathology of endometrial carcinoma. Vet Q 1984; 6:200–208.
12. Enriquez Sr JI, Schydlower M, O'Hair KC, et al: Effect of vitamin B_6 supplementation on gentamicin nephrotoxicity in rabbits. Vet Hum Toxicol 1992; 34:32–35.
13. Flatt RE: Bacterial diseases. *In* Weisbroth SH, Flatt RE, Kraus AL, eds.: The Biology of the Laboratory Rabbit. New York, Academic Press, 1974.
14. Flatt RE, Jackson SJ: Renal nosematosis in young rabbits. Pathol Vet 1970; 7:492–497.
15. Garibaldi BA, Fox JG, Otto G, et al: Hematuria in rabbits. Lab Anim Sci 1987; 37:769–772.
16. Garibaldi BA, Pecquet Goad ME: Hypercalcemia with secondary nephrolithiasis in a rabbit. Lab Anim Sci 1988; 38:331–333.
17. Hillyer EV: Pet rabbits. Vet Clin North Am Small Anim Pract 1994; 24:25–65.
18. Hobbs BA, Parker RF: Uterine torsion associated with either hydrometra or endometritis in two rabbits. Lab Anim Sci 1990; 40:535–536.
19. Hofmann JR, Hixson CJ: Amyloid A protein deposits in a rabbit with pyometra. J Am Vet Med Assoc 1986; 189:1155–1156.
20. Ingalls TH, Adams WM, Lurie MB, et al: Natural history of adenocarcinoma of the uterus in the Phipps rabbit colony. J Natl Cancer Inst 1964; 33:799–806.
21. Johnson JH, Wolf AM: Ovarian abscesses and pyometra in a domestic rabbit. J Am Vet Med Assoc 1993; 203:667–672.
22. Kamphues J: Calcium metabolism of rabbits as an etiological factor for urolithiasis. J Nutr 1991; 121:S95–S96.
23. Kamphues VJ, Carstensen P, Schroeder D, et al: Effekte einer steigenden Calcium- und Vitamin D–zufuhr auf den Calciumstoffwechsel von Kaninchen. J Anim Physiol Anim Nutri 1986; 17:191–208.
24. Karalezli G, Gögüs O, Bedük Y, et al: Histopathologic effects of extracorporeal shock wave lithotripsy on rabbit kidney. Urol Res 1993; 21:67–70.
25. Kojima T, Kobayashi T, Iwase S, et al: Gentamicin nephrotoxicity in young rabbits. Exp Pathol 1984; 26:71–75.
26. Kraus AL, Weisbroth SH, Flatt RE, et al: Biology and diseases of rabbits. *In* Fox JE, Cohen BJ, Loew FM, eds.: Laboratory Animal Medicine. New York, Academic Press, 1984.
27. Lee KJ, Johnson WD, Lang CM, et al: Hydronephrosis caused by urinary lithiasis in a New Zealand white rabbit *(Oryctolagus cuniculus)*. Vet Pathol 1978; 15:676–678.
28. Linsey JR, Fox RF: Inherited diseases and variations. *In* Weisbroth SH, Flatt RE, Kraus AL, eds.: The Biology of the Laboratory Rabbit. New York, Academic Press, 1974.
29. Lipman NS, Murphy JC, Newcomer CE: Polycythemia in a New Zealand white rabbit with an embryonal nephroma. J Am Vet Med Assoc 1985; 187:1255–1256.
30. Lulich JP, Osborne CA, Carlson M, et al: Nonsurgical removal of urocystoliths in dogs and cats by voiding urohydropropulsion. J Am Vet Med Assoc 1993; 203:660–663.
31. Morrell M: Hydrometra in the rabbit. Vet Rec 1989; 125:325.

32. Okerman L: Diseases of Domestic Rabbits. 2nd ed. London, Blackwell Scientific Publications, 1994.
33. Patton NM, Holmes HT, Cheeke PR: Hairballs and pregnancy toxemia. J Appl Rabbit Res 1983; 6:99.
34. Percy DH, Barthold SW: Pathology of Laboratory Rodents and Rabbits. Ames, IA, Iowa State University Press, 1993.
35. Quimby F, Foote R, Profit-Olstad M, et al: Hypercalcemia, hypercalcitoninism, and arterial calcification in rabbits fed a diet containing excessive vitamin D and calcium. Lab Anim Sci 1982; 32:415.
36. Samman S, Fussell SH, Rose CI: Porphyria in a New Zealand white rabbit. Can Vet J 1991; 32:622–623.
37. Soave OA, Dominguez J, Doak RL: *Moraxella bovis*–induced metritis and septicemia in a rabbit. J Am Vet Med Assoc 1977; 171:972–973.
38. Talbot AC, Ireton VJ: Unusual cause of intestinal blockage in the female rabbit. Vet Rec 1975; 96:477.
39. The National Research Council: Nutrient Requirements of Domestic Animals: Nutrient Requirements of Rabbits. 2nd Revised ed. Washington DC, National Academy of Sciences, 1992.
40. Van Herck H, Hesp APM, Versluis A, et al: Prolapsus vaginae in the IIVO/JU rabbit. Lab Anim 1989; 23:333–336.
41. Watson GL, Evans MG: Listeriosis in a rabbit. Vet Pathol 1985; 22:191–193.
42. Weisbroth SH: Neoplastic diseases. *In* Weisbroth SH, Flatt RE, Kraus AL, eds.: The Biology of the Laboratory Rabbit. New York, Academic Press, 1974.
43. Zimmerman TE Jr, Giddens WE, DiGiacomo RF, et al: Soft tissue mineralization in rabbits fed a diet containing excess vitamin D. Lab Anim Sci 1990; 40:212–215.

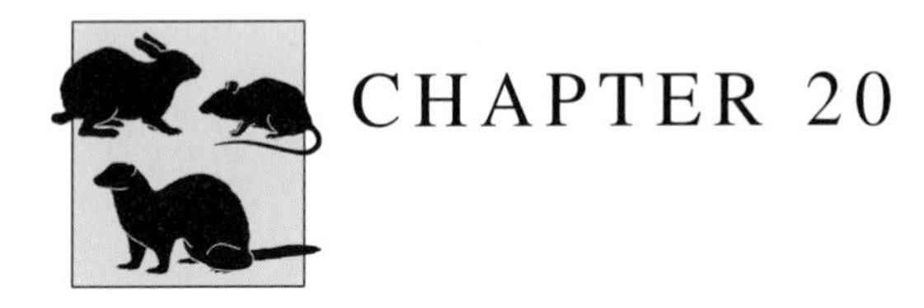

CHAPTER 20

Dermatologic Diseases

Elizabeth V. Hillyer, DVM

SUBCUTANEOUS ABSCESSES

Rabbits can develop abscesses in almost any tissue or organ. Abscesses are probably most commonly the result of bacteremia, but often no obvious trauma or predisposing cause is identified. Abscesses on the head may occur secondary to dental disease, tooth root abscesses, or an oral foreign body (Fig. 20–1). Subcutaneous abscesses, either single or multiple, can occur anywhere on the body but are usually found on the head or limbs. In my experience, *Staphylococcus aureus, Pasteurella multocida, Pseudomonas aeruginosa, Proteus* species, and *Bacteroides* species are the most common isolates from subcutaneous abscesses in rabbits.

Affected animals typically are presented with a swelling reported to have developed over a matter of a day or several days. Some of these rabbits have no past history of bacterial disease; others have a history of snuffles or previous abscessation or a long-term history of medical problems or weight loss. Animals of all ages may be affected. Typically, the swelling is not painful, and there are no associated clinical signs; however, signs of dental disease or lameness may be present with associated abscesses.

Abscesses in rabbits are simple to diagnose but difficult to treat. On physical examination, subcutaneous abscesses are soft to firm swellings that are not freely moveable (although dermal abscesses are moveable). Palpate the involved region carefully to identify a bony swelling that could indicate bone involvement. Run your hands over every part of the rabbit's head, body, and extremities to feel for other abscesses. A complete oral and dental examination is important during any rabbit physical examination; however, it is mandatory for any rabbit with an abscess on the head. Obtain a fine-needle aspirate from the swelling with a 22-gauge needle or larger, and submit samples for cytologic evaluation, Gram's stains, and bacterial culture. Most abscesses contain a creamy, thick, white purulent exudate. Cytologic evaluation and Gram's stains of this material are usually more informative than culture, which may yield negative results.

The prognosis for resolution of the abscess depends greatly on whether underlying bone is involved; therefore, always obtain radiographs of the affected area if bone involvement is a possibility. Depending on location, ultrasound and computed tomography also can be used for characterization and delineation of an abscess. In rabbits with abscesses on the head, thoroughly examine the oral cavity and teeth while the rabbit is sedated for skull radiography. Obtain a blood sample for a presurgical complete blood count (CBC) and, for older animals, submit samples for serum chemistry analysis and urinalysis. If the rabbit has been chronically ill, obtain thoracic radiographs to screen for pneumonia or pulmonary abscesses before taking the animal to surgery.

It is important to educate the owner about rabbit abscesses before proceeding with therapy. This condition can be frustrating to treat because affected rabbits often remain "healthy" while the abscesses tend to recur (in the same place or at other sites) and require multiple surgeries. Rabbits with joint abscesses may develop abscesses in other joints. Some animals require lifelong antibiotic therapy to prevent abscess recurrence. The owner must be prepared to provide nursing care, to return with the animal for frequent clinical visits, and to make the financial commitment required for the treatment of chronic medical conditions.

The optimal treatment for rabbit abscesses is complete surgical excision followed by antibiotic therapy for 2 or more weeks after surgery (see Chapter 22). Abscesses are likely to recur if any infected tissue is left at the surgical site; abscesses also recur if underlying osteomyelitis is present. Therefore, amputation of a limb may be necessary if a joint is involved or if the abscess is too extensive to excise. Most rabbits tolerate the loss of a leg well, even if it is a rear leg. Abscesses that have an identifiable cause, such as a molar point or an oral foreign body, may be easier to treat, especially if the cause can be eliminated and the abscess excised (see Fig. 20–1).

If the situation allows, wait to start antibiotic therapy for the rabbit until the abscess has been cultured. At surgery, take a sample of the abscess wall for culture and sensitivity testing. If total excision of the abscess is not possible, radically débride the area and leave the wound open to heal by granulation, flushing and cleaning it two to three times daily. Simple incision of the abscess for drainage does not work in a rabbit, because the exudate is so thick it will not drain, even with a large opening and optimal drain placement. In fact, surgical drains have performed consistently poorly in the treatment of abscesses in rabbits. One clinician has some success with a Water Pik (Teledyne Water Pik, Los Angeles, CA) used for flushing twice daily with a 10% povidone iodine or a 1% chlorhexidine solution.[7]

For mandibular or maxillary abscesses associated with periapical disease, Remeeus and Verbeek[11] describe a successful treatment procedure that includes external abscess drainage, extraction of any infected teeth, and filling of the abscess cavity with calcium hydroxide paste, which is left in place for 1 week (see Chapter 22). Serial débridements and packing of the abscessed tissue may be needed with this technique. With any technique that is used, do not establish a stoma into the oral cavity for external abscess drainage. Once a stoma or fistula is present, healing is very poor.

The most challenging abscesses to treat are retrobulbar abscesses and those that deeply involve the bones of the skull. The prognosis is very poor for resolution of retrobulbar abscesses, which usually recur even with enucleation, radical débridement, and antibiotic therapy.

For rabbits with abscesses that have recurred after one or more surgeries, long-term, low-level antibiotic therapy can suppress abscess recurrence. Immediately after excising or radically débriding the abscess, start the rabbit on the standard therapeutic dosage of the chosen antibiotic. If the rabbit does well, after 2–4 weeks gradually begin to taper to a low dose given one to two times daily. Enrofloxacin (Baytril, Miles Inc., Shawnee, KS) is a good empirical choice for suppression therapy. Begin by giving the rabbit the standard dosage (5–15 mg/kg q12h PO or SC). Use the SC route for a maximum of 1–2 days if the rabbit is hospitalized. After 2–4 weeks, gradually taper the dosage to 2.5–5 mg/kg q24h PO. It may be necessary to keep the rabbit on this

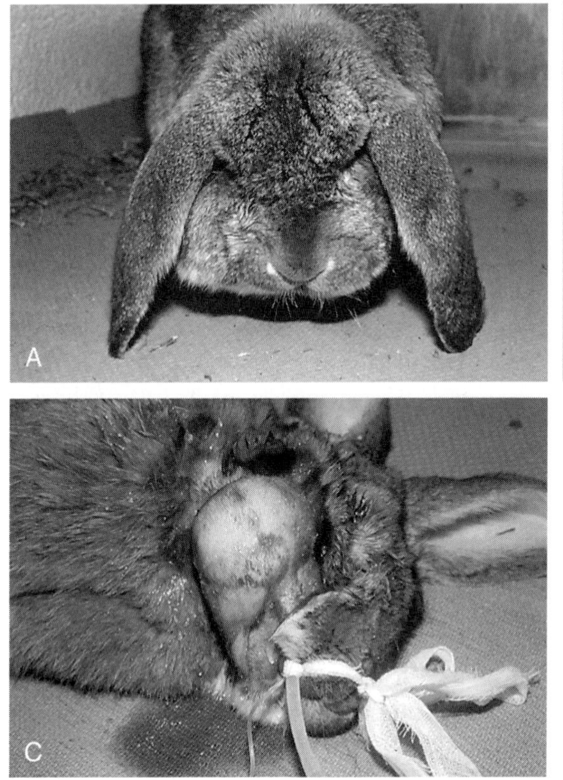

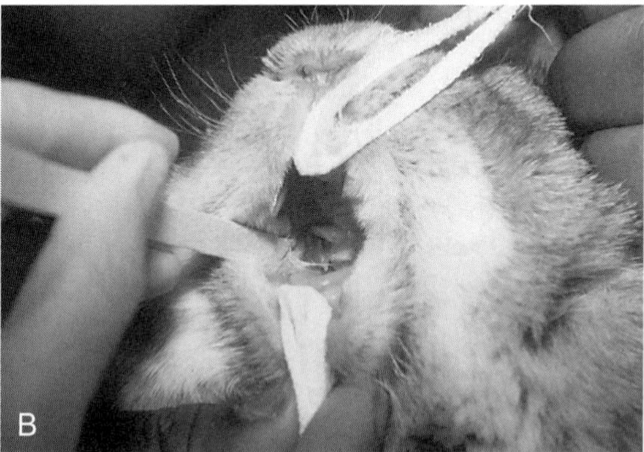

FIGURE 20–1
A, This rabbit presented for inappetence and swelling of the right side of the face. Thick, white, purulent material was found on fine-needle aspiration of the swelling. *B,* On oral examination, the rabbit had a sharp lateral point on the first premolar. The point had lacerated the buccal gingiva and was associated with the right facial abscess. (From Hillyer EV: Approach to the anorexic rabbit. J Small Exotic Anim Med 1992; 1:106–108.) *C,* The rabbit was anesthetized and clipped for surgery. This abscess was successfully treated with complete excision, in conjunction with clipping of the premolar point and administration of an oral trimethoprim-sulfa combination antibiotic for 2 weeks.

regimen lifelong. Always review management for these animals and be sure that they are receiving a well-rounded, high-fiber diet with plenty of leafy greens.

STAPHYLOCOCCUS AUREUS

S. aureus is a common cause of suppurative infection and mastitis in rabbits. Infection with *S. aureus* in pet rabbits is usually sporadic and not accompanied by high mortality; however, a virulent rabbit biotype of *S. aureus* is associated with more serious disease and with heavy losses of young rabbits at rabbitries, particularly in Europe. Okerman and coworkers[9] describe an outbreak of cutaneous staphylococcosis that occurred at one Belgian rabbitry and caused high mortality among neonatal and very young rabbits. Exudative dermatitis with small superficial pustules developed in young rabbits, whereas suppurative mastitis developed in lactating does. Subcutaneous abscesses and an increased incidence of pododermatitis were seen in rabbits of all ages.

ACUTE CELLULITIS

Acute cellulitis has been described in pet rabbits.[7] Affected rabbits develop a febrile illness, typically of acute onset and accompanied by an inflamed, painful, and sometimes edematous area of swelling, most often on the head, neck, or thoracic area. *S. aureus* and *P. multocida* are cultured most frequently from the lesions. Aggressive parenteral antibiotic therapy is necessary. The lesions may mature into an abscess or heal, leaving a large necrotic eschar.

VIRAL SKIN DISEASES

Myxomatosis is caused by several strains of poxvirus. The virus is endemic in European wild rabbits and cottontails *(Sylvilagus* species*)* in the western United States. Wild rabbits develop local skin tumors associated with infection. Domestic rabbits *(Oryctolagus cuniculus)* typically develop severe systemic illness associated with high mortality that begins as lethargy, red eyes and swollen lids, watery ocular discharge, and fever.[4] If the rabbit survives this stage, clinical signs progress to include erythema and swelling around the face and perineal region. There is no specific treatment; supportive care is usually unsuccessful. Keeping rabbits within screened areas prevents entry by mosquitoes, fleas, and other arthropods that serve as vectors of the virus.

A herpesvirus has been seen histopathologically and cultured from several breeder rabbits that died of an acute illness in British Columbia.[10] Clinical signs in these animals included circular, raised, erythematous skin lesions on the head and dorsum.

DERMATOPHYTOSIS

Dermatophytosis (ringworm) is not common in pet rabbits but should be included in the differential diagnosis for scaly alopecic dermatopathies. Lesions appear as dry, crusty patches of hair loss, with or without pruritus. *Trichophyton mentagrophytes* is the most common dermatophyte in rabbits; *Microsporum* species is seen occasionally. The lesions typically occur on the head, legs, and feet. Young animals are affected most commonly, and environmental stressors, such as overcrowding, poor sanitation, malnutrition, and concurrent infection, are predisposing factors. Dermatophytosis in rabbits is usually self-limiting, and rabbits can be asymptomatic carriers.[3] However, ringworm is potentially zoonotic, particularly for children, immunocompromised individuals, and the elderly.

Diagnosis is based on identification of the organism in skin scrapings mounted in 10% potassium hydroxide (KOH) or on culture of the organism on fungal or dermatophyte media. *T. mentagrophytes* does not fluoresce under ultraviolet light from a Wood's light.

Treatment of dermatophytosis in rabbits is based on canine and feline protocols and depends on the extent of the lesions. For small, solitary lesions, use scissors to clip surrounding hair and apply a topical antifungal, such as miconazole cream (Conofite, Mallinckrodt Veterinary, Inc., Mundelein, IL) or clotrimazole cream (Veltrim, Miles Inc., Shawnee, KS). For multiple or widespread lesions, clip the entire haircoat and dispense oral griseofulvin (25 mg/kg PO q24h or divided q12h). Griseofulvin is contraindicated in pregnant animals because it is a teratogen. Recommend that the owner wear gloves while administering treatment. Continue treatment for 2 weeks beyond the resolution of clinical signs. Disinfection of the environment includes vacuuming and cleaning of surfaces with a 1:10 solution of bleach in water.

Eradicating ringworm in large rabbit colonies can be challenging. Franklin and associates[3] were able to significantly reduce the number of *T. mentagrophytes* carriers in a large commercial rabbit colony with either of two topical treatments applied six times over 26 days: a 1% solution of copper sulfate (cupric sulfate pentahydrate, Sigma Chemical Co., St. Louis, MO) applied as a dip, or a spray containing metastabilized chlorous acid/chlorine dioxide (MECA, LD Disinfectant, Alcide Corp., Norwalk, CT) diluted as 1 part base compound to 1 part activator compound to 10 parts water. MECA is a nonirritating, nonmutagenic environmental disinfectant. Griseofulvin administration was impractical and too expensive in this particular situation.

PARASITIC DISEASES OF THE SKIN

Ear Mites

Rabbits infected with *Psoroptes cuniculi,* the rabbit ear mite, develop inflammation and crusting in the external ear canal. The crusts can be very thick and are composed of mites, mite feces, desquamated epithelial cells, serum, and inflammatory cells. Affected rabbits scratch at the ears and shake their head, further traumatizing the lesions. Infection with *P. cuniculi* can become generalized in debilitated animals, involving the perineum, legs, and feet.

A tentative diagnosis of ear mite infestation is possible based on clinical signs and physical findings. Confirmation is by identifying the mite with the naked eye, an otoscope, or under the microscope. Ivermectin is an effective treatment for both localized[1, 2] and generalized infection with *P. cuniculi*. Administer injectable ivermectin (Ivomec, Merck AgVet Division, Rahway, NJ) at 400 μg/kg SC once every 2 weeks for three treatments, or once and repeated in 18 days. The life cycle of the mite is 3 weeks. Adjunctive topical therapy is not necessary, and the infection resolves without the need for cleaning of the ears (Fig. 20–2). In fact, do not attempt to clean out the crusts as the ears are very painful and will bleed. The ears can

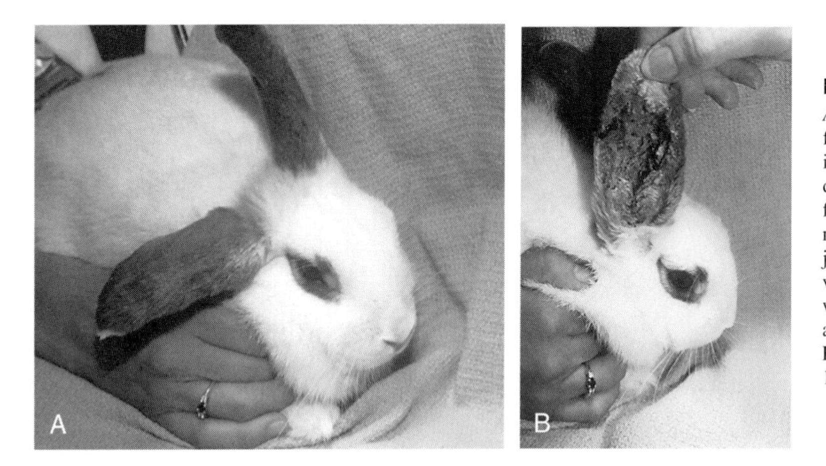

FIGURE 20–2
A, Unilateral *Psoroptes cuniculi* infestation in the ear of a rabbit. Crusting is so heavy that the right ear droops. *B,* Inner surface of the affected ear. This infection resolved rapidly after administration of injectable ivermectin (repeated every 2 weeks for a total of 3 doses). The ear was not cleaned, and no topical therapy was administered. (From Hillyer EV: Pet rabbits. Vet Clin North Am 1994; 24:25–65.)

be cleaned after the mites have been eradicated and the skin lesions have healed if there is residual debris in the ears. Cleaning of the environment (particularly of rabbitries) is important to prevent reinfection.[2]

If ivermectin is not available, alternative therapies include topical application of mineral oil, liquid acaricides, or flea powder in the ears.

Fur and Mange Mites

Cheyletiella parasitovorax is the rabbit fur mite. Infestation with *C. parasitovorax* is not common on the east coast of the United States; however, a clinician in California reports a 15–20% incidence in pet rabbits in the southern part of that state.[7] *C. parasitovorax* is potentially contagious to both humans and other animals, including dogs and cats.

The dermatitis caused by *C. parasitovorax* in rabbits is usually mild and may be inapparent to some owners; other owners complain of their rabbit's "dandruff" or "dry skin." Clinical signs include a white, scaly dermatosis with hair thinning, usually on the rump, dorsum, and dorsal cervical area; sometimes, this is accompanied by pruritus. Diagnosis is based on microscopic examination of superficial skin scrapings, acetate tape preparations (the "Scotch tape test"), or skin and hair debris collected with a flea comb. *C. parasitovorax* mites are relatively large and have hooklike accessory mouth parts.

The life cycle of *C. parasitovorax* lasts approximately 5 weeks. Administer ivermectin (400 μg/kg SC once every 2 weeks) for three treatments. Alternative treatments include once weekly lime sulfur dips for 6 weeks or dusting with a flea powder that is safe for cats twice weekly for 6 weeks. The mite eggs are attached to hair shafts; therefore, treat the environment as well. Flea products should be effective against *C. parasitovorax* in the environment.

Infestations with *Sarcoptes scabiei* and *Notoedres cati* have been reported in laboratory rabbits[8] but are rare to nonexistent among pet rabbits.

Demodex cuniculi is rarely described, and I have never seen it in clinical practice. One author[5] found it to be an apparently normal resident of the epidermis and hair follicles in a small colony of dwarf rabbits in the United Kingdom. Theoretically, active dermatitis associated with *D. cuniculi* in rabbits could occur as in other species—namely, secondary to other disease or a predisposing factor. Base your diagnostic testing and treatment on those for demodicosis in dogs and cats.

Fleas

Pet rabbits can become flea infested, particularly when they are kept in multipet households with dogs and cats. Treat a rabbit with flea infestation as you would a cat, making sure to treat the environment as well.

Myiasis

It is not uncommon to see pet rabbits with myiasis caused by the larvae of *Cuterebra* species flies or maggots of the smaller dipterid flies, particularly in the summer and autumn months. Myiasis is most common in rabbits that are housed outdoors without protective screening or that spend time on the grass;

however, maggots can also infest animals kept indoors in urban areas.

Cuterebra *Larvae*

Species of the genus *Cuterebra* are large, obligate-myiasis flies with three larval stages that are pathogenic and commonly found in wild rabbits and rodents. Human infections with cuterebrid larvae have been reported.[4] The adult *Cuterebra* flies are seen rarely as they have a short life span that is dedicated to breeding.

The large *Cuterebra* larvae usually pupate in the subcutis, typically in the ventral cervical, axillary, or inguinal regions, or on the back or rump. One single larva is typically found within each subcutaneous swelling with its associated air hole (Fig. 20–3). One to several swellings is usually seen on an individual pet rabbit, although heavier infestations are possible. Affected rabbits may show no clinical signs other than the presence of swellings. Other rabbits may show progressive weight loss secondary to chronic infection, debilitation, lameness, or severe toxic shock. Central nervous system signs have been described in dogs and cats secondary to aberrant migration of *Cuterebra* larvae in the nasal passages, middle ear, eye, or brain.[6]

Prepare the area surrounding each swelling for surgery. Remove the larva carefully after gently enlarging the air hole with hemostats. Débride necrotic tissue or completely excise the swelling if it is extensive. Provide supportive care as necessary and administer antibiotics to prevent secondary bacterial infection. Sometimes, surgical excision of the swelling is necessary at a later date if it does not resolve or if it becomes abscessed.

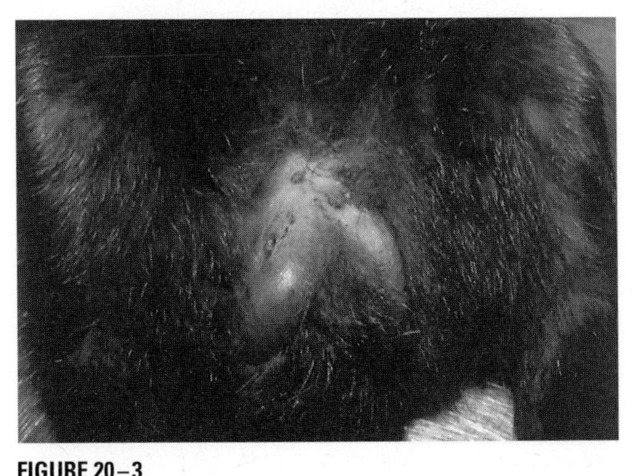

FIGURE 20–3
Cuterebriasis in a male rabbit. An air hole is evident at the cranial aspect of each testicle.

Noncuterebrid Maggots

In my experience, infestations with smaller maggots most commonly begin in the perineal region and then extend dorsally onto the rump. The owner notices the moist dermatitis and hair matting associated with the presence of hundreds of fly larvae. The rabbits that I have treated for maggots have had no history of trauma or wounds; however, these animals had quite extensive dermatitis and open skin wounds at the time of presentation. All were sedentary, overweight, mature rabbits. Perineal dermatitis or urine scald may be a predisposing factor. Moreover, as for other species, maggots can occur on any part of the body in association with an open wound.

Sedate maggot-infested rabbits for a thorough evaluation. Clip the hair carefully over the damaged skin and its periphery. Physically remove any visible maggots, débride necrotic tissue, and flush the wound with copious amounts of sterile saline. Administer one dose of ivermectin (400 μg/kg SC), and start therapy with an antibiotic that has good skin penetration, such as a trimethoprim-sulfa combination. If the wounds are kept clean, dry, and free of maggots, they usually heal rapidly by granulation. Schedule follow-up visits as necessary to recheck the wounds.

OTHER DERMATOLOGIC DISEASES

Barbering and Hair Pulling

Subordinate rabbits may show barbering by dominant ones. The barbering appears as plucked and broken hairs on the head and back. There is no specific treatment other than separation of the two rabbits.

Does in heat and rabbits on low-fiber diets may barber and pull their hair. Pregnant does nearing the end of gestation pull hair from their forelegs, ventral thoracic region, and hips to build a nest.

Moist Dermatitis: Slobbers and Urine Scald

Moist dermatitis in rabbits occurs most commonly under the chin and ventral cervical region and in the perineal area. Chin dermatitis, which has been dubbed "slobbers," usually results from constant drooling associated with dental disease (Fig. 20–4).

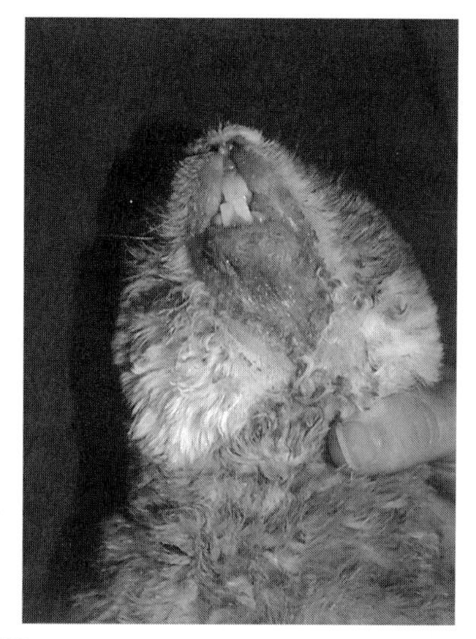

FIGURE 20–4
Moist dermatitis under the chin of a rabbit secondary to drooling because of dental malocclusion. Vertical malalignment of the incisors is an indication of malocclusion of the cheek teeth in this rabbit.

Occasionally, it develops in rabbits that drink from water bowls because the dewlap remains wet. Secondary infection with *P. aeruginosa* may cause the fur to turn green. The treatment for slobbers is removal of the inciting cause—namely, correction of the dental malocclusion or replacement of a water bowl with a water bottle. The skin usually heals uneventfully once it is dry.

Urine scald in rabbits occurs because of constant exposure to urine, either because of excessive urination or urinary incontinence secondary to renal disease, cystitis, or the presence of urinary tract calculi or because of a lack of mobility associated with posterior paresis or obesity (Fig. 20–5). Perform a medical workup, including a CBC, serum chemistry analysis, urinalysis, and abdominal radiography, for rabbits that are polyuric or dribbling urine as well as for those with posterior paresis. The optimal treatment for urine scald is keeping the area dry. Applying ointments and creams only aggravates the problem. Gently clip the hair in the affected area and prescribe an astringent, such as Domeboro (Miles Inc., Consumer Healthcare Products, Elkhart, IN), that is to be applied twice daily to the area. Correct any underlying problems and recommend management changes to help in keeping the area dry. Two surgical procedures that may be useful for correcting the problem in selected cases are described in Chapter 22. Recommend an improved diet (with fewer pellets and low calcium content) and increased exercise if obesity is the problem.

Lumps and Other Dermatologic Conditions

Other differential diagnoses for skin lumps seen in rabbits, in addition to abscesses, myxomatosis, and cuterebriasis, include lipomas, subcutaneous lymphoma, fibromas and other neoplasms, and impacted scent glands. Lipoma and lymphoma are diagnosed by cytologic examination of a sample obtained by fine-needle aspiration; firm lumps are best diagnosed with excisional biopsy. Treatment of lipoma involves surgical excision. Lymphoma carries a poor prognosis; thus, evaluate each rabbit individually. Not enough is known about lymphoma in rabbits for specific treatment recommendations to be made.

Waxy secretions can build up in the perineal scent glands and produce a strong, musky odor. These secretions are easily removed with a cotton-tipped swab.

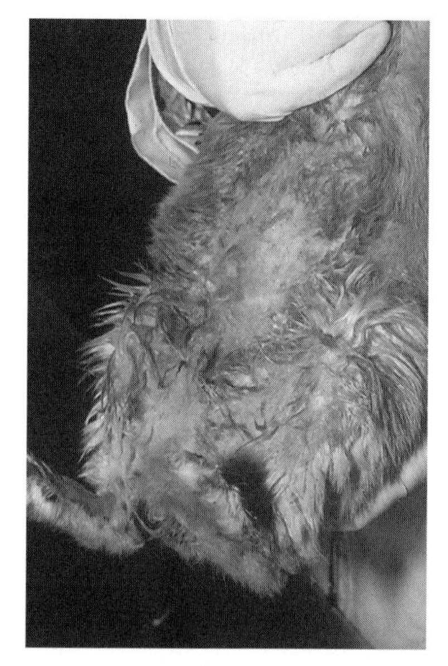

FIGURE 20–5
Severe urine scald in a female rabbit that was polydipsic, polyuric, and constantly soaked with urine. This rabbit was mildly azotemic, and urinalysis revealed isosthenuria and an active urine sediment. A presumed upper urinary tract infection resolved on therapy with an oral trimethoprim-sulfa combination antibiotic for 6 weeks. The urine scald was treated with (gentle) clipping of the hair from the affected area and application of Domeboro astringent solution twice daily as needed.

Venereal spirochetosis, or rabbit syphilis, is associated with crusting and ulcerations around the nostrils, lips, eyelids, chin, external genitalia, and perineum (see Chapter 19). This condition can be confused with dermatophytosis. Ulcerative pododermatitis, or sore hocks, is discussed in Chapter 21.

REFERENCES

1. Curtis SK, Brooks DL: Eradication of ear mites from naturally infested conventional research rabbits using ivermectin. Lab Anim Sci 1990; 40:406–408.
2. Curtis SK, Housley R, Brooks DL: Use of ivermectin for treatment of ear mite infestation in rabbits. J Am Vet Med Assoc 1990; 196:1139–1140.
3. Franklin CL, Gibson SV, Caffrey CJ, et al: Treatment of *Trichophyton mentagrophytes* infection in rabbits. J Am Vet Med Assoc 1991; 198:1625–1630.
4. Harkness JE, Wagner JE: The Biology and Medicine of Rabbits and Rodents. 4th ed. Baltimore, Williams & Wilkins, 1995.
5. Harvey RG: *Demodex cuniculi* in dwarf rabbits *(Oryctolagus cuniculi)*. J Small Anim Pract 1990;31:204–207.
6. Hendrix CM, Cox NR, Clemons-Chevis CL, et al: Aberrant intracranial myiasis caused by larval *Cuterebra* infection. Compend Contin Educ Pract Vet 1989; 11:550–559.
7. Jenkins JR: Skin disorders of the rabbit. J Small Exotic Anim Med 1991; 1:64–65.
8. Kraus AL, Weisbroth SH, Flatt RE, Brewer N: Biology and diseases of rabbits. *In* Fox JG, Cohen BJ, Loew FM, eds.: Laboratory Animal Medicine. San Diego, CA, Academic Press, 1984, pp 207–240.
9. Okerman L, Devriese LA, Maertens L, et al: Cutaneous staphylococcosis in rabbits. Vet Rec 1984; 114:313–315.
10. Onderka DK, Papp-Vid G, Perry AW: Fatal herpesvirus infection in commercial rabbits. Can Vet J 1992; 33:539–543.
11. Remeeus PGK, Verbeek M: The use of calcium hydroxide in the treatment of abscesses in the cheek of the rabbit resulting from a dental periapical disorder. J Vet Dent 1995; 12:19–22.

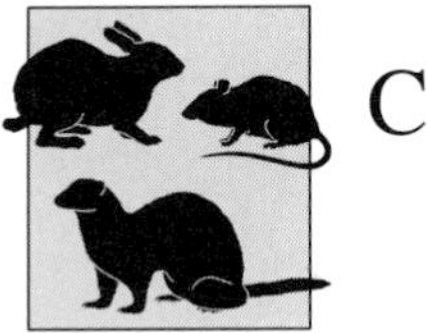

CHAPTER 21

Neurologic and Musculoskeletal Disease

Edward J. Gentz, DVM, and James W. Carpenter, DVM

HEAD TILT

Neurologic, neuromuscular, and musculoskeletal conditions in rabbits, such as head tilt, posterior paresis and paralysis, and generalized muscular incoordination, can be caused by a number of factors. Because practitioners are often presented with pet rabbits displaying such signs, the selection of an appropriate treatment requires assessment and identification of these various differentials.

Vestibular dysfunction causing an ipsilateral head tilt ("torticollis" or "wry neck") can arise either centrally, in the medulla or cerebellum, or peripherally, in the inner ear (Figs. 21–1 and 21–2). Otitis externa or vestibular dysfunction secondary to cranial trauma can be ruled out on the basis of data from a thorough physical examination and radiography for assessing possible skull fractures. Head tilt in dwarf breeds is most frequently caused by *Encephalitozoon cuniculi,* whereas in standard breeds it is more likely to be caused by *Pasteurella multocida.*[23] Head tilt occurs in young rabbits affected with *E. cuniculi* more commonly than in old ones, and it can be accompanied by ataxia and rolling.

Rabbits with suppurative otitis media caused by *P. multocida* often show no clinical evidence of infection. The otitis may extend into the inner ear, resulting in head tilt or torticollis. Occasionally, nystagmus may be present. Affected middle ears are characterized by tympanic bullae filled with thick, yellow pus.[29] Rupture of the tympanic membrane is possible. Diagnostically, *P. multocida* is a non–spore-forming, bipolar, gram-negative rod. Sero-

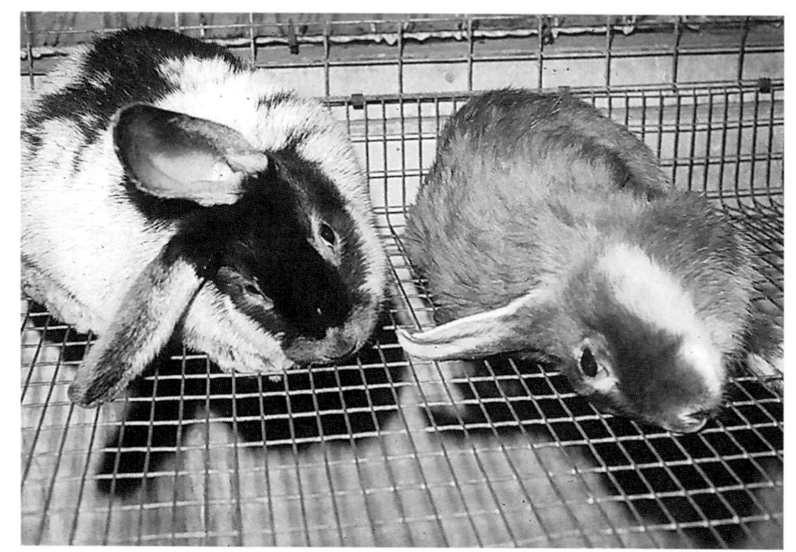

FIGURE 21-1
Head tilt in two rabbits with otitis media interna and associated vestibular infection caused by *Pasteurella multocida.* (Courtesy of George Kollias, DVM.)

logic tests for pasteurellosis, such as ELISA (enzyme-linked immunosorbent assay), are available.[32] Radiographic examination of the skull may show soft tissue density in the bullae, indicating pus-filled bullae. The head tilt in these rabbits has been reported to be irreversible, but its worsening can be prevented with appropriate antibiotic therapy.[14] Other clinicians report a lower incidence of residual head tilt following successful therapy.[16] Prognosis is favorable if a positive response is exhibited within the first week of therapy, and therapy is continued for 1 week after the resolution of clinical signs. Chloramphenicol, enrofloxacin, and trimethoprim-sulfa combinations have been reported to be successful antibiotic choices.[16] However, some authors have found oral chloramphenicol and trimethoprim-sulfa to be ineffective against pasteurellosis,[27] and parenteral administration of enrofloxacin (5–10 mg/kg q12h) to be more efficacious than oral administration.[4] Continued administration of parenteral enrofloxacin can cause skin sloughing; therefore, administer enrofloxacin PO for long-term therapy. For a full discussion of pasteurellosis, refer to Chapter 18.

Central nervous system infection with *E. cuniculi* is another common cause of head tilt in rabbits. *E. cuniculi*, also known as *Nosema cuniculi,* is an obligate, intracellular, microsporidian parasite. Central nervous system lesions (which include focal nonsuppurative granulomatous meningoencephalomyelitis, astrogliosis, and perivascular lymphocytic infiltration) do not normally occur until at least 1 month after infection.[29] Transmission is by ingestion or by oral inoculation of infective spores shed in the urine. Transplacental transmission may also occur.

A positive encephalitozoon titer in conjunction with compatible clinical signs suggests, but is not conclusive for, encephalitozoonosis. Serologic testing by complement fixation, dot-ELISA, India ink immunoreaction, indirect fluorescent antibody, or

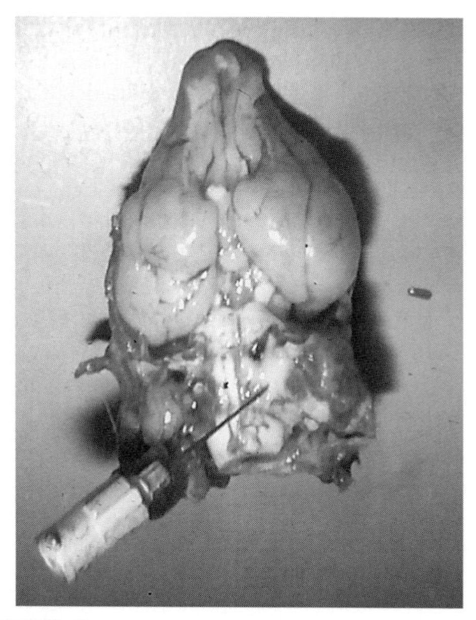

FIGURE 21-2
Purulent exudate (needle) in the brain (cerebellum has been removed) of a rabbit with neurologic signs, including torticollis. (Courtesy of the College of Veterinary Medicine, Kansas State University, Manhattan, KS.)

indirect microagglutination is more commonly used.[3] One source of encephalitozoon testing for the practitioner is the Research Animal Diagnostic and Investigative Laboratory (RADIL) of the University of Missouri.* Definitive diagnosis of encephalitozoonosis requires histopathologic identification of the organism, which is gram-positive and stains positively with carbol-fuchsin.

Although many rabbits infected with *E. cuniculi* are asymptomatic, other neurologic signs may include urinary incontinence, stiff rear gait, and posterior paresis. Infectious motor paralysis in rabbits caused by *E. cuniculi* was first reported in 1922.[36] There is no effective treatment for encephalitozoonosis, and rabbits infected with *E. cuniculi* should be isolated from other rabbits.

Cerebral nematodiasis has been reported in domestic rabbits to be caused by *Baylisascaris procyonis,* the common roundworm of raccoons *(Procyon lotor).*[9, 10, 19, 20] Severe encephalopathy can be caused by just a few *B. procyonis* larvae.[10] Neurologic signs include ataxia, circling, opisthotonos, tremors, and torticollis. These parasites are most commonly acquired by rabbits from hay or bedding that has been contaminated by raccoon feces. Eggs remain infective for at least 1 year. Diagnosis is by postmortem histologic evaluation of the brain. Evidence of larval migration can be found in the cerebrum, cerebellum, midbrain, and medulla and includes multifocal areas of necrosis with aggregations of inflammatory cells (eosinophils, lymphocytes, plasma cells, and macrophages). The Baermann technique can be used to recover larvae from brain tissue. To prevent this disease, guard against fecal contamination of rabbit housing, feed, and bedding by raccoons.[10] Once in the brain, larvae of *B. procyonis* cause destruction of nervous tissue[10] that is basically nonresponsive to medical therapy. Euthanasia is indicated in affected rabbits.

Listeriosis has been reported in domestic rabbits.[34] Although *Listeria monocytogenes* affects rabbits less commonly than cattle or sheep, it has been reported to cause rolling and torticollis associated with brain stem meningoencephalitis.[12] Diagnostically, *L. monocytogenes* is a short, motile, gram-positive, non–spore-forming rod that is catalase-positive. The suspected route of transmission is oral. Antemortem diagnosis is rare, and treatment seldom is attempted. Tetracycline or penicillin/streptomycin combination therapy have been recommended.[12]

*Address: RADIL, 1600 East Rollins, Columbia, MO 65211.

POSTERIOR PARESIS/PARALYSIS

The most common cause of posterior paralysis of acute onset is vertebral fracture or luxation. Fractures are more common than dislocations. The most common fracture site is L7.[21] This injury often results from improper handling but can also occur in caged rabbits that are startled or frightened. Injury occurs when the heavily muscled hindquarters are allowed to twist about the lumbosacral junction, which acts as a fulcrum in the application of leverage to the vertebral column. In addition to paraplegia, neurologic signs may include the loss of skin sensation and of motor control of the urinary bladder and anal sphincter, depending on the amount of compromise to the spinal cord.

Confirm the clinical diagnosis radiographically. If treatment is delayed, rabbits with broken backs can become azotemic or uremic because of the retention of urine in the urinary bladder.[21] Decubital ulcers often develop, and the perineum becomes stained with feces. Occasionally, mildly affected rabbits respond to conservative medical management if the spinal cord is not transected. Supportive therapy must include manual expression of the bladder. However, euthanasia is more often indicated. The extrusion of intervertebral disc material into the vertebral canal, particularly in the area of the lumbar spine, also can cause spinal cord compression and paresis.[2] Both of these conditions can generally be prevented in a physically restrained rabbit by proper support of its hindquarters.

Splay leg, a developmental musculoskeletal condition, is commonly seen in pet rabbits ranging in age from a few days to a few months (Fig. 21–3). These rabbits are unable to adduct from one to all four limbs, and thus they cannot ambulate effectively.[21] The hind limbs are more commonly affected, with femoral neck anteversions, femoral shaft torsion, and subluxation of the hip.[1] The condition is inherited in a simple autosomal recessive pattern. Culling is the most effective long-term management.

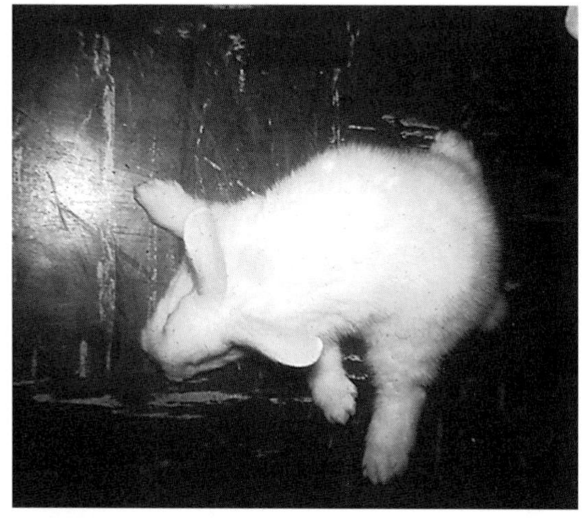

FIGURE 21–3
Splay leg in a rabbit. (Courtesy of the College of Veterinary Medicine, Kansas State University, Manhattan, KS.)

GENERALIZED MUSCULAR WEAKNESS/INCOORDINATION

Toxoplasmosis is an uncommon cause of central nervous system disease in domestic rabbits. Neurologic signs associated with this disease include ataxia, muscle tremors, posterior paralysis, and tetraplegia.[24] Diagnostically, tachyzoites and tissue cysts may be identified in histologic specimens. Serologic tests are available. The immunoperoxidase technique is probably the best test available for diagnosis of toxoplasmosis. Paraffin-embedded sections of the spleen of affected rabbits react with anti–*Toxoplasma gondii* serum but not with anti–*Neospora caninum* serum. Histologically, *T. gondii* can be differentiated from *E. cuniculi* by its strongly positive uptake of hematoxylin stain. *T. gondii* is transmitted primarily by the ingestion of oocysts in infected cat feces. To prevent toxoplasmosis, do not expose pet rabbits to an environment that may have been contaminated with cat feces. Because clindamycin can cause fatal clostridial enteritis in rabbits, treat rabbits with toxoplasmosis with pyrimethamine in combination with a sulfonamide drug such as a trimethoprim-sulfa combination.[11]

Sarcocystosis has been reported in domestic rabbits.[6] The causative agent in rabbits is *Sarcocystis cuniculi,* also known as *S. leporum. S. cuniculi* forms cysts in the skeletal muscle of the rabbit host, especially in the hind legs, flanks, and loins. Intact cysts do not induce an inflammatory response in the muscle; however, degeneration of the cyst wall results in a severe myositis.[28] There is no effective treatment for sarcocystosis. To prevent transmission, isolate pet rabbits from wild cottontail rabbits (*Sylvilagus* species), a common host for *Sarcocystis.*

Several neuromuscular mutations controlled by single gene loci have been reported in domestic rabbits.[25] These include hereditary ataxia, a glycogen storage disorder characterized by neurologic signs such as nystagmus, opisthotonos, and paddling. One type of shaking palsy is characterized by tremors that are exaggerated by sudden noises and are followed eventually by flaccid paralysis. A different form of paralytic tremor that resembles Parkinson's disease in humans is distinguished by a progressive spastic paralysis. Additional neuromuscular mutants include lethal muscular contracture and syringomyelia. Heritable skeletal mutants known to occur in the domestic rabbit include achondroplasia, brachydactylia, chondrodystrophy, dwarfism, distal foreleg curvature, hypoplastic pelvis, osteopetrosis, and spina bifida.[25]

Some neurologic and musculoskeletal diseases in rabbits have a nutritional basis. Nutritional muscular dystrophy in rabbits is caused by hypovitaminosis E and is characterized by degeneration and necrosis of skeletal muscle myofibers.[30] Degenerative changes include hyalinization, swelling, and fragmentation of individual muscle fibers and the proliferation of sarcolemmal and interstitial nuclei. Diagnostically, rabbits with vitamin E deficiency show elevated serum creatine phosphokinase levels[31] and plasma cholesterol levels.[7] Prolonged storage of feed adversely affects the vitamin E content. Feeding pet rabbits only fresh feed, or supplementing the diet with an alternative vitamin E source such as wheat germ,[37] should prevent this problem.

Hypovitaminosis A causes a neurologic disturbance in rabbits characterized by circling, convulsions, opisthotonos, and paralysis.[17] Hydrocephalus has been observed in young born to vitamin A–deficient does. Convulsions can occur in rabbits maintained on a diet deficient in magnesium.[22] Prevent these nutritional disorders from occurring by feeding pet rabbits only a fresh, high-quality diet.

OTHER NEUROLOGIC AND NEUROMUSCULAR CONDITIONS

Seizures in rabbits may be caused by hypoxia secondary to empyema, pneumonia, or metastatic tumor, or may result from the azotemia and electrolyte imbalances associated with renal disease. Bacterial encephalitis, primarily caused by *P. multocida*, can also cause seizures in rabbits. Epilepsy is a rare diagnosis in this species.[8]

Neuromuscular lesions, including skeletal muscle necrosis, peripheral nerve degeneration, and lumbar kyphosis, have been reported in restrained rabbits.[26] Similar lesions are possible in pet rabbits housed in cages that are too small. Cages should be large enough to enable rabbits to move about freely and to turn around completely.

Shope fibromas have been reported in domestic rabbits.[18] Musculoskeletal lesions include subcutaneous nodules and indurations that intimately encompass underlying muscles and tendons. These masses sometimes coalesce and invade underlying skeletal muscle. Rabbits housed outdoors in areas where the Shope fibroma virus exists in the wild rabbit population are at risk of contracting this disease.

Pregnancy toxemia can manifest neurologic signs in rabbits. Although primarily a problem of late gestation, toxemia also occurs in postpartum and pseudopregnant does. Neurologic signs may include weakness, depression, incoordination, convulsions, and coma.[15] Death may occur within a few hours after the signs are first noted. Obesity and fasting are predisposing factors. Dutch, Polish, and English breeds may have an hereditary predisposition. Direct treatment at the correction of the associated ketosis, which involves IV administration of lactated Ringer's and 5% glucose solutions. Prevent toxemia by avoiding fasting and preventing obesity in pregnant does, and by providing a high-energy diet during late gestation.

Rabbits are particularly susceptible to heat stroke or heat stress.[15] Neurologic signs may resemble those of pregnancy toxemia, but evidence of ketosis is not present. Signs are accompanied by an elevation in rectal temperature to greater than 40.5°C (105°F). Slowly reduce the core body temperature of a heat-stressed rabbit by spraying it with or immersing it in tepid water. Give IV fluids and shock doses of corticosteroids if the rabbit is unresponsive. Rabbits that recover from heat stroke should be monitored closely for several days for metabolic abnormalities or renal failure. Rabbits with heat stroke usually do not respond well, and prognosis is poor. Pet rabbits housed outdoors during the summer when the ambient temperature can exceed 29°C (85°F) require shade, good ventilation, and an adequate supply of cool drinking water. Also, rabbits should not be transported during hot weather in cars that are not airconditioned.

Lead poisoning in rabbits may be characterized by subtle neurologic signs, depression, and lethargy; however, anorexia and weight loss are the most common presenting signs.[16] The complete blood count may show the presence of nucleated red blood cells or basophilic stippling of the erythrocytes. Take abdominal radiographs to search for gastrointestinal metallic densities in rabbits with suspected lead poisoning. Institute appropriate therapy in rabbits with blood lead levels greater than 10 μg/dL if clinical signs of plumbism are present. The treatment of choice for lead poisoning is chelation with Ca-EDTA (calcium versenate) at a dosage of 27.5 mg/kg SC q6h for 5 days. Two courses of treatment 1 week apart may be required. Rabbits allowed to wander unrestrained in homes and basements are more likely to encounter a source of lead on which to gnaw.[33] Unsupervised, unrestrained movement of pet rabbits throughout the home should be discouraged.

At least one case of rabies in a pet rabbit has been reported. This case resulted from an encounter with a skunk. Neurologic signs, which developed approximately 1 month after exposure, included blindness and forelimb paralysis.[5] Pet rabbits housed outdoors should be protected from contact with wildlife, especially in areas where rabies is endemic or where a rabies epizootic is underway.

ULCERATIVE PODODERMATITIS

Ulcerative pododermatitis, commonly referred to as "sore hocks," is a musculoskeletal problem frequently seen in pet rabbits. This condition is generally a chronic, ulcerative, granulomatous dermatitis of the plantar surface of the metatarsal area and, less commonly, of the volar metacarpal area.[21] Therefore, the name "sore hocks" is actually a misnomer because the hock is rarely involved.

The lesion initially begins as an ulcer; it then becomes secondarily infected with *Staphylococcus aureus* when the untreated lesion comes into contact with soiled bedding and cage floors.[12] Typical le-

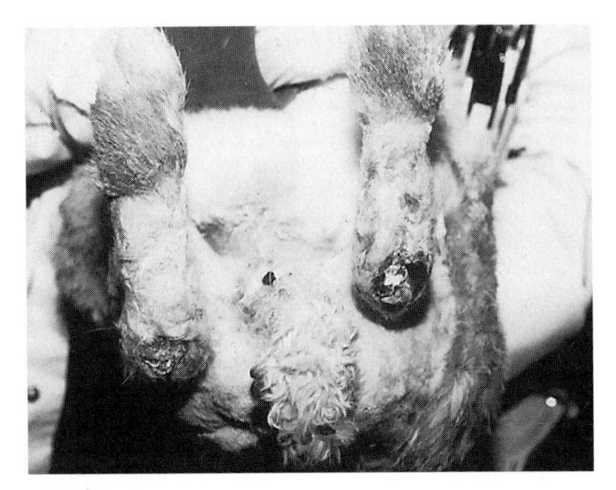

FIGURE 21–4
Bilateral pododermatitis and osteomyelitis in a rabbit. (Courtesy of Karen Rosenthal, DVM.)

sions are roundish and initially ulcerated but later become elevated and hyperkeratotic or have scabbed surfaces.[21] The lesions may become abscessed (Fig. 21–4). Occasionally, the disease extends to the bone, resulting in osteomyelitis and septicemia.[8] Although affected rabbits generally appear healthy, some may show signs of painful, awkward movements, and later, inanition.[21]

The cause of ulcerative pododermatitis is multifactorial. It is generally associated with trauma to or pressure necrosis of the skin.[12] Predisposing factors include abrasions from rough, irregular, or poor-quality cage flooring; frequent thumping and bruising of the foot; lack of movement in a small cage; pressure from excessive weight; soiled cage surfaces; and hereditary factors such as thin furring of the feet.[8, 15, 21] Although this disease occurs most frequently in mature animals housed in cages with wire flooring, pododermatitis has been reported in young animals and can occur in any type of cage or confinement situation.

Treatment of ulcerative pododermatitis in rabbits can be difficult. Clean the lesions with antiseptic solutions and treat them with topical antibiotic ointments. Systemic antibiotic therapy is often clinically useful. Foot bandages are useful but are often not well tolerated by rabbits. The application of a light, protective dressing, such as Tegaderm (3M Medical-Surgical Division, St. Paul, MN) or BioDres (DVM Pharmaceuticals, Miami, FL) may be better tolerated if no active infection is present.[16] Housing an affected animal in a clean cage with dry bedding is essential.

OTHER CONDITIONS

Rabbits are susceptible to a variety of other neurologic and musculoskeletal diseases, including abscesses, arthritis, joint swellings, osteomyelitis, and tumors. Similar to other body systems, the central nervous system and musculoskeletal system can be affected by pasteurellosis, which can cause neurologic signs, osteoarthritis, osteomyelitis, and septic arthritis.[13, 16]

Abscesses are generally associated with either *P. multocida* or *S. aureus* infection. They may occur in muscles, joints, long bones, bones of the skull, and the brain.[15, 16, 29] Osteomyelitis has also resulted from a *Pseudomonas aeruginosa* infection, presumably originating from an ulcerated dermatitis (personal observation). Tumors affecting the musculoskeletal system, including leiomyoma, leiomyosarcoma, osteochondroma, and osteosarcoma, have also been reported in rabbits.[35]

REFERENCES

1. Arendar GM, Milch RA: Splay leg—a recessively inherited form of femoral neck anteversion, femoral shaft torsion and subluxation of the hip in the laboratory lop rabbit. Clin Orthop 1966; 44:221–229.
2. Baxter JS: Posterior paralysis in the rabbit. J Small Anim Pract 1975; 16:267–271.
3. Beckwith C, Peterson N, Liu JJ, Shadduck JA: Dot enzyme–linked immunosorbent assay (dot ELISA) for antibodies to *Encephalitozoon cuniculi*. Lab Anim Sci 1988; 38:573–576.
4. Broome RL, Brooks DL: Efficacy of enrofloxacin in the treatment of respiratory pasteurellosis in rabbits. Lab Anim Sci 1991; 41:572–576.
5. CDC Veterinary Public Health Notes: Rabbit rabies. J Am Vet Med Assoc 1981; 179:84.
6. Cerna Z, Louckova M, Nedvedova H, Vavra J: Spontaneous and experimental infection of domestic rabbits by *Sarcocystis cuniculi* (Brumpt, 1913). Folia Parasitol (Praha) 1981; 28:313–318.
7. Chupukcharoen N, Komaratat P, Wilairat P: Effects of vitamin E deficiency on the distribution of cholesterol in plasma lipoproteins and the activity of cholesterol 7a-hydroxylase in rabbit liver. J Nutr 1985; 115:468–472.
8. Collins BR: Common diseases and medical management of rodents and lagomorphs. *In* Jacobson ER, Kollias Jr GV, eds.: Exotic Animals. New York, Churchill Livingstone, 1988, pp 261–316.
9. Dade AW, Williams JF, Whitenack DL, Williams CSF: An epizootic of cerebral nematodiasis in rabbits due to *Ascaris columnaris*. Lab Anim Sci 1975; 25:65–69.
10. Deeb BJ, DiGiacomo RF: Cerebral larva migrans caused by *Baylisascaris* sp. in pet rabbits. J Am Vet Med Assoc 1994; 205:1744–1747.
11. Dubey JP, Greene CE, Lappin MR: Toxoplasmosis and neosporosis. *In* Greene CE, ed.: Infectious Diseases of the Cat and Dog. Philadelphia, WB Saunders, 1990, pp 818–833.
12. Flatt RE: Bacterial diseases. *In* Weisbroth SH, Flatt RE,

Kraus AL, eds.: The Biology of the Laboratory Rabbit. New York, Academic Press, 1974, pp 194–236.
13. Hago BED, Magid OYA, El Sanousi SM, et al: An outbreak of suppurative osteoarthritis of the tibiotarsal joint in rabbits caused by *Pasteurella multocida*. J Small Anim Pract 1987; 28:763–766.
14. Harkness JE: Rabbit husbandry and medicine. Vet Clin North Am Small Anim Pract 1987; 17:1019–1044.
15. Harkness JE, Wagner JE: The Biology of Rabbits and Rodents. 3rd ed. Philadelphia, Lea & Febiger, 1989.
16. Hillyer EV: Pet rabbits. Vet Clin North Am Small Anim Pract 1994; 24:25–64.
17. Hunt CE, Harrington DD: Nutrition and nutritional diseases of the rabbit. *In* Weisbroth SH, Flatt RE, Kraus AL, eds.: The Biology of the Laboratory Rabbit. New York, Academic Press, 1974, pp 403–433.
18. Joiner GN, Jardine JH, Gleiser CA: An epizootic of Shope fibromatosis in a commercial rabbitry. J Am Vet Med Assoc 1971; 159:1583–1587.
19. Kazacos KR, Kazacos EA: Diagnostic exercise: neuromuscular condition in rabbits. Lab Anim Sci 1988; 38:187–189.
20. Kazacos KR, Reed WM, Kazacos EA, Thacker HL: Fatal cerebrospinal disease caused by *Baylisascaris procyonis* in domestic rabbits. J Am Vet Med Assoc 1983; 183:967–971.
21. Kraus AL, Weisbroth SH, Flatt RE, Brewer N: Biology and diseases of rabbits. *In* Fox JG, Cohen BJ, Loew FM, eds.: Laboratory Animal Medicine. New York, Academic Press, 1984, pp 207–240.
22. Kunkel HO, Pearson PB: Magnesium nutrition of the rabbit. J Nutr 1948; 36:657–666.
23. Kunstyr I, Naumann S: Head tilt in rabbits caused by pasteurellosis and encephalitozoonosis. Lab Anim 1985; 19:208–213.
24. Leland MM, Hubbard GV, Dubey JP: Clinical toxoplasmosis in domestic rabbits. Lab Anim Sci 1992; 42:318–319.
25. Lindsey JR, Fox RR: Inherited diseases and variations. *In* Weisbroth SH, Flatt RE, Kraus AL, eds.: The Biology of the Laboratory Rabbit. New York, Academic Press, 1974, pp 379–382.
26. Mendlowski B: Neuromuscular lesions in restrained rabbits. Vet Pathol 1975; 12:378–386.
27. Okerman L, Devriese LA, Gevaert D, et al: In vivo activity of orally administered antibiotics and chemotherapeutics against acute septicaemic pasteurellosis in rabbits. Lab Anim 1990; 24:341–344.
28. Pakes SP: Protozoal diseases. *In* Weisbroth SH, Flatt RE, Kraus AL, eds.: The Biology of the Laboratory Rabbit. New York, Academic Press, 1974, pp 272–273.
29. Percy DH, Barthold SW: Rabbits. *In* Pathology of Laboratory Rodents and Rabbits. Ames, IA, Iowa State University Press, 1993, pp 179–224.
30. Ringler DH, Abrams GD: Nutritional muscular dystrophy and neonatal mortality in a rabbit breeding colony. J Am Vet Med Assoc 1970; 157:1928–1934.
31. Ringler DH, Abrams GD: Laboratory diagnosis of vitamin E deficiency in rabbits fed a faulty commercial ration. Lab Anim Sci 1971; 21:383–388.
32. Schaeffer DO: Rabbit pasteurellosis. Semin Avian Exotic Pet Med 1993; 2:175–178.
33. Swartout MS, Gerken DF: Lead-induced toxicosis in two domestic rabbits. J Am Vet Med Assoc 1987; 191:717–719.
34. Watson GL, Evans MG: Listeriosis in a rabbit. Vet Pathol 1985; 22:191–193.
35. Weisbroth SH: Neoplastic diseases. *In* Weisbroth SH, Flatt RE, Kraus AL, eds.: The Biology of the Laboratory Rabbit. New York, Academic Press, 1974, pp 331–375.
36. Wright JH, Craighead EM: Infectious motor paralysis in young rabbits. J Exp Med 1922; 36:135–140.
37. Yamini B, Stein S: Abortion, stillbirth, neonatal death, and nutritional myodegeneration in a rabbit breeding colony. J Am Vet Med Assoc 1989; 194:561–562.

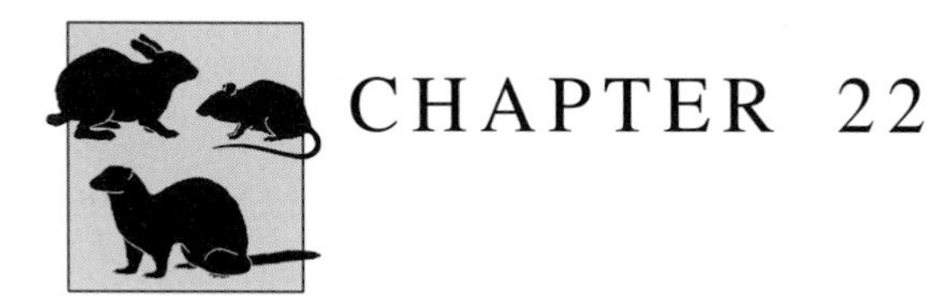

CHAPTER 22

Soft Tissue Surgery and Dental Procedures

Jeffrey R. Jenkins, DVM

The intrinsic physiologic and anatomic differences between rabbits and the species that are more familiar to veterinarians are substantial. Rabbit behavior, such as reaction to stress and pain and to sutures, dressings, and coaptation devices, is unlike that of other pets.

The behavior of rabbits has a strong influence on their suitability as candidates for surgery. Rabbits are timid and submissive. Not uncommonly, rabbits may become anorectic, even to the point of starvation, following a surgical procedure. Rabbits are fractious and may struggle violently if frightened while restrained, resulting in a fractured limb or spine. A frightened rabbit may have very high circulating catecholamine concentrations, which could seriously affect anesthesia. Rabbits are fastidious about their grooming, and this behavior, combined with finely honed incisors, makes short work of most sutures and dressings.

The rabbit is a highly specialized herbivore with a posterior fermentative digestive strategy. A highly complex population of gastrointestinal microflora is responsible for normal digestion. The intricate relationship between the microflora and gut motility is affected by several factors, including diet, antibiotics, and stress. The rabbit has both incisors and cheek teeth that grow continuously, which may lead to problems of malocclusion. The oral cavity is long and curved and opens only a few centimeters, which makes intubation difficult. The stomach pH is significantly more acidic than that of the dog or cat. The small intestine of the rabbit has a small luminal diameter and a relatively thick visceral wall. The cau-

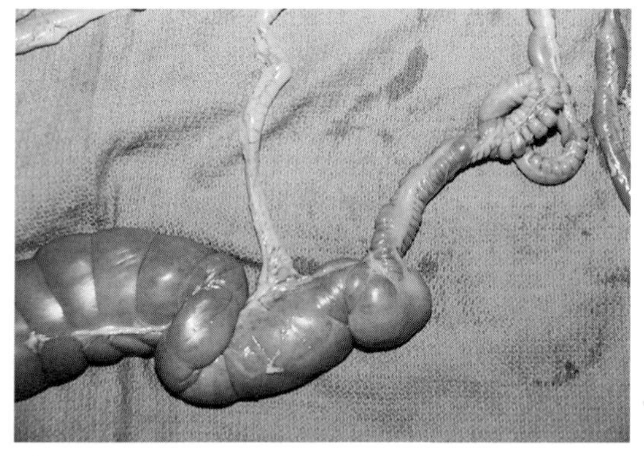

FIGURE 22–1
The caudal end of the ileum of the rabbit is modified to form a round, muscular enlargement called the sacculus rotundus, which is a common site of foreign body impaction.

dal end of the ileum is modified to form a round, muscular enlargement called the sacculus rotundus, which is involved in the direction of material into the cecum or colon. This is a common site of foreign body impaction and a very important structure in normal digestive tract function (Fig. 22–1). The rabbit's cecum is a large, blind-ended sac with a terminal appendix. It is of primary importance in the digestive physiology of the rabbit. The serous membranes of the cecum are extremely thin and delicate compared with those of other sections of the bowel and may tear easily when handled or sutured.

The kidneys are mobile, accessible, and convenient for biopsy. The urinary bladder of the rabbit is tough but thin walled. When greatly distended, it may rupture easily.

EVALUATION OF THE RABBIT AS A SURGICAL PATIENT

Complete a thorough history, including signalment, diet and appetite, and physical examination, including state of hydration and presence of infection, before surgery. Addressing pre-existing problems will improve a patient's prognosis for successful surgery. Make an attempt, through discussion with the owner, observation of the animal, and evaluating clinical data, to assess the level of stress that the animal is experiencing. Sometimes it may be advantageous to postpone surgery until the animal has adapted to its new situation.

EQUIPMENT

Little specialized equipment is required for surgery in rabbits. A short, narrow laryngoscope or an open-style otoscope and a rigid plastic catheter are helpful for intubating the rabbit (see Chapter 32). Equipment to monitor heart rate should be capable of measuring rates of 350 to 400 bpm. A heated surgery table or circulating water blanket and a device to accurately monitor body temperature are necessary during long procedures on small patients. A small Balfour retractor and mechanical suction are needed for surgery of the gastrointestinal tract.

An assortment of sterilized stainless steel spoons of various sizes is helpful for removal of the stomach contents during surgery for hair block or gastric exploratory. Small (baby) Balfour retractors aid in enhancing abdominal exposure, and malleable retractors serve well to hold viscera out of the way without removing them from the abdomen. Skin staples work well for skin closure and cannot be removed by *most* rabbits.

PRESURGICAL TREATMENT

Food, but not water, should be withheld from rabbits for a period of 2–4 hours before surgery. A large volume of stomach ingesta may cause variations in anesthetic dose effects.[4] Rabbits with a low blood glucose concentration after fasting have been shown to have a greater chance of recovery from cerebral ischemia that may result from respiratory or cardiac arrest.* Begin antibiotic therapy in rabbits with systemic or localized bacterial infections, such as those with upper respiratory infections ("snuffles") caused by *Pasteurella* species or with infected wounds. Prophylactic antibiotics may be given if there is a significant chance of bacterial contamination during surgery. Quinolones, trimethoprim-sulfa combinations, sulfa drugs, and aminoglycosides generally do not affect the normal cecal-colic microflora of rabbits. Use caution with beta-lactams, macrolides, or other antibiotics that target gram-positive bacteria.

Parenteral fluids are not indicated in many routine procedures. In rabbits that require supportive fluid therapy or when vascular access is needed,

*Spooner M: Personal communication, 1992.

place a 22- to 26-gauge indwelling catheter in the cephalic or lateral saphenous vein. Peripheral catheters work well during surgery and the immediate recovery period. However, some rabbits do not tolerate a catheter when awake and need to be collared. Cover the catheter and IV line with split-loom tubing or heavily bandage the IV line to keep the rabbit from chewing it. Alternatively, an intraosseous catheter placed within the greater trochanter moves the IV line away from the face of the rabbit and is better tolerated by some rabbits (Fig. 22–2).

Steroids are given only if indicated by the underlying disease process and are generally not given for routine or elective surgery. Give atropine (0.1–0.2 mg/kg SC or IM; see also Chapter 33) or glycopyrrolate to control bradycardia, salivation, or respiratory secretions. These problems rarely occur when isoflurane anesthesia is used. Some rabbits produce atropine esterase, and the dose of atropine may have to be repeated as signs recur.

The combination of thin skin and dense, fine fur makes it easy to cut a rabbit when clipping hair or shaving. Keep the skin spread flat in front of the blade and clip with the blade held flat and close to the skin to minimize nicks and cuts (Fig. 22–3). A fine, #40 blade and an unhurried approach will help to prevent the fine hair from accumulating between the clipper blades, causing them to jam or cut poorly.

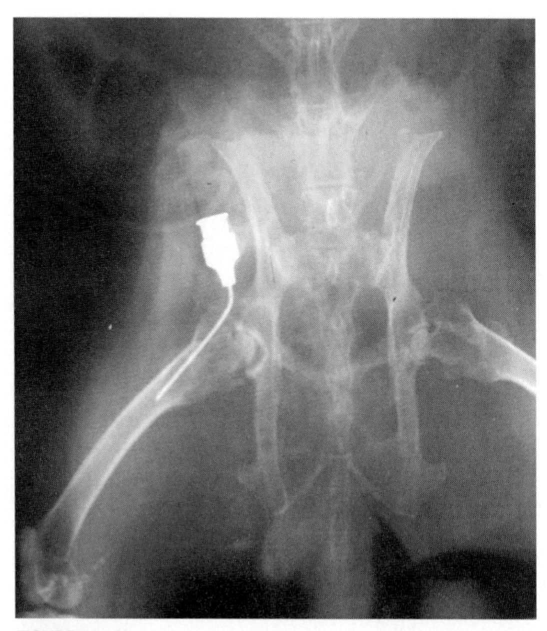

FIGURE 22–2
Radiographic survey film showing an intraosseous catheter placed in the greater trochanter of a rabbit. This moves the catheter away from the face and is better tolerated by some rabbits.

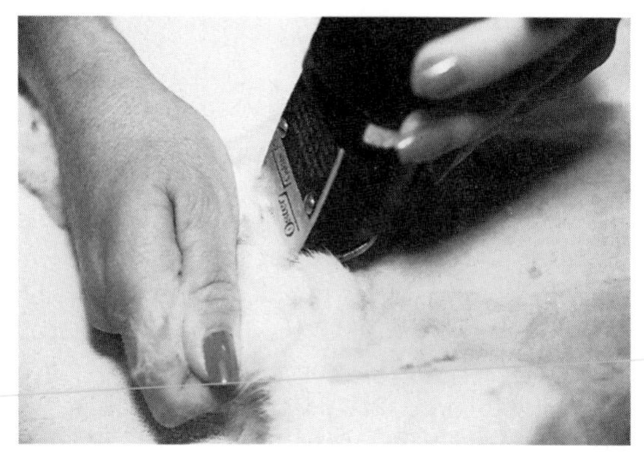

FIGURE 22–3
When clipping fur from the skin of a rabbit, keep the skin spread flat in front of the blade and hold the clipper close to the skin to prevent cutting the skin.

POSTSURGICAL MONITORING

Blood Loss

The blood volume of the rabbit is reported at approximately 57 mL/kg body weight.[6, 8] Most mammalian species experience a drop in arterial pressure and cardiac output with moderate blood loss. Loss of 15–20% of the total blood volume causes massive cholinergic release, with tachycardia and intense arterial constriction that redistributes blood away from the gut and skin. In a 4-kg rabbit, this amounts to 34–45 mL of blood. An acute blood loss of 20–30% of total blood volume, or 45–68 mL in a 4-kg rabbit, is critical.

Pain and Analgesics

The very nature of rabbits is the foremost argument for the use of analgesics. A painful rabbit is inactive, anorectic, and poorly responsive and may grind its teeth. Pain is assumed based on anthropomorphic evaluation of the injury or surgery the animal has experienced. See Chapters 32 and 33 for suggested dosages of analgesics.

SURGICAL TECHNIQUES

Adhesion Formation

Rabbits are used extensively as models for formation of intra-abdominal adhesions. Promising research has been published on the use of calcium channel blocking agents to reduce or prevent adhesion formation in rabbits. In one study, verapamil (Calan, Searle Pharmaceuticals, Skokie, IL), at a dose of 200 μg/kg slowly IV or PO administered to rabbits immediately after surgery and continued every 8 hours for a total of nine doses, was shown to significantly decrease adhesion formation, as compared with untreated controls, with no overt evidence of cardiopulmonary compromise, increased infectious morbidity, or failure of wound healing.[12] My experience mimics these results when I have used verapamil in rabbits in which surgery resulted in damage or irritation of abdominal organs. Studies of nonsteroidal anti-inflammatory drugs[10] or other drugs or methods to prevent adhesion formation may also have clinical applications in rabbits.

Choice of Suture Material

The biologic and physical characteristics of suture material influence wound healing. Rabbits are more negatively affected by suture than other mammals because of the caseous, suppurative response of the rabbit's immune system to foreign material and their proclivity to form adhesions. New absorbable suture material made from polymers that are removed by hydrolytic degradation are much less reactive and cause fewer and weaker adhesions in my experience. I prefer monofilament polyglycolic acid or other similar monofilament synthetic suture for closure of gastrotomy, enterotomy, or colotomy sites, cesarean sections, or other major abdominal surgery. Stainless or tantalum clips (Hemoclips, Dilling Weck, Research Triangle Park, NC) are excellent for vessel and small pedicle ligation with minimal adhesion formation. A recent study of laser anastomosis for sutureless closure of the colon of rabbits has been published[7]; this technique holds potential for the future.

Skin Closures

Rabbits have a great fondness for suture removal and a similarly great dislike of Elizabethan collars. This combination has led to a search for a dependable method of skin closure. All but the smallest of rabbits make short work of stainless steel monofilament. Intradermal closures work very well but are time consuming to place. Cyanoacrylate tissue cement (Vetbond, Medical-Surgical Division/3M, St. Paul, MN) is adequate but is occasionally removed by the rabbit. Skin staples are both reliable and well-accepted by the rabbits and their owners and are my preference.

COMMON PROCEDURES

Ovariohysterectomy

The reproductive tract of the female rabbit is unusual compared with that of the dog or cat. The uterus is bicornuate, and each uterine cornua possesses a cervix (there is no uterine body) and is coiled tightly in the caudal abdomen cranial and dorsal to the urinary bladder. The uterus is easily exteriorized but is more fragile than that of other species. The mesometrium in a healthy doe is a principal site of fat storage (Fig. 22–4), which makes identification and ligation of uterine vessels difficult.

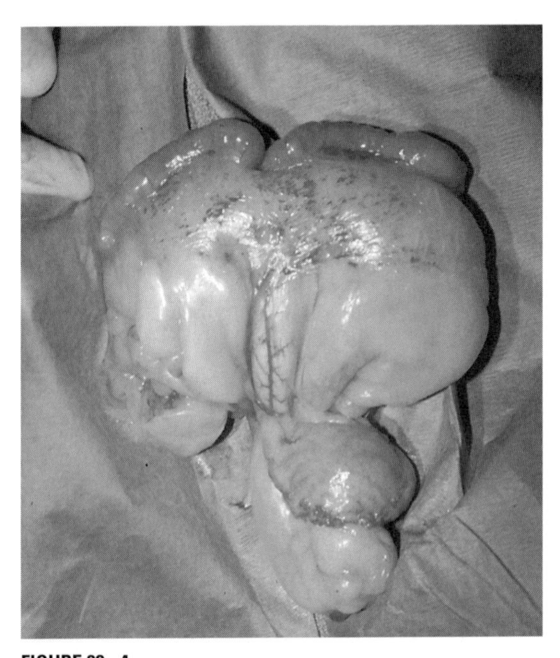

FIGURE 22–4
The mesometrium of a doe is a primary site of fat storage. This makes identification and ligation of uterine vessels difficult during an ovariohysterectomy.

The urethra of the female rabbit empties into the proximal end of a deep vaginal vestibule. Expression of the bladder with the animal in dorsal recumbency often leads to retrofilling of the vaginal vault. This is a possible source of contamination of the peritoneal cavity during uterine surgery and may be confused with the bladder.

With the rabbit anesthetized before surgery, empty the rabbit's bladder by gentle palpation. Shave and prepare the abdominal area, and restrain the rabbit on the surgery table in dorsal recumbency, draped for surgery. Make a 2- to 3-cm midline incision centered over the cranial pole of the bladder about half the distance between the umbilicus and the cranial rim of the pubis. Lift the narrow linea alba from the abdominal contents as you make a stab incision into the abdomen; be very careful when entering the abdominal wall, as the thin-walled cecum and bladder are often pressed firmly against the ventral abdomen. The uterus typically can be seen as it lies dorsal to the cranial pole of the bladder and may be lifted through the incision with forceps. A spay (snook) hook is not necessary, but take care if one is used to avoid damage to the cecum. Follow the uterus to the oviduct and infundibulum. The oviduct is coiled in a large loop that is several times longer than that of a dog or cat, so be careful not to leave a portion of it. The ovarian vasculature is manifold, but vessels are small compared with those of many mammals. Carefully identify vessels and double ligate with transfixing sutures of chromic gut or synthetic absorbable suture. Hemorrhage is seldom a problem. The uterine vessels stand several millimeters off the uterus and may be of significant size in mature does. Double ligate these vessels with transfixing ligatures to the uterus or vaginal serosa. Ligate the uterus just cranial or just caudal to the cervices. Avoid contaminating the abdomen with urine or vaginal contents if a caudal ligature is used. Ligate each uterine horn if removed cranial to the cervix, or carefully ligate at the dorsal vagina if the uterus is removed caudal to the cervices. Closure of the abdomen is routine. Close the skin with surgical staples, an intradermal suture pattern, or tissue cement.

Orchidectomy (Castration)

Sexually active male rabbits (bucks) have obnoxious urine marking behaviors that generally lead to their owners wanting to have them neutered. Furthermore, bucks may become territorial and possessive about their environment and owners, leading to aggressive behavior.

The rabbit's testes are similar to those of the cat but may move freely from the scrotum to the abdomen through an open inguinal canal. Soft tissue herniation and strangulation of bowel loops is prevented by a large mass of fat associated with the epididymis that rests in the inguinal canal when the testicle is in the scrotum.

For castration, anesthetize and restrain the rabbit in dorsal recumbency. Carefully shave the hair from the scrotum and surrounding area, and surgically prepare and drape the area to minimize contamination. Make a 1- to 1.5-cm incision with a #15 scalpel blade through the skin and vaginal tunic on the ventral surface of both sides of the scrotum. Remove the testis from the tunic and carefully tear the ligament of the testicle from the tunic with a dry gauze sponge (Fig. 22–5). Pull the testis caudally to expose a section of the vas deferens and the vascular structures of the spermatic cord, which are then tied in an overhand knot with a small Mayo needle holder or mosquito forceps. Alternately, ligate the duct and vasculature with 3–0 chromic gut or synthetic absorbable suture. Cut the duct and vessels distal to the knot or ligature and return the spermatic cord to the inguinal canal such that it may be recovered if bleeding occurs. Return the tunic to the scrotum and repeat the process for the remaining testis. Observe the rabbit for several hours after the surgery for hemorrhage. Complications most often result from overactivity or sexual activity; therefore, I hospitalize these castrated rabbits overnight for "cage rest."

DENTAL PROBLEMS

Malocclusion

Malocclusion of either the incisors, the cheek teeth, or both is common in rabbits. The causes of malocclusion can be multifactorial and include genetic, traumatic, and infectious causes. The vertical opening of the oral cavity of a rabbit is very restricted; therefore, the chewing action of a rabbit is normally a horizontal as well as a vertical movement, providing a grinding action that keeps the occlusal surfaces evenly worn. Many dental problems in rabbits are the result of a mandible that is too narrow or too short, resulting in misalignment of the teeth.[3] Misalignment of an individual tooth can result from infection of the root or trauma to the tooth.

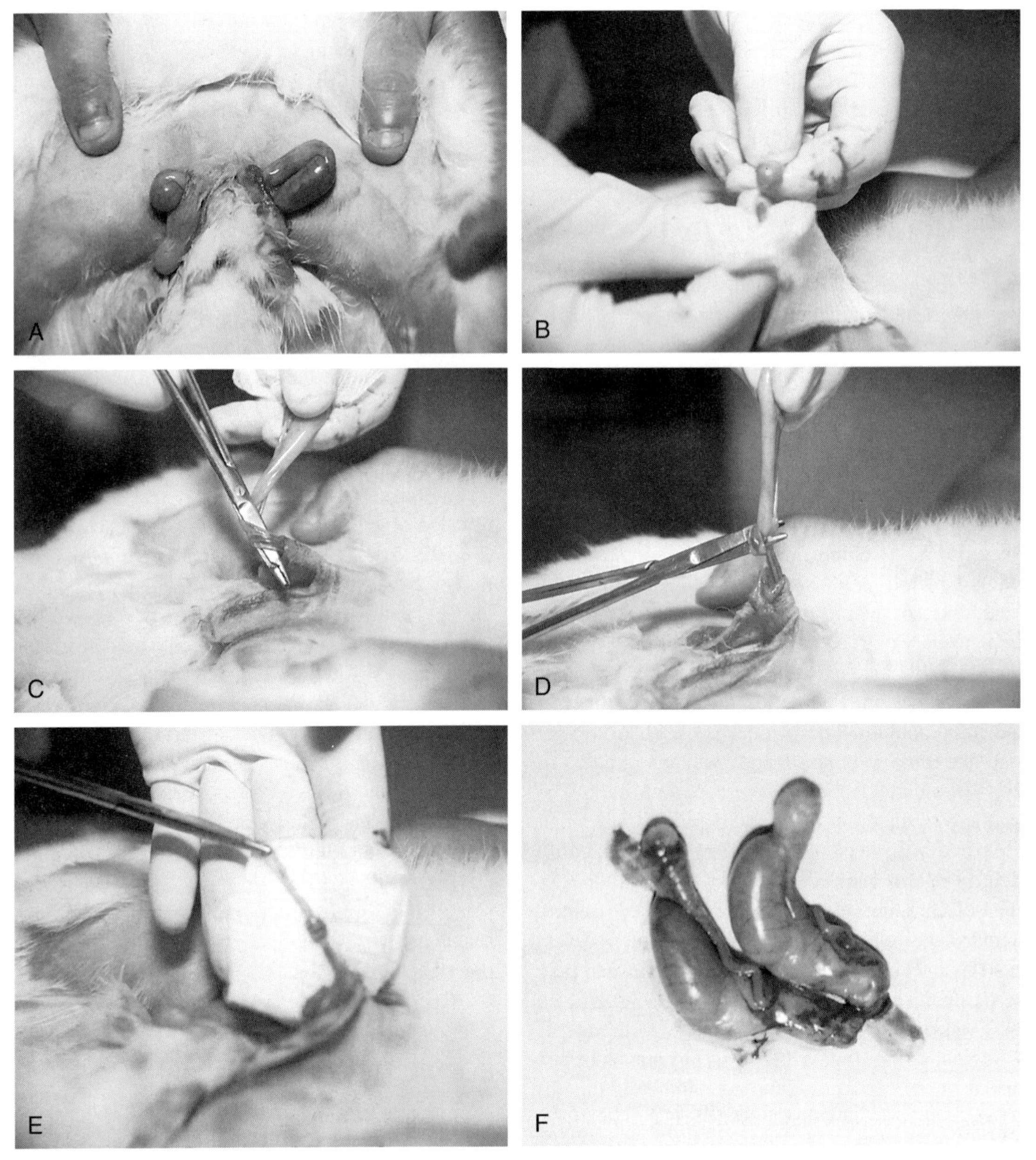

FIGURE 22–5
A technique for castration of a rabbit. After incising the skin and vaginal tunic on both sides of the scrotum, the testes are removed from the vaginal tunic *(A)*. The ligament of the testicle is torn from the tunic with a dry gauze sponge *(B)*. The vas deferens and vessels of the spermatic cord are tied with an overhand knot or ligated *(C, D)*. The testicle is removed by cutting distal to the knot or ligature *(E)*. The testes as removed from a castrated rabbit *(F)*.

Incisor malocclusion is usually apparent at an early age in many rabbits, especially in small breeds. Rabbit owners usually notice the overgrown teeth and present their rabbit to the veterinarian before inability to prehend food becomes a severe clinical problem. Malocclusion of the cheek teeth is not obvious to the owner, and a rabbit with molar malocclusion is usually presented with a history of anorexia and weight loss. Often the rabbit is bright and alert and appears hungry but refuses pellets or drops food from its mouth.

Routine physical examination of every rabbit should include examination of the incisors and the cheek teeth. Use an otoscope or vaginal speculum to obtain a good view of the cheek teeth (Fig. 22–6; see also Chapter 15). Tranquilization of the rabbit is

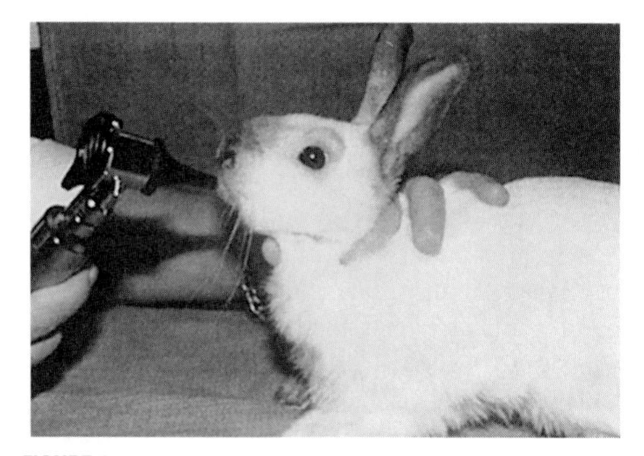

FIGURE 22–6
An otoscope is used to examine the cheek teeth of a rabbit. (From Hillyer EV: Pet rabbits. Vet Clin North Am Small Anim Pract 1994; 24:31.)

sometimes necessary to thoroughly examine the cheek teeth. Use gauze strips looped around the upper and lower incisors to hold the mouth open during the examination (Fig. 22–7). Take care to keep the neck extended and to avoid occluding the nares during restraint, or respiration may be compromised.

Routine Dentistries

Incisors can be trimmed with a dental drill or side-nosed cutters. Avoid the use of a nail trimmer to cut the teeth, as it usually results in splitting the teeth, which may predispose teeth to root infection, and jagged edges. Cutting the teeth with a side-nosed cutter is acceptable but can also result in splitting or jagged edges if not done carefully. This method is done on an awake rabbit and can be demonstrated to the owner for cutting the incisors at home. A high-speed dental drill is the preferred tool for trimming the incisors. However, this method usually requires that the rabbit be tranquilized because any movement by the rabbit can result in cutting the tongue or gums. A small tapered fissure bur with a water coolant is suggested.[3] The incisors usually require trimming every 6–8 weeks.

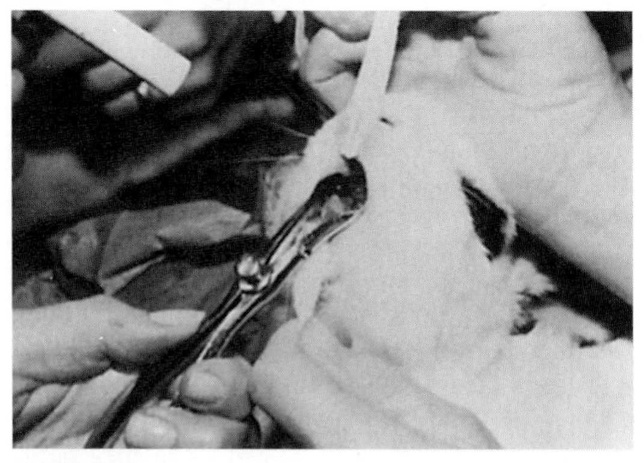

FIGURE 22–7
Examination of the oral cavity of a sedated rabbit. Gauze strips are used to hold the mouth open, and a vaginal speculum retracts the cheeks. (From Hillyer EV: Pet rabbits. Vet Clin North Am Small Anim Pract 1994; 24:50.)

Molar malocclusion usually results in overly long edges of the inner occlusal edge of the mandibular teeth and the outer occlusal edge of the maxillary teeth, the overgrown edges of which are often quite sharp and cause lacerations of the tongue and buccal mucosa, respectively. Often there are one or more very sharp spicules, which cause puncture-like lacerations that are apparently very painful to the rabbit.

Tranquilization or anesthesia is usually necessary for dentistry of the cheek teeth. Restrain the rabbit in a sternal position with the neck extended and the mouth held open with gauze strips, as previously described. Use a vaginal speculum to retract the cheeks for examination of the molars. A vaginal speculum with an attached light source is very useful for this purpose. Trim the molar teeth with a Lempert rongeur or a dental drill. If a dental drill is used, be very careful to avoid lacerating the tongue or buccal mucosa. Retract the tongue with a tongue depressor or cotton-tipped applicator if necessary. Carefully inspect all lateral edges of the upper arcade and the medial edges of the lower arcade. Occasionally it is difficult to see the edges of the most caudal molars; use a probe or cotton swab to check for asymmetric or long edges of these teeth.

Periodontal disease or tooth root abscessation often requires extraction of affected teeth. If a tooth is extracted, consider extraction of the opposing tooth in the opposite arcade or routinely check the tooth to prevent overgrowth of that tooth.

Incisor Extraction

Removal of the incisors is sometimes elected in rabbits with severe incisor malocclusion or incisors that need very frequent trimming. Surgical removal can provide a permanent solution and is usually well tolerated by the rabbit.[2] Occasionally the procedure is not successful because the full root of the tooth is not extracted, resulting in regrowth of the tooth in its original or an aberrant position. Anesthesia is required for this procedure; use either an injectable anesthetic drug combination or isoflurane anesthesia with intubation of the rabbit.

With the rabbit anesthetized, break down the periodontal ligaments of the incisors with a small elevator, pushing in to the gums as deeply as possible on all sides of the teeth.[2] Break the medial ligament, which is the strongest, by inserting the elevator on the medial side of the tooth and gently rotating it. Once the ligament is broken and the tooth is loosened, extract it with a tooth extractor, pulling up and inward in the natural direction of the growth of the tooth as the root is very curved. Remove the lower incisors first, then remove both sets of the upper incisors (the primary incisors and the peg teeth). Inspect the root tip of the extracted teeth; the root tip should be soft and hollow.[2] If the tooth breaks above the root, wait 6–8 weeks to allow regrowth of the tooth, then reattempt extraction of the tooth. After surgery, administer prophylactic antibiotics for 10 days, unless there is evidence of infection of the root. If infection is present, submit a tissue sample for bacterial culture and sensitivity testing, and administer an appropriate antibiotic for 6–8 weeks. Analgesics may be indicated for 3–5 days after surgery.

Dental Abscesses

Abscesses of the cheek teeth are common in rabbits (see Fig. 31–8). Infections may be secondary to food impacted alongside the tooth or into a longitudinal fracture of a tooth or from bacterial contamination of oral lesions. Mixed bacterial infections are sometimes present; however, pure cultures of *Pasteurella multocida* or *Staphylococcus aureus* predominate. Because total excision of the abscess is not possible, the prognosis is guarded, and the owner should be warned of protracted treatment.

Treatment consists of aggressive débridement and curettage of the lesion as well as extraction of the tooth or teeth involved. Leave the area open following débridement and irrigate the area daily with saline or a disinfectant solution using a Water-Pic or lavage. A cream (Kymar Ointment, Schering-Plough Corporation, Kenilworth, NJ) or spray (Granulex, Dow B. Hickam, Inc., Sugarland, TX) containing digestive enzymes (trypsin) may be applied after cleansing the lesion and continued until all purulent exudate is removed and a good granulation bed is established. Continue cleansing and irrigating the area until the wound is well epithelialized. Systemic antibiotic therapy, most often with enrofloxacin or trimethoprim-sulfadiazine combined with good wound management, results in complete healing in some rabbits. Sometimes infection can be "controlled" as long as the rabbit is maintained on antibiotics.

Recent research[9] has shown that packing the abscess with a dental preparation, calcium hydroxide, may greatly improve the chances of complete healing. Ten of 14 rabbits treated in this study healed without recurrence of the abscess. In this technique, the abscess is opened and débrided, and the involved teeth are extracted. The empty abscess cavity is then filled with calcium hydroxide paste, and the wound is left open. The paste is removed after 1 week, and treatment is repeated if purulent material remains. Calcium hydroxide creates an environment with a pH of 12.0, which kills bacteria but does not harm tissue. I have treated a limited number of cheek tooth abscesses with this protocol, with promising results.

GASTROINTESTINAL SURGERY

Gastrotomy

Gastrotomy for removal of gastric trichobezoars (wool block) is rarely necessary, as most rabbits respond well to medical management. Aggressive therapy with parenteral fluids, metoclopramide (0.5 mg/kg q4–8h), force feeding, and a high-fiber diet should always be attempted before surgery. Surgery is indicated in rabbits with suspected gastric foreign bodies or complete gastric or pyloric obstruction, or in those that fail to show clinical signs of improvement after 3–4 days of medical therapy. Rabbits with chronic wool block should be thoroughly worked up, and every effort should be made to return the rabbit to a positive energy balance and to correct fluid and electrolyte imbalances before surgery. A common accompanying lesion with gastric hairballs is severe hepatic lipidosis, presumably as a result of starvation. Correction of the negative energy balance will decrease acidosis and ketosis and the likely complications of fatty hepatopathy.[5]

Compared with hairballs in cats or ferrets, the network of food, fur, and "felt" contained in the stomach of a rabbit with gastric obstruction may be so large as to distend the stomach beyond its normal limits. This mass is intertwined and sometimes can be removed in one piece. The stomach of a rabbit without gastric obstruction may contain loose hair, which will disintegrate when removed. This leads one to suspect that the pathogenesis of the problem is one of abnormal gastric physiologic function rather than simply the presence of hair.

Anesthetize the rabbit, restrain it on a circulating water blanket in dorsal recumbency, shave it from the inguinal to midthoracic area, and prepare it for aseptic surgery. Place a catheter in the cephalic or lateral saphenous vein for fluid administration and vascular access during surgery. Make a midline incision long enough to explore the entire gastrointestinal tract, taking care not to damage the stomach or cecum, which may be pressed tightly against the abdominal wall. Drape lap pads moistened with normal saline along the incision line and use a Balfour retractor to fully expose the abdomen. Explore the abdomen before the gastrotomy to determine whether additional lesions are present. Examine the liver carefully; if it is abnormally pale or yellow, do a liver biopsy and submit the sample for histopathologic examination. Place stay sutures in the greater curvature of the stomach and elevate it into the surgical field. Place additional moistened lap pads around the stomach to prevent contamination of the abdomen with gastric contents. Make an incision in the avascular area between the lesser and greater curvatures, and carefully remove the trichobezoar and any other ingesta with a sterile surgical spoon. Rinse the lumen with a small volume of warm saline and examine it for abnormalities, then gently palpate the pylorus for patency. Close the stomach in a two-layer inverting pattern with 3–0 synthetic monofilament suture or 3–0 chromic gut. Extend the sutures into, but not through, the gastric mucosa. Thoroughly lavage the abdomen with body-temperature isotonic fluids and close it routinely.

Postoperative management is equally critical to the successful outcome of the procedure.[11, 13] Supportive therapy to optimize wound healing and support the patient, prevent further hepatic damage, and promote hepatic regeneration is essential. Furthermore, care must be taken to support the normal gut microflora to prevent complications of stress-induced enteritis complex.

Intestinal Resection, Anastomosis, and Enterotomy

Intestinal resection or enterotomy is most often indicated in rabbits with foreign body ingestion or those with trauma to the intestine. Neoplasia and infiltrative intestinal diseases are uncommon and in my experience consist mostly of metastatic uterine adenocarcinomas. Successful intestinal surgery in the rabbit demands attention to surgical principles. Special attention to preserving the blood supply and luminal diameter must be taken to compensate for the small lumen-to-visceral wall thickness of the rabbit intestine.[1] The bowel must be handled gently to prevent shock and postoperative ileus.

Preparation of the rabbit for surgery and the abdominal incision is the same as that for gastrotomy, with care taken not to damage the cecum while making the incision. Examine the entire gastrointestinal tract before the enterotomy. If resection and anastomosis are necessary, ligate the mesenteric and arcade vessels and apply crushing and noncrushing clamps, as done in other small animals. Incise the intestine at an acute angle to augment the small luminal diameter. I prefer an appositional suture technique with 4–0 to 6–0 synthetic monofilament suture. Linear foreign bodies accompanied by bowel plication or intussusception occasionally occur in rabbits. Multiple enterotomy sites may be required for removal of these foreign bodies. Longitudinal incisions and transverse closures are sometimes used if the luminal diameter is small (Fig. 22–8). If the abdomen is contaminated during the procedure, lavage with warm saline for several cycles of irrigation and suction before closure.

Surgery of the Large Bowel

Surgery of the rabbit colon is seldom done. It is indicated primarily in injuries that result from bite wounds, intraluminal trauma from diagnostic or clinical instrumentation, or trauma secondary to accidents during surgery. Many rabbits with these injuries are seen as referral cases, and the condition may have been present for several days before examination. Neoplasia of the lower bowel, with the exception of rectal polyps and metastatic uterine adenocarcinoma, are rarely seen in my practice. Several areas of the colon and cecum are thin walled and easily torn, and their suturing characteristics are less than optimal. As with the small bowel, incise at an acute angle when doing a bowel resection, and close longitudinal incisions transversely to increase luminal diameter. An interrupted suture pattern is typically used in an appositional or crushing technique for anastomosis of the colon. An inverting suture tech-

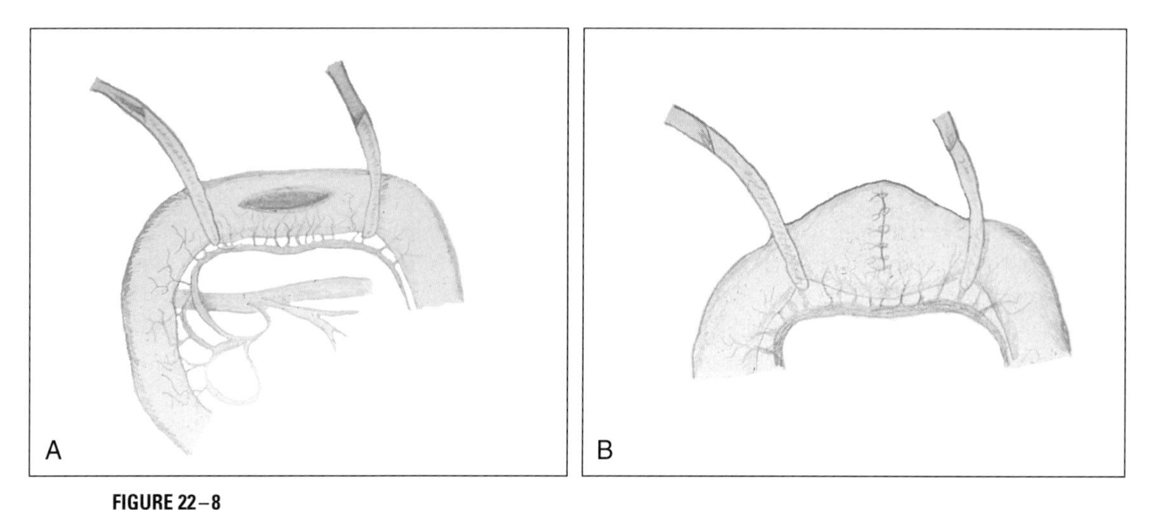

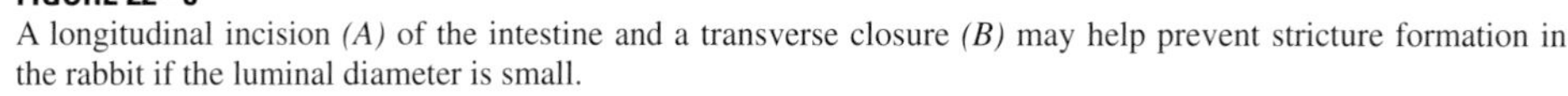

FIGURE 22–8
A longitudinal incision *(A)* of the intestine and a transverse closure *(B)* may help prevent stricture formation in the rabbit if the luminal diameter is small.

nique may be used when closing lesions of the cecum; I prefer a 4–0 to 6–0 synthetic monofilament suture placed at 2- to 3-mm intervals. A segment of omentum can be used to reinforce the anastomosis or incision line. Before closing, lavage the abdomen several times with warm saline or a 1 : 10 povidone iodine/saline solution, followed by suction. Remove any grossly evident ingesta in the abdominal cavity. If contamination of the abdominal cavity occurs, take a swab sample for both aerobic and anaerobic bacterial culture, and treat the rabbit aggressively with antibiotics.

Anorectal Papilloma Removal

Anorectal papillomas are cauliflower-like fungating masses that arise from the anorectal junction. These are benign and not related to the papillomas of skin or the oral cavity. Papillomas arise from the rectal squamous columnar junction and protrude from the anus once they have grown to a sufficient size. Removal of these lesions is usually successful.

The tissue of the papilloma is friable and has a tendency to bleed. The mucosal attachment may be stalklike or broad based. Removal is facilitated by good exposure of the lesion. Position the rabbit in dorsal recumbency with the pelvis slightly elevated. Have an assistant place and hold a human nasal speculum (or a veterinary canine vaginal speculum) in the anus. Alternatively, place several stay sutures around the circumference of the anus so that an assistant can provide gentle traction. Remove the papilloma by sharp dissection or electrosurgery, taking care to remove all of the mass to prevent recurrence. Suture the mucosa with 4–0 to 6–0 absorbable suture material in a simple continuous pattern. Large papillomas may be removed in sections to simplify closure.

ABSCESSES

Rabbits form thick-walled abscesses that contain a caseous purulent discharge in reaction to most bacterial infections. If these abscesses are simply opened and drained, they frequently recur. Therefore, abscesses should be excised with a substantial margin, so that all contaminated tissue is removed. Ligate blood vessels with a small-diameter absorbable suture and close the skin with surgical staples. Excision of large abscesses may require the use of skin flaps to cover the defect. Complete excision is often not possible with foot or dental abscesses, and aggressive surgical débridement must be used. After débridement, the wound is allowed to granulate in, but the prognosis is poor for complete cure. Pododermatitis and the resulting osteomyelitis may cripple a rabbit; these lesions are painful, and the rabbit may be reluctant to stand or walk. In these rabbits, consider amputation as an alternative to more conventional therapy of abscesses. (See Chapter 30.)

DERMOPLASTY AND TAIL AMPUTATION TO CORRECT PROBLEMS OF URINE SCALD

Dermatologic problems that result from urine scald or chronic diarrhea are common in pet rabbits (see Chapter 20). Underlying causes of obesity, dietary indiscretion, urinary tract disease, and spinal cord disease must be addressed; however, correction of the dermatologic problem may depend on the prevention of urine contamination of the perineal tissues. These problems result from repeated urine or diarrhea contamination of the perineal skin and medial surfaces of the hind legs. In obese rabbits, a large fold of skin and fat may partially cover the genital area, interfering with the passage of urine. Alternatively, the rabbit may be unable to rotate its pelvis during urination or defecation to direct the stream of urine caudally, resulting in urine contamination of the skin of the perineum and legs. These problems are compounded because the urine scald causes increased immobility, which further contributes to the likelihood of urine contamination.

I have used two techniques to correct these problems: dermoplasty of the caudal abdomen to remove the fold of skin that interferes with the passage of urine, and a combination of tail amputation and dermoplasty to lift the genital area dorsally, resulting in the passage of urine in a more caudal direction. It must be emphasized that these surgeries are adjuncts and salvage procedures for these conditions; every effort should be made to correct the underlying cause of the problem before surgery. I have obtained excellent results, however, in rabbits when I have used these corrective procedures.

Use systemic as well as topical antibiotics and protectants before surgery to decrease inflammation and infection in the area. For the skin fold resection, position the rabbit in dorsal recumbency, and shave and prepare the area from the midabdomen to the tail, including the medial thigh region to the stifle. Identify a crescent area of skin cranial to the genital area that, when removed, will eliminate any excessive tissue that protrudes over the genital area (Fig. 22–9). Incise along this crescent of skin, avoiding damage to the lateral abdominal vein lateral to the nipple and deep to the glandular tissue of the mammary gland. There may be an advantage in removing some portion or all of the inguinal adipose body that extends from just cranial to the inguinal mammary gland to the genital area and is a primary location for deposition of adipose tissue. Tissue removal should result in the skin of the caudal ventral abdomen being taut with the rabbit in dorsal recumbency but without tension on the incision. I prefer two-layer

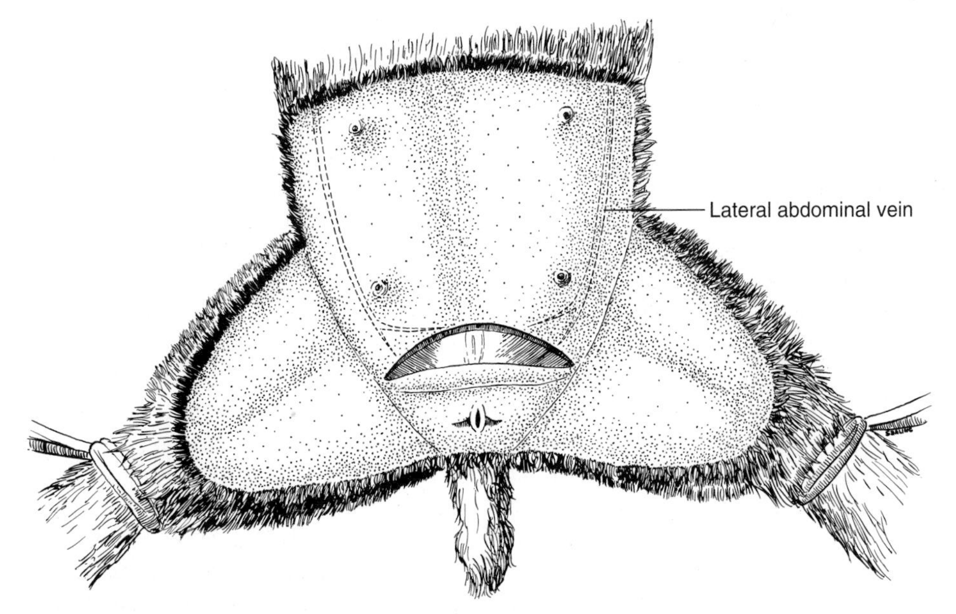

FIGURE 22–9
Illustration of a procedure for ventral skin fold resection in a rabbit. A large fold of abdominal skin may interfere with urine passage in an obese rabbit, causing contamination of the surrounding skin and urine scald. A ventral skin fold resection of the caudal abdomen removes a crescent-shaped area of skin, allowing unimpeded passage of urine.

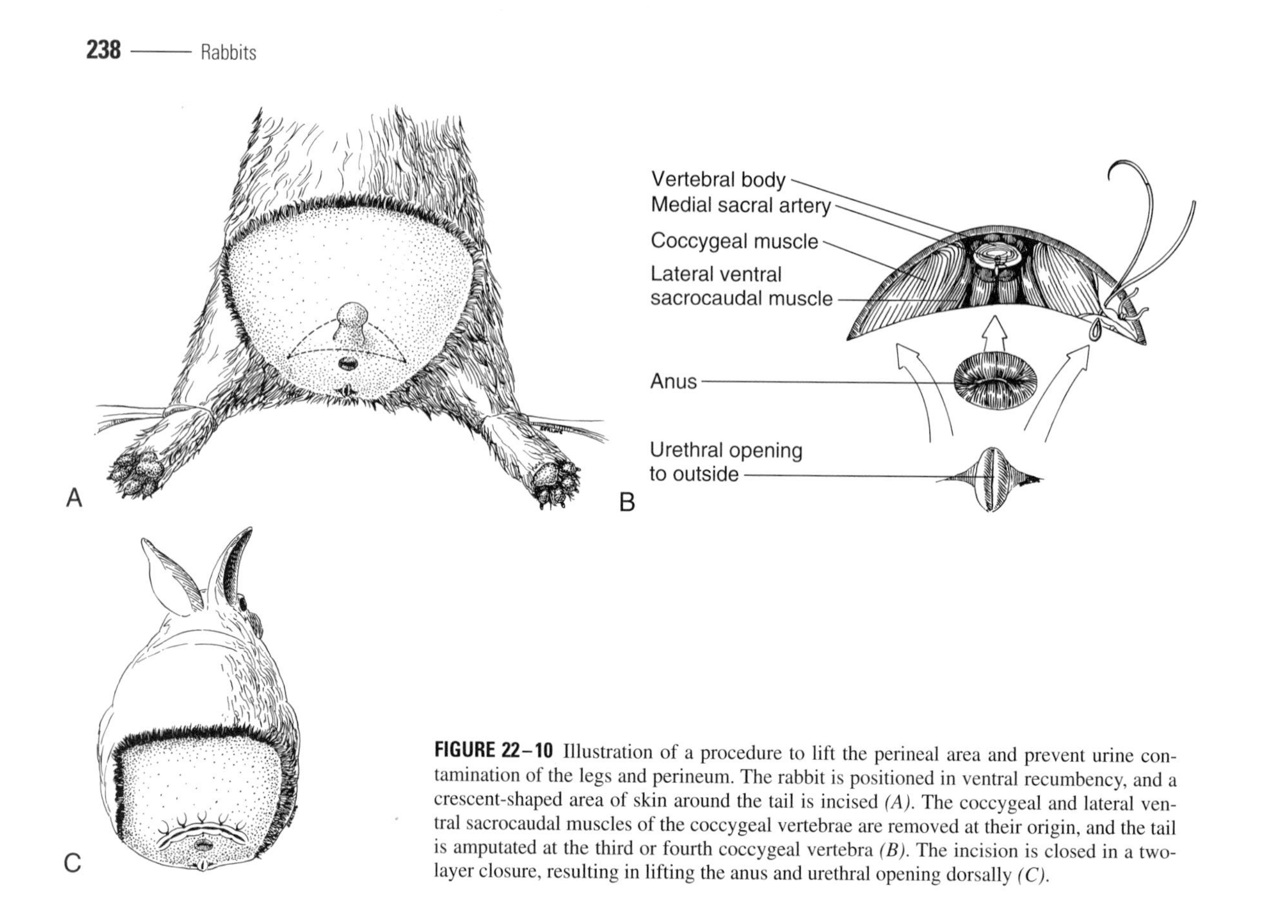

FIGURE 22–10 Illustration of a procedure to lift the perineal area and prevent urine contamination of the legs and perineum. The rabbit is positioned in ventral recumbency, and a crescent-shaped area of skin around the tail is incised *(A)*. The coccygeal and lateral ventral sacrocaudal muscles of the coccygeal vertebrae are removed at their origin, and the tail is amputated at the third or fourth coccygeal vertebra *(B)*. The incision is closed in a two-layer closure, resulting in lifting the anus and urethral opening dorsally *(C)*.

closure, with an absorbable suture in the deep layer and staples in the skin.

The second procedure, developed by Dr. Brian Loudis, is more difficult to perform but very effective for rabbits that urinate on their legs because of an inability to lift their pelvis and direct the stream of urine away from their legs. Position the rabbit for surgery in ventral recumbency with the rear legs extended behind the rabbit. Shave an area extending 3 to 5 inches from the anus and tail and prepare it for surgery. Delineate a crescent-shaped section of skin that, when removed, will lift the anus and urethral opening to a dorsal position at the caudal most extreme of the rabbit. The crescent should extend from a point dorsal to the anus, just beyond the dorsal limits of the external anal sphincter muscle on its ventral curvature to immediately dorsal of the tail, and lateral and ventral to the urethral opening (see Fig. 22–10). Identify the coccygeal and lateral ventral sacrocaudal muscles of the coccygeal vertebrae and remove them from their insertion. In male rabbits the retractor penis muscle must also be identified and, in some cases, carefully dissected from its origin. Amputate the tail at the third or fourth coccygeal vertebra and ligate the medial sacral artery. The coccygeal and (if removed) retractor penis muscles are reattached at or about the dorsocaudal origin of the semitendinosus muscle with polypropylene or strong absorbable suture. Place vertical mattress sutures to position the closure and relieve tension and close the incision in two layers, as in the procedure just described.

REFERENCES

1. Booth HW, Hartsfield SM: Use of the laboratory rabbit in the small animal student surgery laboratory. J Vet Med Educ 1990; 17:16–18.
2. Brown SA: Surgical removal of the incisors in the rabbit. J Small Exotic Anim Med 1992; 1:150–153.
3. Emily P: Problems peculiar to continually erupting teeth. J Small Exotic Anim Med 1991; 1:56–59.
4. Harkness JE, Wagner JE: The Biology and Medicine of Rabbits and Rodents, 4th ed. Media, PA, Williams and Wilkins, 1995.
5. Gillett NA, Brooks DL, Tillman PC: Medical and surgical management of gastric obstruction from a hairball in the rabbit. J Am Vet Med Assoc 1983; 183:1176–1178.
6. Kozma C, Macklin W, Cummins LM, et al: Anatomy, physiology, and biochemistry of the rabbit. *In* Weisbroth SH, Flatt RE, Kraus AL, eds.: The Biology of the Laboratory Rabbit. New York, Academic Press, 1974, pp 50–72.
7. Kuramoto S, Ryan PJ: First sutureless closure of a colotomy: short-term results of experimental laser anastomosis of the colon. Dis Colon Rectum 1991; 34:1079–1084.
8. McGuill MW, Rowan AN: Biological effects of blood loss: implications for sampling volumes and techniques. ILAR News 1989; 31:5–18.

9. Remeeus PGK, Verbeek M: The use of calcium hydroxide in the treatment of abscesses in the cheek of the rabbit resulting from a dental periapical disorder. J Vet Dentistry 1995; 12:19–22.
10. Rodgers K, Girgis W, diZerega GS, Johns DB: Intraperitoneal tolmetin prevents postsurgical adhesion formation in rabbits. Int J Fertil 1990; 35:40–45.
11. Sebesten A: Acute obstruction of the duodenum of a rabbit following the apparently successful treatment of a hairball. Lab Anim 1977; 11:135.
12. Steinleitiner A, Lambert H, Kazensky C, et al: Reduction of primary postoperative adhesion formation under calcium channel blockade in the rabbit. J Surg Res 1990; 48:42–45.
13. Wagner JL, Hackel DB, Samsell AG: Spontaneous deaths in rabbits resulting from gastric trichobezoars. Lab Anim Sci 1974; 24:826–830.

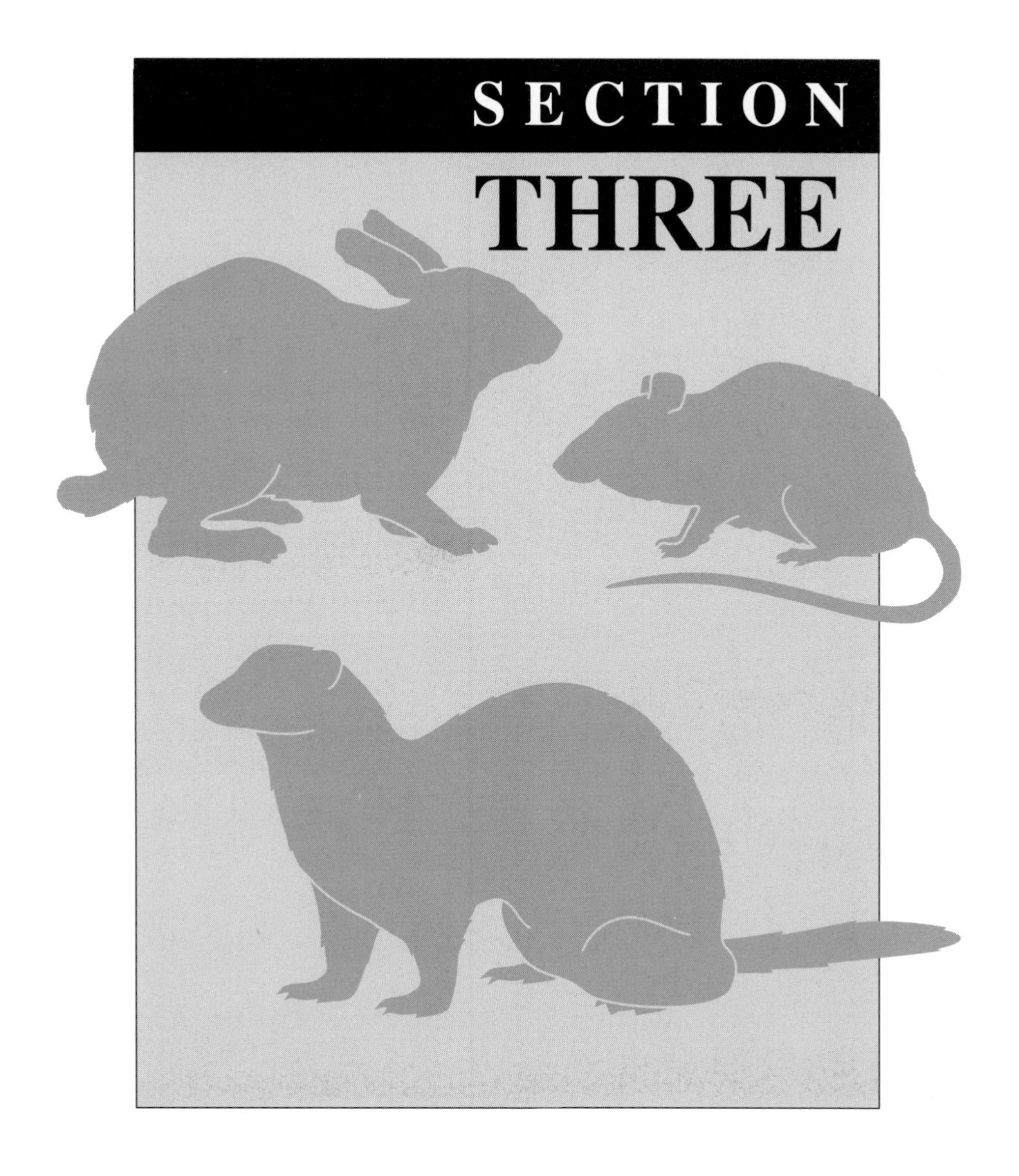

Guinea Pigs and Chinchillas

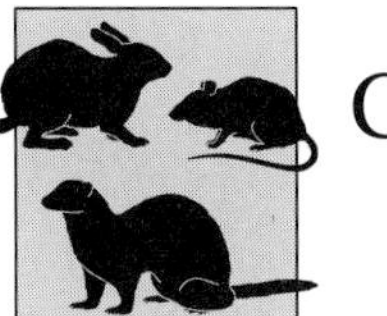

CHAPTER 23

Biology, Husbandry, and Clinical Techniques

Elizabeth V. Hillyer, DVM,
Katherine E. Quesenberry, DVM, and
Thomas M. Donnelly, BVSc

Guinea pigs *(Cavia porcellus)* and chinchillas *(Chinchilla laniger)* are hystricomorph rodents from South America (Fig. 23–1). They share many anatomic and physiologic characteristics, and the approach to their veterinary care is similar. Both species are monogastric herbivores with a large cecum; both produce precocious young after a relatively long gestation period. There are also some important differences between the two species: for example, guinea pigs require a dietary source of vitamin C but chinchillas do not; dystocia is common in guinea pigs but not in chinchillas; and chinchillas require daily dust baths but guinea pigs do not. Both guinea pigs and chinchillas are small, gentle, and lively species that make good pets because they are docile and relatively easy to care for.

In this chapter we summarize the information on basic biology, husbandry, and clinical techniques that is relevant to the medical care of these species as pets. Readers interested in more detailed descriptions of anatomy and physiology of guinea pigs can find these in the references.[4, 27, 31] Guinea pigs have been used as laboratory animals for over 400 years, and there is abundant information available about them; less has been published about chinchillas. Much of the information available on chinchillas concerns their husbandry and breeding and is found in the lay literature. Information on anatomy and physiology of chinchillas is more difficult to find. The contents of this chapter reflect this disparity in knowledge.

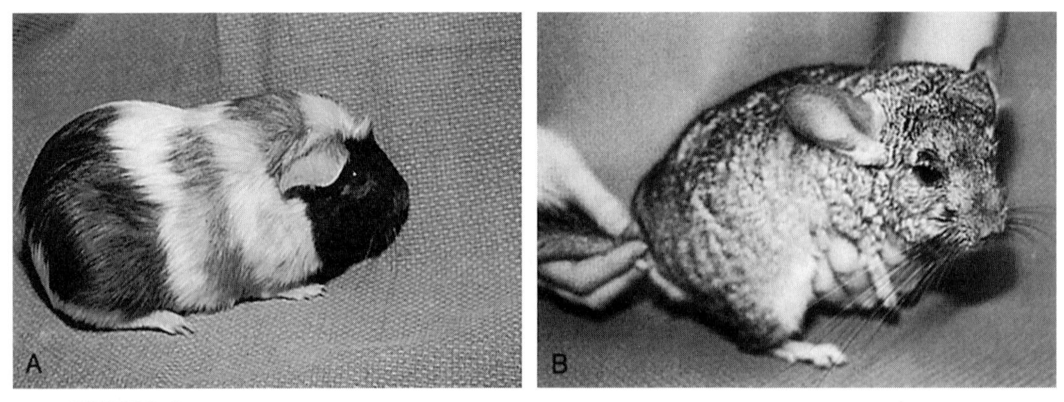

FIGURE 23–1
A, Normal guinea pig. *B,* Normal chinchilla, showing method of restraint. (*B* reprinted with permission from Hoefer HL: Chinchillas. Vet Clin North Am Small Anim Pract 1994; 24:103–111.)

BIOLOGY AND HUSBANDRY OF GUINEA PIGS

Guinea pigs *(C. porcellus)*, also known as cavies, were domesticated in South America by 500–1000 AD and possibly as early as 1000 BC.[37] At the time of the Spanish invasion of South America, guinea pigs were raised by the Incas for food and for use in religious ceremonies.[37] Guinea pigs were brought to Europe about 400 years ago, and, although they never became popular as a food source outside of South America, they have been raised as pets and laboratory animals ever since then.

Several species of wild cavy have been described *(C. aperea, C. tschudii, C. cutleri, C. rufescens,* and *C. fulgida);* according to one source, these may all be different varieties of *C. aperea.*[34] Wild cavies are found today in Colombia, Venezuela, Brazil, Argentina, Paraguay, and Peru.[34, 37] They inhabit a wide variety of habitats, including grasslands, the forest edge, swamps, and rocky areas. Domestic guinea pigs are still raised by the Indians of the altiplano; they are often left uncaged to forage for food about the dwellings.[34, 37]

There are three common types of domestic guinea pigs seen as pets: short-haired English and American varieties, Abyssinian, and Peruvian. The hair of Abyssinian guinea pigs is relatively short and coarse and grows in whorls or rosettes. Peruvians have very long hair (up to 15 cm long); they are sometimes seen as pets but are primarily show animals. Coat colors of guinea pigs include white, red, tan, brown, chocolate, and black; coats can be monochromatic, bicolored, or tricolored. The Himalayan color variety has a white body with black or chocolate nose, ears, and feet. Brindle describes a coat of mixed black and white hairs, while roan describes a coat of mixed black and red hairs. Albino guinea pigs are common in a laboratory setting.

Guinea pigs are lively, responsive, and gentle pets, particularly if handled frequently at a young age. They have some peculiarities, however, of which all persons working with them should be aware. First, their response to perceived danger is freeze or flight (rather than fight or flight). They tend to become immobile if frightened or, alternatively, to make an explosive attempt to escape. Second, guinea pigs do not tolerate dietary or environmental changes. Their food preferences are established early in life, and they often refuse to eat if their food is changed in type or presentation. Moreover, they may become depressed or go off feed when hospitalized; therefore, hospitalization of this species should be minimized, and the attitude and food consumption of all hospitalized animals should be monitored carefully. Third, guinea pigs require a dietary source of vitamin C. Finally, guinea pigs are messy.

Under conditions of good husbandry, guinea pigs are hardy animals with few disease problems. Conversely, inadequacies in diet or husbandry can lead to illnesses that, if not managed early, can be difficult to reverse (Fig. 23–2). Sick guinea pigs do not tolerate clinical procedures very well and have been known to go into cardiac and respiratory arrest secondary to the stress of a diagnostic workup that would be routine in species like ferrets and cats. Handle very sick guinea pigs with "kid gloves." Similar to the approach in birds, concentrate on pro-

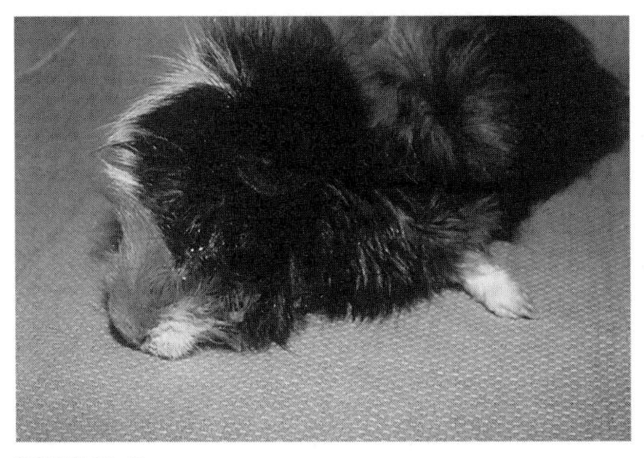

FIGURE 23–2
Very ill guinea pigs appear to lose the will to get better. In addition to specific medical therapy, intensive supportive care and force-feeding in a low-stress environment are necessary to help these animals.

viding good supportive care and maintaining caloric intake in a low-stress environment while slowly working toward a diagnosis and specific therapy for that diagnosis.

Anatomy and Physiology

Guinea pigs have stocky bodies, delicate short limbs, rounded hairless pinnae, and no tail. Males are larger than females, weighing 900–1200 g compared with 700–900 g for females. Obesity is relatively common in pets. The life span of pet guinea pigs is typically 5–6 years. Wild cavies feed at dawn and dusk; they live in small groups (5 to 10 individuals) in burrows or crevices.[34]

The haircoat of guinea pigs is composed of large guard hairs surrounded by an undercoat of fine hairs. Sebaceous glands are abundant along the dorsum and around the anus. The sebaceous glands around the anal area are important for marking, and guinea pigs are frequently seen rubbing or pressing the rump against a surface. Other sebaceous glands secrete directly into the well-developed anal sacs.[4] Both male and female guinea pigs have one pair of inguinal nipples (Fig. 23–3).

Guinea pigs have large tympanic bullae. They have 32 to 36 vertebrae; the vertebral formula is C7, T13(14), L6, S2(3), Cd4(6). There are 13 to 14 pairs of ribs, of which the last one or two are cartilaginous. The small cylindrical clavicle attaches laterally to the coracoid process of the scapula and medially to the manubrium. The pelvic symphysis generally remains fibrocartilaginous,[4] and a gap in the symphysis can be palpated at the time of impending parturition. Guinea pigs have four digits on the front feet and three digits on the rear feet; each digit has a short claw that may require periodic clipping in some individuals (Fig. 23–4).

The spleen is relatively broad in guinea pigs. The thymus in immature animals is located in the ventral cervical area and the cranial mediastinum; a thymic remnant may be present in adults in the cranial mediastinum.[4] Guinea pigs, like monkeys, ferrets, and humans, are considered to be corticosteroid-resistant species because steroid administration is not associated with marked changes in thymic physiology or peripheral lymphocyte counts.

Guinea pigs have no laryngeal ventricle, and their vocal folds are small; nonetheless, they show a wide range of vocalizations. The right lung is composed of four lobes (cranial, middle, caudal, and accessory), whereas the left lung is composed of three lobes (cranial, middle, and caudal). In the heart, as in other mammals, the right atrioventricular valve is tricuspid, while the left atrioventricular valve is bicuspid. There is usually one septomarginal trabeculum (moderator band) within the lumen of the right ventricle but rarely within that of the left ventricle.[4]

Gastrointestinal System

The dental formula of guinea pigs is: $2(I\frac{1}{1}\ C\frac{0}{0}\ PM\frac{1}{1}\ M\frac{3}{3}) = 20$. All teeth are open rooted and grow continuously throughout life. In animals with dental malocclusion, the maxillary cheek teeth tend to overgrow laterally into the buccal gingiva, while the mandibular cheek teeth tend to overgrow in a medial direction, entrapping the tongue. The incisors

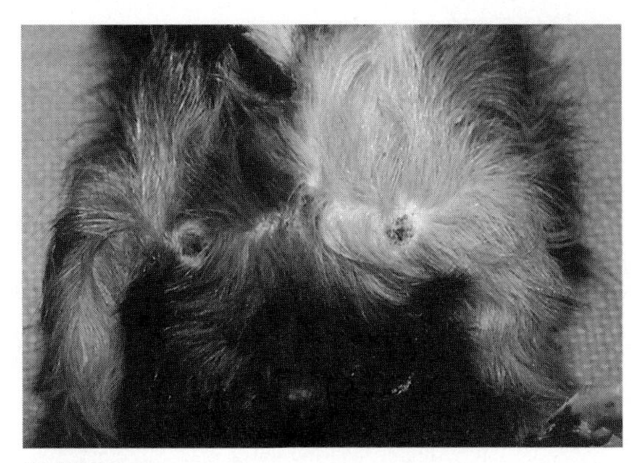

FIGURE 23–3
Guinea pigs have one pair of nipples in the inguinal area.

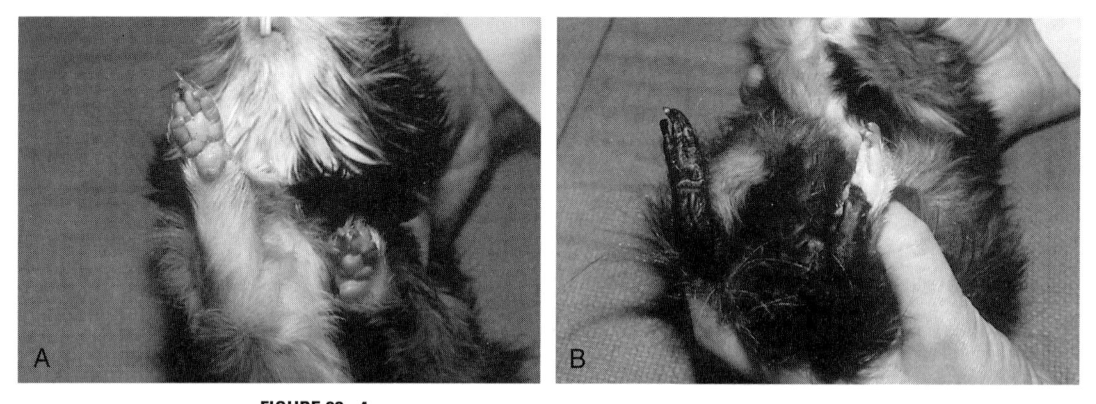

FIGURE 23–4
A, Normal forefeet of a guinea pig. *B*, Normal hindfeet of a guinea pig.

are normally white, unlike those of many other rodents (Fig. 23–5). Between the incisors and the cheek teeth (premolars and molars) is a gap called the diastema.

Guinea pigs have a large tongue and a relatively small, narrow oral cavity. The soft palate is continuous with the base of the tongue. The oropharynx communicates with the remainder of the pharynx through a hole in the soft palate called the palatal ostium.[32] Take care when attempting to pass any instrument, such as a feeding tube, that the instrument passes through the palatal ostium and does not slip to either side of the ostium where it can damage the vascular soft palate.

Guinea pigs have four pairs of salivary glands—parotid, mandibular, sublingual, and molar—the ducts of which empty into the oral cavity near the molars. The entire alimentary tract measures approximately 2.3 m from pharynx to anus.[20] The stomach is lined with glandular epithelium; there is no nonglandular portion as in rats, mice, and hamsters.[4] The small intestine is located on the right side of the abdominal cavity, while the cecum occupies the central and left portions. The cecum is a large, thin-walled sac with many lateral pouches formed by the action of three taeniae coli, which are thick, longitudinal muscular bands running the length of the large intestine. Smooth muscle cells harvested from the taeniae coli of guinea pigs were commonly used in physiologic studies because they can be obtained easily without damaging the gut. The cecum is 15–20 cm long and contains up to 65% of gastrointestinal (GI) contents.[21] The liver has six lobes—right, medial, left lateral, left medial, caudate, and quadrate—and the gall bladder is well developed.

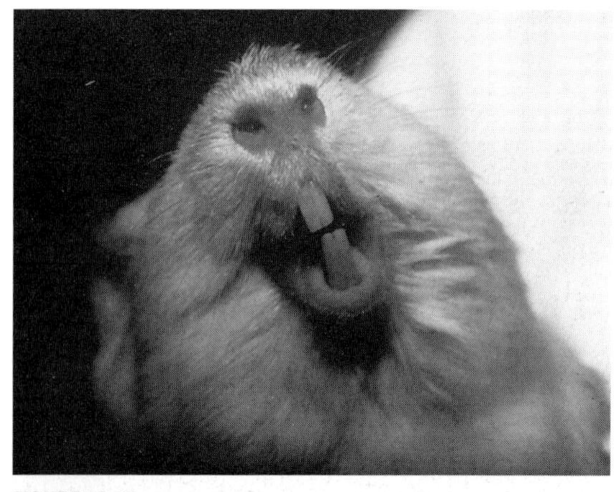

FIGURE 23–5
Normal incisors in a guinea pig. As in other rodents, the upper incisors are much shorter than the lower ones; different from many other rodents, the incisors are white.

The normal gastric emptying time in guinea pigs is 2 hours. Total GI transit time is approximately 20 hours (range 8–30 hours); however, if coprophagy is factored in, the total GI transit time is 66 hours.[20]

Guinea pigs perform coprophagy, or cecotrophy, about 150 to 200 times per day.[10] They eat the soft cecal feces directly from the anus.[29] Obese or pregnant animals may eat them from the floor, and young, unweaned guinea pigs can be seen eating the dam's droppings. Coprophagy appears to be an important function, although its contribution to the nutritional needs of guinea pigs has not been fully characterized. As in rabbits, coprophagy may be a source of B vitamins and a means of optimizing protein utilization.[7] If coprophagy is prevented, guinea pigs lose weight, digest less fiber, and excrete more minerals in the feces.[21]

Geriatric guinea pigs may develop fecal impactions within the anus, perhaps because of a loss of muscle tone or inability to eat feces directly from the anus. One author believes that these impactions are composed of the soft, cecal feces, and that the harder feces can still pass.[29] These impactions can be relieved by gentle manual expression; this procedure may have to be repeated weekly.

Similar to that in rabbits, the GI flora in guinea pigs is primarily gram-positive.[25] Anaerobic lactobacilli are the predominant bacterial species in the large intestine.[7]

Urogenital System

The accessory sex glands of male guinea pigs (boars) include the vesicular glands, prostate, coagulating glands, and bulbourethral glands. The vesicular glands are long, coiled, blind sacs that lie ventral to the ureters and extend 10 cm into the abdominal cavity.[4] Do not mistake these for uterine horns! The testes are located in the open inguinal canals. Guinea pigs have an os penis. A pouch containing two horny styles (slender projections) is located caudoventral to the urethral opening. During erection, the pouch is everted and the styles project externally.

Female guinea pigs (sows) have paired uterine horns, a short uterine body (12 mm long), and a single os cervicis opening into the vagina. Guinea pigs have a vaginal closure membrane that perforates at estrus, parturition, and, in many animals, at day 26 or 27 of gestation.[38]

The renal pelvis is relatively large and has a single longitudinal renal papilla. The alkaline urine is normally thick and cloudy white or yellow. Like that of other herbivores, it contains many crystals.

Sexing

Guinea pigs are easily sexed. Boars have obvious scrotal pouches and large testes (Fig. 23–6*A*). There is a flat area of tissue between the urethral opening and the anus, in which a longitudinal shallow slit may be present, marking the junction of the two scrotal pouches on the midline. The penis can be prolapsed out of the prepuce by placing gentle pressure at its base.

Sows have a Y-shaped depression in the perineal tissues (Fig. 23–6*B*). The top branches of the Y point cranially and surround the urethral opening. The vulvar opening lies at the intersection of the branches, and the anus is located at the base of the Y. In immature males, the penis can be prolapsed out of the prepuce; in immature females, the Y-shaped tissue depression is evident.

Reproduction

Reproductive values for guinea pigs are presented in Table 23–1. Many reported features of the reproductive cycle, such as length of estrus and the estrous cycle, timing of postpartum estrus, and litter size, vary according to the source, presumably because of variations between strains of guinea pigs. The numbers reported here are compiled from several different sources and are referenced accordingly.

Puberty, when defined as age at first conception, occurs at 2 months of age in females and at 3

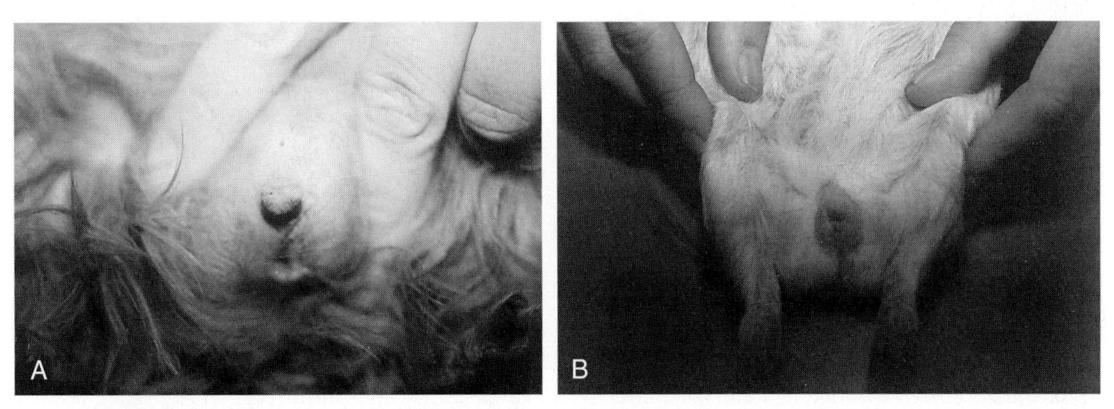

FIGURE 23–6
A, Normal external genitalia of a male guinea pig. *B*, Normal external genitalia of a female guinea pig. Traction on the abdominal skin opens the genitalia slightly to show the transverse slit marking the vaginal opening.

TABLE 23–1
PHYSIOLOGIC VALUES FOR GUINEA PIGS

Usual life span as pet	5–6 y
Adult weight	Males, 900–1200 g; females 700–900 g
Sexual maturity	Females, 2 mo; males, 3 mo
Type of estrous cycle	Nonseasonally polyestrous
Length of estrous cycle	15–17 d
Ovulation	Spontaneous
Gestation period	59–72 d (average, 68 d)
Litter size	1–13 (2–4 is usual)
Normal birth weight	70–100 g
Weaning age	21 d (or at 180 g body weight)
Rectal temperature	37.2–39.5°C (99.0–103.1°F)
Average blood volume	70 mL/kg
Heart rate	240–310 bpm

months in males.[38] Males begin mounting at 1 month of age, and ejaculation is evident at 2 months.[13] The peak reproductive time for females is from 3 or 4 months to 20 months of age; pets may reproduce until 4–5 years of age.[21]

Guinea pigs are polyestrous and breed year-round in a laboratory setting. The estrous cycle in most females is 15–17 days long (range 13–21 days), and ovulation is spontaneous.[21] There is a fertile postpartum estrus that occurs in most females from 2–10 hours after parturition.[31] Females show distinct signs of proestrus and estrus. During proestrus, females become more active and may chase their cage mates; they may sway the hindquarters and utter a distinct guttural sound. Estrus lasts from 6–11 hours, during which time females show lordosis, or the copulatory reflex, an arching and straightening of the back with elevation of the rump and dilation of the vulva. The vaginal membrane is open for approximately 2 days during estrus in mature sows; it closes after ovulation.

COPULATORY PLUGS. Copulation in guinea pigs (and chinchillas) can be confirmed by the finding of the vaginal or copulatory plug, a solid mass of coagulated ejaculate that falls out of the vagina several hours after mating. Rodent copulatory plugs are typically hard and rubbery or waxy in consistency and are the exclusive product of male secretions. So-called copulatory plugs are not restricted to rodents and have been reported in some bats, insectivores, primates, and marsupials.[9]

Voss[33] has advanced five possible functions of rodent copulatory plugs. The copulatory plugs may 1) store sperm; 2) prevent sperm leakage; 3) induce pseudopregnancy; 4) effect sperm transport; or 5) prevent fertilization of the female by subsequent males. Current hypotheses suggest that the primary function of the copulatory plug is chastity enforcement in polygamous breeding rodents. The other functions, especially sperm transport, are regarded as incidental but necessary effects. In guinea pigs, the copulatory plug prevents a second, competing ejaculate from reaching the site of fertilization. This is also the case with chinchillas.

PREGNANCY, PARTURITION, AND LACTATION. Similar to that in humans, the placenta in guinea pigs is hemochorial, meaning that the trophoblasts are in contact with maternal blood. The duration of gestation is 59–72 days (average 68 days) and depends on the strain of guinea pig, parity of the sow, and litter size. Gestation is typically shorter in primiparous sows and in those with small litters. The fetuses can be palpated as early as 15 days of gestation, although they are more evident at 28–35 days of gestation.

Impending parturition is signalled by separation of the pubic symphysis, with a gap of 15 mm palpable about 2 days before parturition that increases in width up to 25 mm or more at the time of parturition.[13] In sows that are bred for the first time after 7–8 months of age, this separation may be smaller, and dystocia commonly results. Other causes of dystocia include obesity and large fetal size. Suspect dystocia in gravid sows showing depression or a bloody or discolored vaginal discharge; an emergency cesarian section is indicated in most cases (see Chapter 25).

Normal parturition is rapid, occurring typically with a few minutes between births. Guinea pigs do not build nests. The average litter size varies according to guinea pig strain and management practices but is typically two to four,[31, 38] with a range of 1 to as many as 13 young reported.[38] Birth weights range from 45–115 g and are inversely related to litter size[21]; young weighing less than 60 g rarely survive.[13] Although otherwise completely herbivorous, guinea pigs are placentophagic. Males and other females may also consume the placenta.

Newborn guinea pigs (typically called pups or young, but not piglets) are precocious, meaning that they are fully furred with eyes open and able to stand shortly after birth (Fig. 23–7). They are not, however, able to fend for themselves at this time.[38] The pups ideally should receive sow's milk for a minimum of 5 days, and the normal lactation period

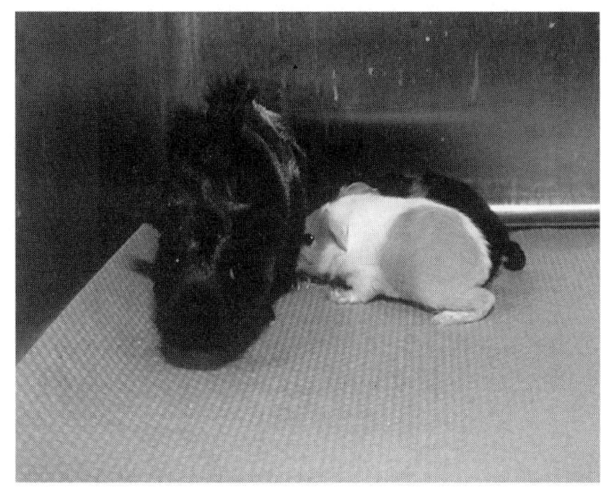

FIGURE 23–7
One-day-old guinea pig young nursing from the dam.

is 3 weeks.[38] Pups often do not survive if they fail to receive sow's milk for the first 3–4 days of life.[13] Guinea pig sows are not very "motherly." They passively allow nursing to occur rather than seek out the young. Lactating sows allow the young of other females to nurse. Licking of the pup's anogenital region by the sow is necessary to stimulate urination and defecation because voluntary micturition does not occur until the second week of life. The young are weaned at a weight of 180 g (15–28 days of age) or at an age of 21 days.[21]

Orphaned guinea pigs should be fostered to a lactating guinea pig if this is feasible. If there is no suitable foster mother, the young can be fed from a dropper or pet nurser beginning at 12–24 hours after birth. One author recommends feeding every 2 hours until 5 days of age, when feeding every 4 hours is sufficient.[29] The hand-rearing formula should approximate guinea pig milk, which contains 4% fat, 8% protein, and 3% lactose.[13] Evaporated milk mixed with equal parts water can be used. Guinea pigs begin nibbling on solid food at 2 days of age, and guinea pig pellets moistened with water or formula can be offered starting at this time.

Behavior

Guinea pigs are social animals that seek physical contact with other guinea pigs when housed together. They often stand side-by-side when resting and crowd together at feeders. However, there is little mutual grooming. Hair pulling can be a form of aggression, and hair pulling and ear nibbling of subordinate animals is seen in crowded or stressful environments.[14]

The vocalizations of guinea pigs have been well characterized. Recognized call types include the chutt, chutter, whine, tweet, whistle (single or in long bouts), purr, drr, scream, squeal, chirp, and grunt.[2, 14] Many guinea pig owners are familiar with the excited squeal emitted by their pet when the refrigerator door is opened or feeding is imminent.

Husbandry

Housing

Housing for guinea pigs should be set up with the knowledge that healthy guinea pigs produce prodigious amounts of feces, often defecate in food and water containers, turn over any unstable container, and are known to inject a premasticated slurry of pellets into the tubes of their sipper bottles. This said, guinea pigs require relatively simple housing.

In a laboratory setting in the United States, the minimum required floor space is 652 cm^2 (101 in^2) per adult animal; however, guinea pigs in a laboratory are often group-housed, and each animal has more than this space. Pets should be provided with at least twice as much floor space. Cages can be constructed of plastic, metal, or wire. Good ventilation is important. If a solid-sided cage, such as an open glass aquarium, is used, the bedding should be changed frequently to minimize ammonia levels in the cage. Guinea pigs do not jump or climb; therefore, the top of the cage does not need to be enclosed. The cage walls should be at least 25 cm (10 in) in height.

The flooring of the cage can be solid or wire mesh, although foot and leg injuries are more common in guinea pigs kept on wire. Guinea pig breeders use a wire mesh 12×38 mm in size to minimize potential for leg injuries.[13] Newspaper, shredded paper, wood shavings, and straw can be used for bedding on solid floors. A small upside-down cardboard box provides a shelter within the cage, although some guinea pigs prefer chewing the box to hiding in it.

The cage should be placed in a quiet area out of direct sunlight. Recommended temperature ranges for guinea pigs are 18–26°C (65–79°F).[13] Guinea pigs tolerate cool temperatures better than heat and should not be exposed to high temperatures and humidity because of their susceptibility to hyperthermia.

For breeding purposes, guinea pigs are usually housed in a harem-style arrangement with one boar and 1 to 10 sows in a single pen.[13] They can also be housed in pairs. In intensive breeding systems, the sow and young are left in the pen so the sow can be rebred at the postpartum estrus. However, removing the sow and young to a nursery area before or shortly after parturition minimizes trampling and ear chewing of the young by other adults.

Nutrition and Feeding

The nutritional needs of pet guinea pigs have not been as well addressed as those of pet rabbits. There is little published information on nutritional needs of adult, nonbreeding, nonlactating, and relatively inactive guinea pigs. Undoubtedly, the dietary recommendations for pet guinea pigs will evolve as our knowledge of these animals as pets increases.

Guinea pigs develop dietary preferences early in life and do not adapt readily to changes in type, appearance, or presentation of their food or water. Even a change in the brand of pelleted feed can result in refusal of food. It may be a good idea to expose new pets while they are still young to small amounts of different guinea pig chows and vegetables so they become accustomed to variety. Always teach clients about this characteristic of guinea pigs, as the knowledge may prevent a potentially dangerous self-imposed fast by a pet guinea pig.

Wild cavies eat many different types of vegetation. Domestic guinea pigs are also completely herbivorous (with the exception of placentophagy). They digest fiber more efficiently than rabbits do.[7] Interestingly, they do not increase their food intake, as do rabbits and many other species, when cellulose or other fiber is used to dilute the diet. This suggests that satiety in guinea pigs is governed more by the distention of the GI tract than by a metabolic energy need.[7] A crude protein level of 18–20% is adequate for growth and lactation, and the recommended minimum level of crude fiber is 10%.[7]

As mentioned previously, guinea pigs require a dietary source of vitamin C (ascorbic acid). This is because they lack L-gulonolactone oxidase, an enzyme involved in the synthesis of ascorbic acid from glucose. Adult nonbreeding guinea pigs require 5 mg/kg per day of ascorbic acid. Higher levels should be provided for growing and pregnant animals; 30 mg/kg per day is recommended during pregnancy.[13]

The recommended diet for pet guinea pigs consists of guinea pig pellets and alfalfa or grass hay supplemented with fresh vegetables. Usually the pellets are offered free choice, although, as for rabbits, some clinicians believe that limiting the quantity of this nutritionally rich food source is best for sedentary adult guinea pigs. A good-quality hay should be available at all times. Guinea pigs enjoy a variety of leafy greens, and these can be offered in handfuls. All fresh foods should be washed and prepared as though for human consumption and removed from the cage, if uneaten, after a few hours. Fruits, rolled oats, and dry cereals should be offered, if at all, only in very small quantities as treats. Any additions or changes to the diet should be made gradually.

Commercially available guinea pig pellets usually contain 18–20% crude protein and 10–16% fiber.[13] Pellets are milled with ascorbic acid; however, this vitamin is very labile and remains active for only 90 days under optimal storage conditions. It is best to assume that the pellets contain no vitamin C and to supply adequate levels of this important nutrient instead in the form of vegetables and fruit or in the drinking water. Foods that contain high levels of ascorbic acid include leafy greens, such as kale, parsley, beet greens, chicory, and spinach; red and green pepper; broccoli; tomatoes; kiwi fruit; and oranges. Vitamin C can be added to the water at 1 g/L.[13] Water should be changed daily to ensure adequate activity of the vitamin.

BIOLOGY AND HUSBANDRY OF CHINCHILLAS

Chinchillas, like guinea pigs, originated in South America. The name *chinchilla* ("little chincha") was coined by the Spaniards in the 16th century after the Chincha Indians, who used chinchilla pelts to decorate their ceremonial dress.[18] Chinchilla pelts were prized by Europeans also, and overhunting almost led to extinction of the species in the late 1800s and early 1900s. In the 1920s, 11 chinchillas were transported to California by Matthew Chapman. From these animals are descended most of the chinchillas in this country today.

Chinchillas are rare in the wild and may be extinct. According to Walker,[34] there is probably only one species of chinchilla *(C. laniger)*. A short-tailed species, *C. brevicaudata,* has been described and is recognized by other authors.[36] The native habitat of

C. laniger is (or was) the Andes mountains of Peru, Bolivia, Chile, and Argentina, where they inhabit the cool, semiarid, rocky slopes at elevations from 3000–5000 m (10,000–16,600 ft) above sea level.[34]

Anatomy, Physiology, and Behavior

Chinchillas have a compact body with delicate limbs, large eyes, large round pinnae, long whiskers, and a bushy tail. They usually weigh between 400 and 600 g, and females tend to be larger than males (Table 23–2). Their life span averages 10 years, which is much longer than that of other pet rodents; some animals are reported to have lived 20 years.[34]

Chinchillas are quiet, shy animals but are agile and enjoy climbing and jumping. They require a relatively large cage compared with their less active cousin, the guinea pig. In their natural habitat they are active at dusk and at night; however, in captivity, they can be active during the day. They readily habituate to humans when handled frequently at a young age. Flight is their defense mechanism; rarely, they bite. Chinchillas are virtually odorless, although one author reports that, when they are frightened, secretions from glands inside the anus give off an odor similar to that of scorched almonds.[24] Moreover, females reportedly may stand up on their hind legs and spray urine at a presumed attacker.

Their haircoat is luxurious, soft, and very dense owing to as many as 60 hairs growing from a single hair follicle.[34] The natural wild-type color is bluish-grey with yellow-white underparts. Breeding has produced color mutations including white, silver, beige, and black. Frequent dust baths are necessary to maintain the health of the fur (see Dust Baths under Husbandry). When frightened, chinchillas can shed patches of fur, a condition known as "fur-slip." The hairless patches take 6–8 weeks to fill in, and it may take several months for these patches to become indistinguishable from surrounding fur.

Chinchillas have four toes on front and rear feet, all with small, weak claws. There is no fur on the palmar and plantar regions of the feet. They have very large, thin-walled auditory bullae, readily visible on radiographs (see Fig. 31–14). The eyes are large and sit in a shallow bony orbit. The iris is densely pigmented with a vertical pupil, both features consistent with the chinchillas' habit of basking in the sun in their high-altitude habitat.[26]

The dental formula of chinchillas is the same as that of guinea pigs: $2\ (I\frac{1}{1}\ C\ \frac{0}{0}\ PM\frac{1}{1}\ M\frac{3}{3}) = 20$. Moreover, as in guinea pigs, all the teeth are open rooted and continuously growing throughout life. The incisors grow 5–7.5 cm (2–3 in) per year and are normally yellow in adult animals.[40] The oral cavity is small and narrow. Like guinea pigs, chinchillas have a palatal ostium, which is an opening in the soft palate through which the oropharynx communicates with the rest of the pharynx.[32]

Chinchillas have a long GI tract. The small and large intestine in one adult animal measured 3.5 m (11.5 ft).[40] The cecum is relatively large and coiled; the colon is highly sacculated. The cecum of chinchillas holds less of the large intestinal contents relative to that of rabbits and guinea pigs. According to one study, in chinchillas, the cecum holds 23% of dry matter content of the large intestine; in rabbits and guinea pigs, the cecum holds 57% and 44%, respectively.[17] In this study, the chinchillas ate food at night and defecated fecal pellets between 3 and 6 AM. They consumed cecotropes between 8 AM and 2 PM. Instead, guinea pigs intermittently and alternately excreted fecal pellets and cecotropes throughout the day.

Urogenital Tract, Sexing, and Reproduction

Females have two uterine horns and two cervices.[30, 36] The vaginal closure membrane is open only during parturition and for 2–4 days during estrus.[38] Chinchillas have three pairs of mammary glands: one inguinal pair and two lateral thoracic

TABLE 23–2
PHYSIOLOGIC VALUES FOR CHINCHILLAS

Usual life span as pet	10 y (up to 20 y reported)
Adult weight	Males, 400–500 g; females 400–600 g
Sexual maturity	8 mo
Type of estrous cycle	Seasonally polyestrous (November to May)
Length of estrous cycle	30–50 d
Ovulation	Spontaneous
Gestation period	105–118 d (average, 111 d)
Litter size	1–6 (2 is usual)
Normal birth weight	30–50 g
Weaning age	6–8 wk
Rectal temperature	37–38°C (98.6–100.4°F)
Heart rate	100–150 bpm

pairs.[38] Several reports in the veterinary literature have erroneously stated that chinchillas have two pairs of mammary glands.

Males do not have a true scrotum. Instead, the testes are contained within the inguinal canal or abdomen, and there are two small moveable sacs (the postanal sacs) next to the anus, into which the caudal epididymis can drop.[36] The inguinal canal is open. The penis is readily apparent below the anus, from which it is separated by an expanse of bare skin. The penis can be manually extruded 1–2 cm when flaccid.

As for other rodents, the anogenital distance is the best criterion for sexing chinchillas, particularly because the relatively large urinary papilla in female chinchillas can be confused with a penis (Fig. 23–8). The anogenital distance is longer in male chinchillas than in females: the penis is approximately 1–1.5 cm (0.4–0.6 in) cranioventral to the anus. This difference between the sexes is evident even at birth, when the urinary papilla is adjacent to the anus in females, and the penis is separated from the anus by a narrow band of tissue in males. Extrusion of the penis from the urethral orifice will confirm the sex of the chinchilla.

Females have a large urinary papilla, at the end of which is the urethral orifice. The structure we call the urinary papilla has been variously called the urethral cone and the clitoris. Immediately caudal to the urinary papilla is the slitlike vulva, which is oriented transversely relative to the craniocaudal axis of the body. The vaginal orifice is difficult to distinguish when closed and is "indicated" by a slightly raised semicircular area. When the vaginal orifice is covered by its closure membrane, the urethral orifice can be mistaken as the genital opening. As previously mentioned, the vulva is closed by a membrane except during estrus and parturition. The anus is located immediately caudal to the vulva.

Chinchillas are seasonally polyestrous in the wild and in captivity, usually bearing two litters of young from November to May, the breeding season in the northern hemisphere.[34] Age of puberty in males, again defined as age of successful conception, is 8 months or more; the average age of puberty in females is 8.5 months (range, 2–14 months).[36] If conception does not take place at the postpartum estrus, the next estrus occurs about 40 days later (see Table 23–2). Estrous cycles range from 30–50 days. An open vulva, often with visible mucus, is an external indication of estrus. There is no vulvar swelling during estrus; rather, there is a change in perineal color, which goes from a dull flesh color to a deep red. The color of the perineum increases dramatically at the time of vaginal perforation and remains intense throughout most of the luteal phase of the estrous cycle.[5]

Chinchillas can be housed in pairs or in polygamous units, with one male per two to six females. The polygamous units used by breeders are set up with separate cages for females, each with a rear door onto a common runway used by the male, which can go through any open door at will. The females wear a collar that prevents exit from their

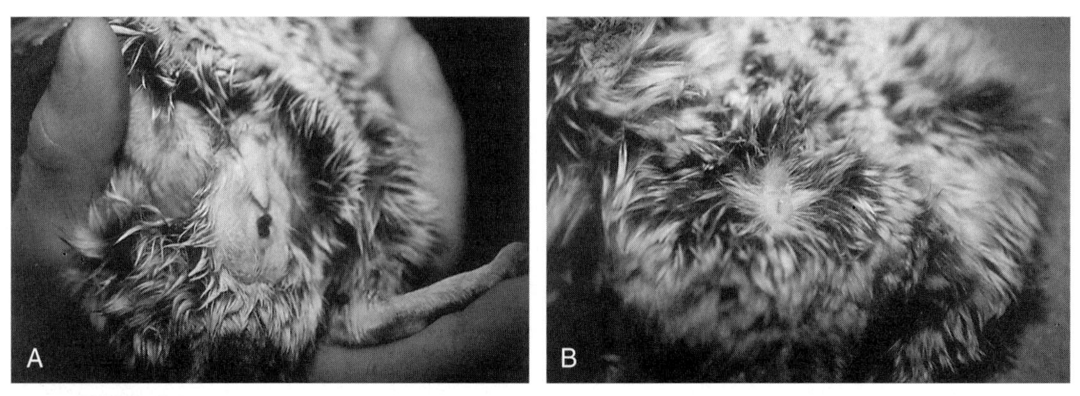

FIGURE 23–8

A, Normal external genitalia of a male chinchilla. *B,* Normal external genitalia of a female chinchilla. Note shorter anogenital distance and presence of the prominent urinary papilla (can be confused with a penis) in the female. (Photos courtesy of Dr. Heidi Hoefer.)

cages. In a polygamous setting, the male is kept out of the female's cage during parturition and raising of the young; however, in a pair setting, the male can often remain with the female during this time if she tolerates his presence.[22] Expulsion of a copulatory plug by the female is a sign that mating occurred the day before (see previous discussion of copulatory plugs in guinea pigs).

Gestation averages 111 days, and there are usually two young in each litter (range, one to six; see Table 23–2).[38] Parturition typically occurs in the early morning, and dystocias are uncommon in well-managed breeding establishments. Although chinchillas do not build nests,[40] the females will learn to use a nest box, which, when heated, prevents the first-born young from becoming hypothermic while the rest of the litter is being born.[24] Chinchillas, like guinea pigs, are placentophagic. Blood on the nose and front paws of the female indicates that she has eaten the placenta and the birthing process is over.[24]

Chinchilla young are precocious, weighing 30–50 g and fully furred with teeth and open eyes and ears at birth. They are able to walk within 1 hour after birth. The dam stands, rather than lying down, while they nurse.[24] If the mother dies after birth, a lactating female will usually accept the newborn young, especially if they are close in age to her own. According to one author, a lactating guinea pig may be an appropriate foster mother in some cases.[35]

Hand-feeding is necessary if no foster mother is available or as supplementary nutrition for litters of four or larger. A formula of equal parts evaporated milk and water can be administered with an eye dropper or pet nurser. One author recommends adding glucose (1 g/15 mL) to this formula.[36] For the first 3–4 days, the young should be hand-fed as often as possible during the day, with no more than 4 hours between feedings, and once or twice at night. After this time, the night feedings can be dropped and the intervals between daytime feedings gradually lengthened.[36]

The young of large litters may fight over access to the teats, and clipping the incisor teeth may be necessary to prevent serious injury to the teats or to siblings. Chinchillas begin to eat solid foods at 1 week of age. To minimize fighting, food bowls should be large enough to accommodate the entire litter simultaneously. Weaning is at 6–8 weeks of age.

Husbandry

Housing

Chinchillas are very active, acrobatic animals and require a lot of space. Ideally, according to one author, the enclosure should be at least 2 × 2 × 1 m (6.6 × 6.6 × 3.3 ft) with a wooden nestbox 30 × 25 × 20 cm (12 × 10 × 7 in).[35] Large, multilevel cages that provide sufficient space for climbing and jumping are excellent for housing pet chinchillas. Because chinchillas chew wooden cages, the cage should be constructed of welded wire mesh 15 × 15 mm, with or without an area of solid flooring. Drop pans below the cage facilitate cleaning.

Chinchillas are shy animals and need a place to hide when in captivity. In the wild, chinchillas will conceal themselves in rock crevices. Polyvinyl chloride (PVC) plumbing pipes, especially elbows and Y and T sections, make ideal hiding places and can be sanitized in a dishwasher. The pipes should be 10–13 cm (4–5 in) in diameter. Alternatively, clay pipes of a similar diameter can be used.

Chinchillas can be housed in pairs, colonies, or polygamous units, although colony housing is not advised for breeding chinchillas.[24] The cage set-up for polygamous units is described in the previous section.

Chinchillas do best in a dry environment at relatively cool temperatures. One recommended temperature range for housing chinchillas is 10–20°C (50–68°F).[35] Temperatures under 18°C (65°F) and relative humidity of less than 50% promote good fur growth.[35] Chinchillas do not tolerate dampness and are prone to heat stroke at environmental temperatures over 28–30°C (82–86°F).

Dust Baths

Access to a dust bath should be provided daily, if possible, or at least several times per week. Sanitized chinchilla dust is available commercially at pet stores. Two commercial dust baths, Blue Cloud (popular in California) and Blue Sparkle (from Kansas), can be obtained from Valentine Rabbit and Chinchilla Supplies (Chicago, IL, [312] 650–9050). Alternatively, a 9:1 mixture of silver sand and Fuller's earth can be used.[19] Fuller's earth is a variety of kaolin containing an aluminum magnesium silicate. The name is derived from the ancient process of cleaning, or "fulling," wool to remove the oil and dirt particles with a mixture of water and earth or clay. Beach or playground sand is not suitable for dust baths.

Some people are allergic to the commercially available powders. It is possible to make a homemade dust bath preparation consisting of perfume-free talc powder (also known as talcum or French chalk) and dietetic-grade cornstarch. Dietetic grades of cornstarch marketed as Maizena and Mondamin are best. Avoid using soluble starch, which is potato or corn starch treated with dilute hydrochloric acid. Some breeders reduce or eliminate the amount of corn starch with nursing mothers because the babies get it up their noses and develop rhinitis. More recently, volcanic ash from Mount St. Helens in Washington has become very fashionable. This is a very fine powder; put it in the box for 3–4 minutes.

The dust is placed at a depth of 2–3 cm (1 in) in a pan, such as a plastic dishpan, big enough for the chinchilla to roll around in it. A chinchilla may spend up to an hour dust bathing—rolling and fluffing its fur.[22] The dust bath is kept clean and free of feces by removing it from the cage after use.

Nutrition and Feeding

In their natural habitat, the relatively barren areas of the Andes Mountains, chinchillas reportedly feed on any available vegetation, eating in the early morning and late evening, holding the food with their forepaws and sitting on their haunches.[34] Work by Farmer[11] nearly 50 years ago showed the importance of grasses and hays in the diet, and it is recommended that chinchillas are given a high-fiber diet. Despite statements made nearly 40 years ago such as, "a great deal of work and clear thinking is required on the nutrition of the chinchilla,"[3] the specific nutrient requirements for chinchillas are still unknown. Commercial chinchilla diets are available (Mazuri Chinchilla Diet, St. Louis, MO) but in reality are mixtures of rabbit, guinea pig, and rodent pellets that provide a diet supplemented with Vitamin C, lower in protein and fat than standard rodent chow, and equivalent in fiber to a rabbit maintenance diet. However, the pellets are longer than rabbit or guinea pig pellets and therefore easier for the chinchilla to hold. The accepted formula for chinchilla pellets is 16–20% protein, 2–5% fat, and 15–35% bulk fiber.[12, 16, 35]

Although very little has been published about the nutritional needs of pet chinchillas, it is safe to assume that growing animals and breeding females require more calories and probably higher levels of calcium, protein, and fat than nonbreeding pet chinchillas. Nonbreeding animals do well on a diet of good-quality grass hay supplemented with small amounts of chinchilla or rabbit pellets, fresh vegetables, and grains.[19] One to two tablespoons of pellets daily should be sufficient for an adult, nonbreeding animal. A pellets-only diet has insufficient roughage and can predispose the chinchilla to enteritis. Chinchillas should take a long time to eat their food because they require bulky food that is high in fiber content.

Treats such as grains, dried apples, raisins, figs, hazelnuts, and sunflower seeds should be limited to not more than one teaspoon a day. As for guinea pigs, all food should be cleaned and prepared as if for human consumption. Any change in diet should be instituted gradually.

Clean fresh drinking water should be available at all times. Chinchillas can be trained to use automated watering devices in a laboratory setting or do equally well with cage-mounted water bottles. Water in a bowl tends to get dirty quickly and can spill.

Hard foods for gnawing can be offered. These may include porous stones such as pumice; young branches of trees such as elm, grapevines, maple, birch, and pieces of bark from apple, pear, and peach trees; and ash. Advise the owner to avoid branches from poisonous trees such as cedar, plum, redwood, cherry, and oleander.

CLINICAL TECHNIQUES FOR GUINEA PIGS AND CHINCHILLAS

Handling and Restraint

Guinea pigs are docile animals that usually need minimal restraint during a physical examination. Most animals will sit quietly on the examination table, with the owner or an assistant placing a hand on the rump so that the animal does not back away. To auscult the heart and lungs and palpate the abdomen, gently pick the animal up in one hand. Turn the animal over on its back while supporting it in your hand to examine the perineal area and genitalia.

Carry a guinea pig by supporting its weight in one hand and cupping its dorsum with the other hand. If the guinea pig is nervous or not used to handling, keep the animal in a carrier as much as possible and avoid excessive handling.

Chinchillas tend to be active at dusk and night; therefore, try to schedule evening appointments. Most pet chinchillas are easy to hold and generally do not bite; however, even a well-mannered pet will give warning nips if distressed, and if frightened, it will bite. A hand-tamed chinchilla will come out of its cage willingly; if it does not, when you or the owner intend to lift it out, you must be fast and on target, because if scared, the chinchilla can lose a patch of fur (known as fur slip) where it is grasped. If the chinchilla escapes from the cage and is loose in a room, it can ricochet off walls like a rubber ball—never try to catch a speeding chinchilla by the tail or you might be left holding the skin of the tail and no chinchilla.[30]

When lifting a chinchilla out of its cage, place one hand under the abdomen or around the scruff of the neck, and hold it by the base of the tail with the other hand (see Fig. 23–1*B*). If you intend to carry a chinchilla, hold the base of the tail with one hand to prevent it from jumping. As for rabbits, the head can be tucked under your arm.

If the chinchilla is prone to bite, two people should hold it. One person should restrain the chinchilla on a table with one hand under the thorax and one hand holding the base of the tail; the examiner additionally holds the animal by the scruff of the neck.

Physical Examination

The initial examination should involve observing the guinea pig or chinchilla in its cage. Focus on its movement, mentation, and rate and rhythm of breathing while in the cage. Healthy guinea pigs have an alert demeanor with clear eyes. The haircoat of short hair varieties should be sleek and shiny. The animal should react to stimuli by moving or vocalizing; some animals will move very quickly. Healthy animals usually eat readily when offered treats or greens.

Healthy chinchillas have a spirited curiosity and a curled tail that is carried high. Sick animals are indifferent and have a dull coat; often their perianal area is stained or covered with feces. An animal that flies around the cage in a frenzy when the owner attempts to capture it has not been socialized to people or other chinchillas and will be difficult to examine without sedation.

Begin the physical examination by measuring the animal's weight; this is also a good time to obtain the temperature before the animal is excited or stressed. Next examine the fur, skin, and mucous membranes. Follow this by auscultating the heart and lungs, and then palpate the abdomen. Check the rectal area for impaction of feces in guinea pigs. Observe the genitalia and note any abnormalities.

Overgrowth of the nails is common in pet guinea pigs. Often a horny growth is present extending from the footpads, especially in older animals. Trim the nails of guinea pigs and chinchillas with nail clippers used for humans or with cat claw clippers. The horny overgrowth can be trimmed back carefully, but avoid causing bleeding.

The oral examination should be done last because it can be stressful for the guinea pig or chinchilla, and the animal may become excited. Guinea pigs will object to examination of their teeth by squealing, and both guinea pigs and chinchillas may struggle or try to escape. For examination of the guinea pig, have an assistant place one hand on the animal's rump, while the other hand is used to gently hold the animal around the shoulder and thoracic area. Use an otoscope to examine the cheek teeth, similar to the method used in rabbits. Chinchillas can be held by the assistant with both hands encircling the thoracic area while restrained on the table, or held with the weight supported in one hand with the other hand restraining the forelimbs. Healthy chinchillas have yellow incisors because of iron deposition on the enamel.

Blood Collection

Venipuncture in guinea pigs and chinchillas can be difficult. The lateral saphenous and cephalic veins are the most accessible but are very small, and only small amounts of blood can be collected from each vein. Shave the fur from the area and wet the skin with alcohol to enhance visibility of the vein. Use an insulin or tuberculin syringe and a small (25- to 27-gauge) needle to prevent collapse of the vein. Venipuncture of multiple veins is often necessary for collection of an adequate volume of blood for analysis.

The jugular vein can be used for collection of large blood samples; however, the restraint required for blood collection can be very stressful for these animals. Guinea pigs especially have short, thick, compact necks, and it is often difficult to locate the jugular vein. For venipuncture, restrain the animal with the forelegs extended down over a table edge

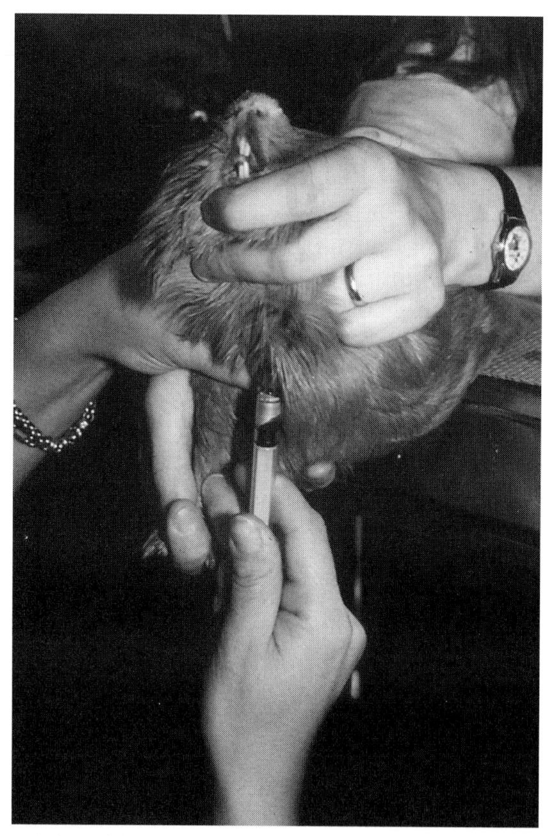

FIGURE 23–9
Jugular venipuncture in a guinea pig. This positioning and blood collection technique is too stressful for very sick guinea pigs.

and the head and neck extended up (Fig. 23–9). Shave the fur from the area if needed to enhance visibility of the vein, and use a small-gauge (22- to 25-gauge) needle and a 3-mL syringe for blood collection. If an animal shows obvious signs of stress or becomes dyspneic during jugular venipuncture, abort the procedure immediately. Observe the animal closely for several minutes after restraint is released to see that the animal recovers. If the animal still appears stressed or dyspneic after several minutes, abandon further venipuncture attempts. Jugular venipuncture can also be done after the animal has been anesthetized with isoflurane or chemically restrained with an injectable tranquilizer.

Venipuncture of the cranial vena cava can be used, but there is a risk of subsequent traumatic bleeding into the thoracic cavity or pericardial sac.[28] Cardiac puncture is not recommended as a blood collection technique unless performed as a terminal procedure during euthanasia, and then only with the animal deeply sedated or under anesthesia.

The blood volume in guinea pigs averages 7 mL/100 g body weight.[31] Approximately 7–10% of the blood volume (0.5–0.7 mL/100 g) can be safely collected from a healthy, nonanemic guinea pig. Similar guidelines can be used in chinchillas.

Cystocentesis

Cystocentesis is sometimes necessary in animals with clinical signs of urinary tract disease. The method used is similar to that used in other small animals, and a small-gauge (25-gauge) needle is used. Anesthesia may be necessary for restraint.

Clinical Laboratory Findings

Reported reference ranges of laboratory values for guinea pigs and chinchillas are depicted in Tables 23–3 and 23–4.[6, 13, 21–23] Published data are readily available for guinea pigs but pertain primarily to laboratory-housed animals, not pets. Published data for chinchillas are sparse. Clinical laboratory values vary according to physiologic state of the animal and laboratory techniques used. Ideally, as for other species, each laboratory should establish normal ranges.

In guinea pigs, the activity of alanine aminotransferase is low in hepatocytes; therefore, it is not sensitive or specific as a marker of hepatocellular injury.[39] Hypercholesterolemia is common in guinea pigs, often in conjunction with fatty infiltration of many tissues, including the liver. When guinea pig serum is stored in plastic, potassium levels are lower than if glass containers are used.[39]

A unique leukocyte of the guinea pig is the Kurloff cell. This mononuclear cell resembles a lymphocyte but contains round or ovoid inclusions termed Kurloff bodies.[31] The origin of Kurloff cells (thymus or spleen) is controversial. The numbers of circulating cells are variable: Kurloff cells are rare in very young animals, numbers are low in males, while numbers in the female are related to the estrous cycle. Kurloff cells are highest in the female during pregnancy and may play a role in a physiologic barrier between the fetus and the mother.[31]

The cellular distribution of bone marrow in the guinea pig is 26.7% erythroblasts, 63.3% myeloid cells, 4.6% lymphocytes, and 5.4% reticulum cells.[1] The myeloid/erythroid (M/E) ratio is 1.5:1[15] to 1.9:1.[8]

TABLE 23-3

REFERENCE RANGES FOR HEMATOLOGY AND SERUM CHEMISTRY VALUES IN GUINEA PIGS

Hematocrit (%)	32–50
Hemoglobin (g/dL)	10–17.2
Red blood cells ($\times 10^6/\mu L$)	3.2–8.0
Sedimentation rate (mm/h)	1.1–14.0
White blood cells ($\times 10^3/\mu L$)	5.5–17.5
Neutrophils (%)	22–48
Lymphocytes (%)	39–72
Monocytes (%)	1–10
Eosinophils (%)	0–7
Basophils (%)	0.0–2.7
Platelets ($\times 10^3/\mu L$)	260–740
Mean corpuscular volume (μm^3)	71–96
Mean corpuscular hemoglobin (pg)	23–27
Mean corpuscular hemoglobin concentration (%)	26–39
Total protein (g/dL)	4.2–6.8
Albumin (g/dL)	2.1–3.9
Globulin (g/dL)	1.7–2.6
Glucose (mg/dL)	60–125
Blood urea nitrogen (mg/dL)	9.0–31.5
Creatinine (mg/dL)	0.6–2.2
Sodium (mmol/L)	120–152
Potassium (mmol/L)	3.8–7.9
Chloride (mmol/L)	90–115
Calcium (mg/dL)	8.2–12.0
Phosphorus (mg/dL)	3.0–7.6
Alanine aminotransferase (U/L)	25–59
Aspartate aminotransferase (U/L)	26–68
Alkaline phosphatase (U/L)	55–108
Bilirubin (mg/dL)	0.0–0.9
Cholesterol (mg/dL)	16–43

Data from Harkness JE, Wagner JE: The Biology and Medicine of Rabbits and Rodents, 4th ed. Baltimore, Williams & Wilkins, 1995; Manning PJ, Wagner JE, Harkness JE: Biology and diseases of guinea pigs. *In* Fox JG, Cohen BJ, Loew FM, eds.: Laboratory Animal Medicine. Orlando, FL, Academic Press, 1984, pp 149–177; Mitruka BM, Rawnsley HM: Clinical Biochemical and Hematological Reference Values in Normal Experimental Animals and Normal Humans, 2nd ed. Chicago, Year Book Medical Publishers, 1981, pp 70–73, 166–177.

The normal pH of guinea pig urine is 9.0.[25] The normal pH of chinchilla urine is 8.5; specific gravity often exceeds 1.045.[22]

Treatment Techniques

Intravenous Catheters

Peripheral IV catheters can be used in these animals but are difficult to place because of the small size and fragility of the veins. Use a small (24-gauge or smaller) indwelling catheter, and place the catheter with the animal under anesthesia. Jugular cutdowns can be done for catheterization of a jugular vein if an indwelling catheter is necessary and placement of a peripheral catheter is unsuccessful. Venous access ports are used in many laboratory animals and are an alternative if long-term IV therapy is anticipated.

Fluid Therapy

Supplemental fluids are usually given by SC administration into the loose skin of the dorsal neck and upper back areas (Fig. 23–10). Normal daily water intake in the guinea pig is estimated at 100 mL/kg per day[21]; base supplemental fluid requirements on

TABLE 23-4

REPORTED AVERAGES AND REFERENCE RANGES FOR HEMATOLOGY AND SERUM CHEMISTRY VALUES IN CHINCHILLAS

Hematocrit (%)	38*
Hemoglobin (g/dL)	11.7–13.5†
Red blood cells ($\times 10^6/\mu L$)	6.6–10.7†
White blood cells ($\times 10^3/\mu L$)	7.6–11.5†
Neutrophils (%)	23–45†
Lymphocytes (%)	51–73†
Monocytes (%)	1–4†
Eosinophils (%)	0.5–2.6†
Basophils (%)	0–1†
Platelets ($\times 10^3/\mu L$)	254–298†
Total protein (g/dL)	5–6
Albumin (g/dL)	2.5–4.2
Glucose (mg/dL)	60–120
Blood urea nitrogen (mg/dL)	10–25
Sodium (mmol/L)	130–155
Potassium (mmol/L)	5.0–6.5
Chloride (mmol/L)	105–115
Calcium (mg/dL)	10–15
Phosphorus (mg/dL)	4–8
Alanine aminotransferase (U/L)	10–35
Aspartate aminotransferase (U/L)	15–45
Alkaline phosphatase (U/L)	3–12
Cholesterol (mg/dL)	40–100

*Data from Williams CSF: Chinchilla. *In* Practical Guide to Laboratory Animals. St. Louis, MO, CV Mosby, 1976, pp 3–11.

†Hematology ranges represent ranges of average figures compiled from several studies by Douglas W. Stone, DVM, and presented in Merry CJ: An introduction to chinchillas. Vet Tech 1990; 11:315–322. Serum chemistry data from The Care of Experimental Animals: a Guide for Canada. Ottawa, Ontario, Canadian Council on Animal Care, 1969, p 438.

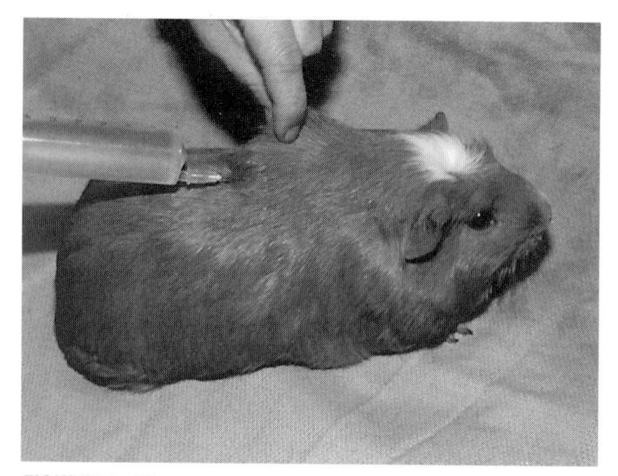

FIGURE 23–10
Subcutaneous fluid administration in a guinea pig.

this estimation plus additional fluids to compensate for dehydration. The total volume can be divided into two to three daily treatments. Volumes of 25–35 mL can be given into each injection site with a 22- to 25-gauge butterfly catheter. Many guinea pigs react painfully when fluids are administered SC and become very stressed. To avoid unnecessary stress, animals that are drinking water readily can be given oral fluids unless they are azotemic or moderately to severely dehydrated.

Use a Buretrol device (Baxter Healthcare, Deerfield, IL) or an injection pump with either continuous or intermittent infusion for IV fluid administration. Monitor fluid volumes closely to avoid overhydration.

Medications

Give parenteral medications by SC or IM injection. The upper back is a common site for SC injection. The skin in this area is thick in guinea pigs and is sometimes difficult to penetrate with a 25-gauge or smaller needle. Give IM injections in the gluteal or biceps muscles. Medications and nutritional supplements are given orally by syringe into the side of the mouth. Administration of tablets to chinchillas is possible if the tablets are hidden in raisins; chinchillas will usually eat them because they are inquisitive.

Force-feed partially anorectic and anorectic guinea pigs and chinchillas a high-energy food supplement such as Nutri-Cal (Evsco Pharmaceuticals, Buena, NJ), softened guinea pig pellets, strained baby food vegetables, or a soy-based liquid enteral formula. Give hospitalized guinea pigs parenteral vitamin C daily.

Guinea pigs do not adapt well to changes in their environment or routine and should only be hospitalized if necessary. Hospitalized guinea pigs should be given supportive care in anticipation of decreased appetite and water consumption.

REFERENCES

1. Baranski S: Effect of chronic microwave irradiation on the blood forming system of guinea pigs and rabbits. Aerosp Med 1971; 42:1196–1199.
2. Berryman JC: Guinea-pig vocalizations: their structure, causation and function. Z Tierpsychol 1976; 41:80–106.
3. Bowden RST: Diseases of chinchillas. Vet Rec 1959; 71:1033–1039.
4. Breazile JE, Brown EM: Anatomy. *In* Wagner JE, Manning PJ, eds.: The Biology of the Guinea Pig. New York, Academic Press, Inc, 1976, pp 53–62.
5. Brookhyser KM, Aulerich RJ: Consumption of food, body weight, perineal color and levels of progesterone in the serum of cyclic female chinchillas. J Endocrinol 1980; 87:213–219.
6. The Care of Experimental Animals: a Guide for Canada. Ottawa, Ontario, Canadian Council on Animal Care, 1969, p 438.
7. Cheeke PR: Nutrition of guinea pigs. *In* Rabbit Feeding and Nutrition. Orlando, FL, Academic Press, Inc, 1987, pp 344–353.
8. Dineen JK, Adams DB: The effect of long-term lymphatic drainage on the lympho-myeloid system in the guinea pig. Immunology 1970; 19:11–30.
9. Donnelly TM: Behaviour and reproduction. *In* Rabbits and rodents: laboratory animal science. Proceedings 142 of the Post-Graduate Committee in Veterinary Science, Sydney, September 1990, pp 381–388.
10. Ebino KY: Studies on coprophagy in experimental animals. Exp Anim 1993; 42:1–9.
11. Farmer FA: A study of the dietary requirements of chinchillas. Nat Chinchilla Breeder Can 1951; 5:11–18.
12. Harkness JE: A Practitioners Guide to Domestic Rodents. Denver, CO, American Animal Hospital Association (AAHA), 1993.
13. Harkness JE, Wagner JE: The Biology and Medicine of Rabbits and Rodents, 4th ed. Baltimore, Williams & Wilkins, 1995.
14. Harper LV: Behavior. *In* Wagner JE, Manning PJ, eds.: The Biology of the Guinea Pig. New York, Academic Press, Inc, 1976, pp 31–48.
15. Harris RS, Herdan G, Ancill RJ, Yoffey JM: A quantitative comparison of the nucleated cells in the right and left humeral bone marrow of the guinea pig. Blood 1954; 9:374–378.
16. Hoefer HL: Chinchillas. Vet Clin North Am Small Anim Pract 1994; 24:103–111.
17. Holtenius K, Bjornhag G: The colonic separation mechanism in the guinea-pig *(Cavia porcellus)* and the chinchilla *(Chinchilla laniger)*. Comp Biochem Physiol 1985; 82A: 537–542.
18. Houston JW, Presturich JP: Chinchilla Care, 4th ed. Los Angeles, Borden Publishing Co, 1962.
19. Jenkins J: Husbandry and common diseases of the chinchilla *(Chinchilla laniger)*. J Small Exotic Anim Med 1992; 2:15–17.
20. Jilge B: The gastrointestinal transit time in the guinea-pig. Z Versuchstierk 1980; 22:204–210.
21. Manning PJ, Wagner JE, Harkness JE: Biology and diseases of guinea pigs. *In* Fox JG, Cohen BJ, Loew FM, eds.: Labo-

ratory Animal Medicine. Orlando, FL, Academic Press, Inc, 1984, pp 149–177.
22. Merry CJ: An introduction to chinchillas. Vet Tech 1990; 11:315–322.
23. Mitruka BM, Rawnsley HM: Clinical Biochemical and Hematological Reference Values in Normal Experimental Animals and Normal Humans, 2nd ed. Chicago, Year Book Medical Publishers, Inc, 1981, pp 70–73, 166–177.
24. Mösslacher E: Breeding and Caring for Chinchillas. Neptune City, NJ, T.F.H. Publications, Inc, 1986.
25. Navia JM, Hunt CE: Nutrition, nutritional diseases, and nutrition research applications. *In* Wagner JE, Manning PJ, eds.: The Biology of the Guinea Pig. New York, Academic Press, Inc, 1976, pp 235–261.
26. Peiffer RL, Johnson PT: Clinical ocular findings in a colony of chinchillas *(Chinchilla laniger)*. Lab Anim 1980; 14:331–335.
27. Popesko P, Rajtová V, Horák J: A Colour Atlas of Anatomy in Small Laboratory Animals. Vol. 1: Rabbit, Guinea pig. London, Wolfe Publishing Ltd, 1992, pp 148–240.
28. Reuter RE: Venipuncture in the guinea pig. Lab Anim Sci 1987; 37:245–246.
29. Richardson VCG: Diseases of Domestic Guinea Pigs. London, Blackwell Scientific Publications, 1992.
30. Ritchey L: The Joy of Chinchillas. Menlo Park, CA (published privately), 1995.
31. Sisk DB: Physiology. *In* Wagner JE, Manning PJ, eds.: The Biology of the Guinea Pig. New York, Academic Press, 1976, pp 63–92.
32. Timm KI, Jahn SE, Sedgwick CJ: The palatal ostium of the guinea pig. Lab Anim Sci 1987; 37:801–802.
33. Voss R: Male accessory glands and the evolution of copulatory plugs in rodents. Occasional Papers of the Museum of Zoology, University of Michigan. Number 689. June 7, 1979.
34. Walker EP: Mammals of the World, 3rd ed. Vol II. Baltimore, Johns Hopkins University Press, 1975.
35. Webb R: Chinchillas. *In* Beynon PH, Cooper JE, eds.: Manual of Exotic Pets. Ames, IA, Iowa State University Press, 1991, pp 15–22.
36. Weir BJ: Chinchilla. *In* Hafez ESE, ed.: Reproduction & Breeding Techniques for Laboratory Animals. Philadelphia, Lea & Febiger, 1970, pp 209–223.
37. Weir BJ: Notes on the origin of the domestic guinea-pig. Symp Zool Soc Lond 1974; 34:437–446.
38. Weir BJ: Reproductive characteristics of hystricomorph rodents. Symp Zool Soc Lond 1974; 34:265–301.
39. White EJ, Lang CM: The guinea pig. *In* Loeb WF, Quimby FW, eds.: The Clinical Chemistry of Laboratory Animals. New York, Pergamon Press, 1989, pp 27–30.
40. Williams CSF: Chinchilla. *In* Practical Guide to Laboratory Animals. St. Louis, MO, CV Mosby, 1976, pp 3–11.

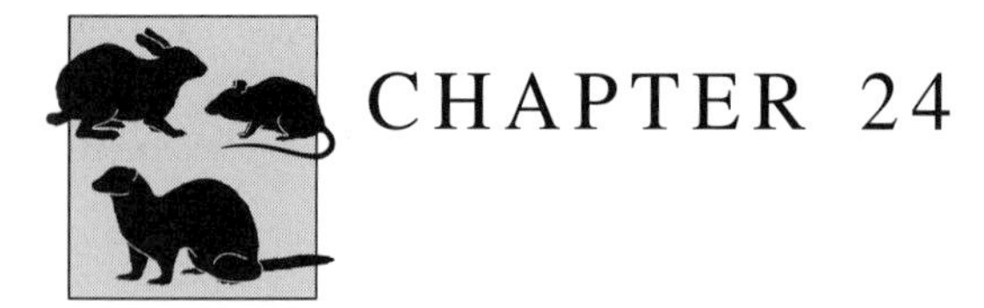

CHAPTER 24

Disease Problems of Guinea Pigs and Chinchillas

Dorcas O. Schaeffer, DVM, and Thomas M. Donnelly, BVSc

Guinea pigs and chinchillas are both New World, montane, hystricomorph rodents. Consequently, they are susceptible to similar diseases. Many disease problems of laboratory guinea pigs have been exhaustively studied; however, disease problems of chinchillas are not as well described. Furthermore, diseases that occur in pet animals and the treatment methods used may differ from those of laboratory animals. Specific treatment information about chinchillas is often not readily available; however, it usually is safe to refer to drug dosages and treatment methods used in guinea pigs.

PART A

Dorcas O. Schaeffer, DVM

GASTROINTESTINAL DISEASES OF GUINEA PIGS

Antibiotic-Associated Enterotoxemia

Guinea pigs possess a predominantly gram-positive gastrointestinal flora and are exquisitely sensitive to antibiotics that eradicate that flora. Drugs such as penicillin, ampicillin, chlortetracycline, clindamycin, erythromycin, and lincomycin will destroy susceptible gram-positive organisms, permitting overgrowth of *Clostridium difficile* and elaboration of its toxin.[11, 48, 65] Toxin production results in a hemorrhagic typhlitis. Clinically, the guinea pig has diarrhea and is anorectic, dehydrated, and hypothermic.[48] Diagnosis is usually based on history, clinical signs, and lesions, since *C. difficile* is difficult to isolate.[5]

Treat antibiotic-associated enterotoxemia symptomatically and with supportive therapy. Place the animal on a recirculating water blanket in an incubator or its cage to correct hypothermia. Administer lactated Ringer's solution or other crystalline fluids IV, IP, or SC to restore hydration. Add daily maintenance fluids at a rate of 100 mL/kg per day to the dehydration deficit until the animal is drinking normally. Administration of a commercial product containing *Lactobacillus* species may help re-establish normal intestinal microflora, but this has not been proved. Transfaunation with a rodent fecal slurry has been done, but use of microflora from healthy guinea pigs rather than mice or rats has proved more successful.[6] Chloramphenicol (50 mg/kg q8h PO) may be effective in suppressing further clostridial overgrowth.[11] In rabbits with clostridial enterotoxemia, daily administration of cholestyramine (an ion exchange resin) in water at a concentration of 2 g per 20 mL resulted in toxin absorption and reduced mortality.[46] This treatment could possibly be of benefit to guinea pigs.

Prevent this disease by treating guinea pigs with appropriate antibiotics. I have used trimethoprim-sulfa (30 mg/kg q12h PO, SC, or IM for 7 days) and chloramphenicol (50 mg/kg q12h PO, SC, or IM for 7 days) effectively. Enrofloxacin (10 mg/kg q12h PO) can also be used successfully without causing enterotoxemia. Sodium ampicillin at a dosage of 6 mg/kg q8h SC for 5 days is well tolerated; however, at 8 mg/kg, it is toxic.[93] Cefazolin (50 mg/kg IM) is well tolerated. However, to be effective against *Bordetella* species (a common guinea pig pathogen) at this dose, it would need to be administered every half hour. Higher doses cause irritation at the injection site and mortality.[23] One author has stated that when antibiotics are used to treat guinea pigs, the animal should also receive a *Lactobacillus* supplement during treatment and for 5 days beyond termination of antibiotic administration.[11] However, this has not been proved conclusively. Administration of a commercial product containing *Lactobacillus* species can be given; alternatively, a live-culture yogurt can be given at a daily dose of approximately 5 mL. If diarrhea develops, stop administration of any antibiotic that is being given, and re-evaluate the animal and the treatment protocol.

Bacterial Enteritis

Salmonella typhimurium and *Salmonella enteritidis* are the most common causes of bacterial enteritis in laboratory guinea pigs. Transmission is usually by fecal contamination of feed. Animals that are stressed, particularly weanlings, pregnant sows, aged animals, and those with nutritional deficiencies, are particularly susceptible.[31] Signs include scruffy haircoat, weight loss, weakness, conjunctivitis, and abortion. Diarrhea may or may not be present. At necropsy, the spleen and liver are enlarged, and yellow necrotic foci may be present in the viscera.[11] In one report, all affected sows that died of salmonellosis had lymphocytic infiltrates in their uteri.[60] Diagnosis of salmonellosis is by bacterial culture of a fecal sample and isolation of the organism. Treatment includes appropriate antibiotic and fluid therapy, but the affected animal could become a subclinical carrier. Prevent salmonellosis by keeping the environment clean, storing food in airtight containers, and thoroughly washing all fresh fruits and vegetables that are offered to guinea pigs. Salmonellosis is a zoonotic disease.

Other causes of bacterial diarrhea in guinea pigs include *Yersinia pseudotuberculosis, Clostridium perfringens, Escherichia coli, Pseudomonas aeruginosa,* and *Listeria monocytogenes.* Like salmonellae these are contracted through fecal contamination of food.[3] Base antibiotic treatment on results of culture and sensitivity testing of a fecal sample, and treat affected animals with supportive therapy.

Tyzzer's disease has been reported in guinea pigs and is caused by *Clostridium piliforme* (formerly *Bacillus piliformis*), an intracellular bacterium. The organism is transmitted by fecal contamination of feed, and young, stressed animals are particularly affected.[82] Clinical signs include diarrhea, an unthrifty appearance, and acute death.[48] In one case, dependent subcutaneous edema and excess serous fluid was reported.[83] At necropsy, lesions included intestinal inflammation and focal hepatic necrosis.[82] Because *C. piliforme* is an intracellular bacterium, it will not grow on routine culture media. Definitive diagnosis is made at necropsy by identifying the organisms on hematoxylin-eosin or silver-stained sections of intestine or liver. Treatment has been unrewarding. Place emphasis on preventing this disease by good husbandry practices and reducing stress, particularly at weaning.

Parasitic Diarrhea

Protozoal diarrhea in guinea pigs is caused by *Cryptosporidium wrairi*, which infects the small intestine.[10] Transmission is by the fecal-oral route; weanlings and immunosuppressed animals are most susceptible.[31] Clinical signs include failure to gain weight, weight loss, diarrhea, and death.[24] Immunocompetent guinea pigs recover within 4 weeks and are resistant to reinfection.[79] The organisms can be seen by examination of a fecal sample or identified by histopathologic examination of the brush border of mucosal epithelial cells.[31] No treatment has proved effective. The oocysts can be destroyed in the environment with a 5% ammonia solution, freezing to below 0°C, or heating to above 65°C.[31] Cryptosporidiosis is a potentially zoonotic disease.

Guinea pigs are hosts to *Eimeria caviae, Balantidium caviae* (protozoa), and *Paraspidodera uncinata* (a roundworm). In rare cases, *E. caviae* will cause diarrhea, and *P. uncinata* can cause bronchoalveolar eosinophilia[12]; otherwise, these organisms cause no clinical disease.

Viral Diarrhea

There is one report of a wasting syndrome in weanling guinea pigs involving diarrhea, anorexia, rapid weight loss, and acute death. Coronavirus-like particles were identified in the feces by transmission electron microscopy; no other organisms were identified.[36]

Malocclusion

Guinea pigs have hypsodontic (open-rooted) incisors, premolars, and molars that grow continuously; therefore, overgrowth of any of these teeth is possible. While there is a strong genetic predisposition to malocclusion, diet, trauma, or infection may also play a role.[31] Maxillary premolars and molars overgrow laterally, abrading the cheeks, and mandibular teeth overgrow medially, abrading the tongue and occluding the oropharynx.[11] Overgrown incisors can be identified on physical examination. Malocclusion of the cheek teeth usually goes unnoticed until the animal appears anorectic, prehends but cannot swallow food, and loses weight. Excess salivation ("slobbers"), wetting of chin and forepaws, and secondary moist dermatitis are also signs of malocclusion.[31, 33]

Diagnose malocclusion by careful examination of

the mouth and teeth. The oral cavity of the guinea pig is narrow with large buccal folds, and examination of the cheek teeth is difficult. Use a vaginal speculum or an otoscope to enhance visibility of the cheek teeth and oral mucosa.[33] Examination is greatly facilitated by first anesthetizing the animal with isoflurane or sedating with a short-acting tranquilizer. Loop gauze strips over the incisors to open the mouth. Trim the teeth with a Dremmel tool or pediatric Lempert rongeurs.[11] Trimming will need to be repeated routinely (every 4–16 weeks) for the remainder of the animal's life. Vitamin C (15–25 mg per guinea pig per day) can be added to the diet of guinea pigs to prevent decreased collagen formation and subsequent tooth movement in the socket.[11] Prevent malocclusion by not breeding affected animals and by feeding a proper diet.

RESPIRATORY DISEASES OF GUINEA PIGS

Bacterial Pneumonia

Guinea pigs are very susceptible to respiratory disease cause by *Bordetella bronchiseptica* and *Streptococcus pneumoniae*. *B. bronchiseptica*, a gram-negative rod, is commonly carried by rabbits, dogs, and nonhuman primates. *S. pneumoniae*, a gram-positive coccus, is also carried inapparently by many species. Stress increases susceptibility to disease, especially in young guinea pigs. The organisms are transmitted by direct contact, aerosolization, and fomites.[31] Clinical signs include inappetence, nasal and ocular discharge, and dyspnea.[48] *B. bronchiseptica* causes a purulent bronchopneumonia with consolidation of lung lobes and exudate in the tympanic bullae. Metritis and abortions have also been described. *S. pneumoniae* causes a fibrinopurulent pleuritis and pericarditis in addition to bronchopneumonia.[31] Torticollis and abortions are seen with *S. pneumoniae*. The combination of *S. pneumoniae* infection and vitamin C deficiency has resulted in septic arthritis.[90]

Diagnosis of bacterial pneumonia is based on clinical signs and results of laboratory testing. Many guinea pigs with pneumonia are very dyspneic and depressed and do not tolerate stress or handling well. Obtaining a blood sample for hematologic testing or doing procedures that require handling may not be possible because of the stress associated with restraint. Therefore, treatment often is based on clinical signs until the guinea pig can tolerate stressful procedures. If possible, submit a blood sample for a complete blood count to determine if the white blood count is elevated or if neutrophilia is present. Submit a sample of any nasal exudate for bacterial culture and sensitivity testing. Radiographs are useful to identify pulmonary changes consistent with pneumonia or pleuritis. Skull radiographs may show bony changes or soft tissue opacity in the tympanic bullae, indicating otitis media.

Antibiotics commonly used to treat bacterial pneumonia in guinea pigs are chloramphenicol (30–50 mg/kg q12h PO), trimethoprim/sulfa (30–50 mg/kg q12h PO), and enrofloxacin (5–10 mg/kg q12h PO or IM). Supportive care includes supplemental fluid therapy, oxygen administration, vitamin C supplementation, and force-feeding as needed.

Vaccination can protect against pneumonia caused by *B. bronchiseptica*. A *Bordetella* bacterin (Bronchicine®, BioCor, Worthington, MN) is given at 0.2 mL IM and repeated in 21 days and 6 months.[77] Good husbandry, minimal stress, and separating guinea pigs from dogs and rabbits will also help prevent pneumonia.

Streptobacillus moniliformis, usually implicated in cervical lymphadenitis, has caused granulomatous pneumonia in guinea pigs.[42]

Viral Pneumonia

A necrotizing bronchopneumonia has been recently described in caged guinea pigs. Animals usually die acutely. An adenovirus may be responsible for this disease.[19]

Pulmonary Neoplasia

Pulmonary adenoma of bronchogenic origin is described as the most common nonhematopoietic tumor of guinea pigs.[31, 48] However, pathologic changes are similar to those of adenomatous hyperplasia, and there is question as to whether these changes are truly neoplastic or are reactive changes associated with foreign bodies or infectious agents.[48]

UROGENITAL DISEASES OF GUINEA PIGS

Urinary Calculi

Urinary tract calculi have been described in guinea pigs.[7, 76] In aged boars, congealed ejaculum can form proteinaceous urethral obstructions and result in urethritis. Females older than 3 years of age appear predisposed to cystitis and cystic calculi.[62] In one report, calcium oxalate uroliths were diagnosed in several guinea pigs suffering from *Streptococcus pyogenes* cystitis. The bacteria formed nidi around which calcium was deposited, resulting in stone formation.[59]

Clinical signs of urolithiasis include hematuria, dysuria, and a huddled, hunched posture. The uroliths can sometimes be palpated; however, definitive diagnosis is most often made by identifying urinary calculi on radiographic survey films.

Initial treatment includes antibiotic administration and relief of urinary obstruction, if present. Trimethoprim/sulfa, enrofloxacin, and chloramphenicol are the antibiotics of choice. Urinary acidifiers are generally not indicated, since the kidneys of guinea pigs cannot easily remove an acid load.[31] Retrograde flushing of the urethra may dislodge a urethral stone and allow urine passage. If this procedure fails, do a cystocentesis for temporary relief of the obstruction. A cystotomy is indicated for urolith removal (see Chapter 25). Uroliths are often recurrent, and multiple surgeries are sometimes needed. Preventative treatment for urolithiasis in guinea pigs is unknown.

Chronic Interstitial Nephritis

Chronic interstitial nephritis is commonly found at necropsy in guinea pigs older than 3 years. It has also been reported in guinea pigs with diabetes mellitus and hyperglycemia.[7] Animals affected by staphylococcal pododermatitis may develop chronic renal amyloidosis and nephritis as sequelae.[31] Secondary interstitial nephritis can be prevented by proper diet, caging, and good sanitation, thereby reducing susceptibility to pododermatitis. Diagnosis of nephritis is based on results of hematologic testing, serum biochemical analysis, and urinalysis. Treatment is supportive, with supplemental fluid therapy and antibiotic administration.

Renal Parasitism

Guinea pigs may harbor *Klossiella cobayae*, a renal coccidian. The organism lives in the epithelial cells lining the renal tubules. Sporocysts are shed in the urine. No clinical disease results from infection, and treatment is generally not recommended.[48] Sulfadimethoxine or trimethoprim/sulfa may be an effective treatment.

Ovarian Cysts

Cystic rete ovarii have been identified in 76% of female guinea pigs between 1.5 and 5 years of age, most commonly in animals 2–4 years of age.[41] Cysts develop spontaneously, range in diameter from 0.5–7 cm, and increase in size as the animal ages. They may be single or multilocular and are usually filled with clear fluid (Fig. 24–1). Both ovaries are normally affected; however, if a single ovary is affected, it is usually the right.[41] Other problems associated with cystic rete ovarii include leiomyomas,[20] cystic endometrial hyperplasia, and endometritis.[41] The most consistent clinical sign of cysts in breeding sows is a decline in fertility in sows older than 15 months. Some affected guinea pigs show bilaterally symmetric hair loss over the flanks and trunk. Cysts can sometimes be detected by abdominal palpation. Diagnosis can usually be confirmed by ultrasonography. An ovariohysterec-

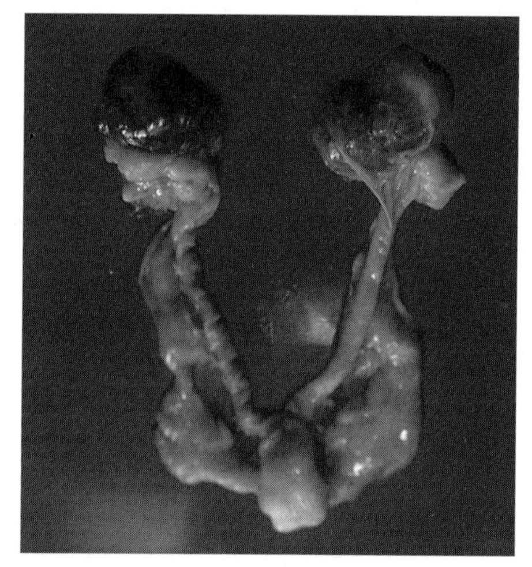

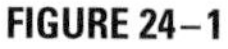

FIGURE 24–1
Ovarian cysts in a guinea pig. Ovarian cysts can develop in up to 76% of female guinea pigs and usually occur in both ovaries. (Courtesy of K. Rosenthal, DVM.)

tomy is the treatment of choice. Medical therapy can be attempted with hormonal therapy with human chorionic gonadotropin (100 IU IM, repeated in 7–10 days), and in some animals, percutaneous drainage of the cyst may be possible (Hillyer EV: Personal communication, 1995). However, medical therapy may cause only temporary improvement, and the cysts may recur.

Vaginitis or Scrotal Plugs

Wet, soiled bedding combined with inguinal sebaceous secretions can become adhered to the penis, scrotum, or vulva. This can result in secondary infection or can obstruct urination and defecation. The condition can be corrected by soaking the affected area in a dilute chlorhexidine solution and gently removing the debris. Give systemic antibiotics if the area appears infected. Prevent this condition by appropriate sanitation and husbandry practices.

Rectal Stool Impactions

Soft impactions of stool in the rectum commonly occur in sick or old guinea pigs (see Chapter 23). The accumulation of stool can become quite large if the rectal area is not cleaned regularly. Use towels soaked in warm water to gently evacuate the stool and clean the area. Topical antibacterial ointments or astringent solutions are occasionally useful if minor skin irritation is present.

Pregnancy Toxemia

Pregnancy toxemia (or pregnancy ketosis) is most commonly seen in primiparous, obese sows during the final 2 weeks of gestation and the first week postpartum. Although pregnancy is a contributing factor, toxemia is not limited to females; boars are also susceptible to this disorder. Obesity and fasting are the most critical predisposing conditions. Dietary alterations, environmental changes, and other stress factors also play a role in precipitating this disease.[22, 48] Onset of signs is abrupt. The guinea pig becomes anorectic and quits drinking, and within 24 hours is recumbent and dyspneic. Convulsions and death can occur within 2–5 days. Clinically, the animal is hypoglycemic (<60 mg/dL), ketonemic, proteinuric, and aciduric (pH 5–6; normal pH = 9).[84] The liver is enlarged and fatty, and the stomach is empty. In pregnant sows, the heavy gravid uterus may compress its own vascular supply, resulting in ischemia, thromboplastin release, and disseminated intravascular coagulopathy.[31, 48] Treatment of pregnancy toxemia is usually unrewarding. Keep the guinea pig warm, administer crystalloid fluids IV or IP, and give glucose PO or IV. If the guinea pig is in shock, treat with short-acting corticosteroids. The stress of treatment combined with anorexia and an empty stomach may also lead to a fatal enteritis.[31]

Prevention is the preferred method of dealing with pregnancy toxemia. Maintain all guinea pigs on a good-quality diet, and monitor food intake to prevent obesity. Supplementing the chow with fresh vegetables conditions the animal to a varied diet and lessens the chance of refusal when new foods are offered. Always provide fresh water free choice, and avoid any environmental, physical, and social stresses, particularly during late pregnancy.

Dystocia

Dystocia is common in guinea pigs. In female guinea pigs, relaxin (a hormone released from the pituitary) causes the fibrocartilage of the pubic symphysis to disintegrate during the last 30 days of pregnancy. The pelvis initially separates about 7–8 mm, but the separation increases dramatically during the last week of pregnancy, resulting in a separation of up to 3 cm.[11, 31, 48] If a sow is not bred for the first time before she reaches 7–8 months of age, her pelvic symphysis may separate less easily during parturition, resulting in dystocia.[31] Obesity, large fetuses, and uterine inertia can also cause dystocia.

Signs of dystocia include contractions and straining (in guinea pigs, pups are normally delivered within a 30-minute period, with a resting period of approximately 5 minutes between pups). Guinea pigs may be depressed and have bloody or greenish-brown vulvar discharge. Diagnosis is based on history and clinical signs. If the pelvic symphysis is wide and the problem is uterine inertia, give oxytocin (0.2–3 units/kg IM) to stimulate contractions.[22] If pups are manually delivered, fetal membranes must be rapidly removed.[11] If oxytocin fails to stimulate contractions, or if the pubic symphysis is separated less than 20–25 mm, *immediate* cesarean section is indicated (see Chapter 25). Guinea pigs do not tolerate the stress of anesthesia and surgery well, and the prognosis for recovery following surgery is guarded.[22] Dystocia is best prevented by breeding guinea pigs before 6 months of age and by preventing obesity.

Mastitis

Mastitis in guinea pigs is caused by infection with *Pasteurella* species, *Klebsiella* species, *E. coli, Staphylococcus* species, *Streptococcus* species, or *Pseudomonas* species.[28] Wet, dirty cages and trauma by pups predispose sows to infection. Organisms enter through the teat canal or through bite wounds to the teats. Clinically, the glands initially appear red and swollen and are warm; later, they can become cool and cyanotic. The milk will often be bloody. The infection can spread systemically and result in the death of both mother and pups.[31] Treat mastitis aggressively with systemic antibiotics, such as trimethoprim/sulfa, enrofloxacin, or aminoglycosides. Hot pack the glands, keep the environment clean, and wean the pups early. If necessary, the mammary glands can be surgically resected.[31]

Mammary Gland Tumors

Mammary gland tumors have been reported in guinea pigs and can occur in males and females. The majority of these tumors are benign fibroadenomas. Approximately 30% are adenocarcinomas, which are locally invasive but rarely metastasize.[11, 48] If tumors are excised, do a *wide* excision including a large amount of normal tissue, and remove local lymph nodes (see Chapter 25).

DERMATOLOGIC DISEASES OF GUINEA PIGS

Dermatophytosis

Guinea pigs are susceptible to ringworm. The dermatophyte most frequently isolated is *Trichophyton mentagrophytes*, although *Microsporum canis* has also been identified. Animals may be inapparent carriers; disease is usually seen secondary to overcrowding, poor husbandry, and other stress factors. Dermatophytes are easily transmitted by direct contact and by fomites. Lesions are pruritic and consist of focal areas of alopecia with crusts. These are usually seen first on the face, forehead, and ears and later spread over the back and down the limbs.[11] Diagnosis is made by identifying fungal organisms on a culture of hair samples. Pluck or scrape hairs and crusts from the periphery of the lesion and place these on dermatophyte test medium or other appropriate culture media. Ringworm can be treated topically with miconazole once daily for 2–4 weeks.[31] A new drug, butenafine, is effective when applied topically once daily for 10 days.[1] Griseofulvin pediatric solution (250 mg/kg PO) given every 10 days for three treatments has been effective.[11] Griseofulvin can also be given daily at a lower dose (25 mg/kg PO q24h) for 3–5 weeks.[33, 86] This drug should not be given to pregnant animals because it is teratogenic.[11] Ringworm is a potentially zoonotic disease.

Ectoparasites

Guinea pigs are susceptible to infestation by mites (*Trixacarus caviae, Chirodiscoides caviae*), lice (*Gliricola porcelli, Gyropus ovalis*), and fleas (*Ctenocephalides felis*). Of these, *T. caviae*, the sarcoptid mite, is the most significant pathogen (Fig. 24–2). This is a burrowing mite and causes intense pruritus. It can also transiently infest humans.[44] Signs of *T. caviae* infestation include intense pruritus with excoriations and secondary infection. Lesions are seen on the thighs and back and can ex-

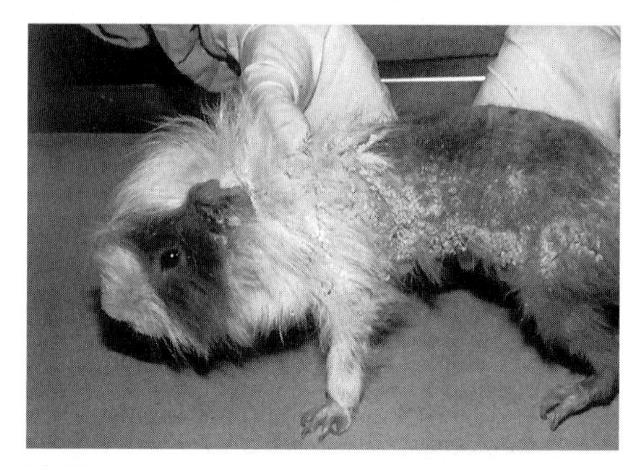

FIGURE 24–2
Sarcoptic mange in a guinea pig caused by *Trixacarus caviae*. (Courtesy of Elizabeth V. Hillyer, DVM.)

tend over the shoulders.[80] Hematologic changes associated with *T. caviae* infestation are leukocytosis, monocytosis, eosinophilia, and basophilia.[70] *C. caviae* is a nonburrowing fur mite and is much less a problem than *T. caviae*. This mite may cause lesions on the perineal and hip area; infestation, however, is normally asymptomatic. *G. porcelli* and *G. ovalis* are debris-feeding lice that attach to the hair shafts (both adults and eggs). Alopecia, crusts, and a rough hair coat are seen with lice infestations.[80] All of these parasites are transmitted by direct contact.

Diagnosis is made by visual identification (fleas), skin scraping (mites), or plucking or combing hairs to look for eggs and adults (lice). Treat fleas with a pyrethrin-based cat flea powder. Lice and *C. caviae* have been treated with ivermectin (0.3–0.5 mg/kg PO or SC), repeated in 10 days.[80] *T. caviae* has been effectively eliminated by treatment with ivermectin (0.5 mg/kg SC),[50] repeated in 7 days. Oral administration of this drug may be equally effective.[66, 87] When treating all ectoparasites, thoroughly clean the environment to prevent reinfestation.

Cervical Lymphadenitis

Cervical lymphadenitis or "lumps" is a disease that commonly occurs in guinea pigs (Fig. 24–3). It is caused most often by *Streptococcus zooepidemicus* Lancefield's group C, a gram-positive coccus. Occasionally, *Streptobacillus moniliformis* is also involved.[48] *S. zooepidemicus* is normally present in the conjunctiva and nasal cavity of guinea pigs. When the animal's oral mucosa becomes abraded from malocclusion, dietary roughage (hay stems), or biting, bacteria can enter through the mucosal abrasions, travel to the cervical lymph nodes, and cause abscessation. Stress increases susceptibility to infection.[31] Clinically, the guinea pig presents with pus-filled, ventral cervical masses. Occasionally, bacteria can spread systemically, resulting in septicemia or pneumonia. Diagnosis is based on physical examination findings and results of impression smears, Gram's stains, and bacterial culture and sensitivity testing of the exudate. Complete surgical excision of the affected lymph nodes is the most effective treatment (see Chapter 25). Alternatively, surgically drain the abscesses and flush the wounds copiously. Begin systemic antibiotic therapy with trimethoprim/sulfa or enrofloxacin. Prevent cervical lymphadenitis by keeping the guinea pig in a clean, stress-free environment and providing a good diet. Isolate affected animals from other guinea pigs until the abscesses are healed.

Bite Wounds

Although guinea pigs are social animals, group housing can lead to bite wounds that occasionally abscess. Treatment consists of draining and flushing the wound and giving appropriate systemic antibiotics, based on results of bacterial culture and sensitivity testing.

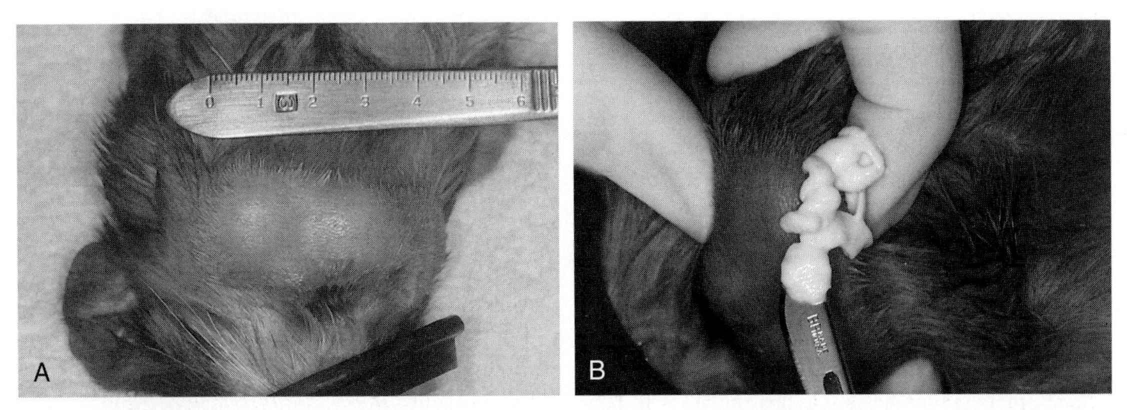

FIGURE 24–3
Cervical lymphadenitis or "lumps" in a guinea pig. Infection is usually caused by *Streptococcus zooepidemicus* and occurs in the ventral cervical lymph nodes (*A*). Nodes are enlarged and filled with a thick, purulent exudate (*B*).

Pododermatitis

Pododermatitis or "bumblefoot" is commonly seen in guinea pigs. Typically, the disease is found in obese animals housed on wire-bottom cages or abrasive bedding. Areas of hyperkeratosis develop on the palmar and plantar surfaces of the feet. These then ulcerate, permitting secondary invasion by *Staphylococcus aureus*.[48] Infection can extend deep into the tissues of the feet, traveling up tendons and into bone, resulting in osteomyelitis. Guinea pigs with pododermatitis appear in extreme pain, vocalize frequently, and are reluctant to walk. Diagnosis is based on clinical signs and identification of lesions. Radiographs may be useful in identifying osteomyelitis. Treatment consists of appropriate systemic antibiotics, surgical débridement of lesions (see Chapter 25), foot soaks, and bandaging the wounds. As with pododermatitis in most species, prognosis is guarded. Prevent pododermatitis by keeping the environment clean and dry, housing guinea pigs on soft, nonabrasive bedding, and avoiding obesity.

Trichofolliculoma

The most common skin tumor in guinea pigs is the trichofolliculoma, which is a benign basal cell epithelioma.[48] Trichofolliculomas appear as solid or cystic masses, most commonly over the lumbosacral area.[11,48] They are easily removed surgically (see Chapter 25).

Alopecia

Alopecia resulting from noninfectious causes is quite common in guinea pigs. Included in this group are barbering, endocrine alopecia, and vitamin deficiencies. Barbering is recognized by close examination of the area of hair loss; broken hair shafts should be present, and the underlying skin should not be inflamed or pruritic.[48] Alopecia over the flank areas indicates self-barbering, which can occur secondary to boredom. Providing hay, other roughage, or chew toys may alleviate this problem. In group-housed guinea pigs, the dominant animal often barbers subordinates. Guinea pig sows in late gestation often experience transient endocrine alopecia, and nursing pups will barber their mother.

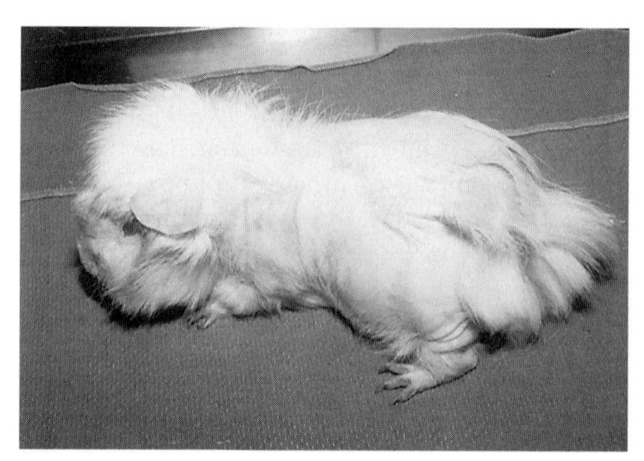

FIGURE 24–4
Alopecia secondary to ovarian cysts in a female guinea pig. (Courtesy of Elizabeth V. Hillyer, DVM.)

Partial alopecia has also been documented in weanlings.[48] Bilaterally symmetric alopecia may occur in guinea pigs with ovarian cysts (Fig. 24–4).

MUSCULOSKELETAL DISEASES OF GUINEA PIGS

Scurvy

Guinea pigs possess a mutated gene for L-gulono-γ-lactone oxidase and therefore cannot produce this enzyme. Without L-gulono-γ-lactone oxidase, guinea pigs cannot convert glucose to ascorbic acid and are thus incapable of endogenous synthesis of vitamin C.[58] Guinea pigs therefore require 15–25 mg/d of vitamin C, and pregnant animals require 30 mg/d.[31] Ascorbic acid is necessary for formation of hydroxylysine and hydroxyproline, which in turn are necessary for collagen synthesis. Therefore, lack of dietary vitamin C results in defective collagen formation in guinea pigs. Collagen is necessary for structural integrity of blood vessels; lack of collagen results in leaky vessels and hemorrhage, particularly in joints and gingiva. Collagen is also necessary to keep teeth anchored tightly in their sockets; without collagen, teeth loosen and malocclusion occurs. Other clinical signs of vitamin C deficiency include rough hair-coat, anorexia, diarrhea, teeth grinding and vocalizing from pain, delayed wound healing, lameness, and increased susceptibility to bacterial infections.[48] Radiographically, long bone epiphyses and costochondral junctions of the ribs appear enlarged. Pathologic fractures may also be evident. Young, growing animals are most susceptible to scurvy, and clinical disease can develop in as little as 2 weeks of ascorbic acid deprivation.[11] Always consider scurvy in young animals with vague clinical signs, such as reduced appetite and decreased activity, and with no definitive physical findings.

Diagnosis of vitamin C deficiency is based on history, clinical signs, and radiographic findings. Serum ascorbic acid levels can be used to confirm the diagnosis. However, a positive response to treatment is often the most practical means of confirmation. Many animals with infectious disease, such as upper respiratory disease, also have subclinical scurvy and benefit from supplemental vitamin C. Begin treatment with parenteral administration of ascorbic acid (50 mg SC); once response is noted, administer vitamin C orally at the same dosage. After recovery, supplement vitamin C daily in the diet. Fresh, good-quality guinea pig (*not* rabbit) chow provides adequate vitamin C if used within 90 days of the *milling* date. Fresh cabbage, kale, and oranges also provide a source of vitamin C. One hundred grams of kale contains 125 mg vitamin C, and 50 g of cabbage contains 30 mg vitamin C.[31] Vitamin C can also be added to the drinking water at a concentration of 200–400 mg/L water.[48] However, deionized or distilled water should be used, and copper watering systems should be avoided, as contact with metal accelerates deterioration of vitamin C. The vitamin C should be added fresh daily, as 50% of the potency remains after 24 hours when plastic or glass containers are used.[84]

Osteoarthrosis

Spontaneous cartilage degeneration and osteoarthrosis of the femorotibial joint of young guinea pigs has been described.[4] No causative factor has been identified, and the disease does not appear to be widespread.

Iatrogenic Muscle Necrosis

Fentanyl-droperidol has been documented to cause muscle necrosis at the injection site in guinea pigs.[31] Ketamine has also been implicated in nerve damage and self-mutilation distal to the injection site in guinea pigs.

NEUROLOGIC DISEASES OF GUINEA PIGS

Lymphocytic Choriomeningitis Virus

Lymphocytic choriomeningitis virus is an arenavirus that causes meningitis and hindlimb paralysis in guinea pigs.[48] Lymphocytic choriomeningitis is more commonly reported in mice and hamsters and is rare in pet guinea pigs. Lesions include lymphocytic infiltrates in the choroid plexus, ependyma, and meninges.[48] The virus is transmitted in the urine through aerosolization, fomites, and biting insects. Transplacental transmission also occurs. Lymphocytic choriomeningitis can cause flulike signs and meningitis in humans. The disease is usually contracted from infected hamsters, which secrete large amounts of virus in their urine. No treatment is currently available.

MISCELLANEOUS DISEASES OF GUINEA PIGS

Heat Stroke

Guinea pigs are susceptible to heat stroke. Guinea pigs housed outdoors have developed heat stroke even in ambient temperatures as low as 70–75°F. Guinea pigs with heat stroke salivate profusely in an attempt to thermoregulate. They exhibit shallow, rapid respiration, pale mucous membranes, elevated rectal temperature, coma, and death.[33] Diagnosis is based on history and clinical signs. Treat guinea pigs with heat stroke supportively with cool water baths, corticosteroids, and parenteral fluids. Prognosis is very guarded.

Metastatic Mineralization

Metastatic mineralization in guinea pigs is normally an incidental finding at necropsy. The cause is unclear, but is possibly related to subclinical mineral imbalances and dehydration. Although normally the disease is clinically inapparent, it can present as muscle stiffness and renal dysfunction.[48] Lesions are seen in animals older than 1 year and include mineralization of kidneys, heart, vessels, stomach, and colon. There is no treatment.

Myocardial necrosis and mineralization have been described in inbred guinea pigs.[26]

Cavian Leukemia

Lymphosarcoma is the most common tumor of guinea pigs and is caused by a type C retrovirus. Affected animals present with a scruffy coat and lymphadenopathy. Hepatomegaly and splenomegaly are occasionally also seen. Leukemic animals have a total white blood cell count of 25,000–500,000/μL.[11] At necropsy, lymph nodes and visceral organs may be enlarged, with infiltration by proliferating lymphoblasts. The course of the disease is 2–5 weeks.[48] Diagnose this disease based on results of a complete blood count, cytologic examination of a smear of a lymph node aspirate, or lymph node biopsy. Abdominal ultrasound may also be helpful in identifying lymphoid infiltration of abdominal organs. The disease has been reported to respond favorably to chemotherapy.[48] However, most guinea pigs do poorly clinically and are usually euthanatized.

PART B

Thomas M. Donnelly, BVSc and Dorcas O. Schaeffer, DVM

Acquiring knowledge about the diseases, diagnosis, and treatment of pet chinchillas has been different than procuring similar information about other exotic rodents. This is because of the paucity of information from laboratory or clinical settings. Although their small size and ease of handling have made them suitable experimental animals, chinchillas have been almost exclusively used in hearing research. They have an auditory sensitivity remarkably similar to that of humans[68] and large bullae surrounded by thin bone that allows easy surgical access to the middle ear. A clinically useful consequence of their use in otitis media research has been establishing the pharmacokinetics of newer antibiotics such as cephalosporins in chinchillas. A good review describing the use of chinchillas in this area of research was done by Goycoolea and others.[25]

The vast majority of the literature on the diseases of chinchillas has come from the fur industry. At a meeting in England in 1959, one speaker contrasted the state of knowledge on chinchilla diseases with mustelid diseases[8] and finished by stating "the chinchilla stood today where the mink (and ferret) had stood six years ago." That analogy is still appropriate today. Only in recent years has a body of information dealing exclusively with the diseases of pet ferrets emerged separately from that of the diseases of laboratory and fur ferrets. The same situation is slowly occurring with pet chinchillas.

In a review of the literature of diseases in chinchillas, only four reports described diseases in pet chinchillas. Two reports described protozoal infections with *Sarcocystis* species[64] and *Cryptosporidium* species,[92] and two reports described lead poisoning in pet chinchillas.[33, 54] Most papers in English that describe diseases in chinchillas were written in the 1950s and early 1960s. In contrast, the majority of papers written after 1980 are in German and Spanish, often without an English summary. Constructive efforts to document health problems in pet chinchillas in English are coming from pet chinchilla breeders,[43, 67] but their information is not readily available through conventional computer searches.

Despite a significant number of publications over the past 50 years on chinchilla diseases, most were printed in fur trade periodicals and newsletters and not in clinical or scientific journals. The situation is further complicated by the misinterpretation of non-English sources such as *Deutsche Pelztierzuchter* (*German Fur-Animal Breeder*) as scientific journals and the referencing of them in clinical reports.

We have emphasized this unusual state of the body of knowledge on chinchilla diseases because many readers may find two aspects of this part of this chapter unusual: 1) there is referenced information that is not necessarily current but has not been cited extensively and may seem "new" and 2) although we describe the same diseases as in recent, brief reviews,[30, 33, 52] we place far greater emphasis on diseases associated with poor husbandry. We consider these problems to be more frequent reasons that an owner of a pet chinchilla seeks veterinary consultation.

GENERAL COMMENTS ON DISEASE PROBLEMS OF CHINCHILLAS

Diseases Likely to Be Seen in Practice

Husbandry and feeding mistakes are the most common causes of disease seen in practice; therefore, it is essential to ask about the husbandry conditions before attempting a diagnosis. Because chinchillas hide symptoms of disease as a survival mechanism, they are usually brought to the veterinarian at a much later stage of disease than a dog or cat, unless the owner is well informed. Owners often follow the recommendations of the pet store before seeking veterinary help, which is another reason why the chinchilla is often seen in a late stage of disease.

DISORDERS ASSOCIATED WITH HUSBANDRY OF CHINCHILLAS

Disorders of the Digestive System

Thirty years ago, the Chinchilla Fur-Breeders Association of England showed that approximately half of all deaths in adult chinchillas were related to disorders of the digestive tract; malocclusion accounted for one quarter of those deaths.[13] Presently, disorders of the digestive tract not associated with infectious disease remain the most frequent problems seen in clinical practice. Inappetence and lethargy are common presenting signs. However, these signs are also associated with infectious and metabolic diseases; therefore, a thorough diagnostic workup is always recommended.

Malocclusion of the Teeth and Slobbers

Like all rodents, chinchillas have open-rooted (hypsodontic) teeth that grow continuously, and malocclusion can occur (Figs. 24–5 and 24–6). Griner reported malocclusion of the incisors and periodontitis with alveolar abscessation of maxillary cheek teeth in one chinchilla and similar mandibular periodontitis and alveolar periostitis in a second.[27] Clinically, chinchillas with malocclusion present with a history of anorexia, weight loss, excess salivation and a wet chin (slobbers), and lethargy. Oral examination and corrective procedures are similar to those in guinea pigs. One reported complication of malocclusion in chinchillas is invasion of the orbit by the roots of the maxillary molars.[18] This may result from a weakening of the periodontal structures by the masticatory stresses of the misaligned molars, which causes the molars to be pushed apically into the maxillary bone. This can also occur in the mandibular molars, resulting in a corresponding exostosis in the ventral border of the mandible.

Choke and Bloat

Like rabbits and rats, chinchillas cannot vomit, and esophageal choke has been described in chinchillas of all ages.[13] Clinical signs include drooling, retching, dyspnea, and anorexia. Choke is more common in animals offered tidbits such as raisins, fruits, and nuts; animals that eat their bedding; and postparturient females that eat their placentas. Bloat or gastric tympany is another problem of lactating females and is associated with overeating hay rich in clover, sudden food changes (especially the addition of fresh greens and fruits), and gastrointestinal inflammation. Affected animals are swollen, lie on their sides, hesitate to stir, and are dyspneic. Treat bloat by decompressing the stomach, either by passing a gastric tube or inserting a needle or trochar transabdominally.

Gastric trichobezoars are often associated with fur-chewing. Clinical signs, including anorexia and lethargy, are similar to those in rabbits. The proteolytic enzymes in pineapple juice or papaya tablets are claimed to help break down fur in the stomach, although their efficacy is questionable. However, pineapple juice and papaya tablets are sweet, and chinchillas may readily lap pineapple juice or eat papaya tablets as a tasty treat. This treatment may not be efficacious but is unlikely to cause harm.

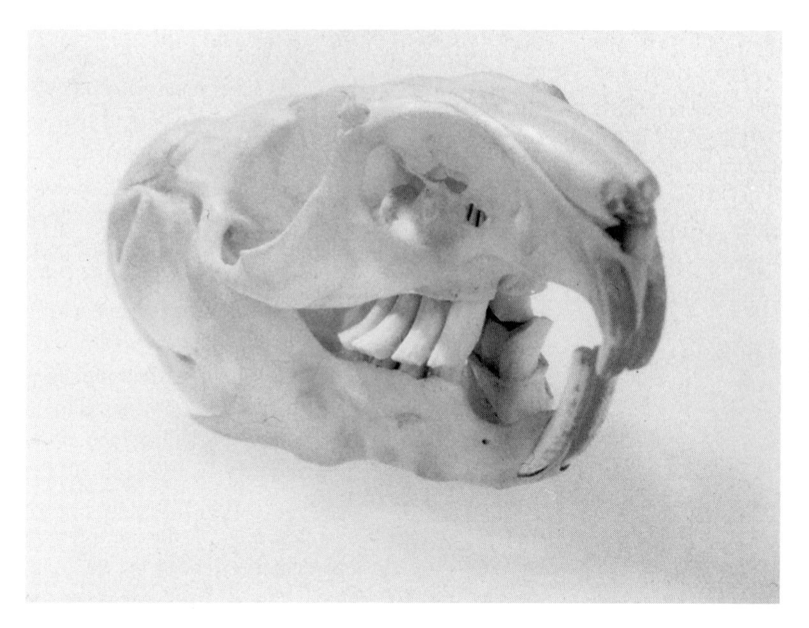

FIGURE 24–5
Skull of a chinchilla with severe molar malocclusion. Note how the upper molars curve outward. (Refer to Fig. 24–6 to see mandible.)

Constipation

Constipation has been described as a more common clinical problem than diarrhea in the chinchilla.[32] Constipation is easily overlooked because owners do not always recognize their pet's normal droppings. Healthy fecal pellets are plentiful and odorless, shaped like large grains of rice, either brown or black, and when fresh are soft and plump.[13] Chinchillas with constipation will strain to defecate, and the few pellets they pass are thin, short, hard, and occasionally blood stained. The usual cause of constipation is feeding too much concentrated diet, which is high in energy and protein, without supplying sufficient roughage or fiber.[13] Therapeutically it is possible to change the diet by simply increasing the fiber. This is achieved by careful addition of small amounts of fresh food such as apples, carrots, or lettuce and omitting treats such as grains or raisins. If the constipation does not improve, laxatives such as those used in cats can be used. Cisapride (0.5 mg/kg q8h PO) (Propulsid, Janssen Pharmaceuticals, Inc, Titusville, NJ) may be useful to enhance intestinal motility if it is determined that intestinal blockage is not present. Some breeders give vegetable oil or sweet butter on a spoon to prevent constipation. Other causes of constipation include obesity, lack of exercise, intestinal obstruction, and intestinal compression secondary to large fetuses.[30]

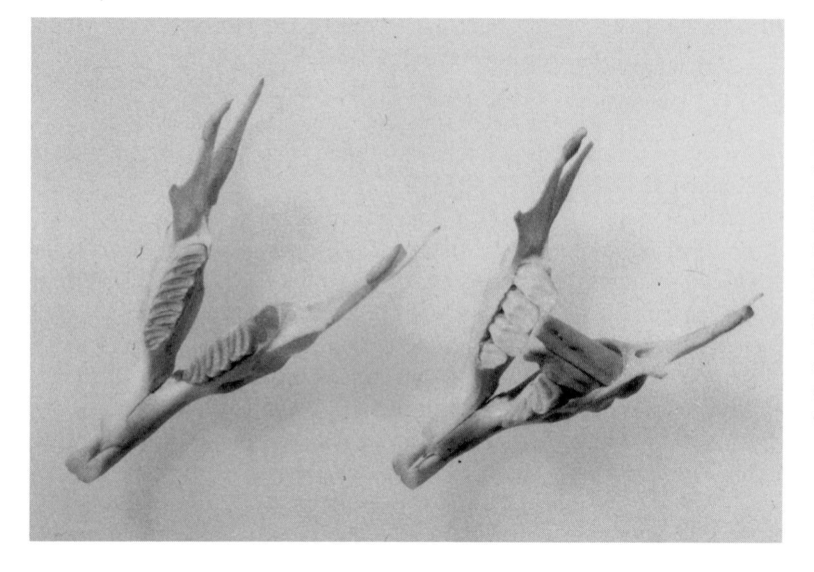

FIGURE 24–6
Two chinchilla mandibles. The mandible on the left shows normal molar occlusion. The mandible on the right is from the skull of the chinchilla in Figure 24–5. Note how the lower molars curve inward in contrast to the upper molars, which curve outward. This is a severe case in which the molars no longer occluded and continued to grow; this led to trauma of the mouth.

Diarrhea

Diarrhea is also a frequent reason for consultation. The most common cause of diarrhea in pet chinchillas is inappropriate feeding. This includes overfeeding fresh green foods and offering damp hay that may be moldy or hay that is too young. Stress and sudden changes of food also seem to predispose chinchillas to diarrhea. The owner may first notice that feces are smeared on the resting board in the cage and the fur around the anus is matted with feces. The diarrhea is acute, and generally the chinchilla does not appear sick. Hartmann recommends withholding food for the first day and adding a palatable oral electrolyte replacement solution to the drinking water.[32] A well-dried, high-quality hay that is older than half a year is offered on the second day, and an electrolyte solution is administered subcutaneously if the animal is dehydrated.

Bacterial and parasitic infections will also cause diarrhea (see later), but generally the owner will describe signs of diarrhea that have been present for a few days. These chinchillas are often lethargic and have dry and dull fur. Fecal staining of the fur is not always apparent, as the animals may camouflage this sign by cleaning their fur. Breeding females and young chinchillas up to 4 months of age are most susceptible to infectious diarrhea.[30]

Intestinal Torsion, Intussusception, and Impaction

Intestinal torsion, intussusception, or impaction of the cecum or colonic flexure can occur in chinchillas with chronic constipation or gastroenteritis.[8, 33, 49] Ileus can be diagnosed radiographically by the presence of severely distended and gas-filled intestinal loops.[71] Animals may sit hunched, stretch out, or roll in an attempt to relieve pain. Use warm, soapy water or mineral oil enemas to correct impaction; intussusception or torsion requires surgery.

Rectal Prolapse

Rectal prolapse may also occur in chinchillas with severe constipation or diarrhea. If diagnosed and treated quickly, the prolapse can be replaced and retained by a pursestring suture. If the tissue is edematous, gently soak it in a concentrated sugar solution, which sometimes reduces the swelling. Address the causative factors of the prolapse to prevent recurrence. Ritchey[67] recommends a bland soft diet of baby food and cereals, except rice cereal, for 10 days after a prolapse has occurred. Gradually return the animal to a normal diet after the sutures are removed.

Reproductive Disorders

Fur-Ring and Paraphimosis

Male chinchillas that groom excessively, produce frequent but small amounts of urine, or strain to urinate and repeatedly clean their penis may have a fur-ring. This is a ring of hair around the penis and under the prepuce that eventually stops the penis from retracting into the prepuce. In severe cases, an engorged penis is seen protruding 4–5 cm from the prepuce, resulting in paraphimosis. The condition not only is painful but also may cause urethral constriction and acute urinary retention. Chronic paraphimosis may culminate in infection and severe damage to the penis, affecting the animal's breeding ability.

Cut or gently roll the fur-ring off the penis after applying a sterile lubricant. In some chinchillas, sedation or anesthesia may be required to remove the fur-ring.

Fur-ring is thought to result from acquiring fur from a female during copulation. However, the fur may come from other males or the same animal, as the condition is also seen in group-housed and single-housed males not exposed to females.[88] Males should be examined for fur-rings at least four times a year. Active stud males should be examined every few days. In some male chinchillas, the penis will continuously hang out of the prepuce and is not engorged. This is not associated with fur-ring but results from overexcitement brought on by separation from its mate or overexhaustion from too many females in the same cage.

Dystocia

Chinchillas usually give birth early in the morning (before 8:00 AM), and only rarely after 12:00 noon.[88] A chinchilla with dystocia is recognized by her extreme restlessness, frequent crying, and constant attention to the genital region. Dystocia is usually associated with the presentation of a single, oversized fetus, or malpresentation of one or more kits.[13] Uterine inertia has also been reported as a cause of dystocia.[63] In uncomplicated dystocias, gentle traction of the fetus with feline obstetric forceps may correct the condition. However, if the chinchilla is in labor for more than 4 hours, then surgical intervention is indicated (see Chapter 25). Chinchillas have been reported to respond well to cesarean section.[38, 63, 78]

Traumatic Disorders and Injuries

Conjunctivitis

Irritation of the eyes that results in conjunctivitis without clinical signs of upper respiratory infection is often caused by excessive dust bathing. Dirty or poor-quality bedding and inadequate cage ventilation also may cause conjunctivitis. Treatment involves restricting dust bath access to 15–30 minutes per day, changing the type of dusting powder (see Chapter 23), and applying a protective ophthalmic preparation such as artificial tears or petrolatum ointment. If the condition does not resolve rapidly, then additional ophthalmic workup is recommended.

Fur Slip

Chinchillas possess a predator avoidance mechanism known as fur slip. When the animal is fighting or handled roughly, it can release a large patch of fur, thus enabling it to escape. A clean, smooth area of skin is left; hair may require several months to regrow.

Bite Wounds

Bite wounds that abscess often occur in group-housed animals, especially during breeding. Female chinchillas are larger than male ones and, like hamsters, are more aggressive; older females may kill a young male housed in the same cage. Female chinchillas are highly selective in their choice of males for mating and will keep "unsuitable" males at bay by urinating, kicking, and biting.[88] Besides abscesses, bite wounds sometimes result in the loss of pieces of ears and toes. Culture of the abscesses often yields *Staphylococcus* species. Jenkins found that surgical removal of the abscess led to significantly greater success than incision and curettage.[37] Treatment with appropriate systemic antibiotics is also indicated.

Fractures

Traumatic fractures of the tibia are commonly seen.[34] The tibia is a long, straight bone with little soft tissue covering it. It is longer than the femur, and the fibula is virtually nonexistent (Fig. 24–7). Tibial fractures are generally either transverse or short spiral and associated with bony fragments. Common causes of fractures are the grabbing of a chinchilla by its hind limb or the animal catching its hind limb in a cage bar.

Similar to those of rabbits, the bones of chinchillas are thin and fragile, and surgical repair can

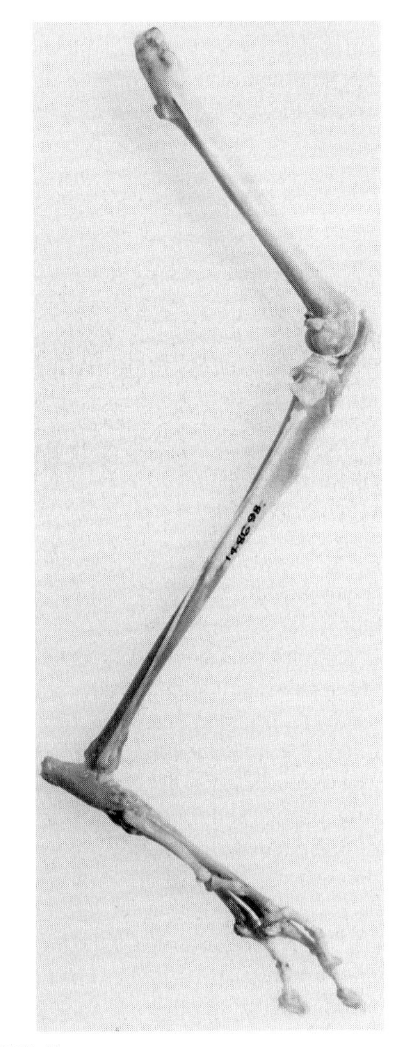

FIGURE 24–7
Hindlimb skeleton of an adult chinchilla. Note how long the tibia is compared with the femur. The fibula is virtually nonexistent. Most traumatic fractures occur in the tibia, and the fragile nature of the bone shows how challenging surgical fixation can be.

be difficult. Soft padded bandages and lateral splints usually do not provide adequate stability for fractures to heal.[34] For best results, surgically repair the fracture with either wire or external fixators and then further stabilize it with bandages (see Chapter 30).

Chinchillas are active animals, and limited mobility is essential for fracture healing to occur. This can be achieved by placing the animal in a small cage. Unfortunately, frequent visits for resetting of the fracture are common. Owners should be advised that nonunion is a possible outcome and will result in a crooked leg.

Dermatologic Disorders

Matted Fur

Chinchillas will develop matted fur if kept in a warm (>80°F), humid environment. They will also develop this condition if they are deprived of a dust bath (see Chapter 23).

Dust baths should be provided daily for approximately 30 minutes a day. Although the dust can be left in for longer periods, it could result in excessive bathing and subsequent conjunctivitis.

Alopecia

Small, scaly patches of alopecia on the nose, behind the ears, or on the forefeet are seen in ringworm infection. Lesions may appear on any part of the body; in advanced cases, a large, circumscribed area of inflammation with scab formation is not unusual. *T. mentagrophytes* is the dermatophyte most commonly isolated, and older reports indicated that there was a rate of 5% latent infection in normal fur-ranched chinchillas.[52] Ultraviolet light is not useful for diagnosis because *T. mentagrophytes* does not fluoresce. Diagnosis and treatment of dermatophytosis are similar to those in guinea pigs. Captan mixed with a dust bath at 1 teaspoon per 2 cups of dust may help control spread of infection.[89]

Fur-Chewing

Alopecia is usually associated with fur-chewing in chinchillas. Chinchillas chew each others' fur, resulting in a moth-eaten coat.

Eidmann contrasted the histologic appearance of selected organs between fur-chewers and healthy chinchillas.[17] There were 39 fur-chewers of different sexes and ages compared with 19 healthy chinchillas. Skin and fur were cultured for bacteria and fungi, feces were examined for parasites, and the number and types of intestinal bacteria were determined. Hematologic tests consisting of a complete blood count and selected serum enzyme measurements were done in all animals. The author concluded that an infectious cause of fur-chewing was unlikely and suggested that affected animals suffer from malnutrition and chew their fur for dietary requirements. The diagnosis of malnutrition was based on histologic and enzymatic evidence of mild, fatty degeneration of the liver and low numbers of cecal bacteria in fur-chewers. However, Eidmann also mentioned the possibility of multiple food factors being involved in this type of malnutrition and that further dietary studies are required. Of particular interest was the correlation of thyroid hyperplasia to the size of chewed fur over the body. This was interpreted as a reactive response of the thyroids to the loss of insulation following fur removal. Both fur-chewers and control animals were found to have large numbers of *Giardia*, but histologic examination of the intestines was not done.

Although a cause of fur-chewing could not be established, the conclusions discredited popular theories supported by scant experimental investigation. Among these theories was the belief that a fungus was the cause of fur breakage.[74] Consequently, some chinchilla fur ranchers regularly add fungicide to the dust bath.[52] Another theory suggested that fur-chewers might have abnormal endocrine activity, as there is increased thyroidal and adrenocortical activity.[81]

A current popular theory suggests that fur-chewing is a behavioral disorder. The vice is often transmitted from mother to offspring. Furthermore, the high incidence of fur-chewing in commercial herds is often suggested as evidence for maladapted displacement behavior. There have been no documented attempts to treat fur-chewers with antidepressants such as fluoxetine hydrochloride (Prozac, Dista Products Co, Indianapolis, IN), despite success with its use in treatment of tail-chasing and lick granulomas of dogs. Based on rabbit and rodent doses,[69] a dose of 5–10mg/kg is suggested for chinchillas.

Neurologic Disorders

Encephalitis

Several disorders result in convulsions or other neurologic signs. In addition to the more common husbandry-associated conditions described here, encephalitis caused by listeriosis, lymphocytic choriomeningitis, and cerebrospinal nematodiasis should also be considered in the diagnostic workup.

Listeria monocytogenes has been reported to cause peracute death in chinchillas.[21] The clinical signs may include ataxia, depression, and enteritis. Animals usually die within 24 hours of onset of clinical signs.[33, 86] Food contaminated by feral rodents and poor husbandry contributes to disease spread. Chloramphenicol (10 mg/oz drinking water) and oxytetracycline (10 mg/kg q12h IM) have been used for treatment but drug efficacy decreases once signs are detected.[33, 85, 86]

Baylisascaris procyonis, the raccoon roundworm, has caused cerebral nematodiasis in chinchillas from aberrant larval migration.[72] The disease is transmitted by ingestion of hay or feed that has been contaminated by feces from an infected raccoon. Parasitism is most common in the northern United States. Clinical signs in chinchillas include ataxia, incoordination, torticollis, paralysis, and tumbling.[73] Necrotic tracts and larvae have been seen in the brain stem of affected animals. Treatment is not effective.[73] The disease is prevented by feeding good-quality feed that has been properly stored. This parasite has also caused infection and mortality in humans.

Lymphocytic choriomeningitis virus has been reported in chinchillas, although it is more common in other rodent species.[85]

Lead Poisoning

Two cases of lead toxicosis in pet chinchillas have been described. A retrospective study described a chinchilla that presented with seizures similar to those in dogs and cats.[54] Although the blood lead concentration was high (660 μg/dL), the authors did not observe nucleated red blood cells or basophilic stippling of the red blood cells in this chinchilla's blood smear. Blood lead concentrations of 25 μg/dL or above are considered indicative of lead poisoning; concentrations of 60 μg/dL or above are diagnostic in companion animals. The affected chinchilla was treated successfully with calcium disodium edetate (25 mg/kg SC, q6h for 5 days), which was diluted to a 1% solution with 5% dextrose water.[55] Hoefer reported lead poisoning in a New York apartment–dwelling chinchilla that presented with acute convulsions and blindness.[33] This animal was also treated successfully with calcium disodium edetate at 30 mg/kg SC, q12h for 5 days.

Both reports described chinchillas with lead toxicosis from cities with poor urban neighborhoods. Morgan showed a positive correlation of lead poisoning in small companion animals that reside in urban neighborhoods where a high percentage of people live in poverty.[55]

Heat Stroke

The ambient temperature range to which chinchillas are adapted is 65–80°F. Exposure to temperatures above their ambient temperature range, especially when coupled with high humidity, can result in heat stroke. A good rule of thumb is to add the unit values of the temperature and humidity and consider any value greater than 150 dangerous (e.g., 85°F + 65% humidity = 150).

Affected animals lie down and exhibit rapid breathing, bright red mucous membranes, thick, stringy saliva, and, sometimes, bloody diarrhea. Owners will often describe animals with engorged ear veins and bright pink or red ears and mucous membranes. Rectal temperature is usually higher than 103°F. Treatment is straightforward and consists of cooling the animal by immersion in tepid water baths and administering intravenous fluids if the animal is in shock. Chinchillas should not be placed in ice-cold water baths, as this can cause seizures. Owners should be alerted not to position chinchilla cages near sunny windows or radiators.

REPORTED INFECTIOUS DISEASES OF CHINCHILLAS

Table 24–1 is a summary of significant reports of infectious diseases in chinchillas over the past 50 years. There are two striking observations: 1) nearly all the reports concern *colonies* of chinchillas raised for fur and involve bacterial diseases, and 2) most of the reports of bacterial disease in colonies are from 20 years ago or longer. There are only two reports in pet chinchillas, and both infections involved protozoa or fungi.

TABLE 24–1
REPORTS OF INFECTIOUS DISEASES IN CHINCHILLAS OVER THE PAST 50 YEARS

	Groups of Animals (Fur; No Laboratory Animal Reports)	Individual Animals	
		Pet	Fur or Laboratory
Reviews	Bowden, 1959 Dall, 1963		
Bacteria	Keagy and Keagy, 1951 Newberne, 1953 Larrivee and Elvehjem, 1954 Wood et al, 1956 Moore and Greenlee, 1975 Finley and Long, 1977 Menchaca and Martin, 1978 Bartoszce et al, 1990a Bartoszce et al, 1990b		Mountain, 1989 Doerning et al, 1993
Protozoa and Fungi	Keagy, 1949	Yamini and Raju, 1986 Rakich et al, 1992	Burtscher and Otte, 1962 Owens et al, 1975
Worms and Larvae	Sanford, 1991		

Recent reviews on the diseases of chinchillas propagate the impression that these animals are very susceptible to infectious disease. However, our impression is that pet chinchillas are equally susceptible as dogs or cats to infectious disease. There are no species-specific viral diseases described for chinchillas. The review by Wallach and Boever on the diseases of exotic rodents gives a good overview of the variety of infectious diseases that may be encountered in groups of rodents, including chinchillas.[85] Opportunistic infections by normal bacterial flora of chinchillas will cause frank disease, either localized to one organ (e.g., *Streptococcus* species, *Pseudomonas* species, and *E. coli*) or as septicemia. Affected animals are generally immunocompromised by age, nutritional status, or husbandry-related stress.

Chinchillas are generally susceptible to many of the same bacterial diseases as guinea pigs. *S. typhimurium* and *S. enteritidis* can cause bacterial enteritis in chinchillas. Other bacteria associated with enteritis in chinchillas include *E. coli, Y. pseudotuberculosis, C. perfringens, P. aeruginosa,* and *L. monocytogenes*.

Parasitic causes of diarrhea include cryptosporidiosis and giardiasis. These diseases are most often associated with poor husbandry, and incidence in pet animals is unusual. *Cryptosporidium* species has been shown to cause severe diarrhea in a chinchilla.[92] Congregations of animals such as in fur ranches and research colonies often have a high prevalence of infection with *Giardia*. Chinchillas normally harbor *Giardia* species in low numbers.[17] Stress and poor husbandry are believed to cause an increase in *Giardia*, resulting in severe diarrhea and death.[11] However, the role of *Giardia* in causing disease in pet chinchillas is difficult to establish, as giardial protozoa are seen in healthy and sick animals. *Giardia* species can be identified on a fresh, fecal smear (Fig. 24–8). The reports of giardiasis in

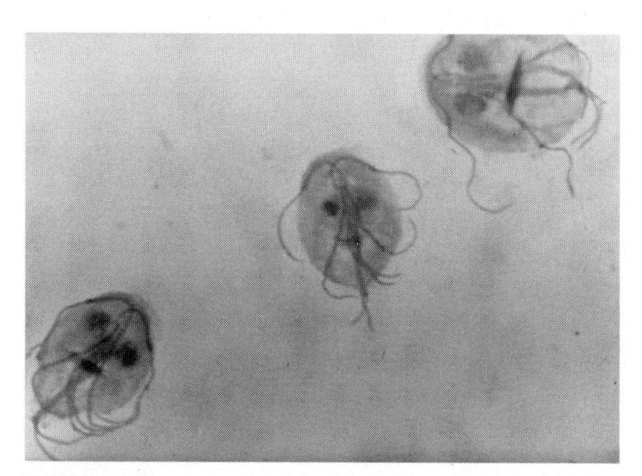

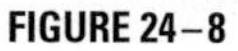

FIGURE 24–8
Wet mount of a fresh fecal sample showing motile trophozoites of *Giardia* species. Notice the prominent pair of nuclei containing a single karyosome of condensed chromatin, flagella running longitudinally between the nuclei, and a pair of curved median bodies. The arrangement of the organelles resembles a wide-eyed face.

pet chinchillas are more frequent on the West coast than the East coast of the United States.[67] Signs of giardiasis in pet chinchillas are reported as cyclic sequence of appetite loss and diarrhea associated with a declining body and fur condition.[67] Until further research on chinchillas is performed, the pathogenicity of *Giardia* species and its association with disease remains controversial. If giardiasis is suspected, it can be treated with metronidazole, albendazole, or fenbendazole (see section on metronidazole toxicity).

Chinchillas are susceptible to pneumonia caused by *Bordetella, Streptococcus, Pasteurella*, and *Pseudomonas* species.[33, 86] Treatment is the same as for guinea pigs.

MISCELLANEOUS DISEASE PROBLEMS OF CHINCHILLAS

Cardiomyopathy

Based on anecdotal reports of cardiomyopathy in two young black velvet females, breeders in the United States have suggested that cardiac problems may exist in chinchillas.[67] Heart murmurs ranging from mild to moderate are described in chinchillas,[67] and murmurs are often auscultated in young chinchillas presented for routine examination.[35] However, there are no reports of cardiac disease in chinchillas, and the relationship of murmurs to cardiac disease is not understood at this time. The exception was a 2-year-old male chinchilla in which a heart murmur was detected as an incidental finding on physical examination.[35] Cardiac ultrasound and electrocardiography revealed a ventricular septal defect and tricuspid regurgitation. (Ultrasound examination of two other animals, one with a murmur and one without, did not reveal abnormalities.) This animal died suddenly, 16 months after initial presentation, during its daily play period. There had been no previous clinical signs. On necropsy there was a marked papillary muscle dysplasia, mitral valve malformation, and a ventricular septal defect. Interestingly, the half-brother of this chinchilla, which also had a heart murmur, died suddenly 1 week before the other animal, but no necropsy was done. Until further investigation is done, ultrasound and echocardiography are probably warranted for any animals in which murmurs are detected. At present, clinical management is empirical.

Metronidazole Toxicosis

Administration of metronidazole has been anecdotally associated with liver failure in chinchillas.[67] It is not known if this was related to toxicity of the drug or a pre-existing condition. Dogs are sensitive to toxic effects of metronidazole and can undergo marked degeneration of Purkinje cells and clinical spasms.[69] These signs have not been reproduced in guinea pigs, mice, rats, or rabbits. Occasional nausea and vomiting are seen in cats on long-term treatment.[69]

Some breeders prefer to use anthelmintic benzimidazoles such as albendazole to treat giardiasis. Interestingly, nitroimidazole drugs such as metronidazole are associated with poor compliance in children compared with adults because the drugs are not well tolerated.[75] Furthermore, recent reports have shown albendazole to be as effective as metronidazole in treating giardial infection in children and with fewer side effects.[16, 29] Until the toxic side effects of metronidazole in chinchillas are established, clinicians may prefer to use albendazole or fenbendazole at a dose of 50–100 mg/kg PO, or 25 mg/kg PO daily for 3 days to treat giardiasis.

Diabetes Mellitus

Diabetes mellitus has been reported in a 5-year-old overweight female chinchilla.[47] The animal had a 3-week history of poor appetite, lethargy, and weight loss. Physical assessment of the chinchilla showed polydipsia, polyuria, and bilateral cataracts. Blood glucose concentration was greater than 400 mg/dL, and urinalysis showed significant glucosuria and ketonuria. Daily treatment with 2 IU insulin was begun, which was increased to 12 IU. The ketonuria and polydipsia resolved, and the blood glucose dropped to 216 mg/dL after 10 days. However, the animal's condition was difficult to stabilize, and hyperglycemia (>400 mg/dL) returned after 2 weeks of therapy. The chinchilla was euthanized, and microscopic examination of pancreatic islets showed prominent vacuolation consistent with diagnosis of diabetes mellitus. Treatment of diabetes mellitus in exotic rodents has been described as difficult.[85] However, regulation of diet is claimed to arrest the disease. High protein, low fat, high complex carbohydrates, and 50 μg of chromium per kilogram of food are suggested.[85]

Neoplasia

Despite the long life span of chinchillas (reported to be up to 20 years) compared with that of other rodents, references on neoplasia in chinchillas are rare. Tumors such as neuroblastoma, carcinoma, lipoma, and hemangioma were listed in the Annual Reports of the San Diego County Livestock Department during the 1950s. Another report in 1953 describes a malignant lymphoma in a chinchilla.[57a] There is, then, a striking absence of reports of neoplasia up to the present. This probably reflects the emphasis on chinchillas as fur producers or research animals.

A 5-year retrospective of chinchillas presented to the Animal Medical Center in New York revealed only one case of a neoplasm, which was an incidental finding at necropsy. A 1-year-old female chinchilla presented for acute onset of neurologic signs caused by chronic otitis media and died shortly after presentation. Necropsy results showed a uterine leiomyosarcoma, and there were no associated metastases. With increasing ownership of pet chinchillas and the increased number of animals being presented for geriatric problems, it is likely that case reports of tumors will be described.

REFERENCES

1. Arika T, Tokoo M, Hase T, et al: Effects of butenafine hydrochloride, a new benzylamine derivative, on experimental dermatophytosis in guinea pigs. Antimicrob Agents Chemother 1990; 34:2250–2253.
2. Bartoszcze M, Matras J, Palec S, et al: *Klebsiella pneumoniae* infection in chinchillas. (letter) Vet Rec 1990; 127:119.
3. Bartoszcze M, Nowakowska M, Rozknowski J, et al: Chinchilla deaths due to *Clostridium perfringens* A enterotoxin. (letter) Vet Rec 1990; 126:341–342.
4. Bendele AM, White SL, Hulamn JF: Osteoarthrosis in guinea pigs: histopathologic and scanning electron microscopic features. Lab Anim Sci 1989; 39:115–121.
5. Boot R, Angulo AF, Walvoort HC: *Clostridium difficile*–associated typhlitis in specific pathogen free guinea pigs in the absence of antimicrobial treatment. Lab Anim 1989; 23:203–207.
6. Boot R, Koopman JP, Kruijt BC, et al: The 'normalization' of germ-free guinea pigs with host-specific caecal microflora. Lab Anim 1989; 23:48–52.
7. Borkowski GL, Griffith JW, Lang CM: Incidence and classification of renal lesions in 240 guinea pigs. Lab Anim Sci 1988; 38:514.
8. Bowden RST: Diseases of chinchillas. Vet Rec 1959; 71:1033–1039.
9. Burtscher H, Otte E: Histoplasme beim Chinchilla (Histoplasma in the chinchilla). Dtsch Tierartzl Wochenschr 1962; 69:303–307.
10. Chrisp CE, Suckow MA, Fayer R, et al: Comparison of the host ranges and antigenicity of *Cryptosporidium parvum* and *Cryptosporidium wrairi* from guinea pigs. J Protozool 1992: 39:406–409.
11. Collins B: Common diseases and medical management of rodents and lagomorphs. *In* Jacobson ER, Kollias GV, eds.: Exotic Animals. New York, Churchill Livingstone, 1988, p. 261–316.
12. Conder GA, Richards IM, Jen L-W: Bronchoalveolar eosinophilia in guinea pigs harboring inapparent infections of *Paraspidodera uncinata.* J Parasitol 1989; 75:144–146.
13. Cousens PJ: The chinchilla in veterinary practice. J Small Anim Pract 1963; 4:199–205.
14. Dall J: Diseases of the chinchilla. J Small Anim Pract 1963; 4:207–212.
15. Doerning BJ, Brammer DW, Rush HG: *Pseudomonas aeruginosa* infection in a *Chinchilla lanigera*. Lab Anim 1993; 27:131–133.
16. Dutta AK, Phadke MA, Bagade AC, et al: A randomised multicentric study to compare the safety and efficacy of albendazole and metronidazole in the treatment of giardiasis in children. Indian J Pediatr 1994; 61:689–693.
17. Eidmann S: Untersuchungen zur Atiologie und Pathogenese von Fellscaden beim Chinchilla (Studies on etiology and pathogenesis of fur damages in the chinchilla). (Thesis [Dr med vet]). Hannover, Tierarztliche Hochschule, 1992.
18. Emily P: Problems peculiar to continually erupting teeth. J Small Exotic Anim Med 1991; 1:56–59.
19. Feldman SH, Richardson JA, Clubb FJ Jr: Necrotizing viral bronchopneumonia in guinea pigs. Lab Anim Sci 1990; 40:82–83.
20. Field KJ, Griffith JW, Lang CM: Spontaneous reproductive tract leiomyomas in aged guinea-pigs. J Comp Pathol 1989; 101:287–294.
21. Finley GG, Long JR: An epizootic of listeriosis in chinchillas. Can Vet J 1977; 18:164–167.
22. Fish RE, Besch-Williford C: Reproductive disorders in the rabbit and guinea pig. *In* Kirk RW, Bonagura JD, eds.: Kirk's Current Veterinary Therapy. Vol XI. Philadelphia, WB Saunders, 1992, p 1175–1179.
23. Fritz PE, Hurst WJ, White WJ, et al: Pharmacokinetics of cefazolin in guinea pigs. Lab Anim Sci 1987; 37:646–651.
24. Gibson SV, Wagner JE: Cryptosporidiosis in guinea pigs: a retrospective study. J Am Vet Med Assoc 1986; 189: 1033–1034.
25. Goycoolea MV, Muchow DC, Goycoolea HG: Otitis media. 16 years of pathogenesis approach. Otolaryngol Clin North Am 1991; 24:967–980.
26. Griffith JW, Lang CM: Vitamin E and selenium status of guinea pigs with myocardial necrosis. Lab Anim Sci 1987; 37:776–779.
27. Griner LA: Pathology of Zoo Animals. San Diego, Zoological Society of San Diego, 1983.
28. Gupta BN, Langham RF, Conner GH: Mastitis in guinea pigs. Am J Vet Res 1970; 31:1703–1707.
29. Hall A, Nahar Q: Albendazole as a treatment for infections with *Giardia duodenalis* in children in Bangladesh. Trans R Soc Trop Med Hyg 1993; 87:84–86.
30. Harkness JE: A Practitioners Guide to Domestic Rodents. Denver, American Animal Hospital Association (AAHA), 1993.
31. Harkness JE, Wagner JE: The Biology and Medicine of Rabbits and Rodents, 4th ed. Baltimore, Williams & Wilkins, 1995.
32. Hartmann K: Haltungsbedingte Erkrankungen beim Chinchilla (Husbandry-related diseases in the chinchilla). Tierarztl Prax 1993; 21:574–580.

33. Hoefer HL: Chinchillas. Vet Clin North Am Small Anim Pract 1994; 24:103–111.
34. Hoefer HL: Chinchillas. *In* Proceedings of The North American Veterinary Conference. Vol 9. Gainesville, Eastern States Veterinary Association, 1995, pp 672–673.
35. Hoefer HL: Clinical management of the chinchilla & hedgehog. In Proceedings of The Avian/Exotic Animal Medicine Symposium. Davis, CA, School of Veterinary Medicine at the University of California, 1966, pp 87–91.
36. Jaax GP, Jaax NK, Petrali JP, et al: Coronavirus-like virions associated with a wasting syndrome in guinea pigs. Lab Anim Sci 1990; 40:375–378.
37. Jenkins JR: Husbandry and common diseases of the chinchilla (*Chinchilla laniger*). J Small Exotic Anim Med 1992; 2:15–17.
38. Jones AK: Cesarean section in a chinchilla (letter) Vet Rec 1990; 126:441.
39. Keagy HF: Toxoplasma in the chinchilla. J Am Vet Med Assoc 1949; 94:15.
40. Keagy HF, Keagy EH: Epizootic gastroenteritis in chinchillas. J Am Vet Med Assoc 1951; 118:35–37.
41. Keller LSF, Griffith JW, Lang CM: Reproductive failure associated with cystic rete ovarii in guinea pigs. J Vet Pathol 1987; 24:335–339.
42. Kirchner BK, Lake SG, Wightman SR: Isolation of *Streptobacillus moniliformis* from a guinea pig with granulomatous pneumonia. Lab Anim Sci 1992; 42:519–521.
43. Kline A: After forty years, Alice Kline talks about chinchillas. Utica, IL, Starved Rock Chinchilla (privately printed), 1990.
44. Kummel BA, Estes SA, Arlian LG: *Trixacarus caviae* infestation of guinea pigs. J Am Vet Med Assoc 1980; 177:9031.
45. Larrivee GP, Elvehjem CA: Disease problems in chinchillas. J Am Vet Med Assoc 1954; 124:447–455.
46. Lipman NS, Weischedel AK, Connors MJ, et al: Utilization of cholestyramine resin as a preventive treatment for antibiotic (clindamycin) induced enterotoxaemia in the rabbit. Lab Anim 1992; 26:1–8.
47. Marlow C: Diabetes in a chinchilla. (letter) Vet Rec 1995; 136:595–596.
48. Manning PJ, Wagner JE, Harkness JE: Biology and diseases of guinea pigs. *In* Fox JG, Cohen BJ, Loew FM, eds.: Laboratory Animal Medicine. Orlando, Academic Press, 1984, p 149–181.
49. McGreevy PD, Carn VM: Intestinal torsion in a chinchilla. (letter) Vet Rec 1988; 122:287.
50. McKellar QA, Midgley DM, Galbraith EA, et al: Clinical and pharmacological properties of ivermectin in rabbits and guinea pigs. Vet Rec 1992; 130:71–73.
51. Menchaca ES, Martin AM: Enfermedades infecciosas de la chinchilla (*Chinchilla lanigera*). III. *Proteus mirabilis* y *Proteus vulgaris* (Infectious diseases of the chinchilla [Chinchilla lanigera]. III. Proteus mirabilis and Proteus vulgaris). Gac Veterinaria 1978; 40:651–656.
52. Merry CJ: An introduction to chinchillas. Vet Tech 1990; 11:315–322.
53. Moore RW, Greenlee HH: Enterotoxemia in chinchillas. Lab Anim 1975; 9:153–154.
54. Morgan RV, Moore FM, Pearce LK, et al: Clinical and laboratory findings in small companion animals with lead poisoning: 347 cases (1977–1986). J Am Vet Med Assoc 1991; 199:93–97.
55. Morgan RV, Moore FM, Pearce LK, et al: Demographic data and treatment of small companion animals with lead poisoning: 347 cases (1977–1986). J Am Vet Med Assoc 1991; 199:98–102.
56. Mountain A: *Salmonella arizona* in a chinchilla. (letter) Vet Rec 1989; 125:25.
57. Newberne PM: An outbreak of bacterial gastroenteritis in the South American Chinchilla. North Am Vet 1953; 34:187–191.

57a. Newberne PM, Seibold HR: Malignant lymphoma in a chinchilla. Vet Med 1953; 48:428–429.

58. Nishikimi M, Kawai T, Yagi K: Guinea pigs possess a highly mutated gene for L-gulono-γ-lactone oxidase, the key enzyme for L-ascorbic acid biosynthesis missing in this species. J Biol Chem 1992; 267:21967–21972.
59. Okewole PA, Odeyemis PS, Oladummade MA, et al: An outbreak of *Streptococcus pyogenes* infection associated with calcium oxalate urolithiasis in guinea pigs (*Cavia porcellus*). Lab Anim 1991; 25:184–186.
60. Okewole PA, Uche EMI, Oyetunde IL, et al: Uterine involvement in guinea pig salmonellosis. Lab Anim 1989; 23:275–277.
61. Owens DR, Menges RW, Sprouse RF, et al: Naturally occurring histoplasmosis in the chinchilla (*Chinchilla laniger*). J Clin Microbiol 1975; 1:486–488.
62. Peng X, Griffith JW, Lang CM: Cystitis and cystic calculi in aged guinea pigs. Lab Anim Sci 1987; 34:527.
63. Prior JE: Cesarean section in the chinchilla. (letter) Vet Rec 1986; 119:408.
64. Rakich PM, Dubey JP, Contarino JK: Acute hepatic sarcocystosis in a chinchilla. J Vet Diag Invest 1992; 4:484–486.
65. Rehg JE, Yarbrough BA, Pakes SP: Toxicity of cecal filtrates from guinea pigs with penicillin-associated colitis. Lab Anim Sci 1980; 30:524–531.
66. Richardson V: Ivermectin in guinea pigs. (letter) Vet Rec 1992; 130:432.
67. Ritchey L, Cogswell M: The Joy of Chinchillas, 3rd ed. Menlo Park, CA (privately printed), 1995.
68. Roberto M, Zito F, Hamernik R: Interazione tra rumore continuo ed impulsivo: valutazione anatomica e funzionale in rapporto al valore energetico dell'esposizione (Interaction between continuous and impulse noise: anatomic and functional evaluation in relation to the intensity of the exposure). Acta Otorhinolaryngol Ital 1992; 12:451–459.
69. Rossoff IS: Handbook of Veterinary Drugs and Chemicals, 2nd ed. Taylorville, IL, Pharmtox Publishing Co, 1994.
70. Rothwell TL, Pope SE, Rajczyk ZK, et al: Haematological and pathological responses to experimental *Trixacarus caviae* infection in guinea pigs. J Comp Pathol 1991; 104:179–185.
71. Rubel GA, Isenburgel E, Wolverkamp P: Atlas of Diagnostic Radiology of Exotic Pets. Philadelphia, WB Saunders, 1991.
72. Sanford SE: Cerebral nematodiasis caused by the raccoon ascarid (*Baylisascaris procyonis*) in chinchillas. Can Vet J 1989; 30:902.
73. Sanford SE: Cerebrospinal nematodiasis caused by *Baylisascaris procyonis* in chinchillas. J Vet Diagn Invest 1991; 3:77–79.
74. Shaull EM: Fur quality and fur breakage in the chinchilla. Chinchilla World 1988; 37:9.
75. Shepherd RW, Boreham PF: Recent advances in the diagnosis and management of giardiasis. Scand J Gastroenterol 1989; 169:60–64.
76. Spink RR: Urolithiasis in a guinea pig. Vet Med Small Anim Clin 1978; 73:501–502.
77. Stephenson EH, Trahan CJ, Ezzell JW, et al: Efficacy of a commercial bacterin in protecting strain 13 guinea pigs against *Bordetella bronchiseptica* penumonia. Lab Anim 1989; 23:261–269.
78. Stephenson RS: Cesarean section in a chinchilla. (letter) Vet Rec 1990; 126:370.
79. Suckow MA, Chrisp CE, Rush HG: Cryptosporidiosis in immunocompetent guinea pigs. Lab Anim Sci 1989; 39:470.

80. Timm KI: Pruritus in rabbits, rodents, and ferrets. Vet Clin North Am Small Anim Pract 1988; 18:1077–1091.
81. Vanjonack WJ, Johnson WD: Relationship of thyroid and adrenal function to fur-chewing in the chinchilla. Comp Biochem Physiol 1973; 45:115–120.
82. Waggie KS, Thornburg LP, Grove KJ, et al: Lesions of experimentally induced Tyzzer's disease in Syrian hamsters, guinea pigs, mice and rats. Lab Anim 1987; 21:155–160.
83. Waggie KS, Wagner JE, Kelley ST: Naturally occurring *Bacillus piliformis* infection (Tyzzer's disease) in guinea pigs. Lab Anim Sci 1986; 36:504–506.
84. Wagner JE, Manning PJ, eds.: The Biology of the Guinea Pig. New York, Academic Press, 1976.
85. Wallach JD, Boever WJ: Diseases of Exotic Animals. Philadelphia, WB Saunders, 1983, pp 135–195.
86. Webb RA: Chinchillas. *In* Beynon PH, Cooper JE, eds.: Manual of Exotic Pets, New Edition. Cheltenham, British Small Animal Veterinary Association, 1991, pp 15–21.
87. Webb RA: Ivermectin in guinea pigs. (letter) Vet Rec 1992; 130:307.
88. Weir BJ: Chinchilla. *In* Hafez ESE, ed.: Reproduction and Breeding Techniques for Laboratory Animals. Philadelphia, Lea & Febiger, 1970, 209–223.
89. Williams CSF: Practical Guide to Laboratory Animals. St. Louis, MO, CV Mosby, 1976, pp 3–11.
90. Witt WM, Hubbard GB, Fanton JW: *Streptococcus pneumoniae* arthritis and osteomyelitis with vitamin C deficiency in guinea pigs. Lab Anim Sci 1988; 38:192–194.
91. Wood JS Jr, Bennett IL Jr, Yardley JH: Staphylococcal enterocolitis in chinchillas. Bull Johns Hopkins Hosp 1956; 98:454–463.
92. Yamini B, Raju NR: Gastroenteritis associated with a *Cryptosporidium* sp in a chinchilla. J Am Vet Med Assoc 1986; 189:1158–1159.
93. Young JD, Hurst WJ, White WJ, et al: An evaluation of ampicillin pharmacokinetics and toxicity in guinea pigs. Lab Anim Sci 1987; 37:652–656.

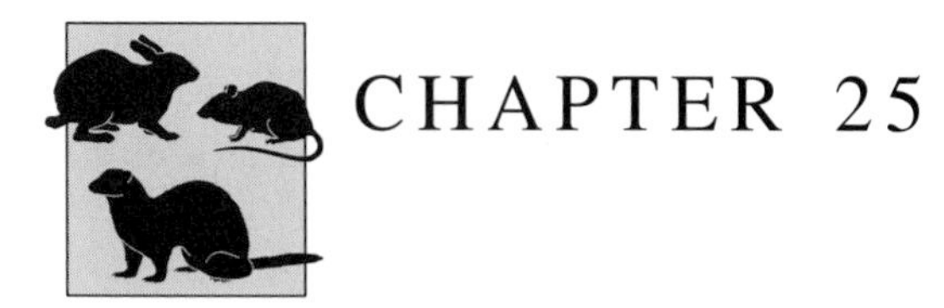

CHAPTER 25

Soft Tissue Surgery

Holly Mullen, DVM

Little clinical information on the surgery of pet guinea pigs has been published; even less information on that of chinchillas is available. Guinea pigs are common and popular pets; pet chinchillas are less common. Both species are members of the order Rodentia and have similar anatomy, disease susceptibility, and surgical conditions. Because of the scarcity of information on chinchilla surgery, this chapter addresses surgery of guinea pigs unless otherwise noted.

Guinea pigs and chinchillas have a thin subcutis and a wide, easily visible linea alba. Guinea pig skin is relatively thicker than that of chinchillas. Although rodents in general have a reputation for chewing at their surgical incisions and sutures, I have found this is uncommon in these two species.

Anesthesia of these species can be challenging. Orotracheal intubation is extremely difficult, if not impossible, in most cases.[1] Inhalation anesthetic can be administered after an injectable anesthetic has been given. I prefer to induce anesthesia with isoflurane by mask or induction chamber and to maintain anesthesia with oxygen and isoflurane by mask for the duration of the procedure.

Respiratory secretions can be thick and copious. Atropine or glycopyrrolate are not usually helpful at controlling these secretions. Guinea pigs also are prone to gastric reflux when under anesthesia and should be fasted for 2–4 hours before induction. For these reasons, and because tracheal intubation is unlikely to occur, I prefer to position the guinea pig so that the head and chest are slightly higher than the abdomen while the animal is recumbent. This position does appear to reduce aspiration and improve respiration during general anesthesia. As with any species, intraoperative and postoperative administration of analgesics is indicated for most procedures. Specific drugs and dosages are given in Chapter 32.

OVARIOHYSTERECTOMY

The uterus is bicornuate in guinea pigs. The ovaries are located caudolateral to the kidneys and are approximately 8 mm in length and 5 mm in width. The uterine body terminates in a single os cervix. A well-developed intercornual ligament also is present.[1,7]

Ovariohysterectomy in guinea pigs is similar to that in ferrets, dogs, and cats. The broad ligaments contain a large amount of fat that can make identification of the ovarian pedicles difficult. The suspensory ligaments are not usually significant. Carefully dissect through the fat to find the ovarian vessels and doubly ligate them with 3–0 or 4–0 absorbable suture material. Strip the broad ligament back to the uterine arteries and uterine body and doubly ligate the vessels with the body. The ovaries and uterus are removed as a unit. Closure of the abdomen is routine; use 4–0 absorbable or nonabsorbable suture for the linea, and 5–0 absorbable suture for the subcutaneous/subcuticular closure. If necessary, use 4–0 or 5–0 nonabsorbable suture or tissue adhesive to close the skin.

PYOMETRA

Pyometra is infrequently reported in guinea pigs and chinchillas. Possible pathogens include *Escherichia coli, Corynebacterium pyogenes,* and *Staphylococcus* and *Streptococcus* species.[8] Affected animals usually are presented with vaginal discharge and may be lethargic and anorectic. One guinea pig owner reported polydipsia and decreased appetite. Treatment is ovariohysterectomy. Recovery is usually uneventful.

UTERINE TORSION

Uterine torsion is uncommon in most domestic pets but has been reported to occur in gravid guinea pigs at greater than 30 days' gestation and in gravid chinchillas.[8] Signs include shock and acute collapse. The mortality rate is high; the diagnosis is usually made post mortem. Treatment is emergency ovariohysterectomy.

DYSTOCIA

Dystocia is common in guinea pigs because of the relatively large fetal size of these animals.[4, 8] Guinea pigs should be bred before they are 6–9 months of age, when bony fusion of the pubic symphysis occurs and fat accumulates in the pelvic canal. If the symphysis fuses before the first litter is delivered, dystocia inevitably results.[4] If a guinea pig delivers a litter before bony fusion has occurred, then cartilaginous fusion is preserved and future litters are possible without dystocia.

Gestation lasts approximately 59–72 days in guinea pigs and 111 days in chinchillas. Average litter size is three to four in guinea pigs and two in chinchillas (range, one to six). Guinea pigs are sexually mature at 60–90 days of age, whereas chinchillas reach maturity later, at 150–270 days.

Approximately 10 days before delivery, the pubic symphysis of the sow (female guinea pig) begins to spread. The symphysis is about 1.5–3 cm wide at birth. This spreading can be palpated externally and is an impending sign of parturition.[4]

If the symphysis is open, or if the sow has had a previous litter without intervention and the sow has been in unproductive labor for longer than 30–60 minutes, 0.1–3.0 U/kg of oxytocin may be given subcutaneously. If no young are delivered after 15 minutes, surgical intervention is necessary.[5]

Dystocia in guinea pigs and chinchillas can be surgically treated by either cesarean section or ovariohysterectomy of the gravid uterus. For either procedure, make a routine ventral midline abdominal incision and exteriorize the gravid uterus. For the cesarean section, pack off the gravid uterus and make a transverse or longitudinal incision in the dorsal or ventral uterine body. Deliver the neonates to your assistants and close the incision with a single interrupted layer or double continuous layer of 3–0 or 4–0 absorbable suture material. Lavage the abdomen and close routinely.

For en-bloc ovariohysterectomy of the gravid uterus, the technique is similar to that of the routine ovariohysterectomy. After ligating and dividing the ovarian pedicles, clamp the uterine vessels and body and transect and remove the gravid uterus. An assistant opens the uterus and removes and revives the neonates. Ligate the uterine pedicle routinely; closure is likewise routine. Viability of the neonates is not affected by this procedure, and contamination of the abdomen by uterine contents is avoided. If the uterus is exceptionally large or engorged with blood and the sow is anemic, the en-bloc technique should probably not be used. If ovariohysterectomy is necessary, a cesarean section should be performed first. The uterus is allowed to involute before removal, returning some blood to the peripheral circulation.

Guinea pig young are precocious at birth. Their eyes are open, they can move about well, and they can eat solid foods; however, they may be allowed to nurse as soon as the sow has recovered from anesthesia.

MAMMARY GLAND NEOPLASIA

Mammary gland neoplasia is uncommon in older guinea pigs and chinchillas and is even rarer in animals younger than 3 years of age.[5] Both male and female guinea pigs have mammary glands located inguinally as a single pair.[7] Neoplasms of the glands, both benign and malignant, have been reported to occur in both sexes. Most mammary tumors in guinea pigs are benign. The most common histologic type is the fibroadenoma. Adenocarcinomas are less common but are the most frequently reported malignant mammary tumor in guinea pigs. A few cases have occurred in males, and metastasis to other organs (lungs, lymph nodes, abdominal viscera) has been reported.[6]

The left and right inguinal mammary glands do not appear to have common blood or lymphatic communication. If a mammary gland tumor is detected in one gland, mammectomy of that gland with removal and biopsy of the gland and associated inguinal lymph node is recommended. Excision should include all mammary tissue on that side. Plan carefully for adequate closure, since there is not an abundance of tissue in this area. Make an elliptical incision around the affected gland and dissect the gland and its deep subcutaneous tissue. Locate and ligate the caudal superficial epigastric artery and vein exiting the inguinal ring and doubly ligate them before they enter the tissue to be excised. Locate and remove the inguinal lymph node. Close the deep subcutaneous and subcuticular layers with 4–0 absorbable suture. Close the skin with 4–0 or 5–0 nonabsorbable suture or with tissue adhesive.

If bilateral mammary tumors are present (these have been rare in my experience), unilateral mastectomies may be done 3–4 weeks apart, as delay facilitates closure of the area. In one case, delay was not possible, and a bilateral mastectomy was done. A rotation flap from the ventral abdomen was used to close the considerable defect. The flap was under moderate tension, but the repair healed uneventfully.

CASTRATION

Castration is performed in pet guinea pigs for population control or to prevent a male (boar) from breeding with intact females for which pregnancy would not be safe (e.g., those with a closed pubic symphysis). No information is available on the incidence of testicular tumors in boars, and I have not encountered a case.

The inguinal rings of the boar are open, and the large testes are easily retracted into the abdomen.[3, 8] Castration is not difficult but must be done by the closed method. Alternatively, the inguinal rings can be closed; however, this requires a more extensive approach and is not necessary if the tunic is closed.

Position the anesthetized boar in dorsal recumbency with the rear limbs spread. Gently shave the hair from the scrotum to allow for a sterile field approximately 3 × 4 cm in size. After sterile surgical preparation, use sterile towels or adhesive drapes to secure the field. I prefer a clear adhesive drape that covers the patient but allows visual monitoring of respirations.

Palpate both testes. Do not confuse the body of the penis with a testicle! The penis can feel similar to a testicle under the skin, especially if one testicle is retained in the abdomen. The testes are wider and rounder than the body of the penis, which is located on the midline and, unlike the testicles, cannot be pushed back into the abdomen. If one testicle is retained in the abdomen, gentle caudoventral pressure results in its prolapse into the scrotum.

Holding one testicle between the thumb and forefinger, make a 1-cm incision through the skin and the subcutis over it approximately 1 cm lateral to the penis. Expose the testicle in its tunic and retract it from the incision. Doubly ligate and transfix the testicular pedicle in a closed fashion with 3–0 absorbable suture. Transect the cord and remove the testicle. The closed stump will retract into the incision. Close the tunic if it is accidentally cut or torn. If it is not possible to close the tunic, the incision must be extended cranially and the inguinal ring closed in order to prevent the herniation of abdominal contents.

Although, the skin incision may be left open, I prefer to close it with 5–0 absorbable suture or tissue adhesive. The procedure is repeated on the other side. Recovery is rapid.

CYSTOTOMY

Cystic calculi are relatively common in guinea pigs. However, urinary tract blockage is rare and occurs mostly in males due to matrix plugs of sperm and seminal vesicle fluid.[7] Guinea pigs have naturally cloudy urine because of the excretion of calcium. Most calculi are calcium oxalates and carbonates.[8] The presence of calculi is the primary differential diagnosis for hematuria in guinea pigs.[3]

Calculi may be found in the urethra, bladder, ureters, and renal pelves. Ureteral calculi are usually located at the distal bend of the ureters as they enter the bladder. If a calculus is obstructing all or part of the ureteral lumen, it should be removed if possible. If the kidney on the affected side is nonfunctional or severely hydronephrotic, it may be necessary to perform a nephrectomy and ureterectomy in order to remove the calculus, which is a nidus for further urinary tract infection. Surgical removal is the treatment of choice for cystic calculi.

Make a caudal, ventral midline incision, exteriorize the bladder, and examine the urinary tract carefully. If possible, place an indwelling urinary catheter in males with multiple small cystic calculi to prevent the lodging of a stone that is too large to pass normograde in the urethra during surgery.

If a distal ureteral stone is present, gently manipulate it toward the bladder, where it can be removed during cystotomy. Ureterotomy should not be done unless the surgeon is experienced in microsurgical techniques. Ureterotomy may be done if the ureter is sufficiently dilated by the presence of the obstructing calculus to allow primary ureteral closure with 6–0 or 7–0 absorbable suture. In my experience, the ureter is not usually dilated, and the calculus cannot usually be moved from its position in the ureter by gentle palpation. In this case, the ureteral calculus is left within the ureter.

Exteriorize the bladder and pack it off from the surrounding viscera with moistened sterile sponges. Make a 5- to 10-mm incision in either the craniodorsal or cranioventral aspect of the bladder and remove the calculi. Culture the bladder mucosa and crush part of a calculus for culture. Submit the rest for calculus analysis.

Flush the bladder and urethra with sterile saline and close with either a single-layer, simple interrupted or a double-layer, continuous, inverting suture pattern. Use absorbable, monofilament 4–0 or 5–0 suture material. Lavage the caudal abdomen. Close the linea, subcutaneous tissue, and skin in routine fashion. Hematuria may persist for several days postoperatively; this is normal. Postoperative dietary management includes limiting access to alfalfa hays.

CUTANEOUS DERMAL MASSES

Skin and subcutaneous tumors are the second most frequently reported neoplasms in guinea pigs.[2, 6] Frequently, these grow considerably before the animal is presented (Fig. 25–1). Most are benign trichofolliculoma, trichoepithelioma, or sebaceous adenoma,

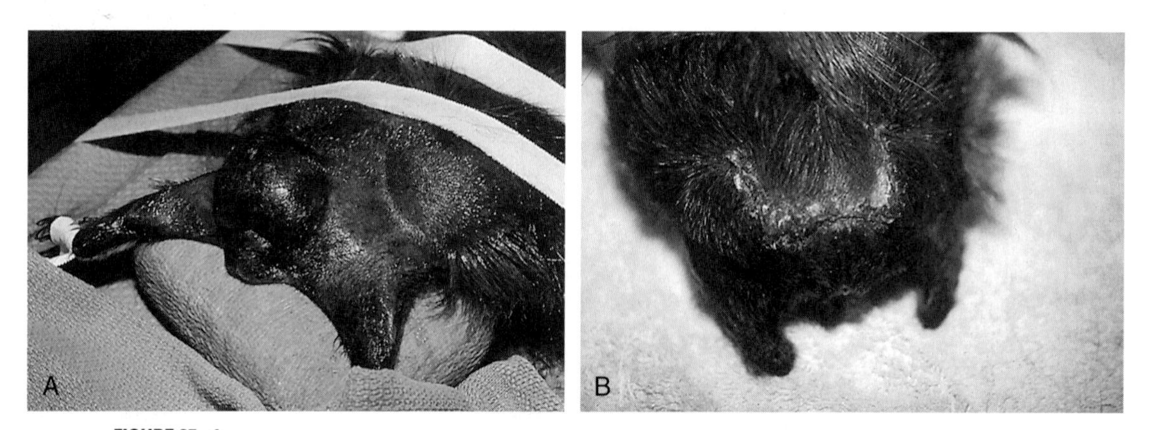

FIGURE 25–1
A, A large sebaceous cyst on the rump of a guinea pig positioned and prepped for surgical removal. *B,* The same guinea pig 2 weeks after surgery.

all of which are typically cystic. These cysts may contain sebum, hair, and keratin debris. Other neoplasms reported to occur in and under the skin include fibroma, fibrosarcoma, fibrolipoma, lipoma, and undifferentiated sarcoma and adenocarcinoma.[6] Aspiration of sebaceous debris from a cutaneous mass suggests the presence of one of the benign cystic neoplasms.

Excision of the mass and definitive biopsy are recommended. Even benign cysts can become infected, and this requires medical management of the sick guinea pig. Guinea pigs have a moderate amount of loose skin over the dorsum, but excision of very large masses may require undermining or skin flaps and creative closure of the defect.

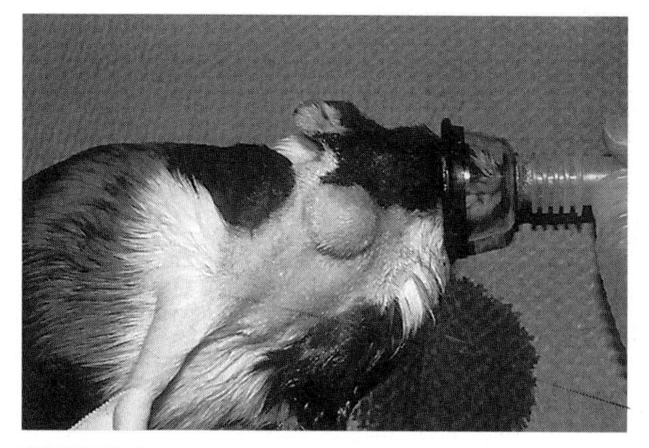

FIGURE 25–2
Cervical lymphadenitis in a guinea pig.

CERVICAL LYMPHADENITIS

Cervical lymphadenitis, a condition known as "lumps" in guinea pigs, is a streptococcal infection of the cervical lymph nodes that is believed to occur secondary to oral mucous membrane trauma and usually results in lymph node abscessation (Fig. 25–2).[5] The optimal treatment is surgical excision of any involved lymph nodes. Provide supportive care and antibiotic therapy based on the results of culture and sensitivity testing of samples taken at surgery. Even with total excision of all grossly infected tissue, the condition can recur shortly after surgery in adjacent tissues. If excision is impossible, lance, drain, and flush all abscesses as in dogs and cats, leaving the wounds open to heal by second intention.

For frustrating cases, a final option to halt recurrence of infection is silver nitrate cautery of open wounds followed by copious flushing with sterile saline. Silver nitrate is very destructive to tissues. Leave the wound open to heal secondarily.

Isolate affected guinea pigs from other guinea pigs until the condition has resolved.

MISCELLANEOUS PROCEDURES

Abdominal exploratory surgery for an abdominal mass in guinea pigs and chinchillas is infrequently performed. Hepatic cyst or neoplasia, uterine neoplasia (Fig. 25–3), ovarian cyst or neoplasia, and gastrointestinal obstruction are the most common reasons for exploratory laparotomy.

Ovarian cysts are seen in middle-aged to older sows. Bilaterally symmetrical, nonpruritic alopecia along the back, flanks, and rump is often present and is the usual reason for presentation by the owner. A fluctuant abdominal mass may be palpable. Ultrasonography aids in differentiation of a cyst from an ovarian tumor. A temporary response may occur with the administration of 100 IU (1000 USP units) of human chorionic gonadotropin administered intramuscularly in two doses given 2 weeks apart.[3] Ovariohysterectomy is the treatment of choice.

Ovarian tumors, most commonly teratomas, may be identified in sows older than 3 years of age.[2] Some of these teratomas may be as large as 10 cm in diameter.[6] They are usually unilateral and rarely metastasize. The most frequent reason for presentation is depression, weakness, or collapse from spontaneous intra-abdominal hemorrhage from the tumor. Acute death from hypovolemia may occur.

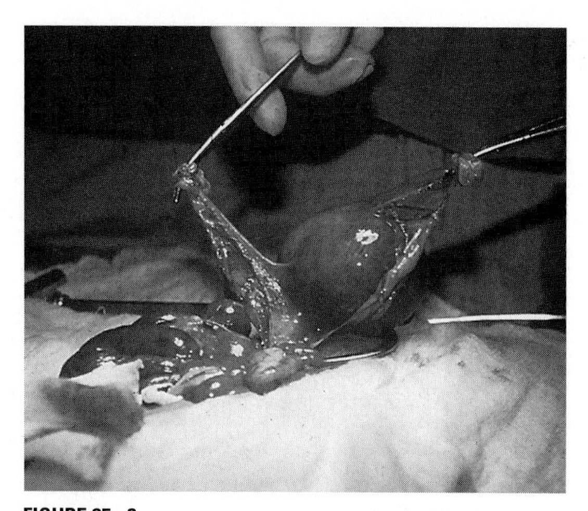

FIGURE 25–3
A right uterine horn leiomyoma in a 4-year-old guinea pig with a palpable abdominal mass.

Ovariohysterectomy is the treatment of choice for these tumors.

Pulmonary tumors are the most common spontaneously occurring neoplasms in guinea pigs. Most primary pulmonary tumors are benign bronchogenic papillary adenomas.[6] Bronchogenic and alveologenic adenocarcinomas are also seen. All of these tumor types tend to start at the periphery of the lung lobe and grow slowly, remaining asymptomatic for a long period. Because routine thoracic radiography is rarely performed, detection of an intrathoracic mass is unlikely in early stages of growth. If a pulmonary mass were detected sufficiently early, lateral thoracotomy performed through the sixth to eighth intercostal spaces (the area of the pulmonary hilus) would allow lobectomy of the affected lung.

Etiology and management of pododermatitis is discussed in Chapter 24. These fibrous granulomas of the plantar surface of the feet are usually seen in guinea pigs kept on wire floors. Prognosis is guarded; many lesions recur following treatment. I have had some success with aggressive excision of the lesions followed by bandaging and open-wound management (allowing the surgical wounds to granulate and re-epithelialize). Bedding material should be changed to a soft substance for the remainder of the animal's life.

REFERENCES

1. Cooper G, Schiller A: Anatomy of the Guinea Pig. Cambridge, MA, Harvard University Press, 1975.
2. Cooper JE: Tips on tumors. Proceedings of the North American Veterinary Conference, Orlando, January 1994, pp 897–898.
3. Hillyer EV: Common clinical maladies of pet rodents. Proceedings of the North American Veterinary Conference, Orlando, January 1994, pp 909–910.
4. Peters LJ: The guinea pig: an overview, part I. Compend Contin Educ Pract Vet 1991; 4:15–19.
5. Peters LJ: The guinea pig: an overview, part II. Compend Contin Educ Pract Vet 1991; 5:20–27.
6. Toft JD: Commonly observed spontaneous neoplasms in rabbits, rats, guinea pigs, hamsters and gerbils. Semin Avian Exotic Pet Med 1991; 1:80–92.
7. Wagner JE, Manning PJ: The Biology of the Guinea Pig. New York, Academic Press, 1976.
8. Wallach JD, Boever WJ: Diseases of Exotic Animals: Medical and Surgical Management. Philadelphia, WB Saunders, 1983.

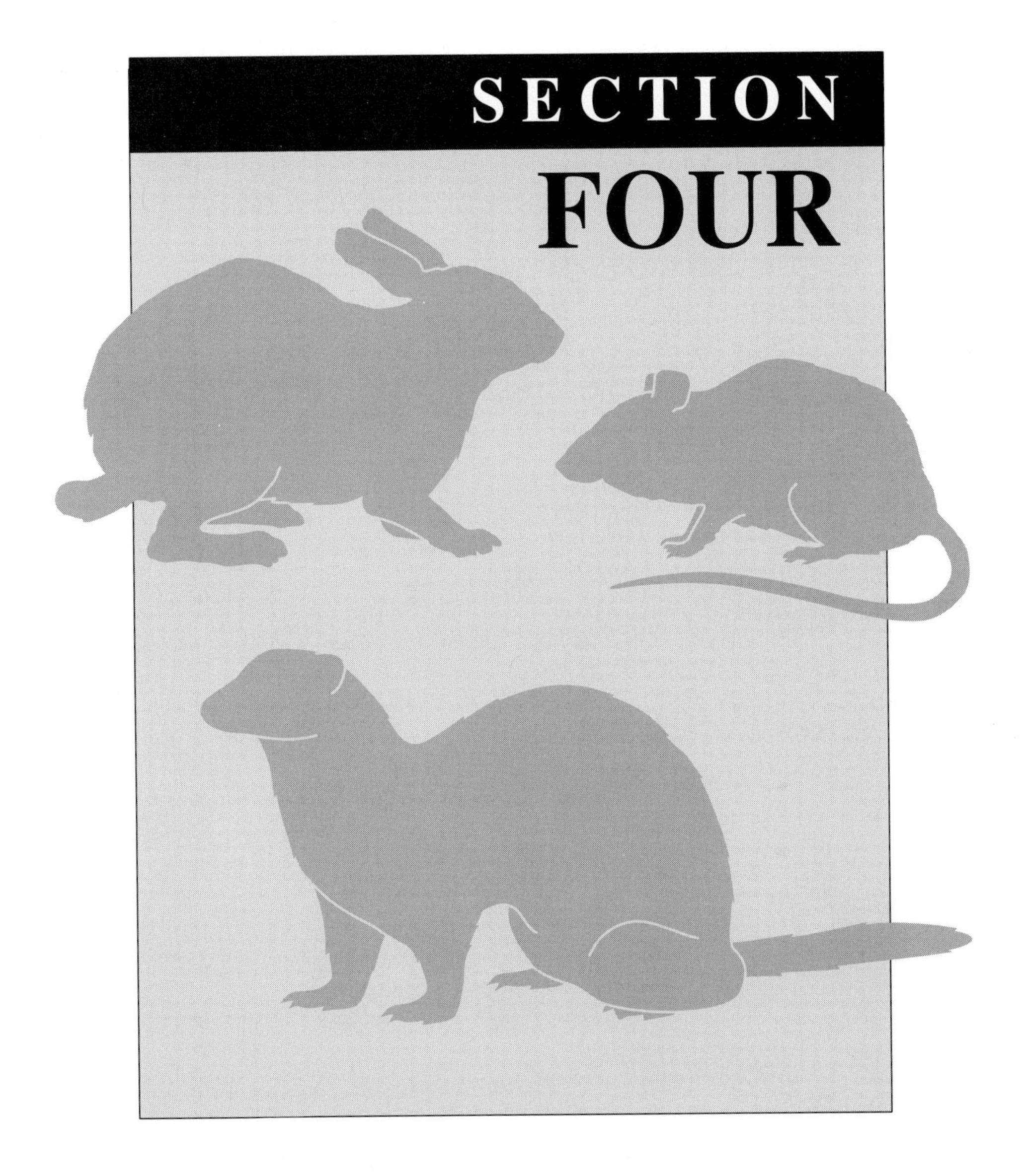

Small Rodents

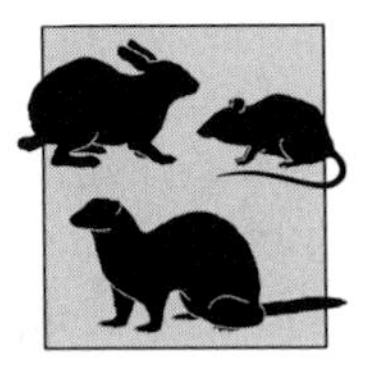

CHAPTER 26

Basic Anatomy, Physiology, Husbandry, and Clinical Techniques

Louise Bauck, DVM
and Craig Bihun, DVM, DVSc

PART I

Louise Bauck, DVM

The traditional small rodent pets such as the golden hamster, the white mouse, the gerbil, and the rat all continue to remain popular but have been supplemented by color and coat varieties not formerly available and by species such as the Siberian or dwarf hamster (*Phodopus sungorus*) (Fig. 26–1), the Chinese hamster (*Cricetus griseus*), the spiny mouse (*Heteromys* species) or rat (*Proechimys* species), the degu (*Octodon* species), the chinchilla (*Chinchilla laniger*), the jerboa (*Jaculus jaculus*), and the African pygmy mouse (*Baiomys* species). Unfortunately, very little specific husbandry and medical information on the newly introduced exotic species is available; however, in general, nutritional requirements and husbandry details are similar for many of these small rodents. Degus and chinchillas are actually hystricomorph rodents related to the guinea pig. Spiny rats and mice have a buff-colored coat with a coarse or spiny appearance, are medium-sized (150–200 g), and are characterized by large, attractive ears. Pygmy mice are among the smallest of mammals (each weighing approximately 10 g). They have a rich brown dorsal surface and white abdomen. They scamper very quickly and for this reason are difficult to catch and handle.

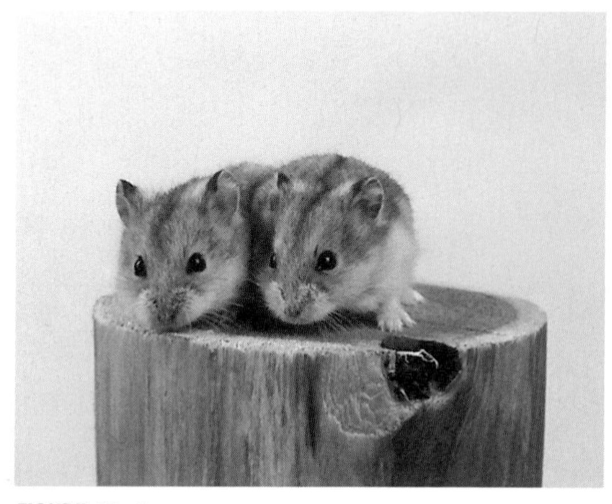

FIGURE 26–1
A pair of dwarf hamsters (*Phodopus* species).

GENERAL CHARACTERISTICS

Mice

Standard laboratory mice (*Mus musculus*) are generally white but also are available in pet varieties, including satin (shining hair coat), long-haired, pied (spotted) (Fig. 26–2), and various solid colors. An adult mouse weighs approximately 30 g. Most mice make good pets for older children (10 years of age and up). Mice rarely bite but may scamper quickly, and thus younger children may not be able to handle them. Mice are largely nocturnal but are easily roused. Female mice are much recommended over males because they are less odorous. Mice are hardy pets and rarely suffer from infectious disease; however, mite infestations are common and are difficult to treat. Mammary tumors may plague older animals. Male mice are aggressive toward each other, but female mice often get along well.

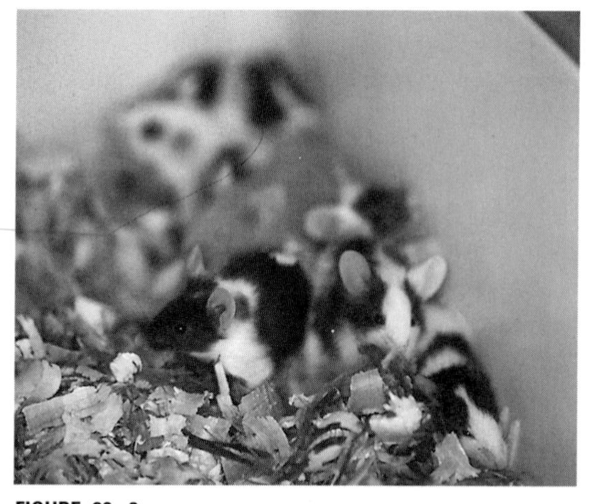

FIGURE 26–2
A group of pied mice.

Rats

Rats (*Rattus norvegicus*) are most popular in the pet market in hooded color varieties, in which the coat color is present only over the head and shoulders. Other color varieties are not as popular. Rats are hardy as young animals but may suffer from obesity, chronic respiratory disease, and mammary tumors when older. Rats are large enough to be easily grasped by children, and they rarely bite. Some may be excitable and run when removed from their cages; however, rats have been known to return to their cage after an "escape."[1] Male and female rats get along well, and males may be present while females are raising a litter. Rats are relatively intelligent and seem interested in humans; they can be trained to come when called for a treat.

Hamsters

The most common hamster kept as a pet is the golden hamster (*Mesocricetus auratus*). Hamsters are the least hardy of the small rodents when newly purchased, and stress-related diseases such as proliferative ileitis are common. Hamsters are usually large and slow enough for children to hold. They are nocturnal, but if they are scooped up gently with two hands, they generally awaken without attempting to bite. Touching a hamster's back with a finger in an attempt to rouse it is likely to provoke a start or a threat response. Excited hamsters often jump from hands or tables, and thus appropriate caution should be used when they are handled. Hamsters are available in many color varieties and in a long-haired ("teddy bear") breed. All hamsters are well known for their ability to escape; most chewing behavior can be attributed to their attempts to escape. Chewed or damaged cage parts should be replaced immediately; if a hamster is cared for by a child, then an adult should regularly check the pet's cage for signs of wear. Teddy bear hamsters may become trapped in exercise wheels if their hair is long enough to reach an axle. Hamsters may be stressed by hot and humid environments; an effort should be made to keep hamsters in a cool area of the house during the summer months. The noise of an exercise wheel may annoy some adults. Plastic exercise wheels that are nearly noise free are available, although some hamsters may chew on them if other materials, such as soft wood blocks, are not available.

Dwarf hamsters (generally, Siberian dwarfs [*Phodopus* species]) are mouse-sized and have a furred short tail, white underparts, and a grayish dorsal surface. They are excitable and more difficult to restrain than other hamsters. Many dwarf hamsters do not hesitate to bite when restrained. Also, they are subject to stress-related enteropathies.

All pet hamsters should be kept singly. Male hamsters fight each other; female hamsters also fight with males and with other females, particularly once they are pregnant.

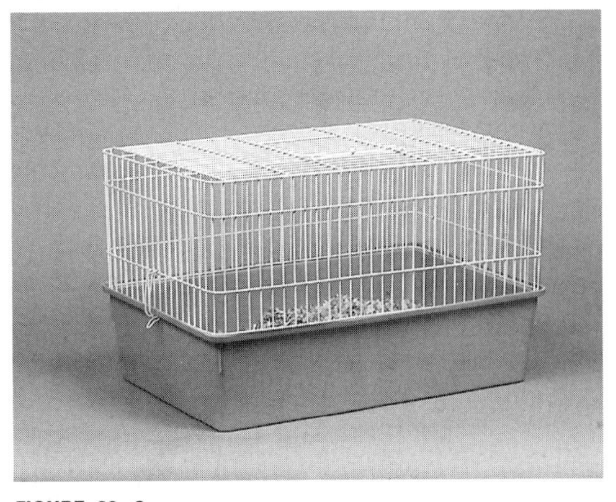

FIGURE 26–3
A cage appropriate for large rodents. It has a lightweight plastic bottom and sides that can contain bedding material.

Gerbils

Gerbils (*Meriones unguiculatus*) are excellent pets for older children. They tend to scamper and may slough their tail skin if picked up incorrectly; thus, they are unsuitable for most children under the age of 10 years. They are more active than hamsters, and their agility in climbing and burrowing makes providing living quarters for them interesting. They are usually gentle when handled correctly. Gerbils are available in white, black, buff, gray, and spotted varieties. Gerbils are territorial in nature and are best kept singly (cannibalism can be the result of attempting to keep incompatible pairs or males together). Gerbils are more disease resistant than hamsters, although older gerbils may suffer from a variety of neoplastic and degenerative conditions. Epilepsy has been reported in the literature but may be uncommon in some strains of pet gerbil.

HUSBANDRY

Housing and Equipment

In general, one of the most important requirements for any cage used for housing pets is that it be easy to clean. Poor husbandry and hygiene frequently result if the cage is heavy or awkward to disassemble. This is particularly true if children are assigned the responsibility for cage cleaning (a practice that is not recommended). Easy-to-clean cages have lightweight plastic bottoms, preferably with sides deep enough to contain bedding (Fig. 26–3). Aquariums are excellent for containing bedding but may be poorly ventilated and are often too heavy to be easily cleaned. However, their large screen tops are easily removed and do allow very easy access to the pet. Conventional cages should have a large door (or doors) to facilitate easy removal of the animal. Screen tops for aquariums should be fitted with a locking mechanism. Solid plastic cages featuring plastic connector tunnels (S.A.M., Pennplax Inc., Garden City, NY; and Habitrail, Hagen Inc., Mansfield, MA) provide an interesting environment for the animal but must be regularly cleaned as ventilation in them may be less than that in cages constructed principally of wire.

Commercial laboratories often use overhead hoppers to provide access to large food pellets or "blocks." This prevents the hoarding and soiling of food with feces. Hoarding, although natural and probably desirable behavior for such pets as hamsters, makes judging the amount of food available to the pet difficult. Hoppers are not widely available for pet rodents, and most owners use small, heavy plastic dishes or crocks.

Water bottles can be easily mounted on or in most conventional cages with the necessary adaptors or fittings. Accidental or negligent water deprivation is a common problem in pet rodents such as the hamster. Although water bottles may look full, sipper tubes can occasionally be blocked by air bubbles, or leaks may lead to the quick emptying out of all the water. Leaks can occur if the rubber fittings are old or if a foreign body such as a wood shaving is present in the sipper tube. Patency of the water bottle should be checked after every installation, and water should be changed *daily* with fresh water so that accidental water deprivation is avoided.

Exercise wheels have been used with most of the small rodent species, including the pygmy mouse and the rat. However, the hamster is best known for its use of the wheel. Some female hamsters are capable of running up to 10 km in a single night.[1] Keep the hair of long-haired hamsters trimmed so that it does not become tangled in the wheel. Check metal wheels for sharp projections. Spherical exercise balls are popular for use with pet hamsters, although owners should be cautioned that stairwells, direct sunshine, small children, and other pets may be hazardous to pets using these exercise devices.

Bedding

Many different beddings are popular for use with pet rodents, including some new beddings, such as recycled paper products, citrus litter, aspen or oak beddings, and a variety of corncob byproducts.

Pine shavings remain the most commonly used bedding for small pet rodents in many parts of North America. Corncob products and recycled paper products are excellent for certain rodents such as gerbils and dwarf hamsters. Cedar shavings also are popular but their use remains controversial. Cedar has been shown to affect microsomal oxidative liver enzymes in rats and mice. Although these changes affect factors such as drug metabolism, no clinical signs associated with them have been documented.[3] Because the changes may interfere with certain aspects of medical research, laboratory rodents are rarely housed on cedar shavings. Although anecdotal reports of respiratory and skin effects in pet species have been published, little is known about the exact mechanism of these effects and about which species might be sensitive. Cedar shavings were originally thought to have allergenic effects in the gerbil (excoriations and ulcers affecting the muzzle and face). However, this was largely disproved when the harderian gland of affected gerbils was found to be involved (abnormal grooming procedures failed to distribute the secretions normally).[1,2] The housing of gerbils on shavings is indirectly involved in the development of facial lesions; sand or dust normally present in the natural environment is absent in cages with shavings, and the dust bathing is thought to be part of gerbils' normal grooming procedure. Sandboxes can be provided for gerbils in much the same way that they are for chinchillas. White, yellow, and red cedar shavings contain one or more aromatic oils and terpenes that may be irritating to animals when present in sufficient quantities. These aromatic oils are reputed to repell insects and other pests; thus, they could conceivably have beneficial effects in certain circumstances. Very aromatic batches of cedar might not be recommended for use with certain species such as dwarf hamsters; there have been anecdotal reports of hair loss and respiratory disease in this species when cedar shavings are used.

Feeding

Seed diets are commonly given to pet rodents; the constant refilling of the feed dish allows pet rodents to select very palatable seeds such as sunflower seeds. These high-fat, low-calcium seeds can be offered as a treat food but should not be fed in excess, particularly to rats and hamsters. Rats may be prone to obesity, whereas hamsters are prone to osteoporosis; the provision of a seed diet may exacerbate these problems. Certain seed diets are composed of hulled seeds with added vitamins and minerals. They are slightly different than the traditional provision of vitamins and minerals in a pelleted vehicle (which is similar in appearance to a rabbit pellet) that is mixed with a variety of seeds. Unfortunately, most pet rodents simply ignore these pellets when they are mixed with seeds.

More uniform nutrition can be provided with the use of formulated-diet, laboratory-style blocks

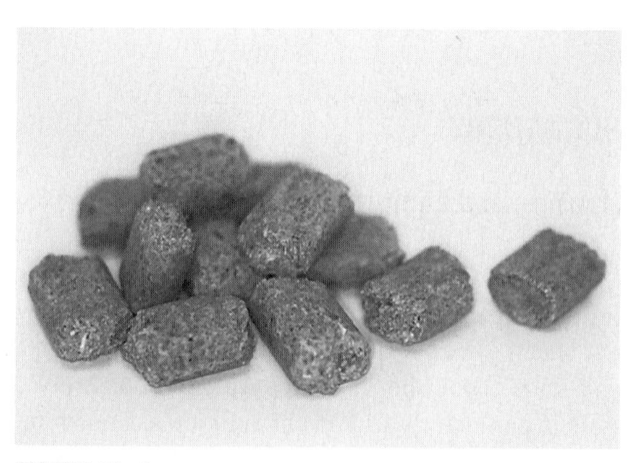

FIGURE 26–4
An example of a block-style rodent diet. This prevents preferential selection of seeds from a mix.

(Fig. 26–4). These blocks are now packaged specially for the pet industry (e.g., Nutri-block, Hagen Inc., Mansfield, MA). These blocks are more visible than are hoarded seeds; thus, although hoppers are not widely available, the blocks are easy to feed and check. Conversion to this type of diet is usually simple because most rodents find them very palatable. Rats might be an exception: they undoubtedly find them palatable, but much like pet birds, they often avoid new foods. A gradual introduction is recommended over a sudden change.

Most of the small rodents have similar nutritional requirements, although minor differences in protein requirements have been noted for gerbils.[1] A typical formulated diet suitable for pet mice, rats, gerbils, and hamsters should have a minimum protein content of 16% and a fat content of 4–5%. The analysis for a seed mix is basically meaningless because feed control authorities require that seed hulls and other discarded items be included in the analysis. Also, rodent pets select certain items from mixes, so that it is impossible to assess the nutritional value of a mixed seed diet. High-protein snacks or treats might occasionally be given to pet rodents. Avoid fatty treats. Offer treats in very small amounts to pets unfamiliar with new items. Reproduction in certain species such as gerbils and rats might require dietary protein levels of 20% or higher.[1]

PART II

Craig Bihun, DVM, DVSc

ANATOMIC AND PHYSIOLOGIC FEATURES

General

Gerbils, hamsters, mice, and rats belong to the largest mammalian order, Rodentia. The word *rodent* is derived from the Latin verb *rōdere,* which means "to gnaw." These particular species have a common dental formula of $2(I^1_1\ C^0_0\ P^0_0\ M^3_3)$. The four prominent, orange-colored incisors are open rooted and therefore grow continuously; in contrast, the molars are fixed rooted. In general, a crown length ratio for the upper to lower incisors is approximately 1:3. Clinicians sometimes mistake the longer length of the lower incisors as overgrowth and clip the teeth; this is to be avoided. The chisel-like occlusal surface of the incisors is the result of differential wearing. The outer convex surface of the incisors is covered by hard enamel, whereas the inner surface is lined only by cementum and dentin. The prominent space between the incisors and molars is referred to as the *diastema* and is occupied by cheek tissue.

The small rodents have bulging, somewhat exophthalmic eyes; this probably accounts for their frequent blinking. An important structure located behind the eyeball is the harderian gland. This gland produces lipid and porphyrin-rich secretions that appear to play a role in ocular lubrication and pheromone-mediated behavior. The porphyrins give the tears a red tinge; when under ultraviolet light, they fluoresce. Normally, the lacrimal secretions are spread over the pelage during daily grooming. However, in stressful situations and in certain disease conditions, there may be an overflow of tears; this can be misinterpreted as bleeding from the eyes and nose.

Hamsters, mice, and rats have four front toes and five hind toes; the opposite is true in the gerbil. The small rodents all have tails, although the length and hair cover of the tails vary. Gerbils, mice, and rats have tails that are longer than their bodies. Hamsters have short, haired tails; the dwarf hamsters' tails are slightly longer and almost prehensile in function. Gerbils' tails are well furred and have a tufted end. Rats' tails are thick, rasplike, and virtually hairless. The tails of mice also are covered only by sparse, fine hair.

Rodents do not possess sweat glands and are unable to pant (panting is an efficient method of heat dissipation). For these reasons, they are prone to heat stress and should not be exposed to extremely high temperatures.

Gerbils, hamsters, mice, and rats have 4, 6–7, 5, and 6 pairs of teats, respectively. Glandular tissue may extend over the shoulders and as far caudad as the perianal region. This is important to remember when a list of differential diagnoses for skin masses is being considered. Mammary tumors or infections can be present anywhere along this tract.

Rodents are monogastric and are usually herbivorous or omnivorous. They are also, to varying degrees, coprophagic; fecal pellets often constitute a significant proportion of what they consume. The fecal pellets presumably provide nutrients, such as B vitamins, that are produced by the colonic bacteria. Regurgitation is difficult in these species because of the presence of a limiting ridge at the junction of the esophagus and the stomach. For this reason and because these small creatures have such a high metabolic rate, preoperative fasting is difficult and is not required or recommended.

Additional data on physiologic parameters, serum biochemistry analyses, and hematology are provided in Tables 26–1 through 26–3, respectively.

The small rodents are polyestrous and spontaneous ovulators. Reproductive problems are not common. Rodents are usually efficient, prolific breeders, and pet owners often become acutely aware of overpopulation problems associated with the housing together of animals of the opposite sex. Vaginal cytologic analysis can be used to determine fairly accurately the stage of the estrous cycle. A small pipette can be used to instill and recover a small volume of normal saline from the vagina. A smear is then prepared with the recovered fluid. In general, proestrus is characterized by the presence of nucleated cells only, estrus by the presence of cornified cells only, metestrus by the presence of cornified cells and leukocytes, and diestrus by the presence of epithelial cells and leukocytes. Mating is confirmed by the presence of a "copulatory plug" within the vagina or on the cage floor. The copulatory plug is a straw-colored gelatinous substance formed by secretions from the accessory sex glands of the male. The presence of sperm in a vaginal smear also is predictive of normal female and male fertility and, indeed, pregnancy.

Other pertinent reproductive parameters are presented in Table 26–4.

Gerbils

Gerbils are adapted to a desert environment, requiring very little water and producing only a small volume of concentrated urine. They can obtain most, if not all, of their water requirements from metabolic

TABLE 26–1
NORMAL PHYSIOLOGIC REFERENCE VALUES*

Value	Gerbil	Hamster	Mouse	Rat
Average life span (mo)	24–39	18–36	12–36	26–40
Maximum reported life span (mo)	60	36	48	56
Average adult weight (g), male	46–131	87–130	20–40	267–500
Average adult weight (g), female	50–55	95–130	22–63	225–325
Heart rate (beats/min)	260–600	310–471	427–697	313–493
Respiratory rate (breaths/min)	85–160	38–110	91–216	71–146
Tidal volume (mL)	NA	0.8	0.15	0.6–1.2
Minute volume (mL)	NA	64	24	220
Rectal temperature (°C)	38.2	37.6	37.1	37.7
Approximate daily diet consumption of adult (g)	5–7	10–15	3–5	15–20
Approximate daily water consumption of adult (mL)	4	9–12	5–8	22–33
Approximate daily urine production (mL)	A few drops	7	1–2	13–23
Approximate daily fecal production (g)	1.5–2.5	2–2.5	1–1.5	9–15
Recommended environmental temperature (°C)	18–22	21–24	24–25	21–24
Recommended environmental relative humidity (%)	45–55	40–60	45–55	45–55

Abbreviation: NA = not available.

*Numbers were compiled by averaging the data obtained from the sources listed in the General References section of this chapter. Note that normal values may not represent the mean or range for certain populations or strains of animals; for this reason, the values should be interpreted as approximations.

TABLE 26–2

SERUM BIOCHEMISTRY AND ELECTROLYTE REFERENCE VALUES*

Value	Gerbil	Hamster	Mouse	Rat
Glucose (mg/dL)	50–135	65–73	174–335	85–132
Urea nitrogen (mg/dL)	17–27	42–60	34–58	32–54
Cholesterol (mg/dL)	90–151	182–237	49–96	46–92
Total protein (g/dL)	4.3–12.5	6.4–7.3	4.2–6.0	6.3–8.6
Albumin (g/dL)	1.8–5.5	3.2–3.7	2.1–3.4	3.3–4.9
Globulin (g/dL)	1.2–6.0	NA	1.8–8.2	2.4–3.9
Aspartate aminotransferase (U/L)	NA	53–124	55–251	39–92
Alanine aminotransferase (U/L)	NA	21–50	28–184	17–50
Alkaline phosphatase (U/L)	NA	8–18	28–94	39–216
Sodium (mEq/L)	NA	128–145	143–150	141–150
Potassium (mEq/L)	NA	4.9–5.1	3.8–10.0	5.2–7.8
Chloride (mEq/L)	NA	94–99	96–111	99–114
Bicarbonate (mEq/L)	NA	30 ± 2.9	NA	NA
Phosphorus (mg/dL)	3.7–7.1	5.3–6.6	8.3–11.2	6.2–11.7
Calcium (mg/dL)	3.6–6.0	10.4–12.3	11.1–12.1	10.7–13.7
Magnesium (mg/dL)	NA	2.2–2.5	NA	2.6–3.11

*Values for hamsters, mice, and rats were adapted from Appendix V in Olfert ED, Cross BM, McWilliam AA, eds.: Canadian Council on Animal Care: Guide to the Care and Use of Experimental Animals. Vol. 1. 2nd ed. Ottawa, Ontario, Canadian Council on Animal Care, 1993, pp. 175–178. Values for gerbils are from Harkness JE, Wagnar JE: The Biology and Medicine of Rabbits and Rodents. 3rd ed. Philadelphia, Lea & Febiger, 1989, pp. 35–36. Note that normal values may not represent the mean or range for certain populations or strains of animals; for this reason, the values should be interpreted as approximations.

processes and from any available fruit or vegetable matter.

The gerbil red blood cell has a life span of approximately 10 days. The rapid turnover of red blood cells is reflected on a stained blood smear as a pronounced basophilic stippling in a high percentage of these cells. Gerbil blood is normally hypercholesterolemic; this characteristic is probably a reflection of their high-fat diet and their love of food such as sunflower seeds.

Gerbils of both sexes have a distinct, orange-tan, oval area of alopecia on the midventral region that is referred to as the *ventral marking gland* or *pad*. This structure is composed of large sebaceous glands that are under the control of gonadal hormones. In the pubescent male, the gland starts to

TABLE 26–3

HEMATOLOGY REFERENCE VALUES*

Value	Gerbil	Hamster	Mouse	Rat
Red blood cells ($\times 10^6/\mu L$)	7.0–10.0	5.0–9.2	7.9–10.1	5.4–8.5
Hemoglobin (g/dL)	12.1–16.9	14.6–20.0	11.0–14.5	11.5–16.0
Hematocrit (%)	41–52	46–52	37–46	37–49
Platelets ($\times 10^3/\mu L$)	NA	300–570	600–1200	450–885
White blood cells ($\times 10^3/\mu L$)	4.3–21.6	5.0–10.0	5.0–13.7	4.0–10.2
Neutrophils ($\times 10^3/\mu L$)	0.3–4.1	1.5–3.5	0.4–2.7	1.3–3.6
Lymphocytes ($\times 10^3/\mu L$)	3.2–9.7	6.1–7.0	7.1–9.5	5.6–8.3
Total blood volume (mL/Kg)	60–85	65–80	70–80	50–65

*Adapted from Appendix IV in Olfert ED, Cross BM, McWilliam AA, eds.: Canadian Council on Animal Care: Guide to the Care and Use of Experimental Animals. Vol. 1. 2nd ed. Ottawa, Ontario, Canadian Council on Animal Care, 1993, pp. 175–178. Note that normal values may not represent the mean or range for certain populations or strains of animals; for this reason, the values should be interpreted as approximations.

TABLE 26–4
NORMAL REPRODUCTION AND GROWTH REFERENCE VALUES

Value	Gerbil	Hamster	Mouse	Rat
Estrogen cycle length (d)	4–7	4–5	4–5	4–5
Estrus (heat) duration (h)	12–18	8–26	9–20	9–20
Length of gestation (d)	23–26	15–18	19–21	21–23
Pups per litter	3–8	5–10	7–11	6–13
Weight at birth (g)	2.5–3.5	1.5–3	1–1.5	4–6
Eyes open (d)	16–21	12–14	12–14	12–15
Optimal weaning age (d)	21–28	19–21	18–21	21
Age of maturation of male (wk)	9–18	8	6	4–5
Age of maturation of female (wk)	9–12	6	6	4–5
Recommended minimum breeding age (wk)	10–14	8	8	9
Chromosome number (diploid)	44	44	40	42

Numbers were compiled by averaging the data obtained from the sources listed in the General References section of this chapter. Note that the normal values may not represent the mean or range for certain populations or strains of animals; as a result, the values should be interpreted as approximations.

enlarge and produces an oily, musk-scented secretion. Gerbils can often be seen rubbing their abdomen on objects; and this is thought to be a form of territorial marking.

Hamsters

Hamsters are short-tailed, stocky rodents and are known for their abundance of loose skin. They have large reversible cheek pouches that are paired muscular sacs extending as far back as the scapula. The pouches are evaginations of the oral mucosa and are used for transporting food, bedding material, and occasionally young. Hamsters also have a distinct forestomach that, similar to a rumen, has a high pH and contains microorganisms.

Hamsters have distinctive hip or flank glands. These dark brown patches are found bilaterally along the costovertebral region. They are poorly developed in the female, but in the mature male they are prominent and become wet and matted during sexual excitement. Secretions from these sebaceous glands play a role in territorial marking and mating behavior.

Female hamsters are unique in that they produce a copious vaginal discharge, particularly around day 2 (just postovulation) of the estrous cycle. These secretions should not be misinterpreted as a bacterial infection of the genital tract. Female hamsters also have paired vaginal pouches that collect exfoliated cells and leukocytes. For this reason, it is difficult to use vaginal cytologic examination to determine the stage of estrus.

Hamsters are permissive hibernators. Low environmental temperatures stimulate them to gather food. At temperatures of around 5°C, they curl up and enter a deep sleep.

Mice

Male mice are typically twice the size of female mice. Like most other male rodents, they have open inguinal canals, an os penis, and a complex urogenital system that contains several prominent accessory glands. Intermale aggression is a common problem, particularly if the males were not raised together or if they are housed in a confined space with mature females. Male mice produce a characteristic, strong odor. Pheromones play an important role in mouse behavior and are mediated through tissues like the vomeronasal (or Jacobson's) organ, which is located in the floor of the nasal cavity. Estrus is suppressed in female mice housed in large groups (the "Whitten effect"). Recently bred mice exposed to a strange male may have impaired implantation (the "Bruce effect").

Rats

An extensive amount of information on rat anatomy, physiology, behavior, and diseases is available because of the popularity of this animal in the biomedical research community. Readers are encouraged to consult any of the references listed at the end of this chapter for additional information. In general, rats are typical rodents, many of the pertinent features of which have already been covered in the general discussion earlier in this chapter. Several other points are useful to remember. Albino strain rats, compared with their pigmented peers, have poor eyesight and rely heavily on their vibrissae for spatial orientation. Rats do not have gall bladders. In old animals, yellowing of the hair coat is normal.

SEXING

In general, measuring the distance between the anus and the genital papilla is a reliable method of determining the sex of young animals. The anogenital distance is greater in the male than in the female. In addition, the genital papilla is usually more prominent and has a round opening in male offspring. Elevating an animal's front end or applying gentle pressure to the abdomen often forces the testicles into the scrotum, further assisting sex determination. Nipples are found only on the females of these species. They are noticeable at around 10 days of age in female mice and rat pups (Fig. 26–5).

Other, more species-specific criteria also can be used. In gerbils, weanling males have a darkly pigmented scrotum; in sexually mature males, the midventral abdominal gland is large. The flank gland in hamsters is androgen-sensitive and therefore appreciably larger in mature males as compared with females. Viewed from above, male hamsters have a rounded perineal profile because of the presence of inguinal canal fat pads that tend to keep the testes in the scrotum. Female hamsters have a flat profile that culminates in a point at the tail.

CLINICAL TECHNIQUES

Handling and Restraint

When handling a small rodent, avoid stressing or physically harming the small patient while at the same time minimizing the risk of being bitten. In general, the key to successful handling is being gentle yet firm and decisive in your actions. Knowledge of the animal's behavior also is helpful because each species reacts somewhat predictably to restraint.

The gerbil is docile in nature and very amenable to being picked up and loosely held in a cupped hand. An excited or threatened gerbil often exhibits a rhythmic thumping of the hind limb; this should be taken into consideration when you approach the animal because it is at this time that it would be more likely to bite. For fully restraining a gerbil, the over-the-back grip or scruff-of-the-neck techniques are recommended. The animal may be initially caught by grabbing the base of the tail; however, caution must be exercised because the skin can tear. Damage is especially apt to occur in young animals or when the more distal segments of the tail are grasped. Allow the forefeet to grasp the edge of the cage or examining table so that the animal directs its efforts to moving away from the restrainer. Approaching the animal from behind, place your fore-

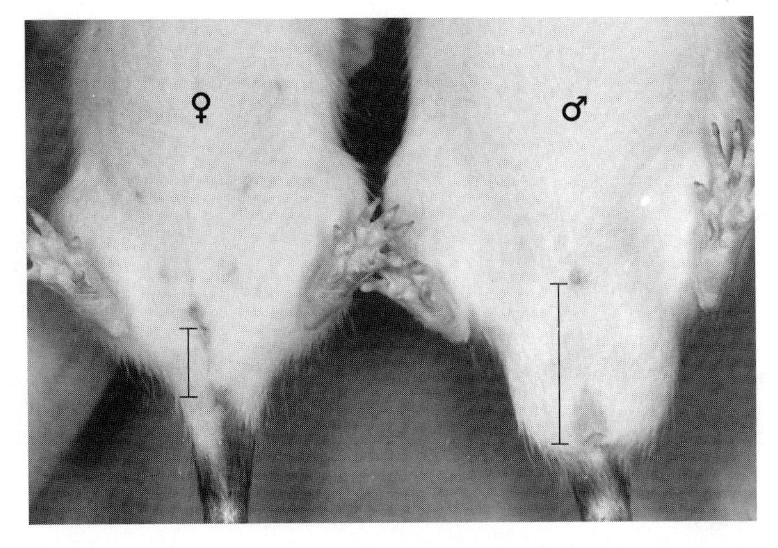

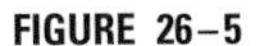

FIGURE 26–5
Male juvenile rat (*right*) and a female juvenile rat (*left*). Note the greater anogenital distance, the prominent presence of the scrotum, and the absence of nipples in the male.

finger and index finger on either side of the neck and exert pressure on the body of the mandible to immobilize the head. Hold the rest of the animal against the palm of your hand with your remaining fingers.

The scruff-of-the-neck technique involves grasping the loose fold of skin along the neck and back (Fig. 26–6). While holding the animal by the tail, use the forefinger and thumb to gently pin down the head; this prevents the animal from turning and biting. Using the same fingers, grasp a sufficient amount of loose skin over the neck. Holding the tail with the little finger of the same hand provides additional support. Both methods of restraint result in good exposure of the head and ventral abdomen and facilitate physical examination and the administration of parenteral or oral drug therapy. Also, restriction of the animal's breathing is minimal as long as the skin is not held too tautly and compression of the chest cavity is avoided.

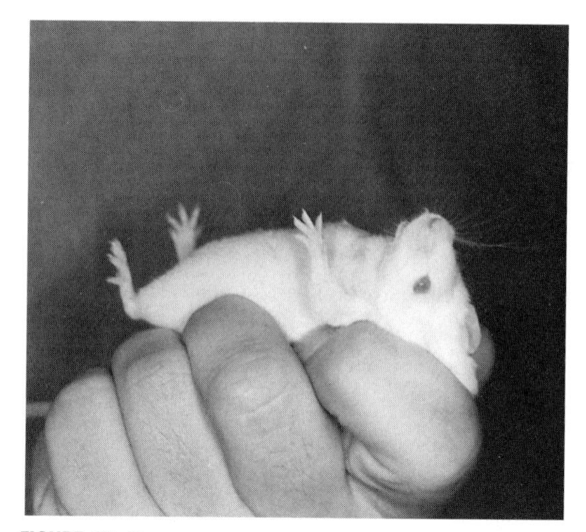

FIGURE 26–6
Scruff-of-the-neck handling technique in a mouse.

Hamsters have a dubious reputation for being biters. They do not tolerate excessive or prolonged restraint as well as do some other rodents. If suddenly awakened from a deep sleep, they usually exhibit typical threatening behavior, such as rolling on their backs or standing on their hind limbs and vocalizing. However, if you avoid startling these animals, they can be quite receptive to being scooped up in the palm of your hand. When full restraint is required, a modification of the scruff grip is required. Because the hamster has an abundance of loose skin over the back and shoulders, a full-handed grip is required for achieving complete immobilization. To do this, grasp the skin between the tips of all four fingers and the base of thumb and lower palm of your hand.

Mice are very active and are quick to jump away from the person handling them. Take precautions to ensure that, if these animals do escape, they do not injure themselves and can be easily recaptured. Mice often bite when being handled; this emphasizes the need for proper restraint of this species. Handle mice as you would gerbils. Initially, grab them by the base of the tail; then, use the scruff-of-the-neck method of restraint (Fig. 26–6).

The majority of pet rats usually are very friendly and do not object to being picked up and gently manipulated. They rarely bite unless they are agitated or hurt. Pick up a rat by grabbing it over the neck and shoulders. Position your forefinger just below the mandible on one side of the head and your thumb on the opposite side, either above or below the forelimb (Fig. 26–7). Provide additional support by holding the tail and hind limbs with the opposite hand. The base of the tail may be used to temporarily catch an animal if it is not receptive to the direct approach; however, if the animal appears to be stressed by the procedure, it is probably best to take a short break and try again later.

Restraint devices for rodents of all sizes may be purchased commercially or custom-made with materials in the clinic. Animals may be simply wrapped in a thin towel or placed in a stockinette. Syringe cases can be modified so that the animal contained within the case can breath through a hole cut in the narrow end. Cone-shaped polyethylene bags that have the tip removed also are designed for this purpose; alternatively, you can modify a clear plastic bag by cutting off one of the corners. This last approach is advantageous because it allows the clinician to observe an animal and, at the same time, permits parenteral drug administration through the plastic.

Blood Collection

The exact technique chosen to collect blood depends on factors such as the species, the volume of blood required, the skill of the technician, and the clinical situation. Certainly, when dealing with the individual pet animal, emphasis is placed on use of the safest, least stressful, and least traumatic method. In order not to unduly compromise the ani-

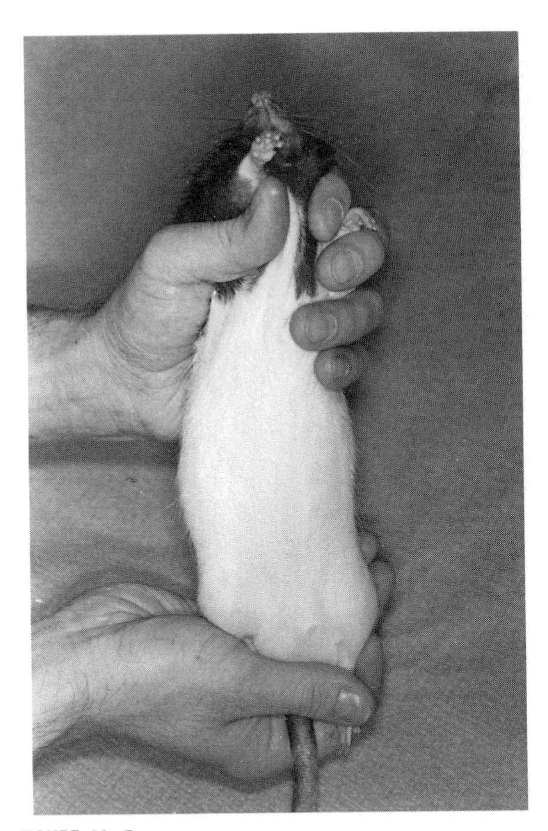

FIGURE 26–7
Over-the-back method of rat restraint.

mal, keep the volume of blood collected close to the minimum required to run the desired test or tests. The general guideline for sampling blood is not to remove more than 10% of the total blood volume. The removal of this volume of blood should have no obvious effect on the healthy subject and can be repeated in 3 to 4 weeks. When collecting samples from clinically ill animals, use discretion and perhaps reduce the volume appropriately. Approximate total blood volumes are provided in Table 26–3. In general, try not to collect more than 0.3, 0.65, 0.14, and 1.3 mL of blood from the adult gerbil, hamster, mouse, and rat, respectively.

In the gerbil, mouse, and rat, the lateral tail veins can be used to collect small to moderate volumes of blood. The veins are located on either side of the tail and are quite superficial; in young albino mice and rats, they can be easily visualized. General anesthesia is not required for this technique, but the animal must be properly restrained. Commercially available or custom-made restrainers that suitably immobilize the animal but provide access to the tail assist in making this a one-person procedure. Dilate the tail vessels by placing the tail in warm water or under a heat lamp (i.e., place the animal 25–30 cm away from a 60-W heating lamp). Incubating the animal at a temperature of 40°C for 10–15 minutes before blood collection also is effective. Occlude the veins by placing a tourniquet around the base of the tail. A rubber band and mosquito hemostat are suitable for this purpose. With a needle of appropriate gauge for the species, enter the skin at a shallow angle approximately one third down the length of the tail. If the initial attempt at collection is unsuccessful, try again at a site closer to the base of the tail. To avoid collapsing the vessel, use a small-volume syringe to withdraw the sample or collect the blood into a microhematocrit tube as it flows freely from the needle hub. A modified butterfly catheter (i.e., all but the proximal 5 mm of tubing removed) also may be used. For repeated intravenous injections or blood sampling in the rat, use a 24-gauge pediatric over-the-needle catheter to catheterize the vessel. After the sample has been collected, remove the needle or catheter and apply gentle pressure to the puncture site until hemostasis is achieved.

The ventral tail artery in the rat is another very accessible vessel from which several milliliters of blood may be easily collected. The artery courses along the ventromedial aspect of the tail, although it is not quite as superficial as the lateral tail veins. Anesthesia is required for this technique, preferably with an anesthetic agent that maintains the animal's blood pressure. Innovar-Vet (Mallinckrodt Veterinary, Inc., Mundelein, IL) at the low dose of 0.13 mL/kg SC, is well suited for this purpose. Place the lightly anesthetized animal in dorsal recumbency. Use a 22-gauge needle and a 3-mL syringe with the plunger removed. Make the first puncture attempt one third down the tail's length. Enter the skin at a 20–30° angle to the tail, with the bevel of the needle facing upward (Fig. 26–8). A perceptible pop usually indicates that the artery has been entered; this is quickly followed by filling of the syringe with blood. The high blood pressure in this vessel negates the need for the negative pressure produced by withdrawal of the plunger. Indeed, the presence of the plunger within the syringe case impairs recognition of correct penetration of the vessel. When the required volume of blood has been collected, withdraw the needle and apply pressure to the puncture site. Note that more time is required to stop the bleeding from the tail artery than that from the tail vein.

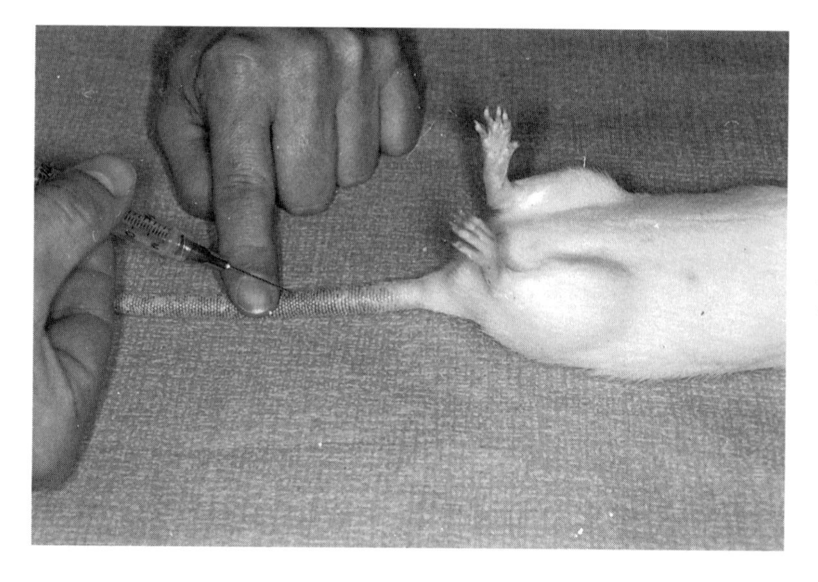

FIGURE 26–8
Tail artery method of blood collection in the rat.

The orbital venous plexus or sinuses are funnel-shaped networks of veins or dilated venous channels located along the caudal one half to two thirds of the rodent orbit. With the animal anesthetized and in lateral recumbency, use a microhematocrit tube to access the sinus by inserting the tube through the conjunctiva along the medial canthus of the eye. Gently rotate the tube along its long axis to overcome any resistance. If the tube is in the correct location, blood will flow freely from the end of the tube. Collect the required volume of blood into the appropriate microcontainer blood collection system. Remove the tube when a sufficient volume has been collected, wipe the excess blood away from the eye with a gauze square, and manually close the eyelids until the bleeding has ceased. The application of sterile ophthalmic lubricant after any anesthetic is highly recommended in these somewhat exophthalmic animals because it helps prevent corneal desiccation. This technique requires minimal skill and is relatively fast. It does require anesthesia and, for aesthetic reasons, should probably not be performed in the presence of the pet owner. In addition, complications are potentially associated with this technique (e.g., damage to the eye or the periocular tissues).

Cardiac puncture is useful for obtaining large volumes of blood. This procedure must be reserved for terminal blood collections because of the inherent risk of lacerating a lung lobe or a coronary vessel. A general anesthetic is always required. Place the animal in dorsal recumbency; with the thumb and fingers of one hand, lightly compress the chest to locate and isolate the heart. Insert the needle at a 30° angle from the horizontal, at a location just underneath but slightly off to the left side of the manubrium. Successful entry into one of the chambers of the heart is signalled by a reduced resistance to insertion and the presence of blood in the needle hub.

Drug Administration

The administration of drugs to small rodents poses some unique challenges to the veterinary clinician. Remember that most drugs are not licensed for use in these animals, and therefore their use must be considered extra-label. In addition, most drug formulations come in a concentrated form. In order to administer an accurate dose and avoid causing tissue damage, it is recommended that the drug be suitably diluted for parenteral use. Ideally, the diluent selected should be the same one in which the drug is currently formulated. Otherwise, an isotonic solution, such as sterile physiologic saline (0.9% sodium chloride), is usually acceptable for most water-soluble compounds.

Table 26–5 summarizes the recommended anatomic sites, maximum volumes to be administered, and needle gauges to be used for the conventional routes of drug administration. As a general rule, select the smallest gauge needle that is compatible with the viscosity of the compound that is being injected; this helps minimize any discomfort to the animal.

TABLE 26–5
RECOMMENDED ROUTES FOR DRUG ADMINISTRATION

Route		Gerbil	Hamster	Mouse	Rat
Intramuscular	Site	Quadriceps, gluteals	Quadriceps, gluteals	Quadriceps	Quadriceps, gluteals, triceps
	Maximum volume (mL)	0.1 per site	0.1 per site	0.03 per site	0.2–0.3 per site
	Needle gauge	≤23-gauge	≤23-gauge	≤23-gauge	≤22-gauge
Intraperitoneal	Site	Lower right quadrant of abdomen	Lower right quadrant of abdomen	Lower right quadrant of abdomen	Lower left quadrant of abdomen
	Maximum volume (mL)	2–3	3–4	1–3	10
	Needle gauge	≤21-gauge	≤21-gauge	≤21-gauge	≤22-gauge
Intravenous	Site	Lateral tail veins	Not recommended	Lateral tail veins	Lateral tail or saphenous veins
	Maximum volume (mL)	0.2–0.3		0.2–0.3	0.5–3 slowly
	Needle gauge	≤23-gauge		≤23-gauge	≤22-gauge
Intragastric	Site	Stomach	Stomach	Stomach	Stomach
	Maximum volume (mL)	NA	NA	5–10 mL/kg	5–10 mL/kg
	Needle gauge	18–22-gauge, 3–4 cm long Bulbed feeding needle	18-gauge, 4–4.5 cm long Bulbed feeding needle	18–22-gauge, 2–3 cm long Bulbed feeding needle	15–18-gauge, 6–8 cm long Bulbed feeding needle or 8-French flexible catheter
Subcutaneous	Site	Neck, back	Neck, back, abdomen	Neck, back, abdomen	Neck, back, abdomen
	Maximum volume (mL)	2–3	3–5	2–3	5–10
	Needle gauge	≤21-gauge	≤21-gauge	≤22-gauge	≤21-gauge

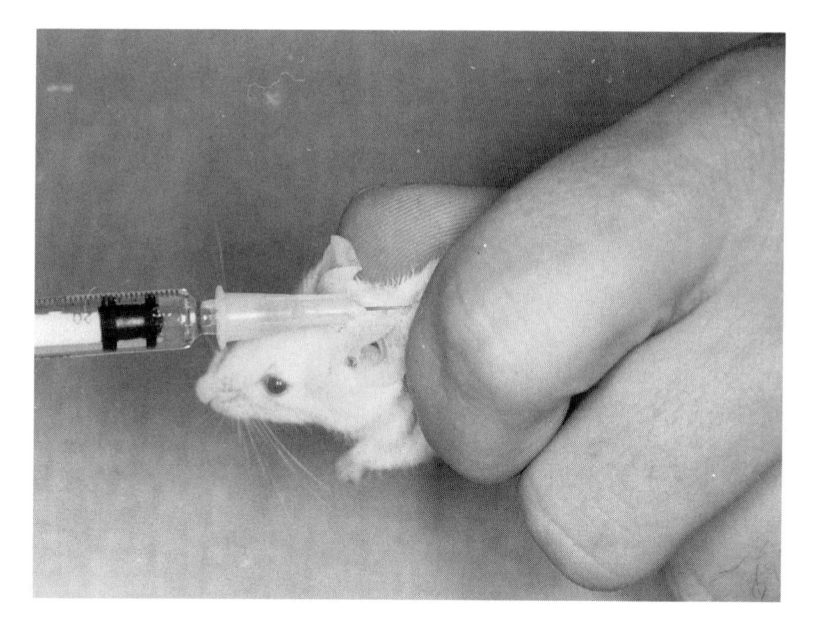

FIGURE 26–9
Subcutaneous injection into the neck skin fold of a restrained mouse.

Subcutaneous injections are preferred for drug administration because they are easy to give and allow the delivery of relatively large volumes. With the animal restrained by the scruff of the neck, make the injection into the tented fold of skin that is held between the thumb and forefinger (Fig. 26–9). If an assistant is restraining the animal, use a fold of skin along the back, flank, or abdomen. Aspirate before injecting to ensure that the syringe has not entered a blood vessel or passed through the skin.

Intraperitoneal injection also is an easy, reasonably safe means of drug administration. Relatively large volumes can be given; thus, potentially irritating solutions can be generously diluted. Additionally, the large surface area of the abdominal cavity and its abundant blood supply facilitate rapid absorption of the compound. One drawback of this and the oral route of administration is that the drug is first absorbed into the portal circulation; therefore, some biotransformation in the liver may take place before the substance reaches the general circulation. To administer an intraperitoneal injection, invert the restrained animal head down so that the abdominal viscera fall forward. Insert the needle into the caudal quadrant of the abdomen, entering the skin at a 20° angle (Fig. 26–10). In gerbils, hamsters, and mice, inject into the right caudal quadrant of the abdomen to avoid hitting the spleen. The left caudal quadrant of the abdomen is recommended in the rat because the cecum occupies the bulk of the right abdominal cavity in this species. Aspirate before injecting to ensure that the intestine or urinary bladder has not been entered.

Small muscle masses restrict the number of practical injection sites and the volume of drug that can safely be given by the intramuscular route. If this route must be used, the quadriceps muscle group,

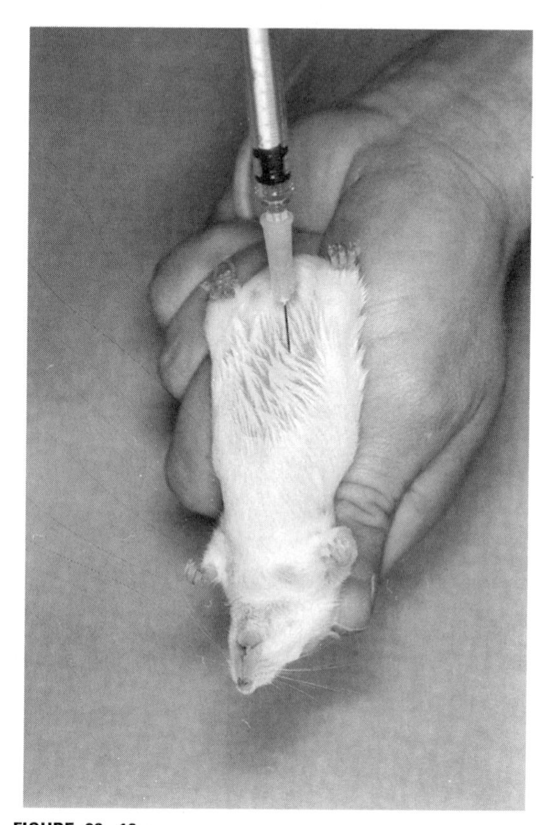

FIGURE 26–10
Intraperitoneal injection into the right caudal abdominal quadrant of an inverted mouse.

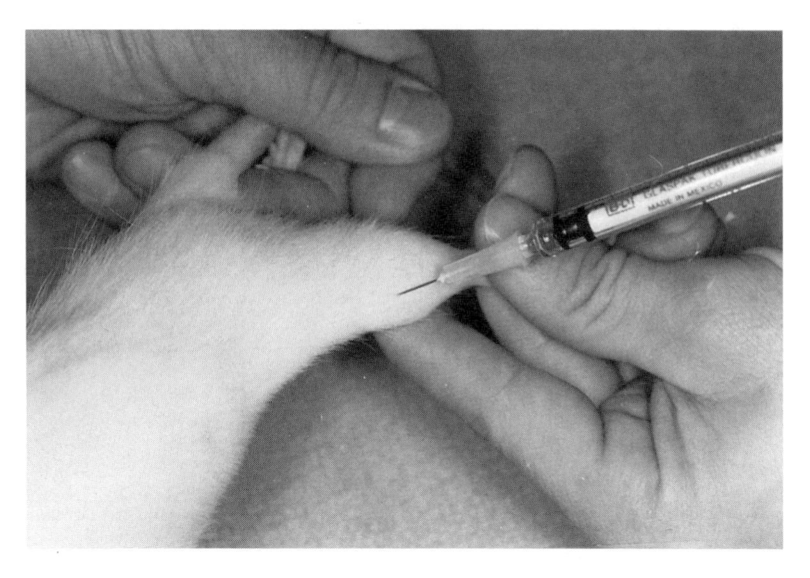

FIGURE 26–11
Intramuscular injection into the anterior muscle mass of the hind limb of a rat.

which covers the anterior aspect of the thigh, or the gluteal muscles of the hip are the recommended locations (Fig. 26–11). Avoid the posterior thigh muscles because the sciatic nerve courses along the back of the femur. Irritating substances that are inadvertently injected in close proximity to this nerve may result in lameness or in the animal's self-mutilation of the affected limb.

Achieving therapeutic blood levels of drugs through the use of medicated food or water is difficult because sick animals usually reduce their food and water consumption. The palatability of medicated food or water often is affected; this too may result in altered food and water intake. If medication is to be given orally in the hospital setting, then intragastric gavage is recommended. Fortunately, intragastric gavage is easy to perform on the conscious animal when a bulbed metal feeding needle or a flexible feeding tube is used. Before intubation, determine the approximate distance that the stomach tube must be inserted by externally measuring the distance from the nares to the last rib. Lubricate the tube with water or a drop of glycerin to facilitate easy passage. Restrain the animal with its neck extended. Insert the tube at the level of the diastema (interdental space) and slowly advance it towards the back of the mouth. In the conscious animal, the tube should pass around the epiglottis and enter the esophagus. Smooth advancement of the tube indicates correct placement; incorrect placement is accompanied by violent struggling and dysphagia. With a flexible catheter, the use of a mouth gag is prudent to prevent the animal from biting through the tube.

Usually, compounding pharmacists can easily prepare oral medications in suitable concentrations for the treatment of pet rodents at home. Most drugs can be compounded into very dilute concentrations in a flavored syrup base. To administer a drug, restrain the rodent as previously described and insert the tip of a small dosing syringe into the lateral cheek pouch. Most rodents readily accept oral medications that taste sweet. Occasionally, a hamster reaches with its front paws in an attempt to push the syringe away. Always show the client how to administer an oral medication to a pet rodent before prescribing a drug to ensure that the client is comfortable performing the procedure.

Many intravenous injection routes have been described; however, the majority require some degree of technical skill or the use of anesthesia. Consequently, this route often is not practical in the pet rodent. If intravenous therapy is imperative, then accessing the lateral tail veins is recommended (see the section on blood collection for more details on this technique).

REFERENCES

1. Harkness JE, Wagner JE: The Biology and Medicine of Rabbits and Rodents. 4th ed. Philadelphia, Lea & Febiger, 1995. 230 pp.
2. Thiessen DD, Pendergrass M: Harderian gland involvement in facial lesions in the Mongolian gerbil. J Am Vet Med Assoc 1982; 181:1375–1377.
3. Weichbrod RH, Cisar CF, Miller JG, et al: Effects of cage beddings on microsomal oxidative enzymes in rat liver. Lab Anim Sci 1988; 38:296–298.

GENERAL REFERENCES

Baker HJ, Lindsey JR, Weisbroth SH, eds.: The Laboratory Rat. Vol. 1: Biology and Diseases. New York, Academic Press, 1979.

Bober R: Technical review: drawing blood from the tail artery of a rat. Lab Anim 1988;17:33–34.

Boorman GA, Eutis SL, Elwell MR, eds.: Pathology of the Fischer Rat: Reference and Atlas. San Diego, Academic Press, 1990.

Buckland MD, Hall L, Mowlem A, Whatley BF: A Guide to Laboratory Animal Technology. London, William Heinmann Medical Books, 1981.

Charles River Technical Bulletin: Basic Husbandry and Production Information for Charles River Animals. Vol 1. No. 1. 1982.

Flecknell PA: Laboratory Anesthesia: An Introduction for Research Workers and Technicians. London, Academic Press, 1991.

Foster HL, Small JD, Fox JG, eds.: The Mouse in Biomedical Research. Vol. III: Normative Biology, Immunology, and Husbandry. New York, Academic Press, 1983.

Fowler ME, ed.: Zoo and Wild Animal Medicine. 2nd ed. Philadelphia, WB Saunders, 1986.

Fox JG, Cohen BJ, Loew FM, eds.: Laboratory Animal Medicine. Orlando, Academic Press, 1984.

Green EL, ed.: Biology of the Laboratory Mouse. 2nd ed. New York, McGraw-Hill Book Co., 1966.

Hoffman RA, Robinson PF, Magalhaes H, eds.: The Golden Hamster: Its Biology and Use in Medical Research. Ames, IA, Iowa State University Press, 1968.

Holmes DM: Clinical Laboratory Animal Medicine. Ames, IA, Iowa State University Press,1984.

Holmes DM: The Mongolian gerbil in biomedical research. Lab Anim 1985;14:23–38.

Inglis JK, ed.: Introduction to Laboratory Animal Science and Technology. New York, Pergamon Press, 1980.

Loeb WF, Quimby FW, eds.: The Clinical Chemistry of Laboratory Animals. New York, Pergamon Press, 1989.

Merck Veterinary Manual. 7th ed. Rahway, NJ, Merck & Co, 1991.

Olfert ED, Cross BM, McWilliam AA, eds.: Canadian Council on Animal Care: Guide to the Care and Use of Experimental Animals. Vol. 1. 2nd ed. Ottawa, Ontario, Canadian Council on Animal Care, 1993.

Percy DH, Barthold SW: Pathology of Laboratory Rodents and Rabbits. Ames, IA, Iowa State University Press, 1993.

Poole T, ed.: The Universities Federation for Animal Welfare on the Care & Management of Laboratory Animals. 6th ed. Essex, UK, Longman Scientific and Technical Publishers; 1987.

Siegel HI, ed.: The Hamster: Reproduction and Behaviour. New York, Plenum Press, 1985.

Svendsen P, Hau J: Handbook of Laboratory Animal Science: Vol. I: Selection and Handling of Animals in Biomedical Research. Boca Raton, FL, CRC Press, 1994.

Van Hossier GL, McPherson CW, eds.: Laboratory Hamsters. Orlando, Academic Press, 1987.

Waynforth HB, Flecknell PA: Experimental and Surgical Techniques in the Rat. 2nd ed. London, Academic Press, 1992.

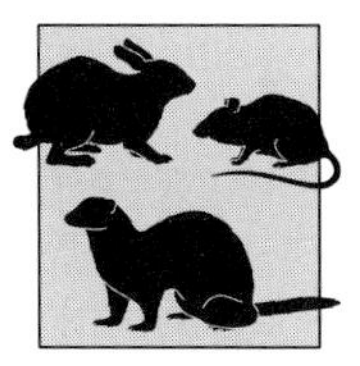

CHAPTER 27

Disease Problems of Small Rodents

Thomas M. Donnelly, BVSc

The most challenging medical diagnoses are those made in areas of discovery. All too often, the animal and its condition are familiar, and the diagnosis and treatment routine. However, some cases involve original investigation in emerging fields of veterinary medicine.

The treatment of rodents as pets is one of these emerging fields, presenting a terrain bristling with complexities for many veterinarians. First among these is the common perception of rodents. Most people do not consider them pets, and they usually are called "vermin." Moreover, almost all scientists consider rodents as experimental tools. Veterinarians are not immune to such prejudices, and some may feel reluctant to examine a fully grown, red-eyed, wheezing rat. Owners of pet rodents often feel the same aversion for unsympathetic veterinarians and as a result travel long distances to see one understanding of their needs. A second area of concern is the unfamiliarity of clinical veterinarians with rodent biology. Although a great deal of information has been accumulated on wild and laboratory rodents, very little of this information pertains to pet rodents. Geriatric diseases, the pharmacokinetics of common drugs, and the beneficial and harmful effects of human handling, contact, and care are a few of the phantom areas that array themselves along the frontier of this field. Yet, the spectrum of problems affecting rodents does not differ greatly from those of dogs and cats.

One of the intents of this chapter is to describe the common diseases of pet rodents seen in practice, so that their relative novelty becomes a challenge and not a stumbling block. The other is to inform clinicians about reasonable methods for accurately diagnosing common diseases of rodents.

THE DIAGNOSTIC CHALLENGE

Pet Rodent Etiquette

Establishing and familiarizing the veterinary staff with a few simple rules of so-called "pet rodent etiquette" can make the physical examination a positive and fruitful experience. This preparation leaves the clinician confident and free of undue anxiety that can arise when presented with a concerned, overprotective owner. The veterinarian should be ready to apply his or her acumen and therapeutic skills to the treatment of the patient. Establishment of a clear and nonconflictual basis for communication between clinician and owner greatly facilitates the rodent's treatment and recovery.

Scheduling an Appointment

Rats and hamsters are essentially nocturnal animals and are only occasionally active during the day. In contrast, gerbils and mice are active during both the night and day.[36] Healthy rodents are generally active during the awake part of their normal circadian cycle. Subtle signs of diseases may be overlooked when a sleep-deprived, drowsy, and irritable animal is brought to the clinician. This is especially the case with hamsters. When possible, receptionists should schedule appointments for rats and hamsters in the early evening hours. Appointment times are not as critical for gerbils and mice. Take the time to explain the reasoning behind appointment scheduling to clients who are unwilling to make an evening appointment. This not only changes their minds but also sets the veterinarian-client relationship off to a good start.

Instruct the client to bring the rodent to the hospital in its own cage. Knowledge of the husbandry and sanitation are essential to a good clinical history. Only by seeing the cage, water supply, feed containers, bedding, and food can the clinician understand the environment in which the rodent lives. Tactfully instruct clients not to clean the rodent's housing in preparation for the appointment because by doing so they may inadvertently destroy information important for diagnosis and treatment.

Reception Area

It is essential that the waiting area for rodents and owners be quiet. Receptionists should avoid planning appointments for natural predators, such as outdoor cats or hunting dogs, when a pet rodent is scheduled for an examination.

The rodent's sense of smell is well developed, and its world is rich in olfactory stimuli and pheromonal cues. Rodents are more sensitive to the effects of heat than of cold. Even though wild golden hamsters and gerbils are desert-dwelling animals, their main method of thermoregulation is to escape from the heat by burrowing or seeking cool places. Mice in particular are very sensitive to the effects of heat. Waiting areas for rodents should be kept relatively cool. The dry-bulb temperature range of 64.4–78.8°F recommended by the National Institutes of Health is ideal for housing rodents. Also, the opportunity for a habituated rodent to nestle next to the familiar smell of its owner can only be afforded in a quiet and safe waiting area.

Educate clients and receptionists about ways to make a trip to the hospital less stressful—it is well worth the time invested. If proper attention is devoted to education, then the veterinarian is likely to see a rodent amenable to examination, instead of one ready to fight, flee, or cringe.

Medical History

Facts about the history and nature of a rodent's problem are generally more useful in reaching a correct diagnosis than is the clinical history for a companion animal. Skill is required to extract a reliable, unbiased history of a pet's disease. Some owners are good at noticing changes and providing important information, whereas others are not.

Find out what owners know about rodents. Have they had rodents as pets before? Where did they obtain their information on caring for their pet? Was it from a book, a pet store, or first-hand experience? Books about rodents for owners of all ages and experience are presented in the Suggested Reading section at the end of this chapter. Although these books are generally available in pet stores or through catalogs, it is my experience that most veterinarians have not seen them. I have found many of these books to be informative on husbandry requirements; however, many provide incorrect or misleading descriptions of diseases. For this reason, the sections on disease must be carefully evaluated. Knowledge of your clients' sources of information further helps you in judging their ability to provide an accurate history.

Do not become unsettled if an owner appears to know more than you do. Such a client can be very informative, enthusiastic, and willing to take an active role in treatment. When discussing a pet's problem with its owner, communicate on a level commensurate with his or her aptitude and background. Parents often present a sick rodent that belongs to their child, who may be the family member most knowledgeable about the pet's habits and behavior. When obtaining a medical history in these cases, the young owner's presence is invaluable.

Ask neutral questions that do not bias responses; for example, "Tell me about your rat's drinking habits." Try to avoid direct or leading questions such as, "Have you noticed that your rat is drinking more water?" because they may influence the response. Pose general questions, such as, "Anything else?" or "What do you mean?" A prompt such as "Tell me more about that" is helpful in encouraging the owner to elaborate on his or her responses. Do not be afraid to say, "I'm not sure what you mean," and never belittle owners' opinions of their pets' illness.

Over the course of the exchange with the owner, answers to the following specific questions should be obtained:

- Where did the pet come from? a pet store? a laboratory?
- How long has the owner had the pet?
- Are there other pets in the household? If so, are they of the same species?
- What food does the owner give to the pet? Where is the food purchased?
- What food does the pet prefer and what does it actually eat?
- Where is the food stored and for how long?
- Who is responsible for feeding and cleaning? How routinely are these tasks done?
- How long have the signs of illness been apparent? Who first noticed them and why?
- Has the pet's condition deteriorated, improved, or remained stable?

Pets isolated from other rodents and household animals, or acquired from private breeders or laboratories, are less likely to suffer from infectious disease than are animals obtained from a pet store. Many diseases are the result of poor or inappropriate feeding. Pet rodents often selectively eat only one ingredient (e.g., sunflower seeds), when offered mixed-seed, vegetable, and fruit diets. In households with children, there may not be a typical feeding pattern, and pets may be inappropriately fed by doting children. Often, owners are ignorant of the availability of specially formulated food for rodents. These diets, which come in the form of pellets, are convenient and nutritionally balanced sources of nourishment.*

Clinical Examination

Seeing the condition of the rodent's living quarters provides information that is helpful in reaching a diagnosis or a reasonable prognosis. Information obtained from a physical examination is limited because of a rodent's size. However, it is only after examination of the animal that the significance of the rodent's history and husbandry can be evaluated. With appropriate handling and a few specialized but simple pieces of equipment, a thorough review of the major organ systems can be conducted. If the same procedure is followed consistently, it eventually requires less and less time to perform.

Observe the pet rodent in its cage for activity, condition of grooming, and the presence of a head tilt or discharges. If dyspnea or depression is seen, be extremely careful when handling the animal as it is probably very sick and could die from the stress of a physical examination. At the same time, warn the owner of your guarded prognosis.

Pet rodents that have been frequently and gently handled usually require minimal restraint. Less cooperative patients need to be more firmly restrained, and the use of a towel or even heavy gloves may be required (see Chapter 26). Although pet rodents do not often bite, their nips can be painful and may elicit an unfortunate reflex response in the handler that results in the pet being pitched onto the floor or at a wall. Besides the po-

*A list of feed manufacturers can be found in the annual Buyers' Guide Directory (December issue) of the journal *Lab Animal* (New York, NY).

tential for traumatic injury, the rodent may escape and become harmed.

The first part of the physical examination that I do is to accurately measure the patient's weight. Weight measurement is essential for calculating appropriate dosages of medications and provides an opportunity for gauging the rodent's temperament before the actual physical examination begins. Rodents are easily weighed in metal or plastic containers placed on a small digital scale or a triple-beam balance.

A binocular loupe and an otoscope are useful for evaluating physical signs. I like to start at the head, examining first the ears, eyes, and nose for discharge and the oral cavity for dentition. The otoscope allows careful examination of the mouth and ears in most rodents except mice. Observe and palpate the lymph nodes and glands of the head for size and consistency. Assessment of the head is probably the most time-consuming part of the examination.

Palpate the abdomen for consistency and the presence of unusual masses. However, do not squeeze the patient too hard because overzealous palpation can result in visceral rupture. Examine the anogenital region for discharges and staining of the fur or skin. When a rodent is picked up, it usually urinates and defecates. Have a dipstick ready to do an immediate urinalysis; feces can be caught in a small tube and examined later, if required. By this point in the examination, I have noted the condition of the fur and have assessed the body in general. I palpate the limbs for tenderness or fractures and pay special attention to the paws, noting the length of the nails and the state of the footpads.

Respiratory and heart rates are difficult to measure because they are rapid in rodents. Instead, look for signs of dyspnea. A sensitive pediatric stethoscope is useful for auscultation in large rodents. Some respiratory infections, such as mycoplasmosis, are clinically silent. These diseases can be better heard than seen; abnormal sounds called "snuffling" in rats and "chattering" in mice are noticeable without a stethoscope.

The value of determining rectal temperature is questionable. A rodent is stressed by the examination, and as a result its body temperature is increased. Furthermore, most thermometers are too big for use in pet rodents, and may cause rectal damage and prolapse because of the patient's small size. However, rectal temperatures can be taken safely with the use of small, semiflexible temperature probes connected to a digital clinical thermometer. YSI Incorporated (Yellow Springs, OH) manufactures the Series-400 temperature probes that can be used for rectal temperature measurement in rodents. These probes are reusable; are available in polyvinyl chloride, nylon, and Teflon; and range in size from 1 to 3 mm in diameter. The probes can be attached to the YSI Model-4000 digital handheld clinical thermometer.

The clinician can obtain a small amount of blood for a smear and microhematocrit from a hind-limb skin stab, nail-clip, or nick of the tip of the tail. Obtaining blood for a complete blood count (CBC) and biochemical analysis often is not practical because of the quantity and quality of blood required. If the saphenous or dorsal metatarsal vein is easily visible, the rodent is often large enough to permit collection of a small amount of blood with a small-gauge needle and syringe. Rats often suffer from chronic renal disease. A blood urea nitrogen (BUN) concentration can be estimated with the use of a blood dipstick, and proteinuria can be detected on urine dipstick analysis.

Technologic advances have made possible electrocardiography and accurate and sensitive recordings of heart rate, respiratory rate, and blood pressure in research rodents. The high cost of the equipment and the invasive procedures that often are necessary to obtain data have not made the use of these testing modalities routine in small exotic animal practice. However, similar advances in high-resolution film screen combinations that require relatively low radiographic exposures, and recent developments in ultrasound have allowed diagnostic imaging to become a useful, ancillary examination. A 1993 review describes the limitations of diagnostic imaging in small pets.[46] The *Atlas of Diagnostic Radiology of Exotic Pets* contains many excellent radiographs of the anatomy of rodents in health and disease; originally published in German, it is now available in English.[42]

DISEASES

General Comments

Diseases of Small Rodents Seen in Practice

The prevalence and types of small rodent diseases seen in practice are quite different from those seen in a research setting. Although this may seem rather obvious, much of the literature describing the maladies of pet rodents has been indiscriminately inferred from conditions seen in laboratory rodents. The diagnosis and treatment of pet rodents involves evaluation and care of an individual animal from a household, not the health management of rodents from a research colony. Derangements likely to be seen in practice include trauma-induced injuries, infectious diseases, and problems related to nutrition and aging; genetic disorders are uncommon. Natural infections that would be considered rare in a laboratory animal colony often are transmitted to pet rodents by other pets and by children; for example, pet animals other than rodents are a major reservoir of dermatophytes,[16] and humans are the main natural host of *Streptococcus pneumoniae* and *S. pyogenes*.[31] Rodents used for research are maintained in tightly controlled environments designed to reduce the impact of unwanted variables in animal experiments.[11] However, pet rodents generally are exposed to temperature, humidity, and light-cycle changes; a broad range of foods; numerous microorganisms borne by animals and humans; and various types of handling. As a result, pet rodents exhibit a wider range of physiologic and pathologic responses than do rodents used for research. Consequently, the disease presentation of many pet rodents does not conform to the classic description of the disease.

Veterinarians must be discerning in their selection of information about rodents. Despite the appearance of an increasing number of articles and books on "pet rodents," or "pocket pets," scientific publications will become a helpful resource for diagnosis only if they deal specifically with this population of rodents. At the moment, I find scientific publications to be more obscuring than elucidating for small exotic animal practice. According to these publications, rodents are treated as part of a herd or as experimental tools, and disease is diagnosed in them on postmortem examination. Successful diagnosis and resolution of disease are not addressed, and it is in this area that our understanding must be broadened.

Significant Diseases and Life Spans

Pet mice, rats, gerbils, and hamsters are subject to a limited number of naturally occurring medical problems. The most common, spontaneous outbreaks of disease are caused, or at least stimulated, by shortcomings in feeding and management. Some of these problems, which are unique to each species, are listed and grouped by the primary organ system affected in Table 27–1. The average life span of each species also is given. Most problems in these species are dermatopathies, enteropathies, or pneumonia. Problems such as malnutrition, hypothermia, and trauma, which also are commonly seen in small exotic animal practice but are not necessarily unique to a species, are not presented.

Prophylaxis for Small Rodents

Prevention of disease in rodents is far more successful than treatment. Disease prevention is primarily based on common-sense husbandry practices, such as purchasing healthy, genetically sound animals; supplying balanced fresh food appropriate in protein and caloric content; providing clean, fresh water; furnishing adequate shelter that includes shade from direct sunlight; avoiding drafts and excessive temperature or humidity changes; keeping cages clean by preventing the accumulation of excess feces and urine; isolating sick animals from a group for treatment; and protecting vulnerable animals from more aggressive members of their group (e.g., young animals from older animals, and male hamsters from female hamsters) or from natural predators living in the same household (e.g., mice from cats). Other sound husbandry practices include housing different species separately in order to prevent interspecies disease transmission (e.g., rats carry *Streptobacillus moniliformis* in their nasopharyngeal cavity, and this pathogen causes septicemia in mice) and reducing obesity by limiting food intake and providing cage accessories that allow play and exploration (e.g., exercise wheels, tunnels, and ramps).

Unlike larger companion animals, pet rodents are not vaccinated; however, a formalin-killed Sendai virus vaccine is available commercially (Microbiological Associates, Bethesda, MD). The introduction of ivermectin, although not approved for use in any rodent species, has allowed routine systemic treatment of pet rodents with pinworms and mites.

Dental problems are commonly seen in pet rodents because of their continually erupting teeth. Overgrown incisors are seen most frequently in rats and mice, and molar malocclusion in guinea pigs and chinchillas. Specially designed cheek dilators, mouth specula, and rasps for the filing of teeth have been available in Europe for several years. This dental equipment is now available in North America (Jorgensen Laboratories, Loveland, CO).

TABLE 27–1
COMMON PROBLEMS OF SMALL RODENTS SEEN IN CLINICAL PRACTICE

	Species (Average Life Span)			
Organ System	*Mice (1.5–2.5 y)*	*Rats (2–3 y)*	*Hamsters (1.5–2 y)*	*Gerbils (3–4 y)*
Integumentary and mammary gland	Alopecia, bite wounds, ectoparasites, mammary neoplasms	Ulcerative dermatitis, mammary neoplasms, ectoparasites, ringtail	Bite wounds, scent gland tumors	Nasal dermatitis, ventral gland lesions, tail-slip
Digestive	Neonatal enteritis, endoparasites	Salivary gland inflammation, incisor overgrowth	Diarrhea, enterotoxemia, weight loss	Enteritis
Respiratory	Chronic respiratory disease	Chronic respiratory disease, pneumonia	Pneumonia	
Urinary	Obstructive uropathies	Chronic renal disease		
Reproductive			Vaginal discharge, maternal cannibalism	
Ocular		Red tears	Exophthalmos	
Cardiovascular			Atrial thrombosis, congestive heart failure	
Endocrine			Hyperadrenocorticism	
Nervous				Epileptic seizures

Clinical Signs and Treatment

Mice

INTEGUMENTARY SYSTEM AND MAMMARY GLANDS

Many of the common problems observed in pet mice are associated with the skin. *Barbering* is a unique condition seen in mice that are housed as a group; in barbering, a dominant mouse nibbles off the whiskers and hair around the muzzle and eyes of cagemates (Fig. 27–1). There are no other lesions, and only one mouse (the dominant one) retains all of its fur. Removal of the dominant mouse stops barbering; frequently, however, another mouse assumes the dominant role. Barbering is often seen in female mice that are caged together. Male mice, except littermates raised together from birth, are more likely to fight and inflict bite wounds on one another, especially over the rump and shoulders.

Sometimes, small patches of alopecia appear on the lateral surfaces of the muzzle. These result from self-abrasion on metal feeders or cage tops. Unlike barbering, dermatitis also may be associated with the alopecic area. Treatment consists of replacing the feeders or providing environmental enrichment toys such as running wheels or hollow tubes in the cage in an effort to stop self-traumatizing behavior. Nursing mice often have ventral abdominal and thoracic alopecia; this is normal and is nearly always associated with the extensive distribution of mammary glands.

Generalized thinning of the hair, especially on difficult-to-groom areas such as the head and trunk, is seen in fur mite infestations (Fig. 27–2). The coat often has a greasy appearance and, in cases of heavy infestation, noticeable pruritus and self-inflicted dermal ulceration may occur. Sometimes, an owner presents a pet mouse with clinical signs of mite infestation but with no known history of recent exposure to other animals. It is my impression that mite

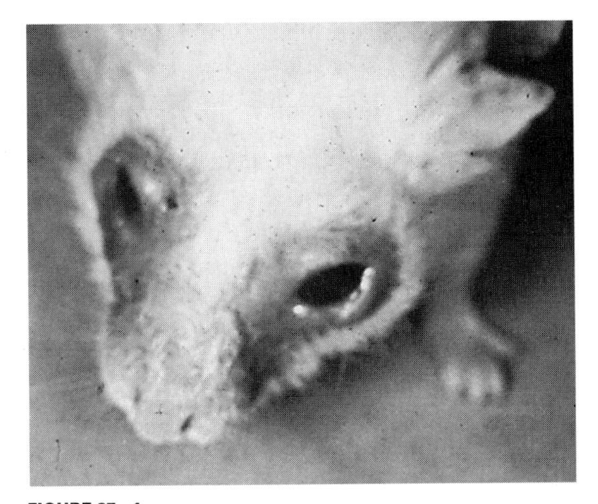

FIGURE 27–1
Barbering in a mouse. Barbering is often seen in mice housed in groups, in which the dominant mouse chews the facial hair and whiskers of its cagemates.

infestation in these cases has been present subclinically for weeks or months before it develops into a clinically recognizable problem. Unless the pet mouse has a known history of exposure to wild mice, only three mites are commonly seen: *Myobia musculi, Myocoptes musculinus,* and *Radfordia affinis*. Clinical disease, diagnosis, treatment, and control are similar for all mice with any of these mites except *M. musculi*. This mite is associated with dermal hypersensitivity in certain inbred strains of black mice and is characterized by severe pruritus, the presence of fine dandruff all over the body, and occasionally ulcerative dermatitis.[15] Infestations usually are caused by more than one species. Mites are spread by direct contact with infected mice or infested bedding. Diagnosis is based on the identification of adult mites, nymphs, or eggs on hair shafts with the use of a hand lens or a stereoscopic microscope. Adults and nymphs appear pearly white and elongate (being about twice as long as they are wide); eggs are oval and seen attached to the base of hairs or inside mature females.

Treat mite infestations with ivermectin (0.2–0.4 mg/kg SC or PO given twice at 10-day intervals). Alternatively, place a few drops of ivermectin solution (diluted to 1:100 in equal parts of water and propylene glycol for three treatments) on the mouse's head to allow spread by grooming and ingestion.[3] Fragrant timber chips such as cedar and pine are high in volatile hydrocarbons and have long been known to have ectoparasiticidal properties. However, the hydrocarbons also induce cytochrome P-450 enzymes in the liver. This results in an increase in the metabolism of many common drugs and a reduction in the anesthetic time of several barbiturates.

Skin swellings usually are tumors or abscesses. Needle biopsy often reveals the nature of the contents and allows diagnosis. Three bacterial species —*Staphylococcus aureus, Pasteurella pneumotropica,* and *Strep. pyogenes*—have been isolated as the causes in various well-described cases.[37] All are considered opportunistic pathogens and can cause abscesses in other organs (e.g., *P. pneumotropica* sometimes is associated with conjunctivitis, panophthalmitis, and swollen eye abscesses). Antibiotic therapy with penicillins or cephalosporins, concurrent with drainage and débridement of the abscess, is effective.

The most common spontaneous tumors associated with the skin are mammary adenocarcinomas, followed by fibrosarcomas. The incidence of

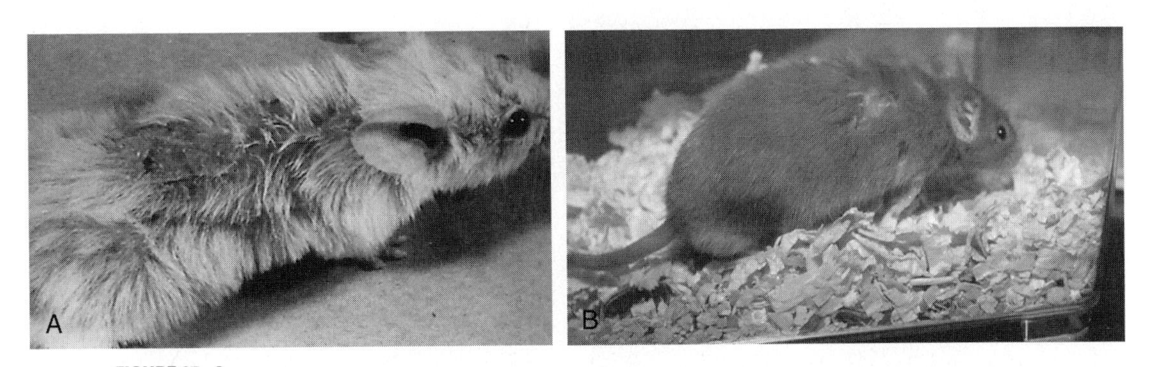

FIGURE 27–2
A, Alopecia is commonly associated with mite infestation in mice. *B*, Noticeable pruritus and self-inflicted dermal ulceration may be observed. Three mite species are commonly seen: *Myobia musculi, Myocoptes musculinus,* and *Radfordia affinis.*

mammary tumors varies according to the mouse strain and the presence or absence of mouse mammary tumor viruses; the incidence is as high as 70% in some strains.[48] In wild and outbred mice, the incidence of fibrosarcomas ranges from 1 to 6%.[21] Subcutaneous tumors are nearly always malignant and often have ulcerated by the time a diagnosis is made. Tumors can be treated by surgical excision, but the chance of recurrence is high and the prognosis is poor. Attempts to treat tumors in mice by radiation or chemotherapy have not been reported.

DIGESTIVE SYSTEM

Diarrhea in neonatal and adult mice is usually of viral origin. Enteritis is more severe in neonates and sucklings than in adults. In addition to more obvious clinical signs such as diarrhea, retarded growth, and dehydration, the absence of milk in the gastrointestinal tract is characteristic of digestive disease in young mice (Fig. 27–3). The most important pathogen is mouse hepatitis virus (MHV), a large group of coronaviruses that naturally infect mice. The research literature on MHV infection is vast, and most of it is not helpful in gaining an understanding of the pathogenesis of natural infections. Numerous factors affect disease expression, such as the virulence and organ trophism of the virus, as well as the age, genotype, and immunocompetence of the mouse; however, the most common clinical form of the disease is severe enteritis in neonates. One of the earlier terms for MHV was *lethal intestinal virus of infant mice*.[27] Affected mouse pups are runted and dehydrated, and no milk is present in the stomach or intestines. A milder form of enteritis in neonatal mice is caused by rotavirus. In contrast to mice with MHV, pups with rotavirus infection have distended abdomens owing to the accumulation of milk in the stomach but not in the intestines (see Fig. 27–3). Varying amounts of watery stool accumulate around the base of a pup's tail, soiling the coats of the young and mother. Affected pups generally survive because they continue to nurse. Treatment involves management of clinical signs and primarily consists of fluid administration.

Endoparasites are relatively common in mice. However, only two parasites regularly encountered in the digestive tract—the closely related protozoa *Spironucleus muris* and *Giardia muris*—are considered pathogenic, even though they are not associated with clinical signs in immunocompetent hosts. Diagnosis is based on the demonstration of characteristic trophozoites in wet mounts of fresh intestinal contents or feces (see Fig. 24–8). Treatment of both parasites is the addition of metronidazole to the drinking water (0.04–0.10% for 14 days), but it does not completely eliminate the infection.[22]

Pinworms are ubiquitous and considered nonpathogenic. Two are commonly encountered in mice: *Syphacia obvelata* and *Aspicularis tetraptera*. Often, the only indication of pinworm infestation is rectal prolapse caused by straining. To establish a diagnosis of *S. obvelata* infestation, make a clear cellophane tape impression of the perianal skin. Adult *S. obvelata* females deposit ova around the anus. *A. tetraptera* does not deposit its ova in this

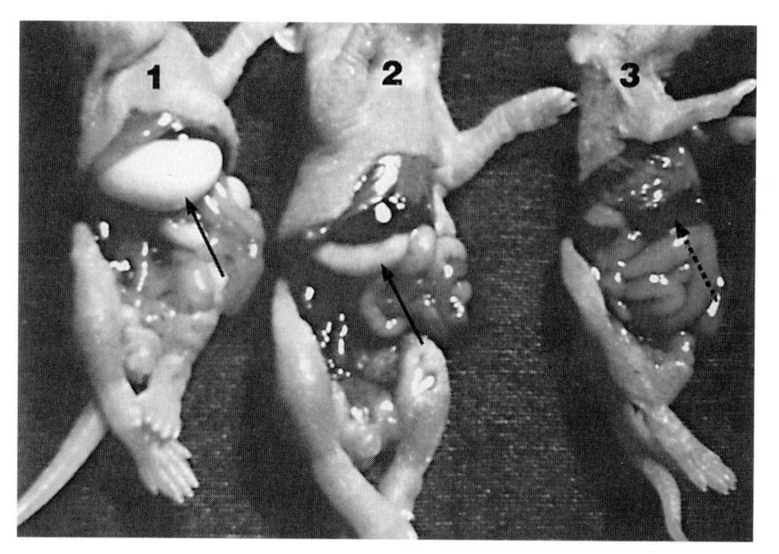

FIGURE 27–3

Two types of enteric viral infection are common in neonatal mice. The three mice shown illustrate (1) rotavirus infection; (2) normal mouse; and (3) mouse hepatitis virus infection. Note that the stomachs either contain milk *(solid arrows)* or are empty *(dashed arrows)*.

area, and a fecal smear or flotation is required for confirmation of a diagnosis. Ivermectin (2.0 mg/kg PO given twice at a 10-day interval) eliminates pinworms from mice. Ivermectin 1% is diluted 1:9 in vegetable oil to establish a concentration of 1.0 mg/mL; affected mice are dosed with a volume of 0.2 mL per 100 g PO.[14] The recommended package label dose for mice with ectoparasites (0.2 mg/kg given twice at a 10-day interval) does not eliminate pinworms.[24]

Diarrhea is not frequently seen in adult mice. Digestive disease in adult mice usually is caused by a varying combination of pathogenic and opportunistic infectious agents. Fecal flotation and fresh wet mounts of feces often yield positive results and do not necessarily give a definitive diagnosis. However, these techniques sometimes are helpful in identifying heavy endoparasite infestations. Treatment is generally directed at clinical signs and consists of the judicious use of antimicrobials and antiparasitics.

RESPIRATORY SYSTEM

Diseases of the upper and lower respiratory tracts are common in pet mice and rats. Animals may be presented with sniffling, sneezing, chattering, and labored breathing. If dyspnea is suspected, do not overhandle the animal during clinical examination as it may die. Collection of tracheal and nasal secretions is not recommended because swabbing is highly traumatic and because the cause of the disease is generally a mixed viral, mycoplasmal, and bacterial infection. Antibiotic treatment is helpful but generally does not eliminate the disease.

The two most common causes of clinical respiratory disease in mice are Sendai virus and *Mycoplasma pulmonis*. Sendai virus is associated with an acute respiratory infection in which mice display chattering and mild respiratory distress. Neonates and weanlings may die. Adults generally recover within 2 months. When respiratory disease exceeds this pattern, the cause is most likely concurrent mycoplasmal infection. *M. pulmonis* is the cause of chronic pneumonia, suppurative rhinitis, and occasionally otitis media. Chattering and dyspnea are caused by accumulations of purulent exudate in inflamed and thickened nasal passages. Survivors develop chronic bronchopneumonia and bronchiectasis, and may develop pulmonary abscesses (this does not happen in rats). Antibiotic therapy may alleviate clinical signs but does not eliminate the infection. A simple and inexpensive treatment is the addition of tetracycline (3 mg/mL) to the drinking water for 7 days. However, tetracycline often alters the taste of water, and some mice do not drink it or are too weak to drink because of their illness. Alternatively, enrofloxacin (10 mg/kg) in combination with doxycycline hyclate (5 mg/kg) given every 12 hours PO for 7 days is helpful.

URINARY SYSTEM

Obstruction of the urethra in male mice has been described as resulting from infections of the preputial glands with *S. aureus* and of the bulbourethral glands with *P. pneumotropica*; accessory sex gland secretions and, rarely, urolithiasis also have been implicated. Mice often are presented to the veterinarian because they mutilate their own penis as a result of these conditions. In addition, occasional injury of the penis is seen in young males from aggressive breeding activity and abrasion on the cage. Treatment involves isolation of the affected mouse, cleaning and débridement of the affected areas, and treatment with antibiotics.

Rats

INTEGUMENTARY SYSTEM AND MAMMARY GLANDS

Ulcerative dermatitis caused by *S. aureus* infection results from self-traumatization associated with fur mite infestation or, more commonly, from scratching of the skin over an inflamed salivary gland. Treatment consists of clipping the toenails of the hindpaws, cleaning the ulcerated skin, and applying a topical antibiotic. Systemic treatment is rarely necessary, as rats have a remarkable ability to resist infection with *S. aureus*.[12]

The most common subcutaneous tumor in the rat is fibroadenoma of the mammary glands. The distribution of the mammary tissue is extensive, and the tumors can occur anywhere from the neck to the inguinal region (Fig. 27–4). Tumors can reach 8–10 cm in diameter and occur in both males and females. The surgical technique for tumor removal is straightforward (see Chapter 28), and survival following mastectomy is good if the tumor is benign.[23] Adenocarcinomas represent fewer than 10% of mammary tumors in rats. The prevalence of mammary tumors, as well as that of pituitary tumors, is significantly lower in ovariectomized rats compared with sexually intact Sprague-Dawley rats.[23] However, the recurrence of fibroadenomas is common in uninvolved mammary tissue, and often several surgeries are needed. In contrast, mammary tumors in mice are nearly always malignant and often are not amenable to surgical removal.

Ectoparasitic infestation is less common in rats

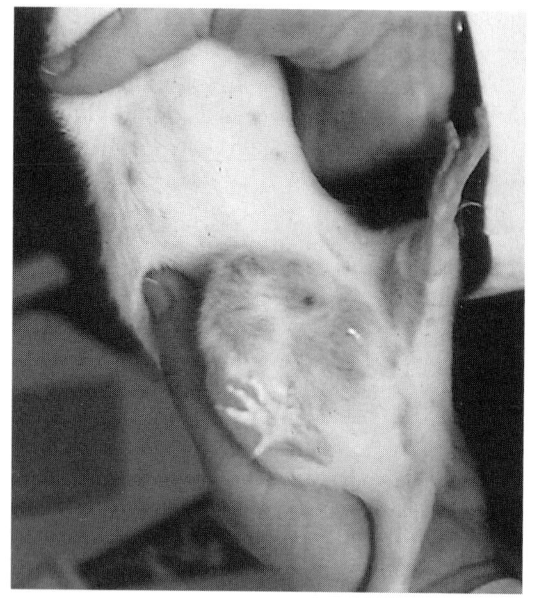

FIGURE 27–4
Mammary fibroadenoma in the inguinal region of a female rat.

than in mice. Occasionally, the fur mite *Radfordia ensifera* is seen. Although *R. ensifera* infestation produces few ill effects, heavy infestation may lead to self-traumatization and ulcerative dermatitis. Other mites, including *Demodex* species, have been described in rats maintained in laboratories[51]; however, they are seldom seen, and no contemporary reports of infestations in pet rats appear in the literature. Diagnosis and treatment are the same as those for mice.

Avascular necrosis of the tail, or *ringtail,* is a highly photogenic lesion of rats and probably for this reason is always described in textbooks and articles on diseases of rats. It occurs primarily in young laboratory rats in low-humidity environments, and often in rats housed in hanging cages; it is rarely seen in pet rats. If ringtail is diagnosed, treatment involves amputation of the tail proximal to the necrotic annular constriction.

DIGESTIVE SYSTEM

Inflammation and edema of the cervical salivary glands is caused by sialodacryoadenitis virus, a coronavirus. Owners of infected rats often describe their pets as having mumps. Sialodacryoadenitis virus infection is highly contagious. It initially causes rhinitis followed by epithelial necrosis of the salivary and lacrimal glands. Cervical lymph nodes also become enlarged. There is no treatment for this disease. Glandular healing follows within 7–10 days, and clinical signs subside within 30 days, with minimal residual lesions remaining. During acute inflammation, affected rats are at high risk for anesthesia-related mortality because of the decreased diameter of the upper respiratory tract lumen; also, ocular lesions such as conjunctivitis, keratitis, corneal ulcers, synechia, and hyphema can occur secondary to lacrimal dysfunction. The eye lesions usually resolve but occasionally progress to chronic keratitis and megaglobus.

Overgrowth of the incisors is common in rats, and their teeth can grow into the nasal cavity (Fig. 27–5). Overgrowth is easily treated by cutting the teeth with rongeurs to correct the overgrown portion. This procedure can be done in a conscious patient. However, it may not produce good long-term results, and problems may arise. The incisor may fracture longitudinally; the fracture may reach the apex and cause the animal discomfort. Bacteria can enter the fractured tooth, track down to the apex, and cause an apical abscess.[13] Also, clipped teeth have jagged edges that may lacerate the tongue and other soft tissues. An alternative technique involves the use of a high-speed drill; the drill cuts through the overgrown incisors without splitting or splintering them, leaving a clean, smooth surface. The rat must be sedated or anesthetized for this procedure. Some owners may prefer not to return their pets regularly for tooth trimming. Extraction of the incisors is an alternative to trimming; however, this procedure is difficult because of the incisors' long roots. Old rats may show yellowing of the cranial aspect of their incisors; this is normal and is caused by iron deposition within the enamel.

RESPIRATORY SYSTEM

Respiratory disease caused by infectious agents is the most common health problem in rats. Five recognized respiratory pathogens cause overt clinical disease: *M. pulmonis, S. pneumoniae, Corynebacterium kutscheri,* Sendai virus, and cilia-associated respiratory (CAR) bacillus. Synergistic interactions are common, and two major clinical syndromes are seen: chronic respiratory disease, which is usually caused by *M. pulmonis* in combination with Sendai virus or CAR bacillus; and acute pneumonia caused by *S. pneumoniae* (Fig. 27–6) but seldom in the absence of some combination involving *M. pulmonis,* Sendai virus, or CAR bacillus. Infection with *C. kutscheri* (Fig. 27–7) results in clinical pneumonia only after immunosuppression. In pet rats, immuno-

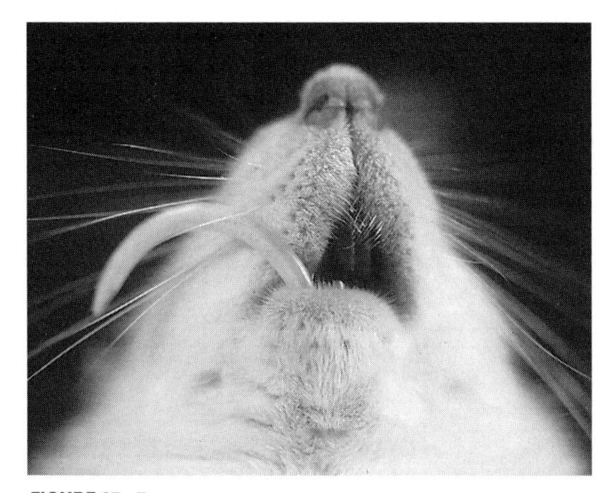

FIGURE 27–5

Overgrown incisors in a rat. Overgrown teeth can be clipped with rongeurs or cut with a high-speed drill.

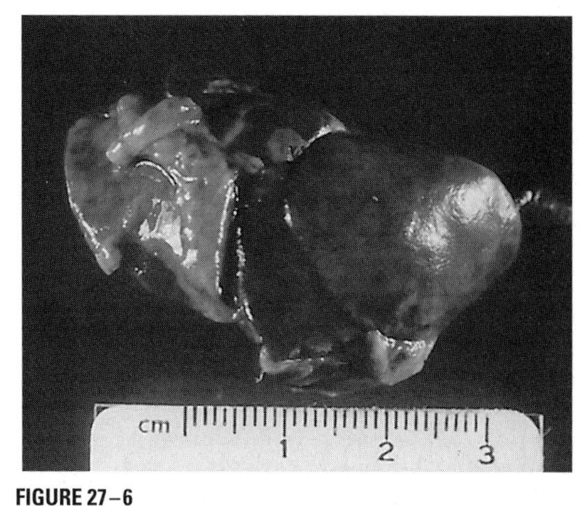

FIGURE 27–6

Fibrinopurulent pneumonia in a rat caused by *Streptococcus pneumoniae*.

suppression can result from diabetes, neoplasia, or dietary deficiencies.

Rats may live 2–3 years with chronic respiratory disease. Clinical signs are highly variable: initial infection commonly occurs without any clinical signs; early signs involve both the upper and the lower respiratory tracts and may include snuffling, nasal discharge, polypnea, weight loss, hunched posture, ruffled coat, head tilt, and red tears.[26, 37] Respiratory mycoplasmosis in rats varies greatly in disease expression because of environmental, host, and mycoplasmal factors that influence the host-pathogen relationship. Examples of such factors include intracage ammonia levels, concurrent Sendai virus, corona-virus (sialodacryoadenitis virus), or CAR bacillus infection, the genetic susceptibility of the host, the virulence of the *Mycoplasma* strain, and vitamin A or E deficiency.[37] For many years, the standard treatment for laboratory rats was the addition of tetracycline (3 mg/mL) to sweetened water. However, this treatment in rats is controversial because antibiotic blood concentrations often are below minimum inhibitory concentrations and because pulmonary tissue concentration of the antibiotic may be noninhibitory. Tetracycline may be considered palliative. In pet rats, I find a better alternative is the daily administration of enrofloxacin (10 mg/kg PO q12h for 7 days) in combination with doxycycline hyclate (5 mg/kg PO q12h for 7–21 days). If the rat responds, there is a good chance that it will exhibit recurrent symptoms because treatment does not completely eliminate the pathogen.

Acute pneumonia caused by *S. pneumoniae* can be of sudden onset. Young rats are more severely affected than are older ones, and sometimes the only sign they exhibit is sudden death. Mature rats may demonstrate dyspnea, snuffling, and abdominal breathing. A purulent exudate may be seen around the nares and on the front paws (from wiping of the nostrils). A tentative diagnosis is based on the identification of numerous gram-positive diplococci on a Gram's stain of the exudate or in a sample submit-

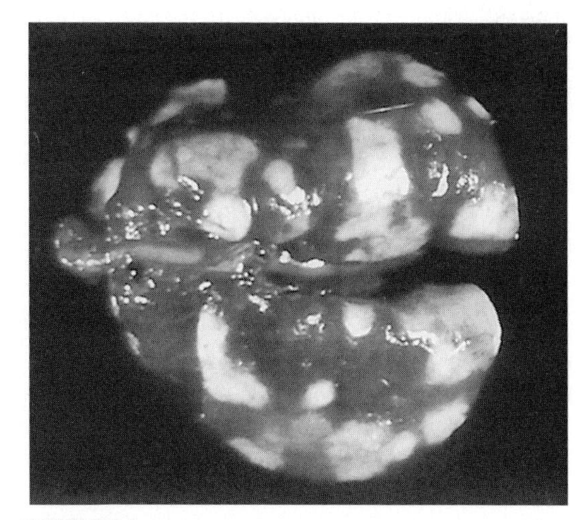

FIGURE 27–7

Gross appearance of the lungs in a diabetic rat with pneumonia caused by *Corynebacterium kutscheri* infection. Lobular pneumonia is the result of the hematogenous spread of the organism. Compare the appearance of these lungs with that of the lungs in Figure 27–6.

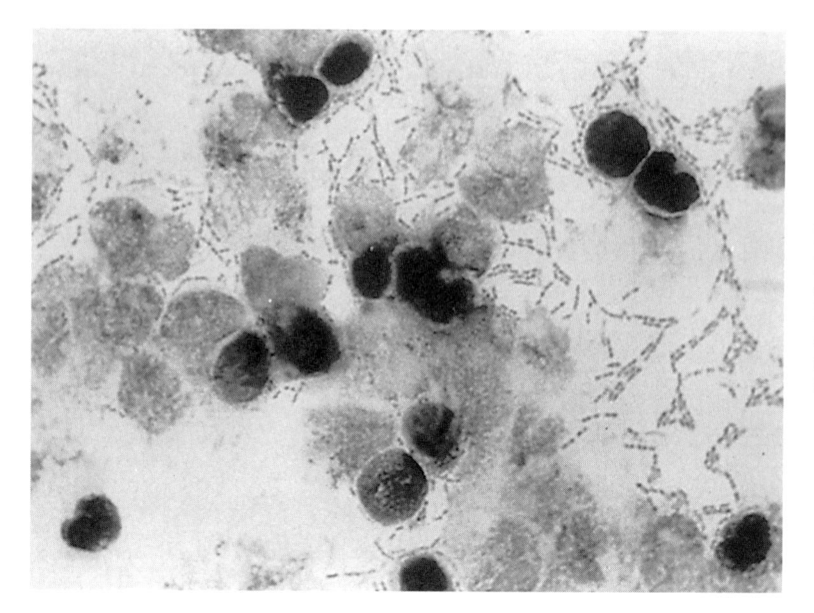

FIGURE 27–8

Photomicrograph of a Giemsa-stained smear from a rat with a nasal exudate. Multiple diplococci characteristic of *S. pneumoniae* are seen. The polymorphonuclear cells characteristic of purulent exudate are clearly visible.

ted for cytologic examination (Fig. 27–8). Severe bacteremia is an important consequence of advanced disease and results in multiorgan abscesses and infarction. Treatment must be aggressive, and the use of beta-lactamase–resistant penicillins such as cloxacillin, oxacillin, and dicloxacillin (all of which can be administered orally) is recommended. There are no published dosages of these drugs for rats, and the dosage is empirical.

URINARY SYSTEM

Chronic progressive nephrosis (CPN) is the best-known age-related disease in rats. In CPN, the kidneys are enlarged and pale and have a pitted, mottled surface that often contains pinpoint cysts (Fig. 27–9). Lesions consist of a progressive glomerulosclerosis and myriad tubulointerstitial disease primarily involving the convoluted proximal tubule[18] (Fig. 27–10). The most striking change in renal function is a proteinuria exceeding 10 mg/d and that increases in severity progressively with age. The features of CPN are qualitatively similar among different strains of laboratory rats, but the onset, incidence, and severity of the disease vary considerably. The disease occurs earlier and is of greater severity in males than in females: urinary protein excretion averaging 137 mg/d has been documented in 18-month-old male Sprague-Dawley rats, whereas excretion averaging 76 mg/d was reported in female rats of the same age.[44] Dietary factors appear to have an important role in the progression of CPN. Caloric restriction, the feeding of low-protein diets (4–7%), and limiting the source of dietary protein reduce the incidence and severity of CPN. The feeding of soybean protein (as opposed to casein) and caloric restriction contribute substantially to a reduction in the incidence and severity of CPN; low-calorie diets that contain high protein levels do not decrease the disease's incidence and severity. CPN also can be exacerbated by drugs and exposure to chemicals. Treatment is supportive and involves feeding a low-protein diet and administration of anabolic steroids.

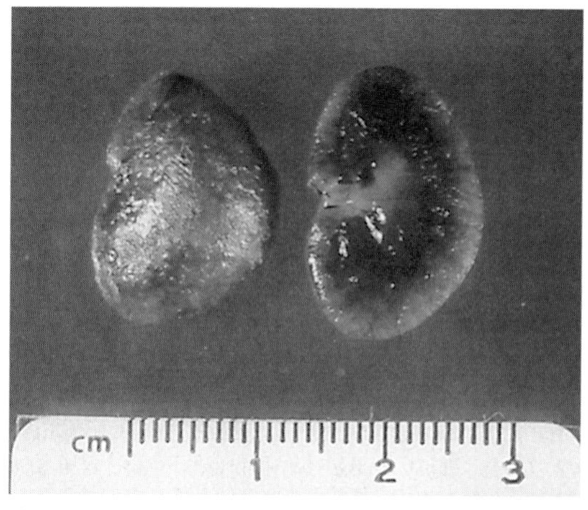

FIGURE 27–9

Enlarged and pale kidneys from a rat with chronic progressive nephrosis. Note the pitted, mottled surface containing pinpoint cysts.

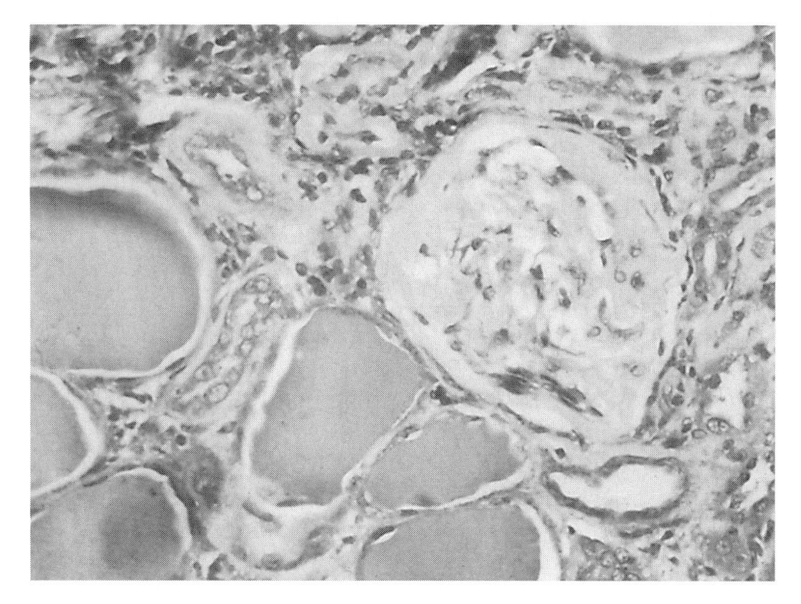

FIGURE 27–10

Photomicrograph of severe glomerulosclerosis in a rat. The proximal tubules are dilated and contain copious amounts of a protein-rich material; this finding is indicative of the deterioration of glomeruli that fail to filter and retain plasma protein.

OCULAR SYSTEM

The harderian glands of rats are located behind the eyes. They secrete various porphyrins that give these animals' tears a reddish color. Harderian gland secretion is increased in response to stress and disease, and the tears themselves dry around the eyes and external nares (the nasolacrimal duct drains into the nasal cavity), resembling crusts of blood (Fig. 27–11). It is common for owners to report bleeding from the eyes and nose of their pet rats. The porphyrins fluoresce under ultraviolet light and can be readily differentiated from blood with a Wood's lamp. The condition is known as *chromodacryorrhea* or *red tears,* and although it is not pathologic, it is a consequence of acute-onset stress such as that caused by pain, illness, or restraint. Red tears often are an indication of a chronic underlying disease, and their discovery warrants a thorough evaluation of the affected pet rat.

Hamsters

Although many types of hamsters live in the wild, only a few types are kept as pets. The most common pet hamster is the golden or Syrian hamster *(Mesocricetus auratus),* which has been kept as a pet since the 1940s. Although two other species of hamsters, the common or European hamster *(Cricetus cricetus)* and the ratlike Chinese hamster *(Cricetulus griseus)* are used in research, they do not make good pets because of their aggressive nature. However, dwarf species such as the Djungarian hamster *(Phodopus sungorus)* and Roborovsky's hamster *(P. roborovskii)* are being seen increasingly as pets because they have a docile disposition, do not attempt to bite or run away, and do well in captivity. Very few reports of spontaneous diseases in these animals have been published; Cantrell and Padovan have prepared the most complete review to date on this subject.[7]

INTEGUMENTARY SYSTEM AND MARKING GLANDS

The most common skin problem seen in hamsters is haircoat roughness. This is a nonspecific sign of fighting, aging, and a variety of diseases. Female

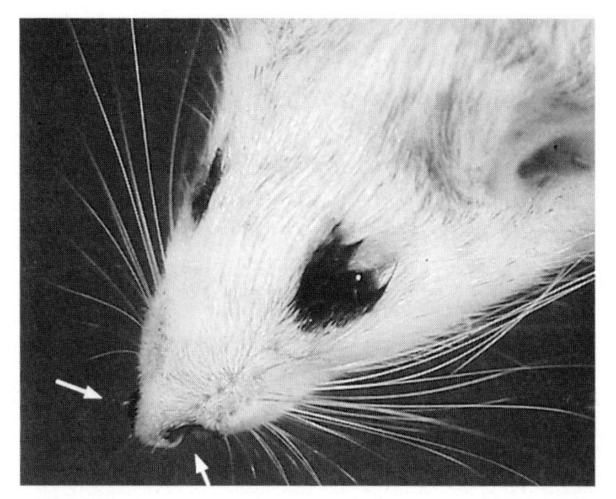

FIGURE 27–11

Chromodacryorrhea or red tears in a rat. The color of the stained fur around the eye results from porphyrin pigments in the harderian gland's secretions, which are also visible around the nares *(arrows).*

hamsters are heavier than males and generally are aggressive, not only toward other hamsters but also their owners and can inflict severe bite wounds on cagemates. Nonestrous females can behave especially aggressively toward young males and may kill them.

Hamsters have distensible cheek pouches that may be mistaken for lesions by the owner.[4] Sometimes, the cheek pouches become impacted, and removal of the material from the pouch with fine forceps is necessary. A radiograph of the head often shows the extent of the impaction.[42] Predisposing causes of impaction, such as malocclusion of incisors or molars, should be investigated. Male hamsters have large, pendulous testes and pigmented sebaceous flank glands, which clients may mistake for "tumors."

DIGESTIVE SYSTEM

The most common problems seen in pet hamsters are enteropathies. Diarrhea may occur in hamsters of any age and is known as "wet-tail," even though this euphemism more frequently is used to describe the disease in young hamsters. Proliferative ileitis is the most significant intestinal disease of 3–10-week-old hamsters and results in high mortality. It is caused by the newly described intracellular bacterium *Lawsonia intracellularis,* which is also responsible for proliferative enteropathy in pigs and ferrets.[34, 39] Treatment must be aggressive and involves the correction of life-threatening electrolyte imbalance, the administration of antibiotics, and force-feeding. Several antibiotic treatments are recommended, including tetracycline hydrochloride (400 mg/L of drinking water for 10 days), tetracycline (10 mg/kg PO q12h for 5–7 days), enrofloxacin (10 mg/kg PO or IM q12h for 5–7 days), and trimethoprim-sulfa combination (30 mg/kg PO q12h for 5–7 days). Symptomatic treatment with bismuth subsalicylate may be given if diarrhea persists. Kuntze recommends giving an electrolyte and glucose injection of 40–60 mL/kg SC q24h and feeding a puree (20–30 mL/kg q24h PO) consisting of baby spinach, apples, carrots, and lettuce mixed in equal parts with a slurry made from rodent pellets.[29] Kuntze also suggests that adding 1 tablespoon of honey to the feed mixture may make it more palatable and that giving slightly salted teas, such as black currant, peppermint, and chamomile, may aid in recovery.[29] Sequelae to proliferative ileitis in surviving hamsters may include eventual obstruction, intussusception, or rectal prolapse (see Chapter 28).[10]

Diarrhea in adult hamsters is associated with *Clostridium difficile* enterotoxemia and, as in guinea pigs, may occur 3 to 5 days after the administration of antibiotics such as penicillin, lincomycin, or bacitracin. Oral administration of bovine antibodies against toxigenic *C. difficile* has been shown to protect hamsters against experimental antibiotic-associated enterotoxemia.[33]

Tyzzer's disease (*Clostridium piliforme,* previously known as *Bacillus piliformis*) was described in hamsters and gerbils obtained from a pet store supplier.[35] The supplier's hamsters and gerbils had a high mortality rate but its rats and mice did not. Affected rodents were depressed and dehydrated and had scruffy coats as well as diarrhea; many animals had no clinical signs before death. The authors concluded that the clinical outbreak was precipitated by severe stress, including that caused by overcrowding, high environmental temperature and humidity, heavy internal and external parasite load, and nutritionally inadequate diets despite the prophylactic treatment of drinking water with oxytetracycline. Tyzzer's disease, first recognized in 1917 by Tyzzer at Harvard in a colony of Japanese waltzing mice,[49] is frequently listed as an infectious intestinal disease of rodents and other animals in laboratory animal textbooks. However, the actual prevalence of the infection in contemporary rodents remains unknown. The report concerning the pet store illustrates the opportunistic nature of *C. piliforme* in immunosuppressed animals. The disease is not seen in healthy immunocompetent animals.

Weight loss is seen in older hamsters and often is associated with hepatic and renal amyloidosis. One research report described amyloidosis in 88% of hamsters older than 18 months of age.[17] Amyloidosis also is reported as the principal cause of death of hamsters in long-term research studies.[43] The same authors reported a higher incidence, increased severity, and earlier age of onset of amyloidosis in female hamsters as compared with male hamsters.[43] There are no descriptions of the incidence or of clinical signs of disease in pet hamsters. However, one would expect edema and ascites caused by hypoproteinemia of hepatic and renal origin. If amyloidosis is diagnosed in a pet hamster, the prognosis is poor and treatment is supportive.

RESPIRATORY SYSTEM

In response to a survey, 6 of 14 laboratories in the United States reported pneumonia as the second most common clinical condition in hamsters after diarrhea.[41] An earlier survey conducted in Germany noted respiratory infections in 8% of all clinical conditions in hamsters.[32] Histologic evidence of bronchopneumonia resembling bacterial pneumonia and of interstitial pneumonia resembling viral pneumonia has been described, but there are no reports of observed clinical cases. Consequently, other authors have stated that respiratory disease is uncommon in hamsters.[20] The true prevalence remains to be established.

Purulent rhinitis associated with pneumonia and gluey eyelids has been described in hamsters and is associated with a poor prognosis.[29] Bacterial pneumonias, especially those caused by *Streptococcus* species may be inadvertently transmitted by children to pet hamsters. Rapid diagnosis can be made with identification of the characteristic gram-positive diplococci on a Gram's stain of nasal and ocular discharges (see Fig. 27–8). Followup culture and treatment with chloramphenicol (chloramphenicol palmitate, 50 mg/kg PO q8h; chloramphenicol succinate, 30 mg/kg IV or IM q8h) are recommended until antibiotic sensitivity results are available.[1]

REPRODUCTIVE SYSTEM

Female hamsters have a 4-day estrus cycle with a characteristic copious postovulatory discharge at the end. The discharge is creamy white and has a distinctive odor; it fills the vagina and usually extrudes through the vaginal orifice (female hamsters have three orifices: urinary, genital, and anal). Its stringy nature is distinctive, and if touched it can be drawn out as a thread of about 4 to 6 inches in length. Owners often describe the discharge as pus and mistakenly believe it to be abnormal.

Pyometra has been observed clinically—although rarely*—in pet hamsters. A tentative diagnosis is made by cytologic examination of the discharge and ultrasound examination of the abdomen, if possible. Ovariohysterectomy is the treatment of choice.

Cannibalism of young is common among hamsters. Most reports describe cannibalism among group-housed female hamsters.[19] Instruct owners of pet hamsters to provide the mother with ample food and water and to leave it alone in a quiet place for at least 1 week or preferably 2 weeks. Disturbing the mother by handling of the young or nest, as well as not providing adequate nesting material, food, or water, most likely results in litter desertion and cannibalism.

*Quesenberry K: Personal communication, 1995.

CARDIOVASCULAR SYSTEM

Atrial thrombosis has been described in aging research hamsters by many authors,[25] and in certain strains it occurs with a high incidence (up to 73%).[8] Most thromboses develop in the left atrium secondary to heart failure and lead to a consumptive coagulopathy (Fig. 27–12). Although the incidence does not differ between the sexes near the end of their respective life spans, atrial thrombosis occurs on average at a younger age in females (13.5 months) than in males (21.5 months).[8] Aged pet hamsters present with clinical signs of cardiomyopathy such as hyperpnea, tachycardia, and cyanosis. In untreated hamsters, death usually follows within a week after these signs are evident. The incidence of atrial thrombosis is influenced by the endocrine status of the animal, and especially by the amount of circulating androgens. Thus, the castration of male hamsters is linked to an increase in the prevalence of atrial thrombosis.[45]

Cardiomyopathy should be suspected in aged pet hamsters (older than 1.5 years) that present clinically with signs of tachypnea, lethargy, anorexia, and cold extremities. Diagnosis of cardiomyopathy in hamsters is based on clinical signs and results of radiography and ultrasound examination of the heart. Treatment of heart disease is symptomatic and involves empirical use of digoxin, diuretics, angiotensin-converting enzyme (ACE) inhibitors, and prophylactic anticoagulants. I have not come across published, recommended dosages of these drugs; I recommend basing dosages on those used in ferrets and monitoring response closely. Verapamil, a calcium antagonist, given to a group of 1-month-old fe-

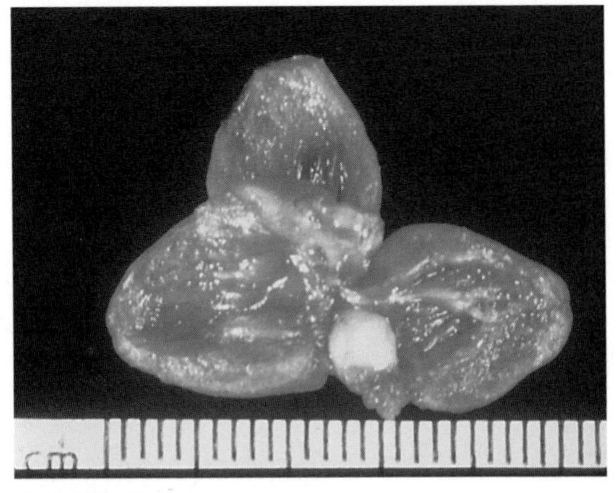

FIGURE 27–12

Thrombosis in the atria of the heart of a hamster secondary to cardiomyopathy. (Courtesy of Heidi L. Hoefer, DVM.)

male myopathic hamsters (0.25 mg–0.50 mg q12h SC over 4 weeks) prevented the development of severe myocardial lesions that were found in the untreated group of animals.[30] However, withdrawing drug treatment caused the return of severe myocardial lesions. This study suggests that continuous treatment with verapamil in hamsters may be protective against the development of cardiomyopathy. A clinical trial remains to be done.

A white, inbred strain of hamsters having an early and severe onset of cardiac failure has been developed as an animal model of muscular dystrophy. When these animals are acquired from laboratories as pets, they present with severe clinical signs of congestive heart failure or experience sudden death.[6] I occasionally see such pet hamsters in children's schools.

ENDOCRINE SYSTEM

Surveys of spontaneous lesions in laboratory hamsters describe a high incidence of adrenocortical hyperplasia and adenoma.[43] However, despite extensive histopathologic study, there has been only one clinical report of hyperadrenocorticism or Cushing's disease in three hamsters, with high serum cortisol concentrations documented in only one of the three animals.[2] This report documented high serum cortisol concentrations in only one of three pet hamsters presented because of alopecia and hyperpigmentation of the skin. Hamsters with clinical signs resembling those of Cushing's disease are occasionally seen in practice (Fig. 27–13). Diagnosis is based on identification of classic signs seen in dogs, such as a history of polydipsia, polyuria, and polyphagia; clinical signs of alopecia and hyperpigmentation; and high concentrations of plasma cortisol and serum alkaline phosphatase. Normal hamster cortisol concentrations are low compared with those of other species and range from 0.5 to 1.0 μg/dL in normal males and females.[52] Research has suggested that hamsters may secrete both cortisol and corticosterone.[38] Therefore, meaningful measurement of plasma cortisol concentrations in hamsters is empirical at present. If hyperadrenocorticism is suspected, the cause, such as hypersecretion by a functional tumor, primary adrenal hyperplasia, or excess adrenocorticotropic hormone production, often is more difficult to determine. Hamsters respond to exogenous adrenocorticotropic hormone stimulation.[52] The treatment of hamsters described in the clinical report by Bauck and coworkers indicated that one hamster receiving metyrapone (8 mg PO q24h for 1 month) responded well; another hamster receiving mitotane (5 mg PO q24h for 1 month) did not improve, and was then given a similar dose of metyrapone, also without success. Further research needs to be done on this syndrome.

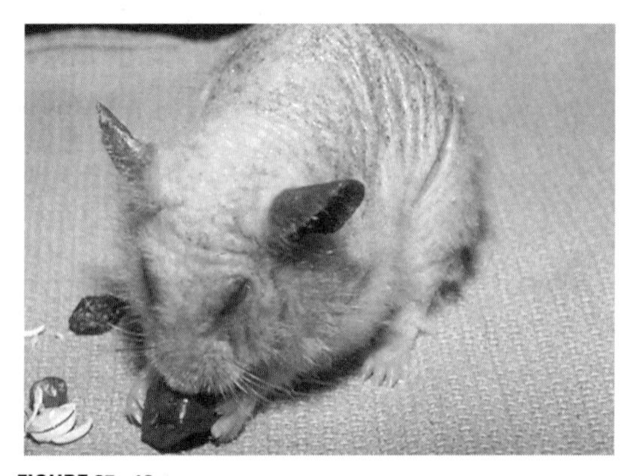

FIGURE 27–13
Generalized alopecia associated with adrenocortical hyperplasia in a hamster.

OCULAR SYSTEM

Protrusion of one or both eyeballs is commonly seen in hamsters and usually occurs as a result of ocular infection, trauma to the periorbital area, or inappropriate restraint. Hamsters with sialodacryoadenitis may develop keratoconjunctivitis sicca and subsequent exophthalmos. Occasionally, a hamster's eye is displaced forward if the skin at the back of the neck is held too tightly when the animal is restrained. Treatment of the hamster soon after the exophthalmos occurs generally results in a good prognosis for saving the eye. Cleanse the ocular area gently with an ophthalmic wash, and lubricate the eye with sterile ophthalmic lubricant. Gently retract the lid margins around the globe until the eyeball returns to its normal position. Treat the eye with an antibiotic ophthalmic ointment for a minimum of 7–10 days. Occasionally, tarsorrhaphy is needed to prevent recurrence. Enucleation may be necessary if the eye cannot be replaced or if significant trauma to the proptosed eyeball has occurred.

Gerbils

INTEGUMENTARY SYSTEM AND MARKING GLANDS

Facial eczema, sore nose, and *nasal dermatitis* all describe a common skin condition seen in gerbils. Clinical lesions adjacent to the external nares appear erythematous initially; these lesions progress to localized alopecia and then to an extensive moist dermatitis (Fig. 27–14). The cause is believed to be an

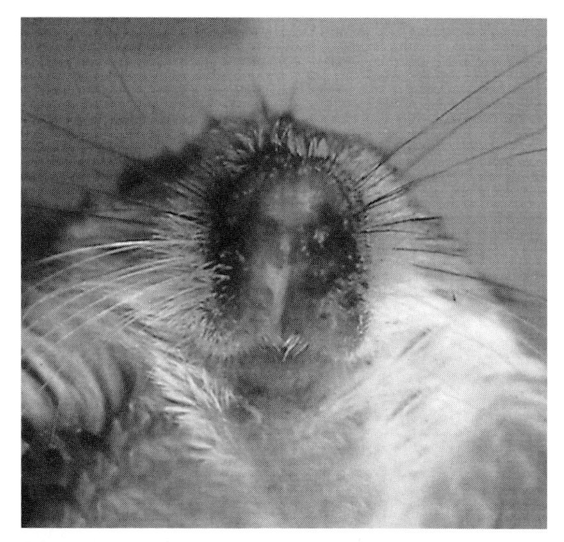

FIGURE 27–14

Sore nose (facial eczema, nasal dermatitis) in a gerbil. This condition may result from an increase in harderian gland secretion complicated by infection with *Staphylococcus* species.

increase in the secretion of porphyrins by the harderian gland (as in chromodacryorrhea in rats), which act as a primary skin irritant. Various staphylococcal species (*S. aureus* and *S. xylosus*) may act synergistically to produce the dermatitis.[5, 47] Stress may induce excessive harderian gland secretion. Two examples of stress are overcrowding and exposure to an environmental humidity of greater than 50% (in this case, the furcoat stands out and appears matted instead of lying sleekly against the body). Keeping the gerbil in a dry environment, cleaning its face, and providing soft clay or sand bedding instead of abrasive wood chip bedding usually alleviate the problem. Use topical or parenteral antibiotics (except streptomycin) in gerbils with severe dermatitis.

The tail of the gerbil is covered by thin skin. Unlike rats or mice, if a gerbil is picked up by the tip of its tail, the skin often slips off, leaving a raw, exposed tail that eventually becomes necrotic and sheds (Fig. 27–15). If the tail skin is lost, surgically amputate the bare tail where the skin ends (see Chapter 28). The tail usually sloughs if it is left untreated. When picking up a gerbil, take care to avoid grasping the tail unless it is gently held at the base. The best holding technique involves placement of the palm of the hand over the gerbil's back and encircling the body with thumb and fingers. Gerbils bite if they are not handled securely, despite the claim in many reviews that they rarely bite human handlers regardless of provocation.

Gerbils have large, ventral, abdominal marking glands that are androgen dependent (Fig. 27–16). Owners may mistake this normal ventral gland for a tumor. In aged animals, the gland may become infected or neoplastic. Local débridement and the topical application of ointments are indicated for treatment of infected glands. Do a wide excisional

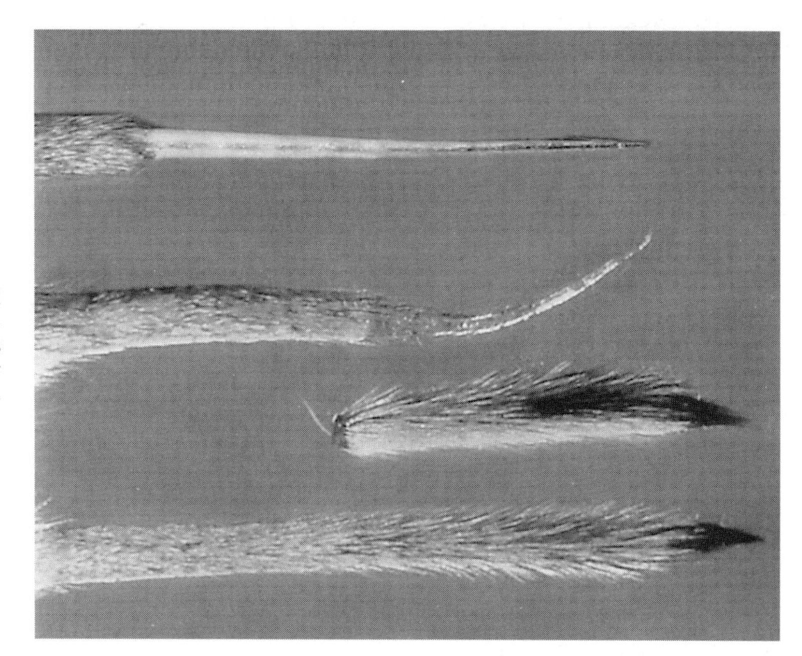

FIGURE 27–15

One normal gerbil tail and two gerbil tails with varying degrees of tail-slip. Immediately next to the middle tail is its displaced skin. Tail-slip frequently results from lifting a gerbil by its tail.

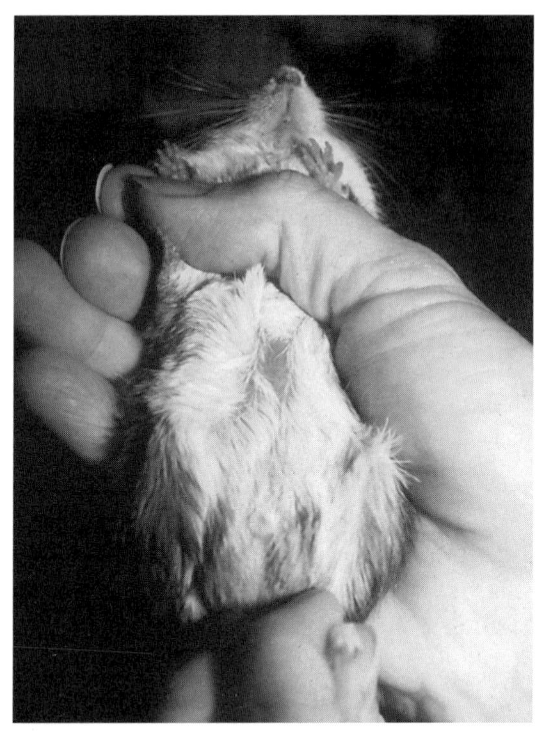

FIGURE 27–16
A ventral marking gland on the abdomen of a male gerbil. Owners sometimes mistake this gland for a tumor.

biopsy if you suspect a tumor such as an adenocarcinoma.

DIGESTIVE SYSTEM

Five reports of naturally occurring Tyzzer's disease have appeared in the literature.[9, 28, 35, 40, 53] It is the most frequently described fatal infectious disease of gerbils. Common findings in all cases were sudden death or death after a short period of illness, and the presence of necrotic foci in the liver. Diarrhea and necrotic lesions (gross and microscopic) were variably present in the intestinal tract. Experimentally induced Tyzzer's disease in gerbils has confirmed that these animals are extremely susceptible to infection[50]; the probable route of infection is oral. Gerbils exposed to infected bedding contract the disease.

CENTRAL NERVOUS SYSTEM

Approximately 20–40% of gerbils develop reflex, stereotypic, epileptiform (clonic-tonic) seizures from around 2 months of age. The susceptibility is inherited and is seen in selectively bred lines. There is no treatment. The animals hopefully outgrow the problem with time. The seizures generally pass in a few minutes; they may be mild or severe and have no lasting effects.

Medication and Antibiotic Therapy in Pet Rodents

Because of the small size of pet rodents, even pediatric-strength medications often must be diluted for use in these species. Knowing the precise bodyweight of the animal, diluting medications, and administering medications with a tuberculin or insulin syringe permit increased accuracy of dosing. Medication often is given by mixing it into feed or water. However, rats do not drink if they find the taste of their water objectionable. Ball-ended dosing needles are ideal for gavage, but always carefully calculate the volume of the dose and depth of penetration when using the dosing needle to prevent gastric rupture. IV injections are difficult to administer, and the substitution of IV administration with intraperitoneal injection (for anesthetics) and IM or SC injections is common.

Exercise caution when administering antibiotic therapy to rodents. Streptomycin and procaine are toxic in mice; nitrofurantoin causes neuropathologic lesions in rats; and gerbils cannot tolerate dihydrostreptomycin and streptomycin. Hamsters are similar to guinea pigs in their susceptibility for the development of clostridial enterotoxicity when they are given penicillins, erythromycin, or lincomycin. Many antibiotics are added to the drinking water of pet rodents, but the water must contain high concentrations and fresh solutions must be prepared daily if therapeutic blood levels are to be achieved. An example is tetracycline, which often is added to the drinking water of rats and mice at a dose of 5 mg/mL for the treatment of respiratory mycoplasmosis. Rats often do not drink the medicated water because of its unpleasant taste. Some researchers have added sugar to the water to encourage drinking, but such supplementation is controversial. Tylosin at a dose of 0.5 mg/mL has been reported to be palatable to rats and achieves inhibitory concentrations against *M. pulmonis*.

Antibiotics that are apparently safe to use in rodents (especially guinea pigs and hamsters) include enrofloxacin, ciprofloxacin, trimethoprim-sulfa combinations, and chloramphenicol. Other sulfonamides, tetracycline, and piperacillin should be used sparingly in hamsters, and ampicillin and amoxicillin should be avoided. (See also Chapter 26 for discussion of antibiotic therapy in rodents.)

EDUCATION

Client Education

Most clients purchase books on pet rodents in pet stores. They often rely on the recommendations of the pet store owner before asking for advice from a veterinarian. Unfortunately, many of the available owner's manuals are not familiar to veterinarians. Having some knowledge about pet rodents from these handbooks, clients often raise questions about what they have read, and clinicians may not appear well informed from the client's perspective if they are unfamiliar with their references. The rodent owners then often return to the pet store owner for guidance; unless their animals are very sick, the owners do not return to the veterinarian for advice on husbandry and diseases. At this point, the prognosis for very ill pets is poor.

Familiarity with the pet hobbyist literature breaks the cycle of mistrust and ignorance. Many hobby books on pet rodents are highly entertaining and informative about the husbandry and biology of the animals; some are not. In any case, the medical information in these books should be carefully reviewed by the veterinarian. Purchasing some of these books and then recommending them to pet rodent owners is an effective method not only of educating clients, but also of establishing a good rapport with them.

These books are generally inexpensive when compared with veterinary textbooks, and they are written for a range of age groups (e.g., children and parents) and levels of interest. TFH Publications, Barron's Educational Series, and Dorling-Kindersley are three reputable publishers of such books, which are readily available. Some of the titles available are listed according to age and interest level in the Suggested Reading section at the end of this chapter.

Veterinary Education

I find that there are two types of veterinary books on rodents. The first are clinical and practice-oriented texts that provide treatments and drug dosages. These books are generally written in an informal style and are reasonable in price. The second are research-oriented books that generally do not provide treatments or readily accessible drug dosages; however, they do contain detailed information and photographs. These books generally are written by multiple authors, are somewhat encyclopedic, and are expensive. (An exception is the National Research Council's *Companion Guide to Infectious Diseases of Mice and Rats*.) The Suggested Reading section at the end of this chapter also provides the titles of eight veterinary books about rodents. These texts provide useful additional reading for the veterinarian who wishes to learn more about rodents.

REFERENCES

1. Anderson NL: Basic husbandry and medicine of pocket pets. *In* Birchard SJ, Sherding RG, eds.: Saunders Manual of Small Animal Practice. Philadelphia, WB Saunders, 1994, pp 1363–1389.
2. Bauck (Brouwer) L, Orr JP, Lawrence KH: Hyperadrenocorticism in three teddy bear hamsters. Can Vet J 1985; 25:247–250.
3. Baumans V, Havenaar R, Van Huch H, et al: The effectiveness of Ivomec and Neguvon in the control of murine mites. Lab Anim 1988; 22:243–245.
4. Bivin WS, Olsen GA, Murray K: Morphophysiology. *In* Van Hoosier GL, McPherson CW, eds.: Laboratory Hamsters. Orlando, Academic Press, 1987, pp 10–41.
5. Bresnahan JF, Smith GD, Lentsch RH, et al: Nasal dermatitis in the Mongolian gerbil. Lab Anim Sci 1983; 33:258–263.
6. Budman L, D'Amico T: Heart lesions in a white hamster. Lab Anim 1994; 23:17–18.
7. Cantrell CA, Padovan D: Other Hamsters: Biology, Care and Use in Research. *In* Van Hoosier Jr GL, McPherson CW, eds.: Laboratory Hamsters. Orlando, Academic Press, 1987, pp 369–387.
8. Carlton WW: Spontaneous cardiac lesions. *In* A histopathology seminar on the cardiovascular system of laboratory animals (Session B). International Life Sciences Institute Histopathology Seminar, Orlando, December 1991.
9. Carter GR, Whitenack DL, Julius LA: Natural Tyzzer's disease in Mongolian gerbils *(Meriones unguiculatus)*. Lab Anim Care 1969; 19:648–651.
10. Cunnane SC, Bloom SR: Intussusception in the Syrian golden hamster. Br J Nutr 1990; 63:231–237.
11. Donnelly TM: Variables in animal experimentation. *In* Rabbits and Rodents: Laboratory Animal Science. Proceedings 142. Post Graduate Committee in Veterinary Science of the University of Sydney, Sydney, Australia, September 1990, pp 191–201.
12. Donnelly TM, Stark DM: The susceptibility of laboratory rats, hamsters and mice to wound infection with *Staphylococcus aureus*. Am J Vet Res 1985; 46:2634–2638.
13. Emily P: Problems peculiar to continually erupting teeth. J Small Exotic Anim Med 1991; 1:56–59.
14. Flynn BM, Brown PA, Eckstein JM, et al: Treatment of *Syphacia obvelata* in mice using ivermectin. Lab Anim Sci 1989; 39:461–463.
15. Friedman S, Weisbroth SH: The parasitic ecology of the rodent mite, *Myobia musculi*: IV. Life cycle. Lab Anim Sci 1975; 25:440–445.
16. Georg LK: Animal ringworm in public health. Washington, DC: Public Health Service; 1960. US Department of Health, Education and Welfare publication PHS 727.
17. Gleiser CA, Van Hoosier GL, Sheldon WG, et al: Amyloidosis and renal paramyloid in a closed hamster colony. Lab Anim Sci 1971; 21:197–202.

18. Gray JE: Chronic progressive nephrosis, rat. *In* Jones TC, Mohr U, Hunt RD, eds.: Monographs on pathology of laboratory animals, urinary system. Berlin, Springer-Verlag, 1986, pp 174–178.
19. Haley J: Cannibalism in hamsters. Am Small Stock Farmer 1965; 35:10–11.
20. Harkness JE: A Practitioner's Guide to Domestic Rodents. Denver, American Animal Hospital Association, 1993.
21. Heider K, Eustis SL: Tumors of the soft tissues. *In* Turusov V, Mohr U, eds.: Pathology of Tumors in Laboratory Animals. Vol. 2. Tumors of the Mouse. 2nd ed. Lyon, International Agency for Research on Cancer Scientific Publications, 1994, pp 611–631.
22. Herweg D, Kunstyr I: Effect of intestinal flagellate *Spironucleus (Hexamita) muris* and of dimetridazole on intestinal microflora in thymus-deficient (nude) mice. Zentralbl Bakteriol Parasitenkd Infektionskr Myg 1979; 245:262–269.
23. Hotchkiss CE: Effect of surgical removal of subcutaneous tumors on survival of rats. J Am Vet Med Assoc 1995; 206:1575–1579.
24. Huerkamp MJ: Correspondence. Lab Anim Sci 1990; 40:5.
25. Hubbard GB, Schmidt RE: Noninfectious diseases. *In* Van Hoosier Jr GL, McPherson CW, eds.: Laboratory Hamsters. Orlando, Academic Press, 1987, pp 169–178.
26. Kohn DF, Barthold SW: Biology and diseases of rats. *In* Fox JG, Cohen JB, Loew FM, eds.: Laboratory Animal Medicine. Orlando, Academic Press, 1984, pp 91–122.
27. Kraft LM: An apparently new lethal virus of infant mice. Science 1962; 137:282–283.
28. Koopman JP, Mullink JW, Kennis HM, et al: An outbreak of Tyzzer's disease in Mongolian gerbils *(Meriones unguiculatus).* Z Versuchstierk 1980; 22:336–341.
29. Kuntze A: Praxisrelevante Erkrankungen bei Meerschweinen und Goldhamster. Monatsheft Veterinarmedizin 1992; 47:143–147.
30. Kuo TH, Ho KL, Weiner J: The role of alkaline protease in the development of cardiac lesions in myopathic hamsters: effect of verapamil treatment. Biochem Med 1984; 32:207–215.
31. Lancefield RC: Group A streptococcal infections in animals: natural and experimental. *In* Wannamaker LW, Matsen JM, eds.: Streptococci and Streptococcal Diseases: Recognition, Understanding and Management. New York, Academic Press, 1972, pp 313–326.
32. Lindt VS: Über Krankheiten des syrischen Goldhamsters *(Mesocricetus auratus).* Schweiz Arch Tierheilkd 1958; 100:86–97.
33. Lyerly DM, Bostwick EF, Binion SB, et al: Passive immunization of hamsters against disease caused by *Clostridium difficile* by use of bovine immunoglobulin G concentrate. Infect Immun 1991; 59:2215–2218.
34. McOrist S, Gebhart CJ, Boid R, et al: Characterization of *Lawsonia intracellularis* gen. nov., sp. nov., the obligately intracellular bacterium of porcine proliferative enteropathy. Int J Syst Bacteriol 1995; 45:820–835.
35. Motzel SL, Gibson SV: Tyzzer disease in hamsters and gerbils from a pet store supplier. J Am Vet Med Assoc 1990; 197:1176–1178.
36. Muridae: Rats, Mice, Hamsters, Voles, Lemmings and Gerbils. *In* Nowak RM, ed.: Walker's Mammals of the World. 5th ed. Vol. II. Baltimore, Johns Hopkins University Press, 1991, pp 643–968.
37. National Research Council: Infectious Diseases of Mice and Rats. Washington DC, National Academy Press, 1991.
38. Ottenweller JE, Tapp WN, Burke JN, et al: Plasma cortisol and corticosterone concentrations in the golden hamster *(Mesocricetus auratus).* Life Sci 1985; 37:1551–1558.
39. Peace TA, Brock KV, Stills HF Jr: Comparative analysis of the 16S rRNA gene sequence of the putative agent of proliferative ileitis of hamsters. Int J Syst Bacteriol 1994; 44:832–835.
40. Port CD, Richter WR, Moize SM: Tyzzer's disease in the gerbil *(Meriones unguiculatus).* Lab Anim Care 1970; 20:109–111.
41. Renshaw HW, Van Hoosier GL, Amend NK: A survey of naturally occurring diseases of the Syrian hamster. Lab Anim 1975; 9:179–191.
42. Rübel GA, Isenbügel E, Wolvekamp P: Atlas of Diagnostic Radiology of Exotic Pets. Philadelphia, WB Saunders, 1991.
43. Schmidt RE, Eason RL, Hubbard GB, et al: Pathology of Aging Syrian Hamsters. Boca Raton, FL, CRC Press, 1983.
44. Short BG, Goldstein RS: Nonneoplastic lesions in the kidney. *In* Mohr U, Dungworth DL, Capen CC, eds.: Pathobiology of the Aging Rat. Vol. 1. Washington, DC, International Life Sciences Institute Press, 1992, pp 211–225.
45. Sichuk G, Bettigole RE, Der BK, et al: Influence of sex hormones on thrombosis of the left atrium in Syrian (golden) hamsters. Am J Physiol 1965; 208:465–470.
46. Silverman S: Diagnostic imaging of exotic pets. Vet Clin North Am Small Anim Pract 1993; 23:1287–1299.
47. Solomon HF, Dixon DM, Pouch W: A survey of staphylococci isolated from the laboratory gerbil. Lab Anim Sci 1990; 40:316–318.
48. Squartini F, Pingitore R: Tumors of the mammary gland. *In* Turusov V, Mohr U, eds.: Pathology of Tumors in Laboratory Animals. Vol. 2. Tumors of the Mouse. 2nd ed. Lyon, International Agency for Research on Cancer Scientific Publications, 1994, pp 47–100.
49. Tyzzer EE: A fatal disease of the Japanese waltzing mouse caused by a spore-bearing bacillus *(Bacillus piliformis N. sp.).* J Med Res 1917; 37:307–338.
50. Waggie KS, Ganaway JR, Wagner JE, et al: Experimentally induced Tyzzer's disease in Mongolian gerbils *(Meriones unguiculatus).* Lab Anim Sci 1984; 34:53–57.
51. Walberg JA, Stark DM, Desch C, et al: Demodicidosis in laboratory rats *(Rattus norvegicus).* Lab Anim Sci 1981; 31:60–62.
52. Wardrop KJ, Van Hoosier GL: The hamster. *In* Loeb WF, Quimby FW, eds.: The Clinical Chemistry of Laboratory Animals. New York, Pergamon Press, 1989, pp 31–39.
53. White DJ, Waldron MM: Naturally-occurring Tyzzer's disease in the gerbil. Vet Rec 1969; 85:111–114.

SUGGESTED READING

Children Ages 4–8 Years

TFH Publications' Your First Series: Gerbil; Guinea Pig; Hamster; Mouse; Rabbit. Paperback, 32 pp, $2.00.

Barron's First Pets: Hamsters; Rabbits. Paperback, 24 pp, $4.00.

Children Ages 8 Years and Up

TFH Publications' Step by Step Series: Chinchillas; Gerbils; Guinea Pigs; Hamsters; Dwarf Rabbits; Rabbits. Paperback, 64 pp, $4.00.

Barron's Young Pet Owners Guides: Taking Care of Your Gerbils; Guinea Pig; Hamster; Rabbit. Paperback, 32 pp, $5.00.

Dorling-Kindersley's ASPCA Pet Care Guides for Kids: Guinea Pigs; Hamster; Rabbit. Hardback, 32 pp, $10.00.

Adults: Beginner

TFH Publications' As a Hobby Series: Gerbils; Guinea Pigs; Hamsters; Mice; Rats; Dwarf Rabbits. Hardback, approximately 96 pp, $8.00.

TFH Publications' As a New Pet Series: Gerbils; Hamsters; Guinea Pigs; Mice; Rabbits; Dwarf Rabbits. Paperback, approximately 64 pp, $6.00.

Adults: Intermediate

TFH Publications' Complete Introduction (KW) Series: Chinchillas; Gerbils; Guinea Pigs; Hamsters; Rabbits. Hardback, approximately 96 pp, $6.00.

TFH Publications' Proper Care Series: Gerbils; Guinea Pigs; Dwarf Rabbits; Fancy Rats. Hardback, 256 pages, $15.00.

Barron's Owners Manuals: Chinchillas; Gerbils; Guinea Pigs; Hamsters; Mice; Rats; Rabbits; Dwarf Rabbits. Paperback, 64–80 pp, $6.00.

Publisher Addresses

TFH Publications, Inc.
One TFH Plaza
Third and Union Avenues
Neptune, NJ 07753
tel.: (908) 988-8400

Barron's Educational Series, Inc.
P.O. Box 8040
250 Wireless Boulevard
Hauppauge, NY 11788
tel.: (516) 434-3311

Dorling Kindersley Publishing, Inc. (UK)
Distributed in the United States by:
Houghton Mifflin Company
222 Berkley Street
Boston, MA 02205
tel.: (617) 350-5956

Clinical and Practice-Oriented Books

Harkness JE, Wagner JE: The Biology and Medicine of Rabbits and Rodents. 4th ed. Baltimore, Williams & Wilkins, 1995. Paperback, 372 pp.

Harkness JE: A Practitioner's Guide to Domestic Rodents. Denver, American Animal Hospital Association, 1993. Paperback, 82 pp.

Quesenberry KE, Hillyer EV, eds.: Exotic pet medicine II. Vet Clin North Am Small Anim Pract 1994; 24:1–224. Hardback.

Williams CSF: Practical Guide to Laboratory Animals. St. Louis, CV Mosby, 1976. Paperback, 178 pp.

Research-Oriented Books

Fox JG, Cohen JB, Loew FM, eds.: Laboratory Animal Medicine. Orlando, Academic Press, 1984. Hardback, 538 pp.

Percy DH, Barthold SW: Pathology of Laboratory Rodents and Rabbits. Ames, IA, Iowa State University Press, 1993. Hardback, 229 pp.

Universities Federation for Animal Welfare (Poole T, ed.): The UFAW Handbook on the Care and Management of Laboratory Animals. 6th ed. New York, Churchill-Livingstone, 1987. Hardback, 931 pp.

National Research Council: Companion Guide to Infectious Diseases of Mice and Rats. Washington, DC, National Academy Press, 1991. Paperback, 95 pp.

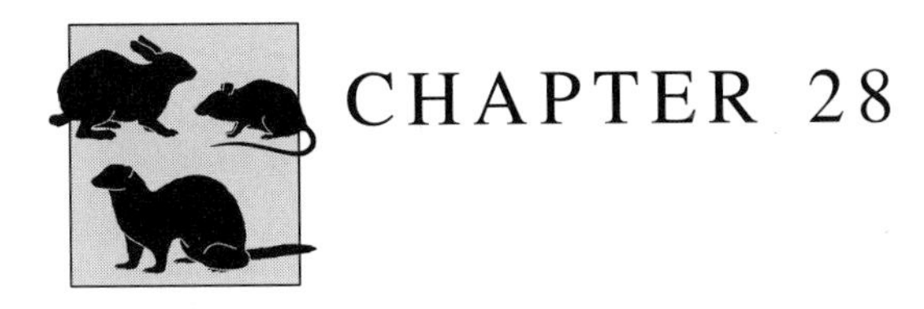

CHAPTER 28

Soft Tissue Surgery

Holly Mullen, DVM

Small rodents such as hamsters, gerbils, mice, and rats are popular pets. They may be the first pets that a child owns or the only pet an apartment dweller is allowed to have. Despite their small size and relative low cost, their owners are frequently as emotionally attached to them as they would be to a dog or cat. This attachment often leads owners to request surgical and medical treatments that have costs much greater than the actual cash value of an animal. The veterinarian involved in these situations must refrain from passing judgment on an owner who wants to "do everything" for a pet. Also, we may need to reassure owners that it is okay to value their rodent pets as highly as any other pets, contrary to the opinions of friends and relatives (who might say, "You could buy 20 more of those for what you're spending on Mickey!").

Hamsters, gerbils, rats, and mice share a very similar anatomy. All are monogastric, have a bicornuate uterus, and have testicles that are usually descended in the scrotum but which can be easily retracted into the abdomen through the open inguinal canals. Rats and mice have a long, hairless tail; gerbils have a long, haired tail, and hamsters have a very short, lightly haired tail. Hamsters have large cheek pouches in which to store food.

The subcutis in these small rodents is relatively thick and holds subcuticular sutures well. I prefer to use 5–0 to 7–0 absorbable suture material to close the subcutis and to avoid the use of skin sutures. If necessary, tissue glue also may be used to facilitate skin closure. Rodents tend to chew at skin sutures and can chew out wire sutures as well as nylon ones.

Anesthesia of small rodents is safely accomplished by chamber or face mask induction with isoflurane, and anesthesia can be maintained by face mask administration. Intubation of the small rodents is impractical and difficult, although some larger rats may be intubated with a 5- or 6-French soft feeding tube trimmed to the proper length. Patency of the tube must be carefully watched because very small endotracheal tubes are prone to blockage by respiratory secretions. I prefer to mask all rodents to save time and to prevent the laryngeal trauma caused by attempts at passing a tube. In a respiratory emergency, endotracheal intubation via tracheostomy may provide an adequate airway for patient ventilation.

OVARIOHYSTERECTOMY

Ovariohysterectomy may be performed for population control when groups of male and female rodents are housed together. Pyometra is rare but may occur in any species. Female hamsters have an odorous, mucoid vaginal discharge at estrus, and this discharge should not be mistaken for pyometra.[3]

Ovariohysterectomy may be used to treat cysts as well as ovarian and uterine tumors in small rodents. Benign and malignant tumors of the uterus and ovaries are reported.[4] Ovarian tumors tend to be benign in hamsters and gerbils. Uterine tumors tend to be benign in rats and malignant in hamsters and gerbils.

Restrain the anesthetized rodent by taping the feet to the surgical table (Fig. 28–1). Make a caudal, ventral midline abdominal incision. Gerbils of both sexes have a sebaceous gland located midventrally on the abdomen near the umbilicus.[3] If this interferes with the abdominal incision, make an elliptical incision and remove the gland during the abdominal approach.

The uterus and ovaries are easily located within the abdominal cavity. The ovarian ligaments are easily stretched. Doubly ligate the ovarian pedicles and the uterine body with 4–0 or 5–0 monofilament, absorbable suture, and then remove them. Close the linea with 4–0 or 5–0 suture and the subcutis with 5–0 to 7–0 absorbable suture. If necessary, use tissue glue to complete the skin closure.

Postoperative analgesics are indicated as they are in all except relatively minor surgical procedures. Recovery is routine.

CASTRATION

Castration is done for population control, to decrease male aggressiveness, and for the removal of testicular neoplasia. Tumors of the testicles are rare in the small rodents but have been reported most frequently in rats. The majority of rat testicular neoplasms are benign-behaving interstitial (Leydig) cell tumors.[4]

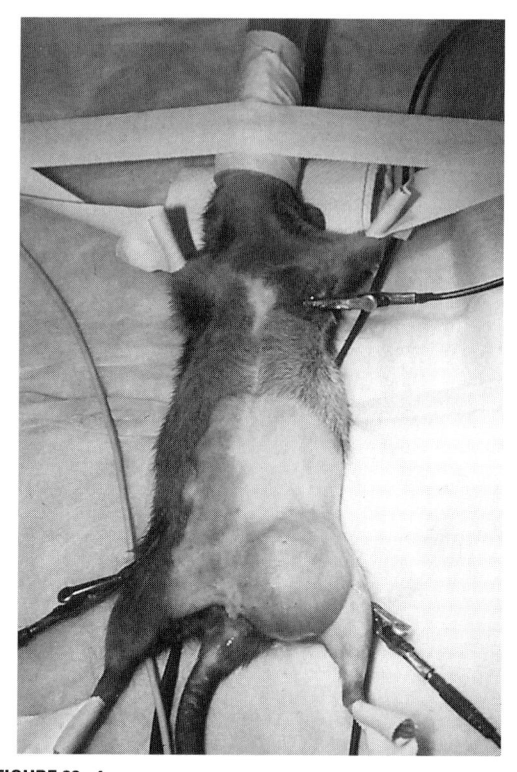

FIGURE 28–1
A rat with a left caudal gland mammary mass positioned for surgery, with its limbs taped down.

The procedure for the castration of rats, mice, gerbils, and hamsters is virtually the same.[6] The testicles are located caudoventrally in the inguinal area and are readily retracted into the abdomen. They can be easily propulsed back into the scrotum with a gentle rolling pressure on the caudal abdomen, in a caudal direction just in front of the pubis.

Make an incision in the scrotal skin over the testicle and elevate it from the sac. Use a closed castration method to prevent the herniation of abdominal contents through the incision. Closure of the inguinal rings is not necessary as long as the tunic is closed. Repeat the procedure for the other testicle. I prefer to close the scrotum with a drop of tissue glue rather than leave it open. By nature of their location, the wounds will be in contact with the cage flooring as the animal moves around and might be kept open or otherwise traumatized.

MAMMARY GLAND NEOPLASIA

Mammary gland neoplasia is probably the most common spontaneous neoplasia found in mice and rats.[2, 4] Although reported, it appears to be rare in hamsters and gerbils. The majority of mammary gland tumors are benign in rats and hamsters. The opposite is true in mice and gerbils.[2–4, 6] Rat mammary tumors are known to be sensitive to hormone stimuli,[4] and ovariectomized Sprague-Dawley rats have a lower incidence of mammary tumors than do intact rats (see Chapter 27).

Mammary gland tissue is extensive in rats and mice, extending from the cervical to the inguinal region ventrally and as high as the shoulders and flanks laterally. Mammary gland tumors may be found anywhere in these areas and grow rapidly to large sizes (see Fig. 28–1). Mammary tissue is confined to the ventral thorax and abdomen of hamsters and gerbils.

Treatment of mammary tumors in all small rodents consists of excision of the tumor and associated mammary gland. Pay careful attention to hemostasis because some tumors can have a well-developed vascular supply. Subcuticular closure is routine.

MISCELLANEOUS ABDOMINAL PROCEDURES

Laparotomy is indicated for the treatment of cystic calculi and for the exploration of abdominal masses. Cystic calculi are uncommon in small rodents. Cystotomy is performed as for any other species, except that the suture material and needle must be small, and delicate tissue handling is required. Close the cystotomy incision with 6–0 or 7–0 absorbable suture in a single-layer, simple interrupted pattern. Abdominal closure is routine. Calculi are usually calcium-based and may respond to dietary management.[6]

Abdominal masses can arise from any organ. Hamsters are prone to polycystic disease; the cysts can become quite large and are most often found in the liver and kidneys. Hamsters are also prone to the development of lymphosarcoma. In addition to involvement of the peripheral lymph nodes, tumors may be found in the liver, kidney, spleen, and bowel.[4]

Gerbils have a high incidence of spontaneously occurring neoplasia, especially if they are older than 2 years of age. Tumors of the ovaries, liver, pancreas, and spleen have all been described.[4]

Renal tumors have been reported in rats. Nephroblastoma is seen most often in young rats; older rats with renal neoplasia usually have renal tubular adenoma or adenocarcinoma. These tumors are often bilateral.[2, 4]

Cystic ovaries have been reported in all of the small rodents, but most often in hamsters and gerbils. These cysts may become very large without causing significant signs of discomfort (Fig. 28–2).

ABSCESSES

Abscesses are not uncommon in the small rodents, particularly hamsters, and they usually occur secondary to a bite wound or other trauma. Some affected animals are systemically ill as a result of the abscess; except for having abnormal swelling, others are asymptomatic. Administer supportive care as necessary.

Abscesses are easily diagnosed by finding pus on fine-needle aspiration. If possible, excise the abscess in its entirety, flush the wound, and close the subcutis and skin as previously described. If the abscess is not amenable to resection, lance it, drain it, and flush the wound with copious amounts of sterile saline; then manage the open wound as in dogs and cats. In either case, submit a portion of the abscess wall for culture and sensitivity testing. Administer a broad-spectrum antibiotic, such as a trimethoprim-sulfa combination drug, until test results are available; then, adjust the antibiotic regimen, according to culture results and the animal's clinical progress.

FACIAL ABSCESS IN HAMSTERS

Hamsters are very prone to periodontal disease and dental caries.[1, 5] A facial abscess located ventral or rostral to the eye may be caused by a tooth root abscess that is secondary to dental disease. These facial abscesses need to be flushed and drained; however, they will recur if the underlying cause, the abscessed tooth root, is not addressed.

As in most rodents, the roots of the teeth are long and deeply seated in the skull. By the time a facial abscess has formed, the tooth root is usually so loosened by decay that extraction is not too difficult. Remove the tooth by elevating the periodontal membrane while alternately and steadily retracting the

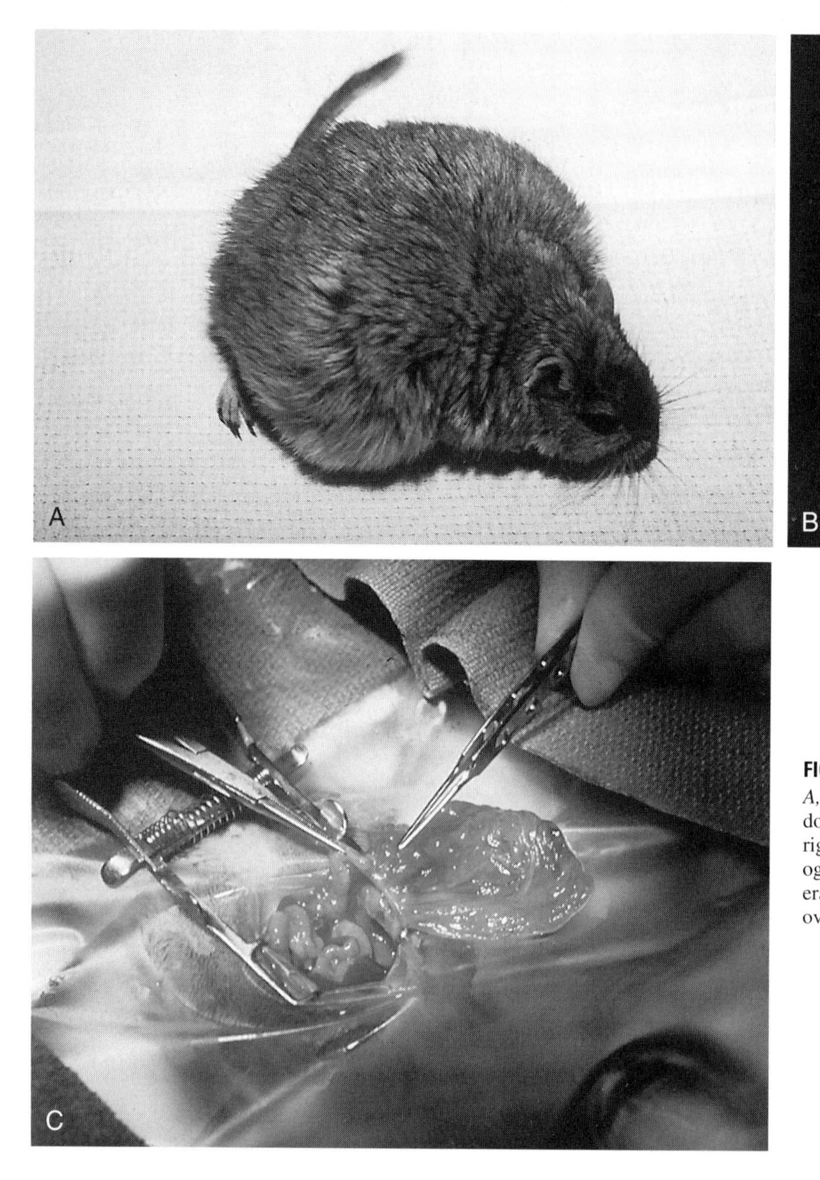

FIGURE 28–2
A, A 2-year-old female hamster with abdominal distention caused by a large right ovarian cyst. *B,* Ventrodorsal radiograph of the same hamster. *C,* Intraoperative view of the drained cyst before ovariohysterectomy.

exposed tooth. Close the defect in the gingiva with a single absorbable suture. Clean the facial abscess area several times daily until the wound has granulated in.

CHEEK POUCH EVERSION IN HAMSTERS

Hamsters have well-developed bilateral cheek pouches that are lined by a thin epithelial membrane that may be everted.[1, 3, 5] These pouches are used to store extra food. One or both pouches can spontaneously evert, and if so, they will need to be replaced. Re-eversion is common unless the pouch is sutured in place.

Sedate the affected hamster and gently replace the everted pouch with a cotton-tipped applicator swab. Place a single, full-thickness, percutaneous suture into the cheek pouch, using 4–0 or 5–0 monofilament, nonabsorbable suture material and a small needle (Fig. 28–3). Recovery is uneventful, and the hamster is able to eat right away. Remove the suture in 10–14 days. The cheek pouch should not evert again after this procedure.

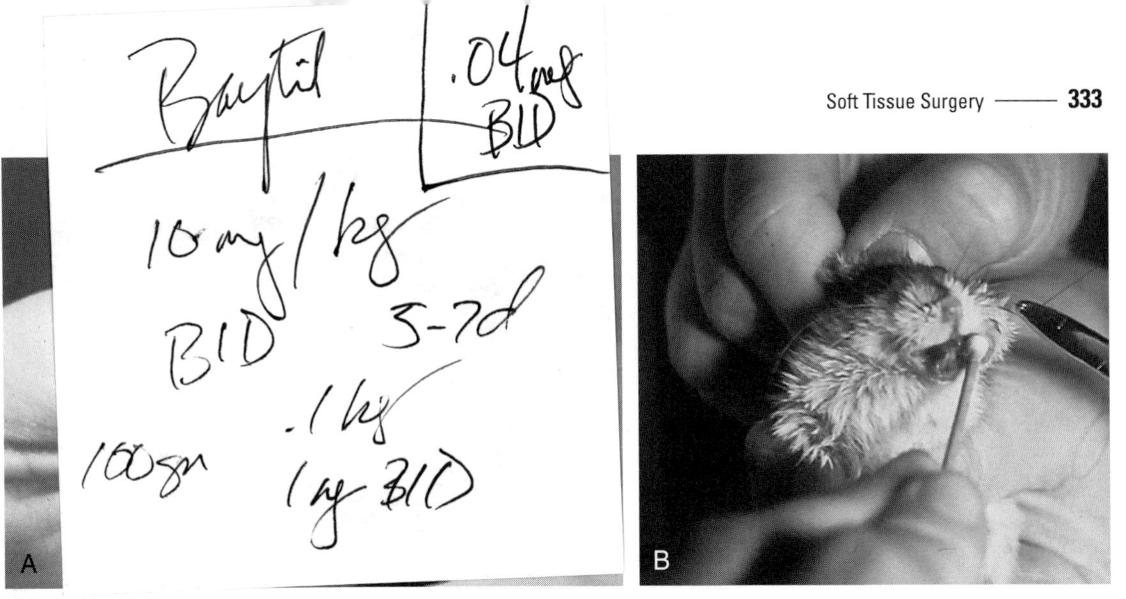

FIGURE 28–3
A, An everted cheek pouch in a Russian dwarf hamster. *B,* Surgical repair. A cotton-tipped applicator swab is used for holding the cheek pouch in position while a full-thickness percutaneous suture is placed.

PROLAPSED BOWEL IN HAMSTERS

Hamsters are prone to proliferative ileitis ("wet tail," regional enteritis), a disease characterized by excessive glandular proliferation in the epithelium of the ileum.[5] Signs seen with this disease include diarrhea (sometimes containing blood) and tenesmus. Intestinal neoplasia of the colon and small intestine can cause similar signs and must be differentiated from proliferative ileitis. Prolapse of the small intestine, colon, or rectum can result from the excessive straining seen with both of these conditions. Other conditions causing tenesmus, such as parasitization and diet-induced diarrhea, can also lead to prolapse.

Hamsters presenting with bowel prolapse are usually sick and should receive necessary medical treatment that includes the administration of fluids, dextrose, and antibiotics before they undergo emergency surgery. It is very important to ascertain what segment of bowel is prolapsed before surgery. A non-necrotic rectal prolapse can be replaced with a pursestring suture. A necrotic rectal prolapse must be amputated and sutured, whereas a small intestinal or colonic prolapse (intussusception) requires abdominal exploration. All of these conditions are considered surgical emergencies.

Determine what has prolapsed by carefully examining the tissue. If there is an orifice at the end of the tissue, it is a section of bowel. If the tissue is solid, it may be a rectal mass or polyp that has extruded on a stalk. Once you have determined that the bowel has prolapsed, gently pass a small, blunt-ended probe (e.g., a tomcat urinary catheter or cotton-tipped miniapplicator) on either side of the prolapsed tissue. If this probe does not pass very far in, it is a rectal prolapse. If the probe passes easily alongside the prolapse for a distance greater than a centimeter, it is an intestinal or colonic prolapse (Fig. 28–4).

Lubricate a simple, non-necrotic rectal prolapse and gently replace it, using a cotton-tipped miniswab or a soft urinary catheter. Pursestring-suture the anus with 5–0 nonabsorbable suture material, so that the anus is snug but not tight over a 5-French catheter. The pursestring suture can be removed in 3–5 days; meanwhile, treat the medical condition causing the prolapse.

Amputate a necrotic rectal prolapse by incising full-thickness through the prolapse at its healthy junction with the remaining rectum, 180° around the prolapse. Suture healthy rectum to healthy anus, using 6–0 absorbable synthetic suture in a simple interrupted pattern. Amputate the remaining prolapsed tissue and close the second half of the anastomosis in the same fashion. A pursestring suture is not needed (Fig. 28–5).

A hamster with intussuscepted, prolapsed bowel has a poor prognosis for survival because it is usually in a debilitated condition from the primary disease causing the prolapse. Anesthesia places such an animal at risk; also, underlying disease processes such as proliferative ileitis and malignant intestinal neoplasia carry a grave prognosis. The opportuni-

A

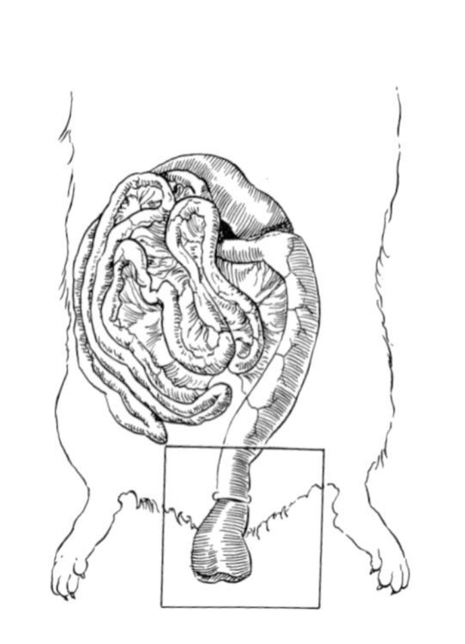

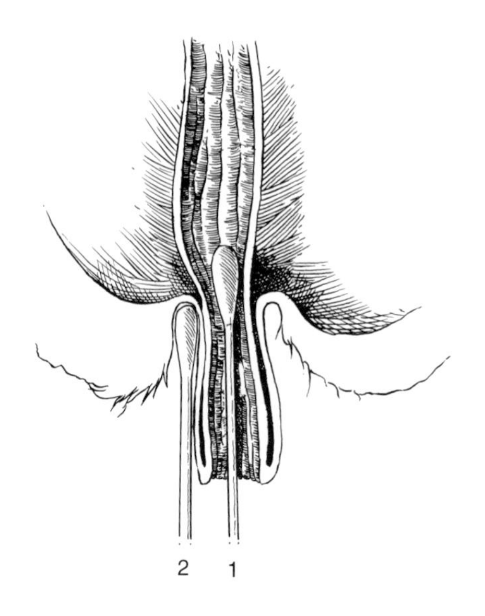

B

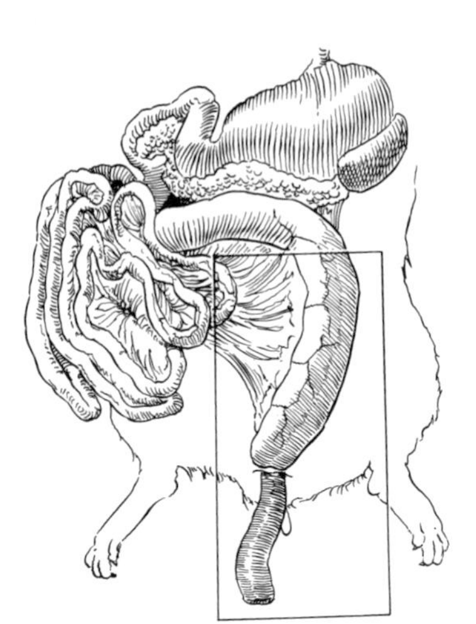

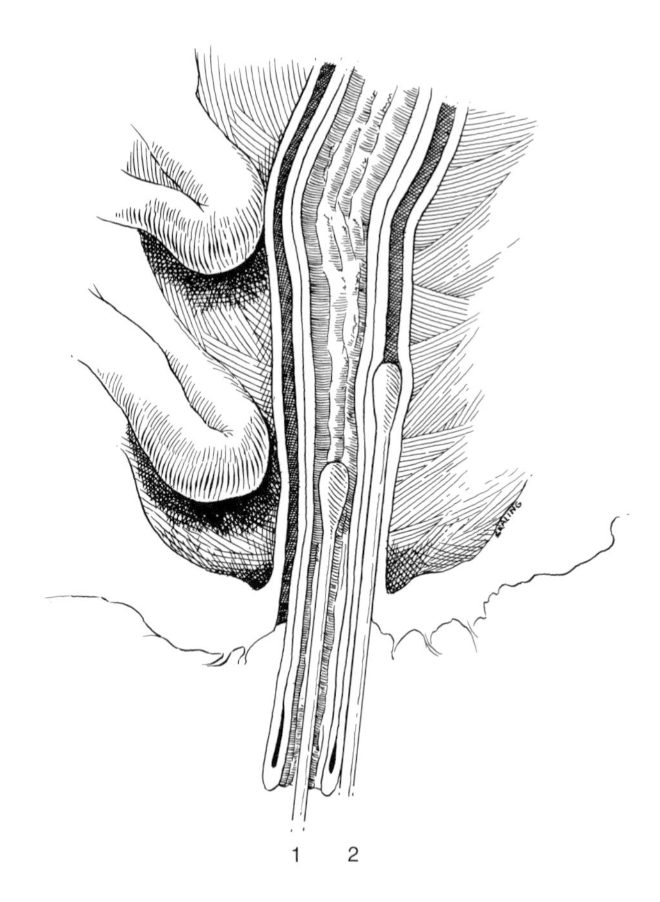

FIGURE 28–4

A, Rectal prolapse in a hamster, sagittal section. A probe is shown passing into the rectal lumen (1) but not on either side of the prolapse (2). *B,* Intestinal prolapse. The probe is shown passing into the intestinal lumen (1) as well as to either side of the prolapse (2).

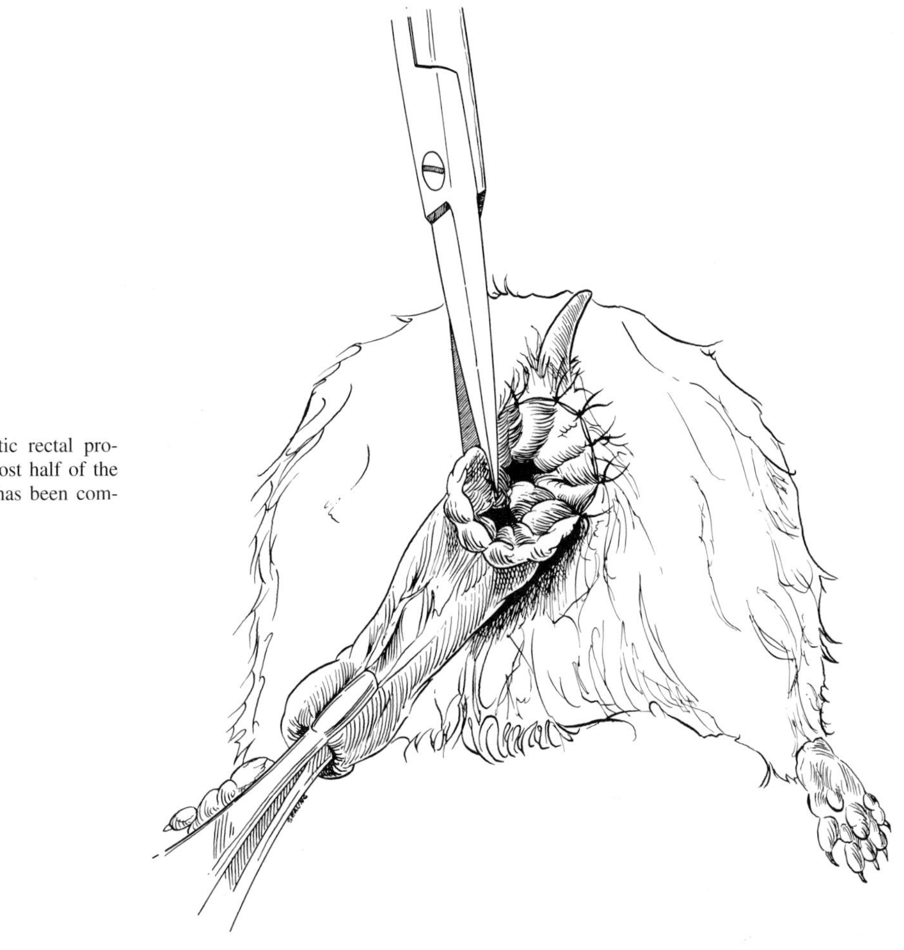

FIGURE 28–5
Amputation of a necrotic rectal prolapse in a hamster. Almost half of the rectocutaneous closure has been completed.

ties to perform exploratory surgery on these patients may be limited because of the understandable reluctance of most owners to pursue surgical treatment.

I have performed resection and anastomosis for intestinal intussusception and prolapse in two hamsters. One animal died 3 hours after surgery, having never fully recovered from anesthesia. The other hamster died during abdominal closure at the completion of the procedure. Both animals had a nonspecific enteritis on biopsy. Death was probably due to the extremely debilitated body condition of both hamsters, leading to shock and the inability to tolerate the stress of anesthesia and surgery. Despite this, I would attempt the procedure again if an owner was willing and if the condition of the animal indicated the possibility of success (since the alternative to surgery is euthanasia).

To surgically treat a prolapsed intestine, do a routine ventral midline abdominal exploratory examination. Identify the intussuscepted segment and gently reduce it if possible. Resect the necrotic portion of intussusceptum, preserving the blood supply to the viable bowel. If it is not possible to reduce the intussusception, amputate it internally and withdraw it externally by applying traction on the segment protruding from the anus. Do an end-to-end anastomosis of the healthy bowel, using 6–0 or 7–0 monofilament suture material. Six to eight simple interrupted sutures are usually needed to close the anastomosis. Test the site for leaks by gently milking intestinal contents past it. Close the defect in the mesentery with 6–0 absorbable suture material. As in dogs and cats, plicate the bowel with 6–0 nonabsorbable, monofilament suture material to prevent recurrence of the intussusception (Fig. 28–6).

Follow proper technique for enteric surgery, which includes the changing of gloves and in-

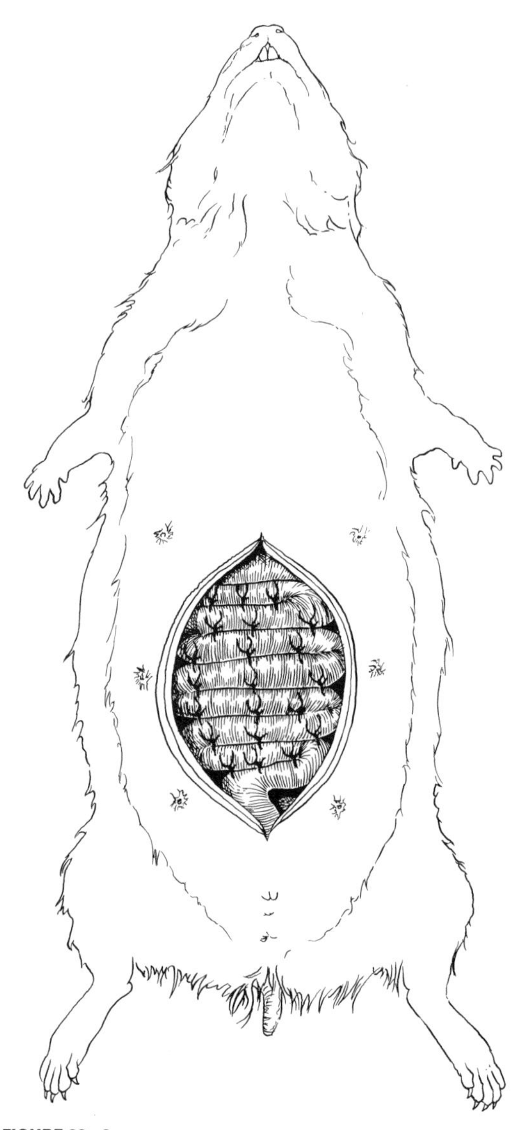

FIGURE 28–6
Plication of the small intestine with suture for the prevention of reintussusception of bowel in a hamster.

struments after completion of the anastomosis, followed by lavage of the abdomen and subcutaneous tissues during routine abdominal closure. Withhold food from the patient for 12–24 hours after surgery.

TAIL AMPUTATION IN GERBILS

Degloving injury to the long tail of a gerbil is common. The skin over the tail is thin and easily pulled off during restraint (never restrain a gerbil by its tail!) or if it becomes caught. A gerbil's tail can be mutilated by a cage mate if the animals do not get along. The skinless tail will eventually slough off, but may be painful or serve as a handy snack for the affected gerbil while it remains on the body. Along with the possibility of infection, these are good reasons for amputation of a degloved tail.

The procedure is simple. Place the anesthetized gerbil in ventral recumbency and suspend the tail with tape away from the body while the surgical site is prepared. Freshen the edges of the torn skin by excising at least 5 mm back from the wound. Disarticulate the tail by cutting between the most cranial coccygeal vertebrae visible when the skin is retracted proximally from the tail. This allows adequate soft tissue coverage of the stump. Bleeding from the coccygeal arteries and veins is easily controlled with pinpoint cautery. Close the subcutis with 5–0 or 6–0 absorbable suture and close the skin with either suture or tissue glue. Sensation to the tail stump can be blocked with the injection of a drop of bupivacaine or lidocaine several millimeters proximal to the site. Self-induced trauma to the amputation site is rare if gentle tissue handling and minimal cautery are employed.

REFERENCES

1. Battles AH: The biology, care, and diseases of the Syrian hamster. Compend Contin Educ Pract Vet 1985; 7: 815–824.
2. Cooper JE: Tips on tumors. Proceedings of the North American Veterinary Conference, Orlando, January 1994, pp 897–898.
3. Hillyer EV: Common clinical maladies of pet rodents. Orlando, Proceedings of the North American Veterinary Conference, January 1994, pp 909–912.
4. Toft JD: Commonly observed spontaneous neoplasms in rabbits, rats, guinea pigs, hamsters and gerbils. Semin Avian Exotic Pet Med 1991; 1:80–92.
5. Van Hoosier GL Jr, McPherson CW: Laboratory Hamsters. Orlando, FL, Academic Press, 1987.
6. Wallach JD, Boever WJ: Diseases of Exotic Animals: Medical and Surgical Management. Philadelphia, WB Saunders, 1983.

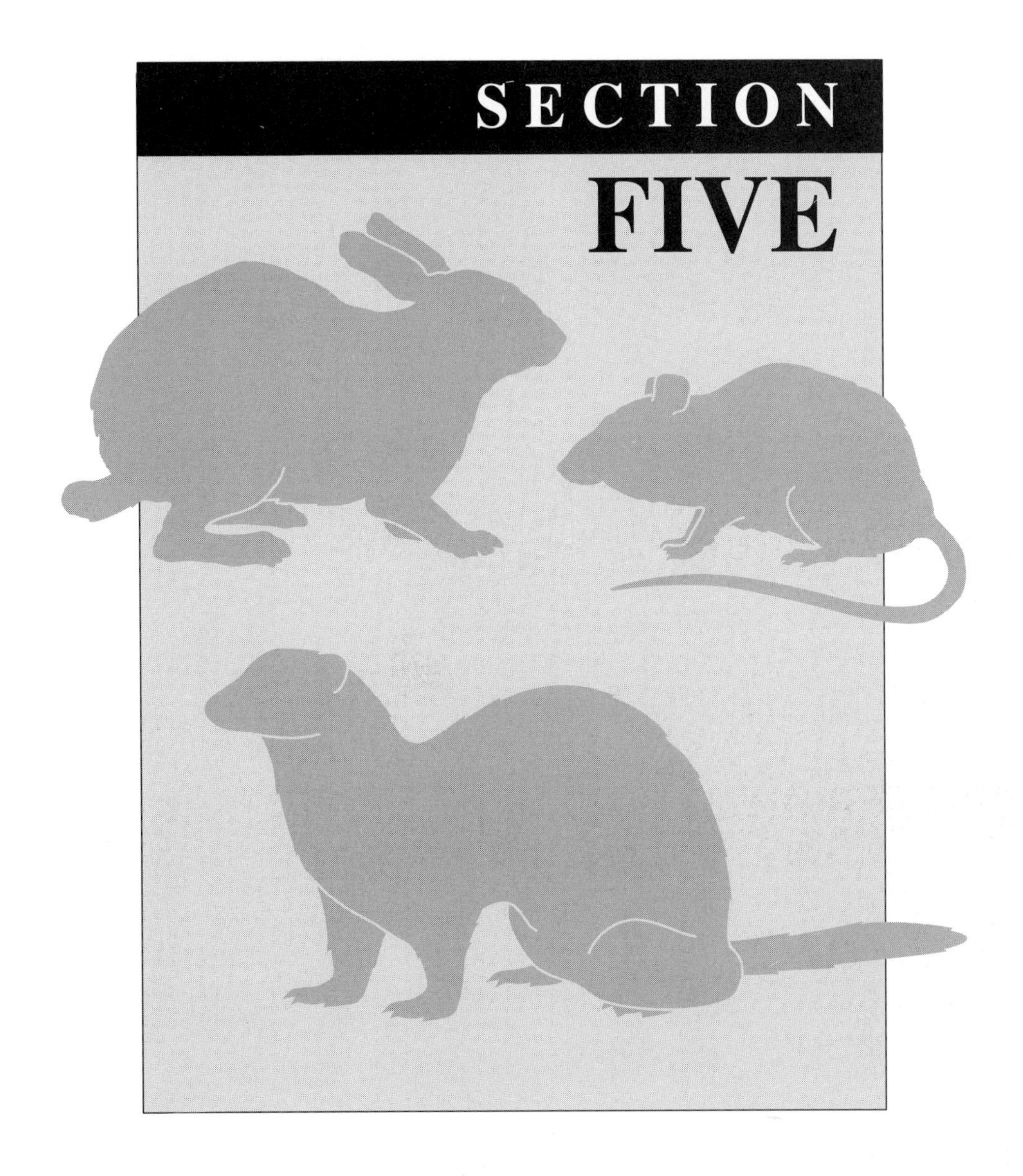

Other Topics

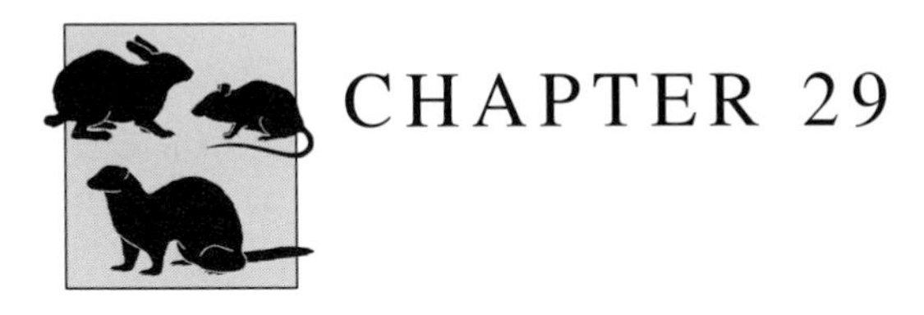

CHAPTER 29

Ophthalmologic Diseases in Small Mammals

Susan E. Kirschner, DVM

RABBITS

Conjunctivitis and Dacryocystitis

Rabbits are prone to inflammatory and infectious diseases of the conjunctiva and nasolacrimal drainage system. Although *Pasteurella* species, including *P. multocida*, are sometimes the causative agents,[7] *Staphylococcus aureus*, poxvirus, myxomatosis virus and allergies have also been implicated.[4, 5, 12, 15, 17, 18] One study showed that most rabbits with conjunctivitis and upper respiratory infection were infected with *S. aureus*, with smaller numbers being infected with *Pasteurella* species.[17] In early stages, rabbits present with epiphora and reddened eyelid margins. Later, white threads of mucus or pus appear at the medial canthus or in the ventral conjunctival cul-de-sac (Fig. 29–1). Because the infection may arise from chronic rhinitis,[7] conjunctivitis can be frustrating to treat if only topical antibiotics are used.

Examine both conjunctivae and the nasolacrimal puncta. The rabbit has only one nasolacrimal punctum for each eye[5] (Fig. 29–2). It is located in the conjunctiva between the lower lid and the nictitans, and it is quite large (2–4 mm in diameter). Elevating the nictitans by pressing on the globe through the upper lid makes the punctum easier to find. Rabbits tolerate cannulation of the puncta with topical anesthesia and do not need sedation. Flush the nasolacrimal system daily (if possible) or weekly, depending on the severity, in any rabbit with

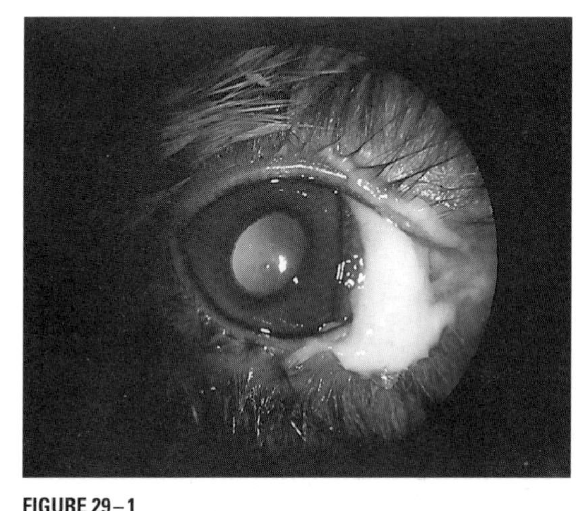

FIGURE 29–1
Rabbit with dacryocystitis. This disease is commonly mistaken for simple conjunctivitis. Rabbits with dacryocystitis have discharge at the medial canthus and purulent debris in the lacrimal puncta.

chronic conjunctivitis or dacryocystitis. Use a standard nasolacrimal cannula and flush with saline with or without added antibiotics. Most rabbits need both topical antibiotics and systemic antibiotics for clearance of the infection. If pasteurellosis is suspected, administer enrofloxacin PO (Baytril, Miles Inc., Shawnee Mission, KS) and topical ciprofloxacin ophthalmic solution (Ciloxan, Alcon Laboratories, Inc., Fort Worth, TX). Remind owners that this syndrome is often recurrent, especially in rabbits with concurrent rhinitis. In long-standing cases of conjunctivitis and dacryocystitis, the punctum may progressively narrow and be replaced with scar tissue until it is lost. This results in permanent epiphora. Entropion is another occasional sequela to chronic conjunctivitis. Repair entropion with the same techniques that are used in dogs.

Schirmer tear test results are variable in rabbits. The New Zealand white rabbit wets a standard strip at a rate of about 5 mm/min, whereas dwarfs and lops wet at up to 12 mm/min.[1] Other breeds tear at a rate between these two extremes. Thus, the diagnosis of keratoconjunctivitis sicca must be based on a combination of Schirmer tear test results and clinical signs of a dry, granular corneal surface; a sticky, dry conjunctival surface; and blepharospasm. Treat with a combination of topical antibiotics and artificial tears. The use of cyclosporine to treat dry eye problems in rabbits has not been studied.

Corneal Diseases

Rabbits are quite prone to corneal ulcers. These ulcers may be sterile or infected. Sterile ulcers are superficial and cause focal gray opacities that may be quite subtle. In contrast, infected ulcers are yellow and cause significant conjunctival and lid margin hyperemia. Most do not cause craters or pits as are typical in dogs or cats, and they more closely resemble stromal abscesses. In choosing an appropriate antibiotic, it may be helpful to do Gram's staining on samples obtained from a corneal scraping. Use a topical anesthetic and a No. 15 scalpel blade to collect corneal cells and bacteria from the ulcer or abscess. Infected ulcers should be treated topically with a broad-spectrum bactericidal antibiotic q1–4h. Remember that rabbits absorb some topically applied medication into the systemic circulation, so watch for development of gastrointestinal or renal disease. Atropine is needed only rarely. Sterile ulcers usually heal readily with only minimal use of topical antibiotics. However, ulcers occasionally are refractory to antibiotic therapy. If this occurs, débride the cornea with dry cotton swabs to remove any necrotic epithelium. Scraping the surface with a scalpel blade can be a helpful adjunctive technique.

Rabbits can acquire cholesterol or other lipids in their corneas. These have a variety of appearances, ranging from white perilimbal arcs to clouding of the ventral or medial cornea.[8, 16, 20] Lesions can be quite faint or can be dense, raised, and vascularized. Most are caused by excessive oil or fat in the diet ingested in the form of vitamin or protein supplements. For example, a protein supplement of fish meal has caused lipid keratopathy in a colony of rabbits.[20] Diagnosis is made on the basis of biopsy results. Make sure that the pathologist knows that lipid keratopathy is suspected because special processing for lipids is required.

Rabbits can have primary corneal dystrophy, which manifests as curved or blotlike, soft, gray opacities in the central cornea. Primary corneal dystrophy is caused by epithelial and basement membrane thickening and disorganization.[16] No treatment is needed.

Poxvirus can cause pink or yellow masslike lesions on the cornea. Diagnosis is based on biopsy results. Another unusual corneal disease that is sometimes seen is corneal occlusion syndrome (Fig. 29–3). This appears as a progressive creeping of

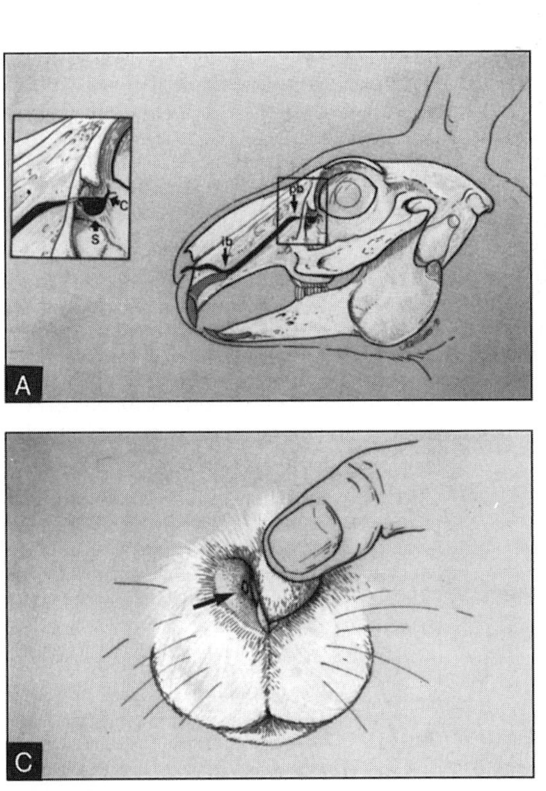

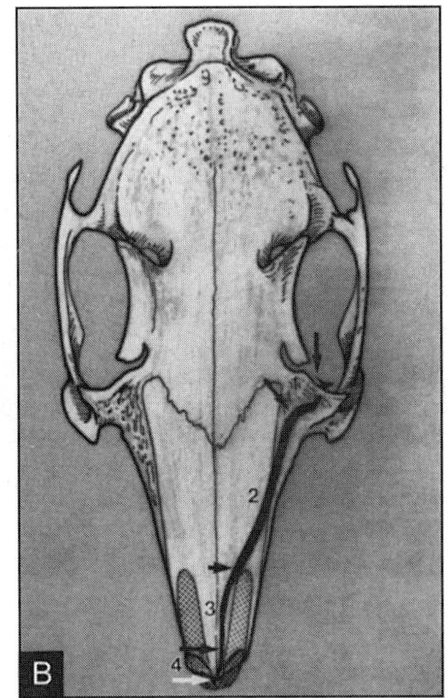

FIGURE 29–2

Diagram of the rabbit nasolacrimal duct. *A*, Lateral view with inset. The two sharp bends, the proximal maxillary bend (pb), and the bend at the incisor tooth (ib) are indicated. The inset shows the canaliculus (C) and the lacrimal sac (S). *B*, Dorsoventral view. 1 = proximal portion of the duct extending from the punctum through the proximal maxillary curve; 2 = portion of the duct extending from the proximal maxillary curve to the base of the incisor tooth; 3 = portion of the duct extending from the base of the incisor tooth to the end of the lacrimal canal; 4 = distal portion of the duct extending from the end of the lacrimal canal to the nasal meatus. *C*, The nasal meatus of the nasolacrimal duct (*arrow*). The opening is enlarged for diagrammatic purposes. (From Burling K, Murphy CJ, da Silva Curiel J, et al: Anatomy of the rabbit nasolacrimal duct and its clinical implications. Prog Vet Comp Ophthalmol 1991; 1:33–40.)

conjunctiva over the cornea.[3] However, in these rabbits, the conjunctiva is not adhered to the cornea. This loose conjunctiva can eventually cover the entire corneal surface. The cause is unknown. Surgical removal is initially successful, but the condition recurs in virtually all affected rabbits.

Uveitis, Glaucoma, and Diseases of the Lens

Uveitis in rabbits can present as focal abscesses in the iris or as a diffuse inflammation (panophthalmitis) of the eye, with hypopyon, corneal edema, and severe episcleral infection. Control focal abscesses with topical antibiotics. Chloramphenicol penetrates best through an intact cornea. Cure is unlikely. Treat panophthalmitis with topical antibiotics q1–4h and with long-term systemic antibiotics. Intravitreal antibiotics may also be helpful. Prognosis is grave; most globes become phthisic (atrophied) or require enucleation.

Glaucoma is hereditary in New Zealand white rabbits, but can be seen in any breed. Hereditary glaucoma begins as a progressive buphthalmos, starting at 3–6 months of age, with intraocular pressures ranging from nearly normal to 10–20 mm Hg above normal.[21] In other breeds, glaucoma

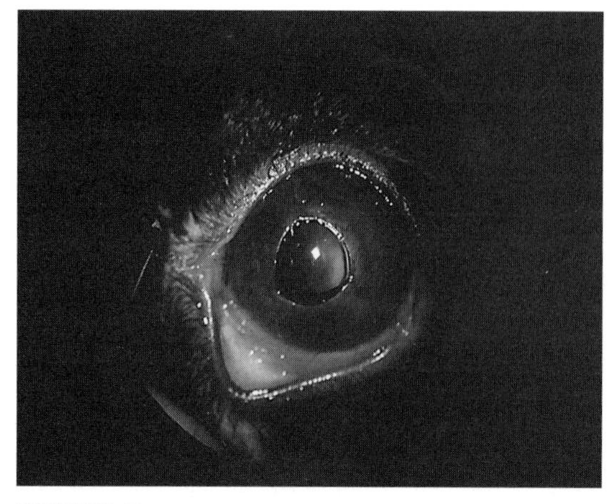

FIGURE 29–3
Corneal occlusion syndrome in the rabbit. The "pupil" is actually the only portion of the cornea not covered by nonadherent conjunctiva.

usually begins in the adult rabbit but rarely causes buphthalmos and is slowly progressive. Often, it begins with only unilateral signs, but most cases become bilateral with time. Watch for decreasing pupillary light responses accompanied by a slowly progressive white haze, often beginning at the perilimbal cornea. Only in later stages is diffuse corneal edema observed. At this point, vision is usually lost. Treat glaucoma with timolol or betaxalol, 0.25% q12–24h. Some rabbits require low-dose dichlorphenamide PO (1–2 mg/kg per day) for the maintenance of normal intraocular pressure.

Spontaneous lens capsule rupture and resultant phacoclastic uveitis associated with *Encephalitozoon cuniculi* is seen sporadically, usually in young rabbits (younger than 2 years of age).[23] Affected rabbits have capsular rupture and uveitis and no history of ocular trauma. The lesion appears as a white mass originating at the lens capsule, with inflammation centered around the break in the capsule. The posterior segment is unaffected. Intralenticular organisms consistent with *E. cuniculi* closely associated with the lens epithelium have been described in reported cases. Associated inflammation is progressive and unresponsive to therapy, and enucleation is eventually needed. The pathogenesis is unknown, but in utero infection is considered likely. *E. cuniculi* has also been implicated as the cause of bilateral cataracts in a laboratory rabbit.[2]

Retina and Optic Nerve

The fundus of rabbits is unlike that of other commonly examined animals. The tapetum is absent, and the background pigmentation is either brown or pink, depending on eye color. The optic nerve appears deeply cupped, and medial and lateral wings of myelinated nerve fibers extend outward from the nerve. Retinal vessels extend along these myelin wings and for a short distance above and below the nerve. The nerve is set relatively high in the fundus, and you must position yourself below the head to see it.

Developmental disorders of the eye occasionally occur in rabbits. These include optic nerve coloboma, retinal folds, and persistent hyaloid artery or persistent hyperplastic primary vitreous.[6] Retinal degeneration is rare but has been reported in one laboratory rabbit breed.[19]

Rabbits may contract chorioretinitis, which may appear as white or yellow foci or as indistinct blurred areas, often near the optic nerve. Differential diagnosis includes systemic pasteurellosis or staphylococcal septicemia. Treat the patient with systemic antibiotics until retinal lesions have resolved.

Orbit

The most common cause of exophthalmos or proptosis in rabbits is orbital disease. This must be differentiated from the buphthalmos seen in rabbits with glaucoma.

The most common cause of exophthalmos in rabbits is retrobulbar abscess. Diagnosis is based on ultrasound examination results. Do not aspirate or drain these through the mouth because an extremely extensive venous sinus surrounds the medial, lateral, ventral, and posterior aspects of the globe.

Retrobulbar abscesses cannot be cured, but the disease process can be slowed with the use of systemic antibiotics. Surgical treatment is by an orbitotomy and involves flapping the zygomatic process posteriorly. However, the abscess can only rarely be entirely removed. Alternatively, remove the eye, its venous sinus, and associated tissues by the more common anterior approach.

Occasionally, enucleation for other diseases is necessary in rabbits. The subconjunctival/sub-Tenon capsule approach is the only approach that does not rupture the venous sinus. Stay very close to the sclera or substantial hemorrhage will result. If hemorrhage occurs, pack the orbit for several minutes and then proceed; the venous sinus cannot be ligated. Also, remove the harderian gland, medial and ventral to the globe.

RATS, MICE, HAMSTERS, AND GERBILS

The term *sialodacryoadenitis complex* refers to a coronaviral infection of the many lacrimal glands that surround the globe of rodents. It usually affects young animals but can appear at any age. Initial signs are blinking, red tears, and exophthalmos or proptosis. Chronic infection results in keratoconjunctivitis sicca, corneal neovascularization, and anterior synechiae at the nasal limbus. In its most severe form, it can result in retinal degeneration, retinal detachment, endophthalmitis, or phthisis bulbi (atrophy of the globe).

In older animals, red tears and associated conjunctivitis and blepharitis can be associated with excessively long lower incisors. Trimming the teeth improves the condition. In gerbils, poor grooming can cause blepharitis and facial lesions secondary to the accumulation of tears on the lids and facial skin.[22] Encourage grooming by bedding gerbils on sand or chinchilla dust.

Older rodents commonly develop calcification of the cornea. This causes the appearance of white patches in the central cornea and may result in punctate corneal ulcers. Rodents of any age can have traumatic corneal ulcers. These lesions respond to topical antibiotics.

Transient cataracts are common in anesthetized rodents. They are theorized to be caused by changes in the aqueous humor composition or temperature secondary to the eye's being open and nonblinking. They resolve when the animal awakens. Rats and mice may have cataracts associated with microphthalmia. Cataracts have been reported in the Chinese hamster model for diabetes mellitus.

Rats, mice, hamsters, and gerbils have a holangiotic retina, with 5–10 radiating retinal vessels that extend from the disk, like spokes in a wheel. The tapetum is absent. The retina can be viewed with the use of a direct ophthalmoscope set at about +8 diopters. One percent tropicamide dilates an albino rodent's pupils in a few minutes. In pigmented rodents, atropine applied every few minutes for 10 minutes is needed for adequate dilation of the pupil, and dilation is usually not as complete as in albinos.

In young rodents, it is extremely common for the hyaloid artery to persist up to the age of 3 months. This persistence commonly causes vitreal hemorrhages, which resolve over time. Other congenital abnormalities that are occasionally seen include optic nerve hypoplasia or coloboma and myelinated retinal nerve fibers. The latter causes the appearance of white, streak-shaped patches on the retinal surface. Diagnosis of retinal degeneration is based on recognition of narrowing of the retinal vessels along with mottling of the background choroidal pigmentation. Differential diagnosis for retinal degeneration includes genetic predisposition, chorioretinitis secondary to inflammation of the orbital lacrimal glands (Fig. 29–4), and phototoxicity. The retinas of rodents, especially those of albino rodents, are extremely susceptible to damage by light. Even 24 hours of continuous light exposure can damage the retina in an albino unless the animal's housing allows escape from the light.

GUINEA PIGS

Blepharitis is manifested by swelling, redness, flaking, crusting, or alopecia of the lids. Vitamin C deficiency, resulting from either dietary deficiency or metabolic disease, can cause the appearance of a flaky discharge on the lids. Ringworm can also be localized to the lids. Treat ringworm with the application of miconazole cream.

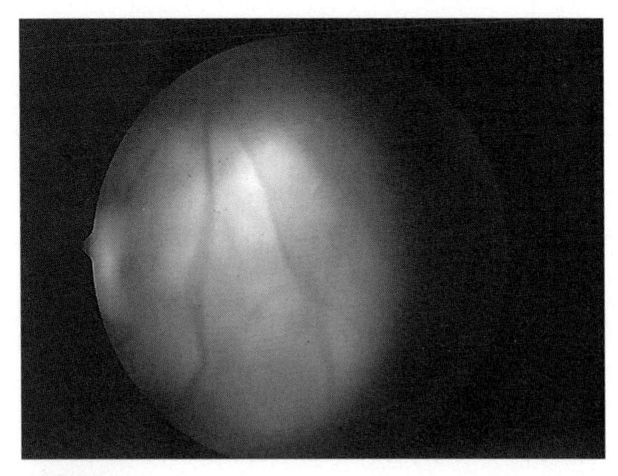

FIGURE 29–4
Chorioretinitis in an albino rat. The normal background color of the albino rat fundus is pink. The white patch represents focal retinal atrophy. A common cause of this is the sialodacryoadenitis complex.

Conjunctivitis can be caused by bacteria, especially *Pasteurella* or *Streptococcus* species or *Chlamydia psittaci*. Conjunctivitis is often seen associated with upper respiratory infections. Most cases respond to topical antibiotics. Guinea pigs are also subject to the development of yellow subconjunctival fatty deposits, a condition that is commonly called "pea eye."[3] No treatment is needed.

Guinea pigs may develop white opaque growths in the anterior chamber; sometimes, these growths are associated with cataracts.[10] Histologically, these growths are osseous choristomas or benign growths containing bone. This may be a form of ectopic mineralization, which is common in other tissues in guinea pigs.

Guinea pigs have a paurangiotic retina, with a fully developed choroidal vasculature but only a few tiny retinal vessels close to the disk. The tapetum is absent. In albino guinea pigs, the fundus background is normally red; retinal degeneration causes the fundus to look more white. In pigmented guinea pigs, the fundus background normally is a mottled reddish-brown; retinal degeneration causes the fundus background to become more mottled.

FERRETS

Anatomically, the ferret eye is similar to the canine eye, except that the pupil is a horizontal slit, which some clinicians believe corresponds to the horizontal retinal visual streak. Ophthalmoscopically, the ferret fundus is similar to the canine fundus, and in general, the eye diseases in ferrets are similar to those in dogs.

The central visual pathways have been extensively studied because ferrets experience significant photoperiodism that influences their endocrine and reproductive systems. They have a direct retinohypothalamic pathway that affects the activity of the sympathetic nerves; these innervate the pineal gland, such that there is increased activity during hours of darkness. Blind ferrets do not have normal estrous cycles because estrus is usually stimulated by long-day photoperiods.[9]

The visual pathways of the ferret have also been a useful tool for the study of visual development, since the visual pathways are immature at birth. Ferrets are mostly monocular; they have very little binocular vision.

The earliest signs of distemper, which is usually fatal in ferrets, are ocular: conjunctivitis, swollen and inflamed eyelids, and corneal ulcers or keratoconjunctivitis sicca.[6] The influenza virus (*Orthomyxoviridae*) can also cause conjunctivitis as well as photophobia.[9]

Vitamin A deficiency has been reported to cause conjunctivitis, cataracts, and night blindness, whereas riboflavin deficiency can cause corneal vascularization.

A zygomatic salivary gland mucocele that caused exophthalmos, with a soft, fluctuant swelling caudal and dorsal to the eye, has been reported.[14] Salivary mucoceles are occasionally seen clinically, and periocular swelling resolves once the mucocele is surgically drained.

Corneal ulcers are commonly seen in ferrets and are treated with antibiotics, as in other species. Old minks (8 years of age and older) are susceptible to the development of cloudy, edematous corneas secondary to corneal endothelial degeneration.[11] However, they do not experience the ulcers and keratitis (bullous keratopathy) that so often afflict dogs with endothelial degeneration.

Cataracts are quite common in ferrets and may be hereditary, secondary to dietary factors, or idiopathic.[13] Because of the risk of genetic transmission, ferrets with cataracts should not be bred. Mature cataracts in ferrets commonly result in cataract-induced uveitis, which causes miosis, mild corneal edema, and squinting. Sometimes, the uveitis can be severe, with keratic precipitates. I have seen cataract-induced uveitis cause either glaucoma, anterior lens luxation, or both.

Carefully examine eyes with mature cataracts for signs of uveitis and treat with either topical corticosteroids (e.g., prednisone acetate, 1% q12–24h in mild cases, q6–8h in severe cases) or topical nonsteroidal anti-inflammatory drugs (e.g., flurbiprofen or suprofen). Remember that cataract-induced uveitis may be chronic and may require long-term treatment (months to years) if complications are to be prevented. If long-term treatment is needed, nonsteroidal anti-inflammatory agents are recommended because they are associated with fewer systemic side effects. Cataract surgery has been done successfully in ferrets; however, intraocular lens implants cannot be placed because currently available lenses are too large.

Retinal degeneration also is commonly seen in ferrets and causes the same clinical and ophthalmoscopic signs as progressive retinal degeneration in the dog. In early stages, night blindness and mild narrowing of retinal vessels, along with mild to moderate tapetal hyperreflectivity, are seen. As the disease advances to cause blindness, the vessels narrow until they are no longer seen, and the tapetum becomes very hyperreflective. Again, ferrets with retinal degeneration should not be used for breeding because retinal degeneration is often hereditary.

REFERENCES

1. Abrams KL, Brooks DE, Runk RS, Theran P: Evaluation of the Schirmer tear test in clinically normal rabbits. Am J Vet Res 1990; 51:1912–1913.
2. Ashton N, Cook C, Clegg F: Encephalitozoonosis (nosematosis) causing bilateral cataract in a rabbit. Br J Ophthalmol 1976; 60:618–631.
3. Bauck L: Ophthalmic conditions in pet rabbits and rodents. Compend Contin Educ Pract Vet 1989; 11:258–266.
4. Buckley P, Lowman DMR: Chronic non-infective conjunctivitis in rabbits. Lab Anim 1979; 13:69–73.
5. Burling K, Murphy CJ, da Silva Curiel J, et al: Anatomy of the rabbit nasolacrimal duct and its clinical implications. Prog Vet Comp Ophthalmol 1991; 1:33–40.
6. Davidson MG: Ophthalmology of exotic pets. Compend Contin Educ Pract Vet 1985; 7:724–736.
7. DiGiacomo RF, Garlinghouse LE, Van Hoosier GL: Natural history of infection with *Pasteurella multocida* in rabbits. J Am Vet Med Assoc 1983; 183:1172–1175.
8. Fallon MT, Reinhard MK, DaRif CA, Schoeb TR: Diagnostic exercise: eye lesions in a rabbit. Lab Anim Sci 1988; 38:612–613.
9. Fox JG: Biology and Diseases of the Ferret. Philadelphia, Lea & Febiger, 1988.
10. Griffith JW, Sassani JW, Bowman TA, Lang CM: Osseous choristoma of the ciliary body in guinea pigs. Vet Pathol 1988; 25:100–102.
11. Hadlow WJ: Chronic corneal edema in aged ranch mink. Vet Pathol 1987; 24:323–329.
12. McLeod CG Jr, Langlinais PC: Pox virus keratitis in a rabbit. Vet Pathol 1981; 18:834–836.
13. Miller PE, Marlar AB, Dubielzig RR: Cataracts in a laboratory colony of ferrets. Lab Anim Sci 1993; 43:562–568.
14. Miller PE, Pickett JP: Zygomatic salivary gland mucocele in a ferret. J Am Vet Med Assoc 1989; 194:1437–1438.
15. Millichamp NJ, Collins BR: Blepharoconjunctivitis associated with *Staphylococcus aureus* in a rabbit. J Am Vet Med Assoc 1986; 189:1153–1154.
16. Moore CP, Dubielzig R, Glaza SM: Anterior corneal dystrophy of American Dutch Belted rabbits: biomicroscopic and histopathologic findings. Vet Pathol 1987; 24:28–33.
17. Okuda H, Campbell LH: Conjunctival bacterial flora of the clinically normal New Zealand White rabbit. Lab Anim Sci 1974; 24:831–833.
18. Petersen Jones SM, Carrington SD: *Pasteurella* dacryocystitis in rabbits. Vet Rec 1988; 122:514–515.
19. Reichenbach A, Baar U: Retinitis-pigmentosa–like tapetoretinal degeneration in a rabbit breed. Doc Ophthalmol 1985; 60:71–78.
20. Sebesteny A, Sheraidah GA, Trevan DJ, et al: Lipid keratopathy and atheromatosis in a SPF laboratory rabbit colony attributable to diet. Lab Anim 1985; 19:180–188.
21. Tesluk GC, Peiffer RL, Brown D: A clinical and pathological study of inherited glaucoma in New Zealand white rabbits. Lab Anim 1982; 16:234–239.
22. Thiessen DD, Pendergrass M: Harderian gland involvement in facial lesions in the Mongolian gerbil. J Am Vet Med Assoc 1982; 181:1375–1377.
23. Wolfer J, Grahn B, Wilcock B, Percy D: Phacoclastic uveitis in the rabbit. Prog Vet Comp Ophthalmol 1993; 3:92–97.

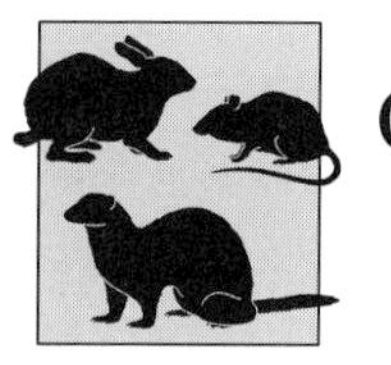

CHAPTER 30

Orthopedics in Small Mammals

Amy Kapatkin, DVM

Orthopedic problems in rabbits, ferrets, and small rodents can be successfully managed by a surgeon who adheres to basic orthopedic principles and who understands the considerations unique to each species.

FRACTURE MANAGEMENT AND FIRST AID

Orthopedic trauma in rabbits, ferrets, and small rodents is often the result of household accidents, including injury from a falling object, a closing door, or an owner's stepping on an animal. Also common are accidents caused by poor cage design, such as trapped limbs in inappropriately sized wire mesh flooring. In cities with tall apartment buildings, we sometimes see ferrets with "high-rise syndrome." Their injuries tend to be similar to those of cats that have fallen from heights, whereas their survival rates tend to be intermediate between those of cats and dogs.[11, 14, 34]

The first consideration is assessment of these animals as trauma patients. Shock, respiratory problems, abdominal emergencies, and bleeding disorders need immediate attention. Once these parameters have been controlled, perform a thorough orthopedic and neurologic examination. Orthopedic trauma is never a medical emergency unless the patient has a spinal fracture that may result in paralysis if surgery is not performed immediately. If this is the case, the veterinarian and owner must weigh the importance of anesthetic safety against that of neurologic competence.

After a patient has been treated for shock, its open

fractures need immediate attention. Clip and clean the wound and place a sterile dressing over it. Ideally, a support splint should be placed. However, these small patients are often difficult to handle without sedation, and they may not be sufficiently stable to undergo sedation. In particular, rabbits with open fractures do poorly because they tend to develop osteomyelitis, which is extremely difficult to cure in this species.

Keep the patient comfortable and quiet, and give analgesics until the patient can tolerate anesthesia and definitive orthopedic treatment. Rabbits, ferrets, and small rodents usually must be sedated or anesthetized before radiography can be performed; thus, imaging is often postponed for 24–48 hours until an animal becomes stable.

The preoperative plan for orthopedic surgery in rabbits, ferrets, and small rodents is distinct from that in dogs and cats in several ways. Although it is easy to confine these animals after surgery, it is not always easy to prevent them from being active in their cages. Assume that rabbits and small rodents will chew at their skin sutures; thus, the use of subcuticular sutures and perhaps tissue glue is preferred. Skin sutures should be avoided because of the difficulty involved in putting an Elizabethan collar on these animals. However, collars for small rodents are commercially available from laboratory animal supply companies if needed.

When considering an external splint or external fixation, keep in mind that most animals will chew on the apparatus and can destroy it or cause self-injury. Many of the surgical implants that veterinarians are accustomed to using are too large for these small species. Also, the application of such large implants can overprotect the bone, leading to bone resorption and the failure of repair.

The expense of each possible surgical repair option must be considered. This includes the cost of the initial surgery and that of subsequent implant removals or bandage changes.

FRACTURE CLASSIFICATIONS

Fractures are classified as either open or closed and according to the direction and location of the fracture line (Table 30–1). *Closed fractures* are those that do not communicate with the external environment; *open fractures* are those that do. Open fractures are further divided into three subgroups on the basis of the severity of the soft tissue injuries[3, 6]:

TABLE 30–1
FRACTURE CLASSIFICATION

Fracture Type	Description
Transverse	Fracture at a right angle to the long axis of the bone
Oblique	Fracture line diagonal to the long axis of the bone
Spiral	Fracture line curved around the bone's long axis
Comminuted	More than two pieces of bone in the fracture
Segmental	Fractures in three or more segments that do not meet anywhere
Avulsion	Tendon insertion is detached because of the pull of the fracture
Physeal	Fracture at the growth plate
Condylar	Fracture through a condyle
Intercondylar	Fracture between two condyles

Adapted from Brinker WO, Piermattei DL, Flo GL: Handbook of Small Animal Orthopedics and Fracture Treatment. 2nd ed. Philadelphia, WB Saunders, 1990, p 5.

Grade I fractures result from the penetration of bone fragment to the environment. If soft tissue trauma is minimal and can be surgically débrided, these fractures can be handled like closed fractures.

Grade II fractures result from external trauma to the soft tissues and are associated with significantly more damage to the soft tissues.

Grade III fractures result from external trauma and are characterized by a high degree of bone contamination and soft tissue destruction. Both grade II and grade III open fractures must be surgically handled as open fractures, even after surgical débridement.

Open fractures are quite common in rabbits, ferrets, and small rodents in the limbs below the elbow and stifle, where there is minimal soft tissue to protect the bone from exiting to the environment. Grade I open fractures are more common than those of other grades except in ferrets with high-rise syndrome, which often have more severe limb trauma.

Rabbits that present with open fractures are difficult to manage. Careful clipping of the very fine underfur is necessary to avoid tearing of the delicate skin. A surgical clipper is the best tool for removing rabbit fur. Be patient and take care not to further complicate the wound.

When handling all open fractures, wear sterile gloves and use aseptic technique, even if the wounds are grossly contaminated. Ideally, take samples for aerobic and anaerobic cultures from open fractures. Then, start broad-spectrum antibiotic therapy. Carefully débride the wound and perform copious sterile lavage. If definitive fracture repair is not planned at this time, place a sterile bandage and splint. If the fracture is above the elbow or stifle, it is not advisable to place a splint unless it is a spica splint (over the shoulder or hip). In rabbits, ferrets, and small rodents, this is difficult because of the animals' size and body conformation.

Regardless of the fracture type, schedule fracture fixation as soon as anesthesia is safe for the patient. Definitive fixation maximizes the patient's comfort and improves bone's ability to heal properly. Fracture stabilization allows the blood supply to aid in healing and increases bone's resistance to infection.[3]

METHODS OF FIXATION

The method of fixation for fracture repair in rabbits, ferrets, and small rodents is chosen according to the basic rules outlined below. No one fixation method or approach can be used in every situation. An orthopedic surgeon must be knowledgeable about and have the equipment to perform multiple different techniques. An investment in small instruments is worthwhile if you anticipate working often with exotic small mammals.

External Coaptation

External coaptation in rabbits, ferrets, and small rodents can often be used quite effectively as a definitive orthopedic treatment for closed fractures. It works best for simple fractures affected by bending and rotational forces that cause bone ends to interdigitate with manipulation and to remain reduced. Fractures affected by compressive or shear forces, such as short oblique fractures, are poorly immobilized with external coaptation.[8]

While trying to reduce a fracture in these small animals, take care not to damage soft tissues and the blood supply. Palpation is often sufficient to determine whether reduction has been achieved; however, radiography is still recommended for detecting a potential rotational or angular deformity. Apply standard splinting principles—namely, maintain the affected limb in normal position, immobilize a joint above and below the fracture, and achieve at least 50% cortical contact on reduction of the fracture.[8]

Standard materials used for splints and casts in dogs and cats are not usually applicable to the management of rabbits, ferrets, and small rodents. Occasionally, a rabbit is large enough to tolerate an aluminum rod with a light Robert Jones bandage. However, I find that this type of splint often causes irritations and complications.

Three products that work well for splinting rabbits, ferrets, and small rodents are available. Orthoplast (Johnson & Johnson, New Brunswick, NJ), Caraform (Carapace, Inc., Tulsa, OK), and Hexcelite (AOA, a division of Kirschner Medical, Timonium, MD) are all castlike materials that are very light in weight, thin, and easy to use. They are softened in boiling water and conform to any shape when molded and allowed to cool. They work best when used for a half cast with a light Robert Jones bandage so they do not cause excessive pressure on the limb (Fig. 30–1). Although the cost of these materials is greater than that for routine casting materials, such a small piece of material usually is required that the final cost is reasonable. Caraform is available in two thicknesses and is easier to manipulate and mold than Orthoplast. It also has the advantage of not returning to its original flat shape if placed back into boiling water, with the result that its contour can be "fine-tuned." Both Caraform and Hexcelite can be layered so that splint thickness and stiffness can be increased, if desired. All three products are very resistant to chewing by the animal. They will not cause any oral trauma or break apart and cause a gastrointestinal obstruction.

Monitor splints and casts weekly to prevent complications. Common complications include soiling, which leads to the formation of pressure sores or local skin infections, and swelling, which results from excessive activity or from the splint's being too tight. Joint laxities and stiffness from the coaptation are also commonly seen.[16, 30]

Intramedullary Pinning

Intramedullary pinning in rabbits, ferrets, and small rodents is a technique that is available to most practice situations. The implants and equipment are relatively inexpensive. Intramedullary pinning is a biomechanically sound technique in these species because the implant shares the load with the bone instead of bearing all of the load. It has been shown

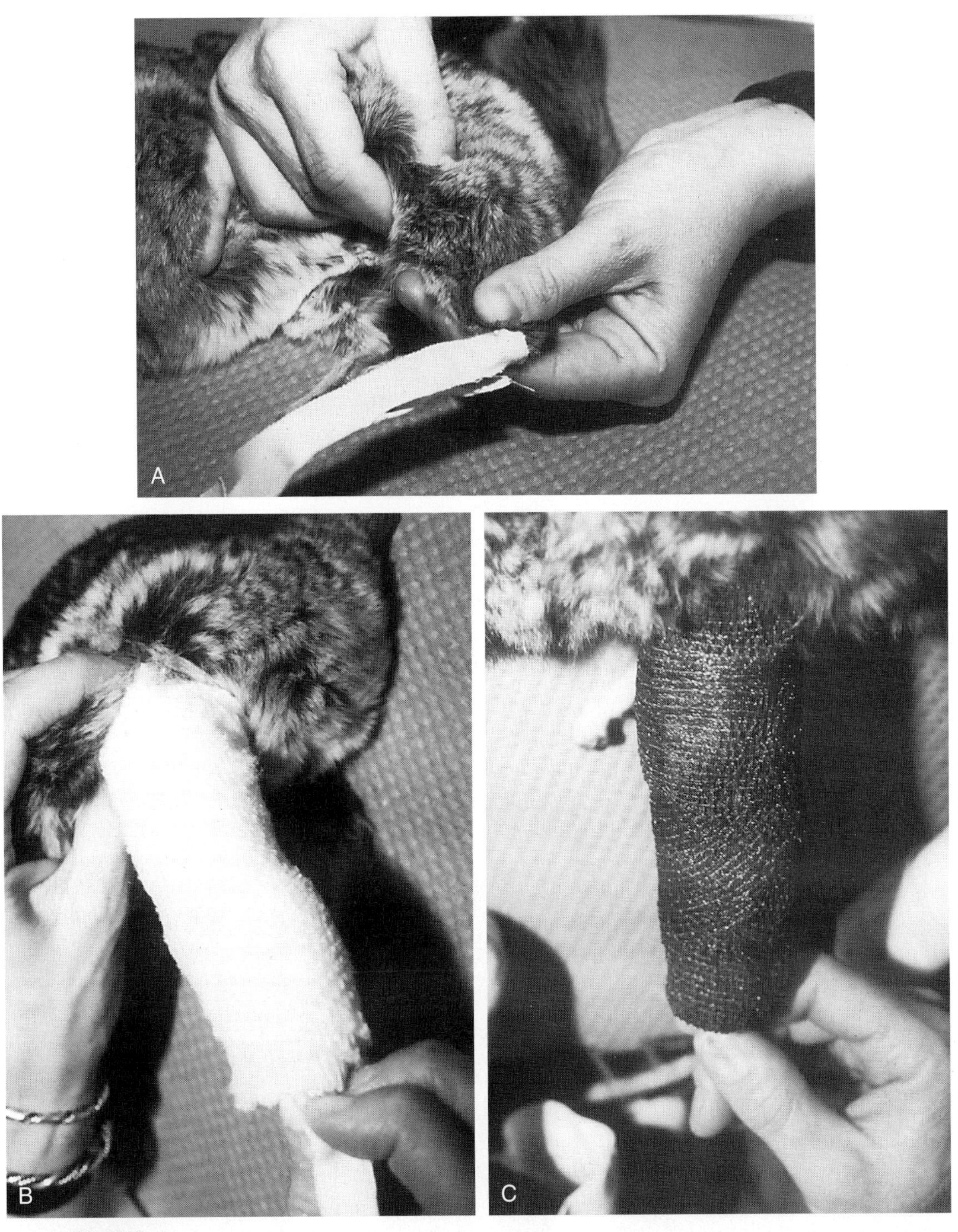

FIGURE 30–1
Splinting of a fractured tibia/fibula in a chinchilla. *A*, Tape stirrups placed on the fractured limb. *B*, Padding complete. *C*, Completed splint.

in a laboratory situation that if the implant does all of the load-bearing, healing will be delayed beyond 12 weeks.[19, 32] Biodegradable pins made of polydioxanone materials are under investigation. They are biomechanically stiff enough to allow fracture healing, and they resorb gradually by 24 weeks, when the bone is remodeling and no longer needs the support. This allows transfer of the forces from the implant to the bone without the need for a second surgery for removal of the implant.[19, 32]

Standard principles for intramedullary pinning are used in rabbits, ferrets, and small rodents. The pin diameter should occupy at least 60–70% of the medullary cavity.[3] In these small species, anything larger than Kirschner wires, which are available in diameters of 0.028, 0.035, 0.045, and 0.062 inches, can rarely be used. Intramedullary pins are smooth, partially threaded, or fully threaded. Use only smooth intramedullary pins to avoid breakage at the thread interface.[23]

Use the pins to obtain good axial alignment and to limit bending and rotational forces. In order to achieve this biomechanically, it is necessary to pack the pins in the medullary cavity as much as possible for the length of the bone (Fig. 30–2). Normograde placement of the pin is advantageous for avoiding penetration into the joints and for enabling custom direction of the pin.[23]

Bone Plating

Bone plating has very limited clinical use in rabbits, ferrets, and small rodents. Extensive research has been done in rabbits with bone osteotomies repaired with rigid plate fixation. The purpose of these studies was determination of the ideal fracture fixation, the type of bone healing, and the point in time when the stiffness advantage of the plate becomes a disadvantage in regard to load-sharing of the bone. In experimental repair of transverse bone osteotomies, it appears that bone heals faster than was previously thought. In dogs and cats, it is assumed that the remodeling stage of bone healing lasts 8–12 months and that a plate implant should not be removed before that time. It has been shown in rabbits that the optimal time for plate removal is 6–8 weeks after surgery. However, this was determined on the basis of results of osteotomy repair in which the blood supply to the bone was not damaged and the fracture was not comminuted. In a clinical situation, optimal plate removal is probably 3–4 months after fixation.[15, 18, 25, 27]

In certain situations, the use of a plate is appropriate for fracture repair in a rabbit or ferret. Open fractures of the humerus or femur can be difficult to manage with an external fixator because of the conformation stance of these species. Since grade II or III open fractures should have one of these two repairs, plating is sometimes the best choice. If plating is chosen, the usual implants employed are 1.5-mm and 2.0-mm cuttable plates (Synthes, Ltd., Wayne, PA). The cuttable plates offer the surgeon flexibility in choosing the appropriate length and stiffness of plate. The standard size AO plates are too large and stiff for use in these small species. Orthopedic principles of AO bone plate application are covered in other texts.[5, 9]

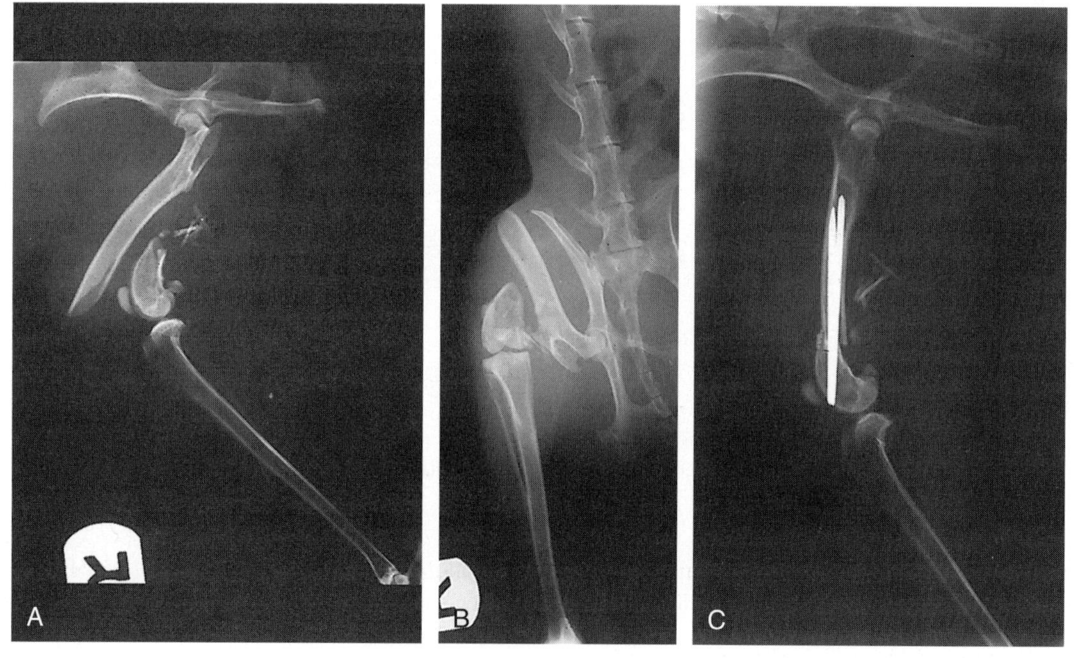

FIGURE 30–2
A and B, Radiographs of a supracondylar femoral fracture in a rabbit. *C,* Dynamic cross-pin repair of the fracture.

There are some specific problems with the use of plating in these species. The bones of rabbits have extremely thin cortices that make screw placement difficult without stripping of the cortex. I have experienced complete collapse of the bone while trying to place a screw. In a clinical setting, rabbit fractures are rarely without comminutions. The blood supply is already compromised to the bone, predisposing the rabbit to osteomyelitis and nonunion. Placing a bone plate with removal of the remaining periosteum and soft tissues only worsens this problem. As has been indicated in research articles, plating often overprotects a fracture, preventing load-sharing and causing subsequent delay or nonunion. If a plate is used, the animal will require staged plate removal, which is costly and unpopular with the owner. Another disadvantage is the high cost of equipment and implants.

As for pins, biodegradable plates and screws have been evaluated, and their successful application looks promising. These implants degrade over time; thus, they do not overprotect the bone from stress and do not need to be removed.[29]

External Skeletal Fixation

External skeletal fixation is probably the most common method of repairing fractures in rabbits, ferrets, and small rodents. External fixators provide rigid stability, can be adapted for use in these small species, and cause minimal soft tissue damage.

The nomenclature of external fixators is outlined in Table 30–2. Type Ia fixators are useful for counteracting rotational forces but are subject to bending. Type Ib fixators are useful for counteracting craniocaudal bending forces. Double connecting bars can be added for limiting compressive forces, but this is never needed in these small species.[10, 31] Type II splints are resistant to compressive and rotational forces. Their use is limited to bones below the elbow and stifle.[10, 31] The type III configuration is very stiff and resists all forces. Its use is rarely indicated in rabbits, ferrets, and small rodents.[10, 31]

Basic principles for applying external fixators are similar in all species. The pins should be inserted with low rotational speed (150 rpm). Manual insertion causes wobble and leads to premature loosening of the pins. High-speed drilling can cause bone necrosis, which also leads to premature loosening of pins. Predrilling with a drill bit is an acceptable technique if smooth pins are used and also is the correct method for inserting threaded and positive-profile pins. However, it would be unusual to use threaded or positive-profile pins in rabbits, ferrets, and rodents because of their small bone size and short healing time. When smooth pins are used, the pins should be angled at about 70° to the longitudinal axis of the bone so that pullout of the pins is prevented. Try to place the pins in the center of the bone so that bone–pin interface stability is increased.[10, 31]

Before repairing a fracture with an external fixator, decide whether a limited open approach or closed placement of the pins is best. In these species with limited soft tissue coverage, it is advantageous not to destroy the tissues by opening the fracture. Therefore, in simple fractures, I place the external fixator with a closed technique. With highly comminuted or open fractures that need débridement, I use a limited open technique for achieving reduction and placing pins.

Rabbits, ferrets, and small rodents are usually too small for their pins to be connected with external fixator clamps and bars. Bone cement and acrylics can be used as fixator bars. Biomechanically, these materials are as rigid as the metal bars and clamps (if used at an appropriate thickness) and are resistant to chewing by the animals. Sometimes, it is very difficult to make a bar light while maintaining rigidity in very small animals. In these patients, I sometimes use Caraform or Hexcelite as the connecting bars. Both materials can be easily shaped and layered if necessary.

Place the fixator pins approximately 1 cm away from the fracture line. The ideal number of pins per bone segment for maximum stiffness is four. Additional pins increase stiffness insignificantly. In these small species, four pins may provide too much stiffness; therefore, I usually use three pins per segment. The fixator pin diameter should not exceed

TABLE 30–2
NOMENCLATURE FOR EXTERNAL FIXATORS

Type I	Unilateral connecting bar(s) with fixation pins penetrating one skin edge and two bone cortices
	Type Ia, uniplanar
	Type Ib, biplanar
Type II	Uniplanar with bilateral connecting bars and fixation pins that pass through two skin surfaces and two bone cortices
Type III	Combination of types I and II, namely, bilateral and biplanar

20% of the bone diameter, so K-wires usually are used. Position the connecting bar about 1 cm away from the skin. Placing the bar too far away from the skin decreases the stiffness and strength of the external fixators. Remember to allow for swelling when placing the bars. Spread out the pins evenly across the fracture segment to achieve maximum strength. Also remember to place the pins through a separate stab skin incision and not through the fracture opening or original incision[10, 31] (Fig. 30–3).

Bone healing in rabbits with fractures stabilized by external fixation has been well studied in the laboratory. The current belief in external fixation is to stage the removal of the apparatus such that bone is allowed to take over load-bearing at a fairly early stage of fixation. This process has been termed "dynamization."[10, 31] The ideal time of removal of external fixators in rabbits was 6 weeks when tibial osteotomies were used as the model. The strength and stiffness of the bone was greater if the fixator was removed at 6 weeks than if it was left in place for 12 weeks.[26, 28] Clinically, many factors affect optimal removal time of a fixator, such as the age of the animal, the type of fracture, and the degree of vascular structure disruption.[10, 31] Therefore, the key is to perform a follow-up examination of these patients postoperatively every 2–3 weeks and to stage removal when there are indications that the fracture has regained normal stiffness even though strength may not be normal.[26] Removal at 4 weeks caused some loss of reduction experimentally and is probably not advisable, even in perfectly reduced fractures.[26]

FRACTURE HEALING AND POSTOPERATIVE MANAGEMENT

Bone healing in rabbits, ferrets, and small rodents is the same as it is in other mammals. There are two major categories of bone healing: direct and indirect. *Direct bone healing* takes place without periosteal or endosteal callus. This occurs when there is anatomic reduction of the fracture and rigid stability. The two types of direct healing are contact healing and gap healing. With *contact healing,* bone union and haversian remodeling occur together. *Gap healing* takes place when a gap smaller than 800 μm is present. Layers of bone are laid down on two surfaces of the fracture. This transverse lamellar bone is then remodeled longitudinally through osteons and haversian remodeling.[12, 20] *Indirect bone healing* is "classic" bone healing. Bony union is preceded by an inflammatory stage, a reparative stage (with formation of soft and hard callus), and a remodeling stage. For further details on bone healing, refer to other texts.[7, 12, 20, 22]

Postoperative management of rabbits, ferrets, and small rodents includes confinement, good husbandry, and frequent monitoring and maintenance of the fixation apparatus. Animals with closed fractures only need perioperative antibiotics (a dose intravenously and intramuscularly at the time of surgery), but open fractures require extended antibiotic therapy. Ideally, the antibiotic is chosen according to the sensitivity pattern of the bacterial culture taken initially.

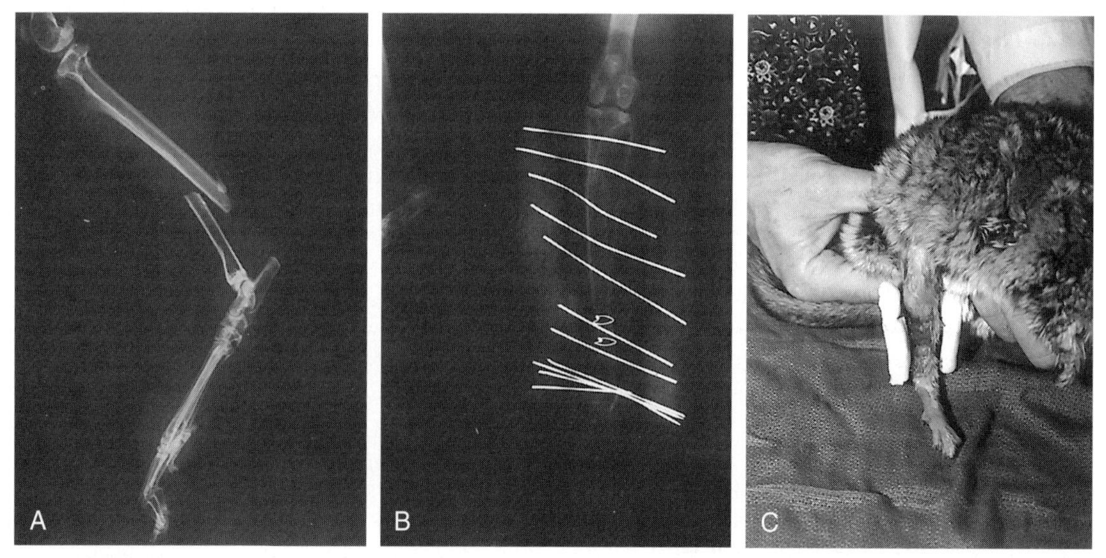

FIGURE 30–3

A, Radiograph of a tibia/fibula fracture in a rabbit. *B,* Postoperative radiograph of the fracture with an external fixator. *C,* Example of polymethyl methacrylate bar fixation in a chinchilla.

Some of the techniques used in the management of open fractures in dogs and cats are not feasible in small mammals. Placing drainage systems or treating open wounds daily with sterile flushes and bandages is extremely difficult. Animals chew excessively at bandages or reach the wound unless a hard splint made of one of the previously discussed casting materials has been placed on the limb. Daily flushes can only sometimes be managed with heavy tranquilization or anesthesia. This is expensive and stressful, especially for rodent species. Therefore, wound management should be definitive at the time of surgery, if at all possible.

Instruct the owner to keep his or her pet confined and quiet. Good husbandry is extremely important for the pet experiencing the added stress of recovery. Instruct the owner how to force feed if the pet is anorectic.

If a splint is present, review bandage care with the owner. The toes should be checked for swelling or discharge. These species often chew at splints even if they appear comfortable. Extreme discomfort in a pet usually manifests as quietness and anorexia. I recommend rechecking splints at least every 2 weeks after a first recheck within a few days of splint placement.

Evaluate the fracture radiographically every 3–4 weeks. In these species, this usually requires heavy sedation or anesthesia. Good palpation of the fracture is also important because radiographic findings often lag behind clinical healing. Depending on the type of fixation, changes can be made in the apparatus as healing becomes evident on radiographs.

COMPLICATIONS

The ultimate goal in fracture repair is bony union. Unfortunately, this does not always occur despite our use of sophisticated treatments. A delayed union, nonunion, or malunion can result.

Delayed Union

Fractures with delayed union do not heal in the expected time period compared with similar fractures under similar circumstances. Causes of delayed union include infection, inadequate blood supply to bone and soft tissues, excessive distraction or compression of the bone ends, excessive loss of bone, poor immobilization at the fracture site, excessive stress protection of the fracture, interposition of soft tissue at the fracture ends, too much weight-bearing by the patient, and systemic factors.[13, 21, 24]

The first step in treating delayed union is identification of the cause. Noninfected delayed union can sometimes be treated conservatively with the addition of a splint for greater stability or with a change in a patient's activity level. Sometimes, a highly comminuted fracture shows delayed union because of an extreme loss of blood supply, which resolves if given additional time. If gross misalignment, instability, loosening of implants, or infection has occurred, surgical intervention usually is necessary. Infected bone heals if kept rigidly stable, but this is extremely difficult in these species.[13, 21, 24]

Nonunion

In fracture nonunion, the fracture has not healed and, without surgical intervention, will not heal. The causes are the same as those of delayed union. Nonunion fractures have been classified by Weber and Cech as either viable (vascular) or nonviable (avascular).[33] Clinical characteristics of a nonunion are movement and pain at the fracture site. The patient is non–weight-bearing lame and usually has severe disuse atrophy of the muscles. On radiographs, either excessive callus (viable nonunion) or no callus (avascular nonunion) may be seen. The clinician can visualize an increased gap between the bone ends, obliteration of the marrow cavity, osteopenia from disuse, or excessive callus with no bridging across the fracture. Regardless of the inciting cause of the nonunion, additional surgery is needed. Rigid stability and a bone graft are necessary for the stimulation of bone production. If infection is still the inciting cause, aggressive wound management also is indicated.[13, 21, 24]

Malunion

Malunions are fractures that heal in an abnormal position. This can result in an abnormal or painful gait secondary to limb shortening or angular or rotational deformity. Degenerative joint disease can occur from abnormal joint alignment or weight-bearing forces. The usual causes are improper alignment or loss of alignment at the time of fracture fixation; this underscores the need for close monitoring of the fracture postoperatively.

Malunions may be nonclinical and may not need any intervention. If correction will improve the function of the limb, surgery is indicated. This may involve osteotomizing the bone in different fashions or using distraction osteogenesis if shortening of the limb is severe.[2, 13] Remember that these species are small and that ring fixators are usually impractical. Due to their small size, light bodyweight, and locomotive stance, these animals seem to tolerate severe deformities with minimal difficulty.

Post-Traumatic Osteomyelitis

Post-traumatic osteomyelitis is another potential complication of fractures in rabbits, ferrets, and small rodents. This is a post-traumatic or postoperative infection of the bone that is due to wound contamination, bone avascularity, and the presence of a suitable environment (e.g., hematoma). An infected wound needs more than 10^5 organisms per gram of tissue for induction of post-traumatic osteomyelitis. Therefore, good surgical débridement and copious lavage is very important in the management of open fractures. Adherence to strict sterile surgical technique, careful wound handling, hemostasis, and anatomic closure help to prevent post-traumatic osteomyelitis.[4]

Post-traumatic osteomyelitis is fairly common in rabbits. Radiographically, rabbits with post-traumatic osteomyelitis show periosteal reactions, osteolysis, and sometimes, an involucrum[35] (Fig. 30–4). I find that the organisms most commonly found on culture are *Pseudomonas* species. Rabbits develop caseous, nondraining abscesses; thus, typical drainage techniques are not useful. Surgically débride the thick abscess and surrounding tissues. Then, either leave the wound open for daily lavage or close it, depending on the location of wound and the thoroughness of the débridement. In my experience, success in treating this condition in rabbits is very limited, with healing occurring in fewer than 5% of wounds.

A similar type of abscess can occur in small rodents, but the incidence of post-traumatic osteomyelitis appears to be low. Ferrets with post-traumatic osteomyelitis have manifestations similar to those of affected dogs and cats. Therefore, treatment and the use of drainage systems can be similar.

Antibiotic therapy is important in post-traumatic osteomyelitis. Collect samples for aerobic and anaerobic bacterial cultures and administer an appropriate antibiotic.

When treatment for post-traumatic osteomyelitis is unsuccessful, which it almost always is in rabbits, amputation of the limb is the only option. This is a salvage procedure that is reserved for only those animals whose prognosis for successful treatment is very poor.

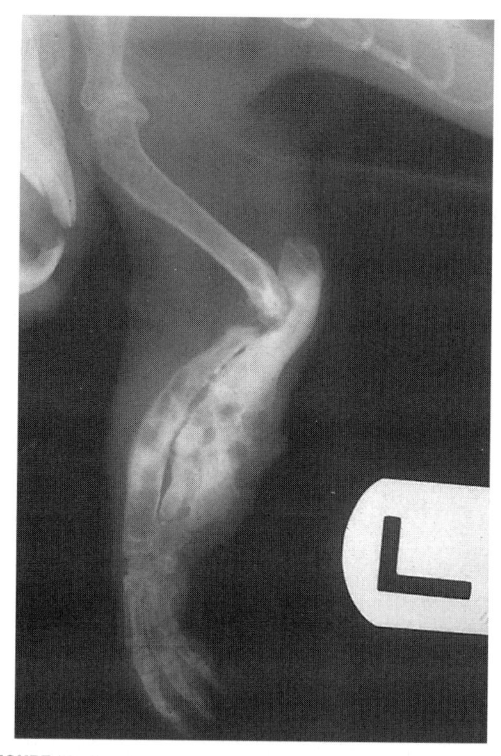

FIGURE 30–4
Severe post-traumatic osteomyelitis in the radius and ulna of a rabbit.

AMPUTATIONS

Amputation is indicated in rabbits, ferrets, and small rodents when orthopedic trauma is so severe that it is unmanageable or when treatment of post-traumatic osteomyelitis is unsuccessful. It is also an option if the owner has severe financial constraints and cannot afford necessary follow-up bandage care and radiography. Fortunately, these species are very adaptable to amputation of a single limb and ambulate well on three legs. Even large rabbits can adapt to the loss of a rear leg.

The level of amputation chosen depends on where the injury has occurred. In the foreleg, it is easier and more cosmetic to remove the scapula instead of amputating at the scapulohumeral joint. Some surgeons prefer to leave the scapula because it

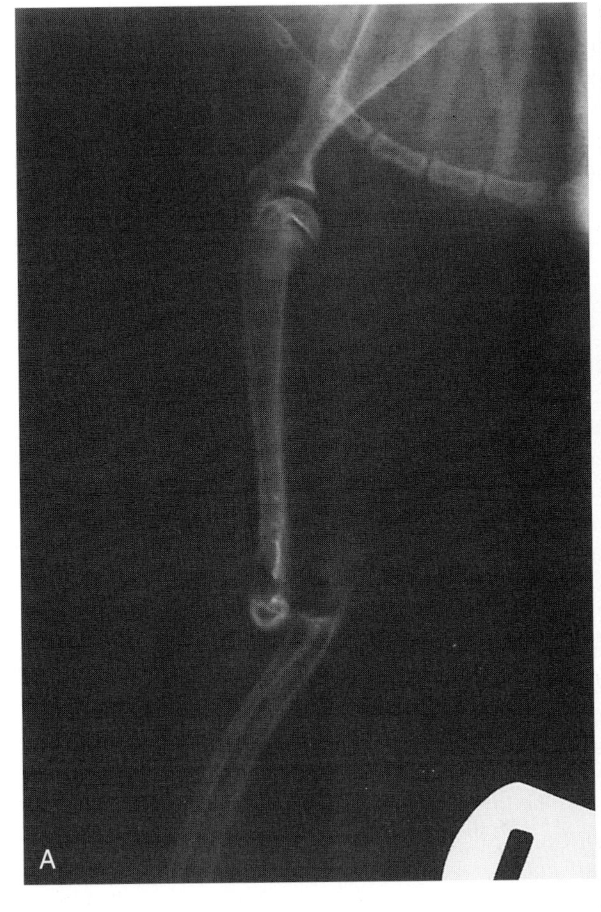

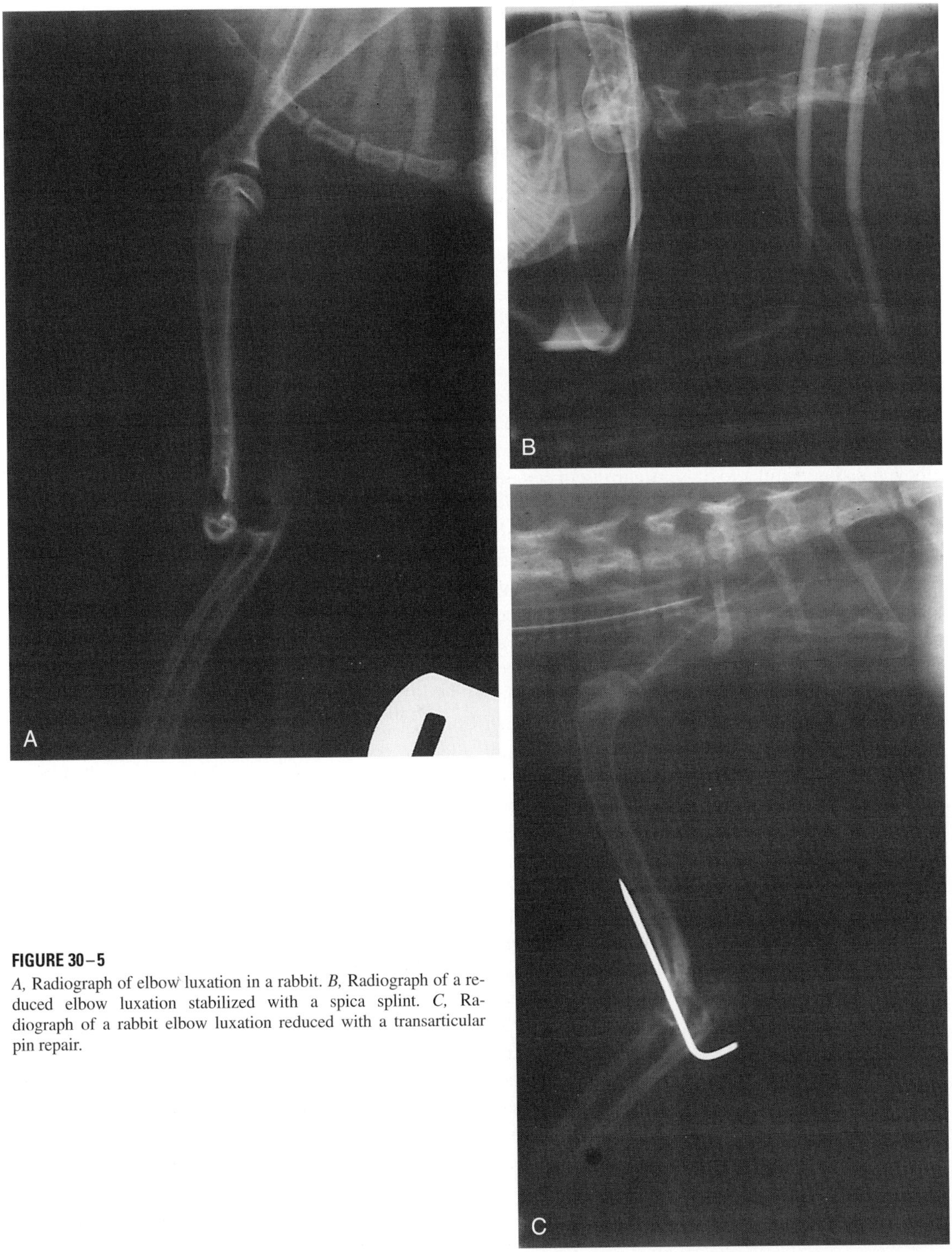

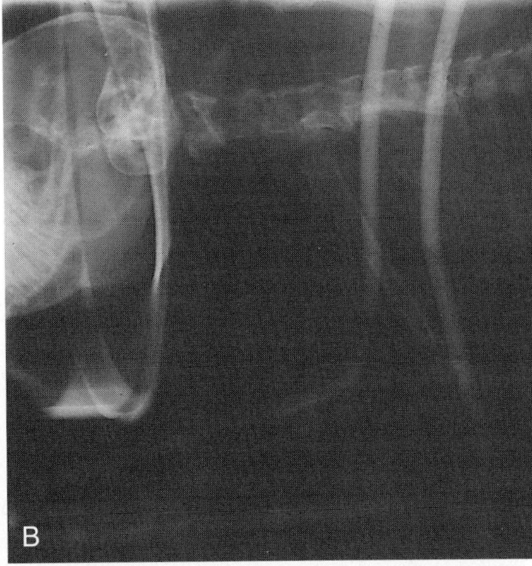

FIGURE 30–5
A, Radiograph of elbow luxation in a rabbit. *B*, Radiograph of a reduced elbow luxation stabilized with a spica splint. *C*, Radiograph of a rabbit elbow luxation reduced with a transarticular pin repair.

serves as a protective barrier to the chest wall. A hindleg amputation is more cosmetic if the amputation is midfemoral rather than at the coxofemoral joint. I disarticulate the limb at the coxofemoral joint only if the infection or injury is so close to the joint that a good resection is not possible.

Surgical approaches to amputation of the limbs are very similar to those for other domestic animals.

The bone in rabbits has such thin cortices that it will shatter if it is cut with a bone cutter. I suggest using either Gigli-saw wire or a power saw to make a straight bone cut. Take care to leave enough soft tissue coverage of the remaining bone for closure. Refer to anatomic texts for locations and variations of the soft tissues in these species.[1, 17]

ELBOW LUXATIONS

Elbow luxations are another common condition seen in rabbits (Fig. 30–5*A*). Animals present with non–weight-bearing lameness of the limb and a very painful, swollen elbow joint. Although this can result from trauma, there may be no known trauma history. Rabbits may have a predisposition for elbow luxations similar to those occurring in certain breeds of dogs.

Treatment consists of reducing the elbow and then keeping it reduced in extension while the soft tissues scar down to keep it in place. Sometimes, this can be achieved with closed reduction with the patient under anesthesia and with the placement of a splint made from Caraform or an aluminum rod (see Fig. 30–5*B*). It is very difficult to immobilize the shoulder joint in a rabbit, although immobilization is the proper technique for this type of injury in other mammals. It is possible to achieve success with a splint placed at the midhumerus, but such a splint must be monitored closely. Joints that reduce easily also reluxate easily.

Many elbow luxations need internal fixation in order to heal. I place a transarticular pin through the joint and then place a light Caraform splint (see Fig. 30–5*C*). The transarticular pin keeps the joint reduced while the splint prevents full weight-bearing by the rabbit. The pin must be removed in about 3 weeks. Usually, the splint is needed for support for another 2–3 weeks after pin removal. Elbow luxation repair is usually successful with this technique; if it is not, a transarticular external fixator can be placed.

REFERENCES

1. An NQ, Evans HE: Anatomy of the ferret. *In* Fox JG, ed.: Biology and Diseases of the Ferret. Philadelphia, Lea & Febiger, 1988, pp 14–31.
2. Anson LW: Malunions. Vet Clin North Am Small Anim Pract 1991; 21:761–780.
3. Anson LW: Emergency management of fractures. *In* Slatter D, ed.: Textbook of Small Animal Surgery. 2nd ed. Vol 2. Philadelphia, WB Saunders, 1993, pp 1603–1610.
4. Braden TD: Posttraumatic osteomyelitis. Vet Clin North Am Small Anim Pract 1991; 21:781–811.
5. Brinker WO, Hohm RB, Prieur WD: Manual of Internal Fixation in Small Animals. New York, Springer-Verlag, 1984, pp 21–80.
6. Brinker WO, Piermattei DL, Flo GL: Handbook of Small Animal Orthopedics and Fracture Treatment. 2nd ed. Philadelphia, WB Saunders, 1990, p 5.
7. Brown SG, Kramers PC: Indirect (secondary) bone healing. *In* Bojrab MJ, ed.: Disease Mechanisms in Small Animal Surgery. 2nd ed. Philadelphia, Lea & Febiger, 1993, pp 671–677.
8. DeCamp CE: External coaptation. *In* Slatter D, ed.: Textbook of Small Animal Surgery. 2nd ed. Vol 2. Philadelphia, WB Saunders, 1993, pp 1661–1676.
9. DeYoung DJ, Probst CW: Methods of internal fracture fixation. *In* Slatter D, ed.: Textbook of Small Animal Surgery. 2nd ed. Vol 2. Philadelphia, WB Saunders, 1993, pp 1610–1640.
10. Egger EL: External skeletal fixation. *In* Slatter D, ed.: Textbook of Small Animal Surgery. 2nd ed. Vol 2. Philadelphia, WB Saunders, 1993, pp 1641–1661.
11. Gordon LE, Thacher C, Kapatkin A: High-rise syndrome in dogs: 81 cases (1985–1991). J Am Vet Med Assoc 1993; 202:118–122.
12. Kaderly RE: Primary bone healing. Semin Vet Med Surg (Small Anim) 1991; 6:21–25.
13. Kaderly RE: Delayed union, nonunion, and malunion. *In* Slatter D, ed.: Textbook of Small Animal Surgery. 2nd ed. Vol 2. Philadelphia, WB Saunders, 1993, pp 1676–1685.
14. Kapatkin AS, Matthiesen DT: Feline high-rise syndrome. Compend Contin Educ Pract Vet 1991; 13:1389–1394.
15. Laftman P, Nilsson OS, Brosjo O, et al: Stress shielding by rigid fixation studied in osteotomized rabbit tibiae. Acta Orthop Scand 1989; 60:718–722.
16. Leighton RL: Principles of conservative fracture management: splints and casts. Semin Vet Med Surg (Small Anim) 1991; 6:39–51.
17. McLaughlin CA, Chiasson RB: Laboratory Anatomy of the Rabbit. 2nd ed. Dubuque, IA, William C. Brown, 1979, pp 7–31.
18. Paavolainen P, Karaharju E, Slatis P, et al: Radiographic evaluation of fracture healing after rigid plate fixation: experiments in the rabbit. Acta Radiol [Diagn] (Stockh) 1981; 22:697–702.
19. Papagelopoulos PJ, Giannarakos DG, Lyritis GP: Suitability of biodegradable polydioxanone materials for the internal fixation of fractures. Orthop Rev 1993; 22:585–593.
20. Perren SM: Primary bone healing. *In* Bojrab MJ, ed.: Disease Mechanisms in Small Animal Surgery. 2nd ed. Philadelphia, Lea & Febiger, 1993, pp 663–670.
21. Robello GT, Aron DN: Delayed and nonunion fractures. Semin Vet Med Surg (Small Anim) 1992; 7:98-104.
22. Schelling SH: Secondary (classical) bone healing. Semin Vet Med Surg (Small Anim) 1991; 6:16–20.
23. Schrader SC: Complications associated with the use of Steinmann intramedullary pins and cerclage wires for fixation of long-bone fractures. Vet Clin North Am Small Anim Pract 1991; 21:687–703.
24. Summer-Smith G: Delayed unions and nonunions, diagnosis, pathophysiology, and treatment. Vet Clin North Am Small Anim Pract 1991; 21:745–760.
25. Terjesen T: Bone healing after metal plate fixation and external fixation of the osteotomized rabbit tibia. Acta Orthop Scand 1984; 55:69–77.
26. Terjesen T: Healing of rabbit tibial fractures using external fixation: effects of removal of the fixation device. Acta Orthop Scand 1984; 55:192–196.

27. Terjesen T: Plate fixation of tibial fractures in the rabbit: correlation of bone strength with duration of fixation. Acta Orthop Scand 1984; 55:454–456.
28. Terjesen T, Johnson E: Effect of fixation stiffness on fracture healing: external fixation of tibial osteotomy in the rabbit. Acta Orthop Scand 1986; 57:146–148.
29. Thaller SR, Huang V, Tesluk H: Use of biodegradable plates and screws in a rabbit model. J Craniofac Surg 1992; 2:168–173.
30. Tomlinson J: Complications of fractures repaired with casts and splints. Vet Clin North Am Small Anim Pract 1991; 21:735–744.
31. Toombs JP: Principles of external skeletal fixation using the Kirschner-Ehmer splint. Vet Clin North Am Small Anim Pract 1991; 6:68–74.
32. Wang GJ, Dunstan JC, Reger SI, et al: Experimental femoral fracture immobilized by rigid and flexible rods (a rabbit model). Clin Orthop 1981; (154):286–290.
33. Weber BG, Cech O: Pseudoarthrosis: Pathology, Biomechanics, Therapy, Results. Bern, Switzerland, Hans Huber, 1976.
34. Whitney WO, Mehlhaff CJ: High-rise syndrome in cats. J Am Vet Med Assoc 1987; 191:1399–1403.
35. Worlock P, Slack R, Harvey L, et al: An experimental model of post-traumatic osteomyelitis in rabbits. Br J Exp Pathol 1988; 69:235–244.

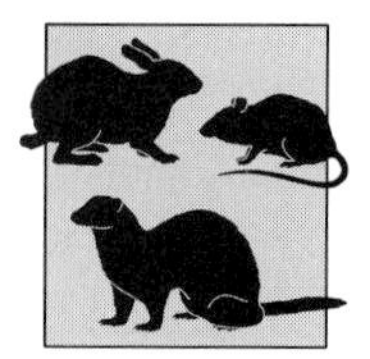

CHAPTER 31

Small Mammal Radiology

Joseph D. Stefanacci, VMD
and Heidi L. Hoefer, DVM

Radiography of exotic pets is challenging and exciting. Small patient size and unique physiologic characteristics, such as rapid respiratory rate, can present technical dilemmas to the practitioner. However, with modern radiologic equipment and a better understanding of the use of anesthetics in these patients, the practitioner can radiograph most animals. Proper restraint and positioning are essential for ensuring correct radiographic interpretation. The use of special x-ray cassettes in combination with the appropriate film provides the necessary radiographic detail and minimizes radiation exposure to personnel and patient.

Rigid restraint is paramount to the production of diagnostic films. Several factors must be considered when you prepare an animal for radiography: the area to be radiographed, the temperament of the animal, and the general state of health of the patient. Most small mammals tolerate radiographic procedures well, but be careful with the very stressed or debilitated patient. Treatment and stabilization of the patient are the primary concerns, and radiography may often be postponed in order to minimize patient risk. Place dyspneic animals in an oxygen cage first; when radiographing them, consider using injectable agents or isoflurane and an oxygen face mask.

RESTRAINT

For screening whole-body ventrodorsal and lateral films, manual restraint sometimes can be used. However, ferrets and small rodents can be difficult to restrain for any length of time, and very often they need to be sedated for radiography. The choice of anesthetic agent varies with the individual practice and the area of radiographic interest. Isoflurane delivered through a face mask is convenient and safe in most animals. In excitable or fractious animals, induce anesthesia in an induction chamber and use a face mask for maintenance. Injectable anesthetic agents can be used for radiography of the head and neck area. Intubation may be preferable for lengthy procedures, such as a skull series, but it can be difficult or impossible to perform in the small species. Anesthesia and sedation are discussed in detail in Chapter 32.

EQUIPMENT AND RADIOGRAPHIC TECHNIQUE

Since motion artifact is a common problem, the use of x-ray generating equipment capable of producing 300 mA in 1/120 (0.008) second is a minimum requirement.[1] Larger, three-phase generators that can produce 1000–1200 mA are ideal because timestops are even shorter. Most radiographs can be exposed for 1/120 (0.008) to 1/60 (0.016) second with excellent results. Incremental adjustments of kilovoltage are necessary through a range of 40–70 kilovolts peak (kVp). A telescoping x-ray tube stand that can be moved along the x-ray table and whose height can be adjusted is helpful. The ability to change the focal-film distance (distance from the x-ray tube to the film) is useful because it aids in the production of magnified views of anatomic areas of interest.[1] A tubestand that can rotate 90° is important for production of a horizontally directed x-ray beam. This allows standing lateral radiographs to be obtained when gravity-dependent and non–gravity-dependent physiologic substances, including gas and fluid, are evaluated.

Fine or detail intensifying screens/cassettes can be used for radiographing most species (e.g., Curix Fine, Agfa, Orangeburg, NY; Quanta Detail, E.I. DuPont, Wilmington, DE; Lanex Fine, Eastman Kodak, Rochester, NY). These screens, combined with the proper x-ray film (Curix Detail RPIL, Agfa; Cronex 10, E.I. DuPont; TMG film, Eastman Kodak) maximize anatomic detail (bone, lung) while minimizing exposure time. Ultrafine detail in exotic pet radiography can be accomplished with the use of the Min R mammography system (Eastman Kodak). We use Min R single intensifying screen cassettes with Min R single emulsion film for best results. This system requires similar settings but a lower kVp range (40–50 kVp). With any film/screen combination, animals less than 10 cm in thickness should be positioned directly on the x-ray cassette, whereas those thicker than 10 cm can be positioned on the x-ray table, with the film/cassette placed in the Bucky tray, under a grid.

The standard radiographic views are the lateral and the ventrodorsal (or dorsoventral). Because of the relatively small patient size, whole-body radiography can usually be done. This is often the easiest way of accomplishing a study and allows for quick examination of the entire patient. Special radiographic projections, such as oblique and magnified views, can be attempted for certain body parts of interest, such as the skull. Thorough technical knowledge and familiarity with anatomy are necessary for successfully obtaining these more difficult views.

CONTRAST RADIOGRAPHY

Contrast radiography can be done in small mammals. Although sometimes technically difficult to perform, this procedure provides important information that can support a clinical diagnosis. Gastrointestinal disease such as mechanical obstruction due to foreign body ingestion or hairball impaction in ferrets and rabbits can be delineated in an upper gastrointestinal examination. Administer 10–15 mL/kg of barium sulfate liquid (Novopaque 30% w/v, Picker Int., Highland Heights, OH) PO or by stomach tube. Make sequential radiographs at 15- to 30-minute intervals until all of the barium is in the large bowel. Extra care should be taken with rabbits when gastric tubes are used; the small oropharynx and short neck of rabbits make this procedure difficult. Esophageal structure and function can be evaluated with the use of barium sulfate paste (Esophotrast Cream, Rhone-Poulenc Rorer Pharmaceuticals, Inc., Collegeville, PA). Megaesophagus in ferrets is easily assessed with this technique.

For urinary tract problems such as cystic, ureteral, urethral, or renal calculi in rabbits, guinea pigs, and ferrets, use of 2 mL/kg of an intravenous iodinated contrast agent produces a good excretory urogram. Calculus location or renal function before surgery can be determined in this way. Iothalamate sodium or meglumine (Conray, Mallinckrodt Medical, St. Louis, MO) is a standard injectable agent for this purpose. If a urinary catheter can be placed, inject meglumine through it for cystography. Expanding the urinary bladder to palpable turgidity allows detection of filling defects, diverticulae, ruptures, or aberrant bladder location.

RADIOGRAPHIC INTERPRETATION

Radiographic interpretation for exotic pets follows guidelines similar to those applicable for all other animals. Note changes in the roentgen signs of size, shape, number, location, margination, and opacity for each projection during the evaluation of the radiograph, taking into account the small body size and described anatomic variations.[2] Knowledge of normal anatomy is required; it is important to understand, for example, that the thorax of rabbits and rodents is not clearly visualized because of its small size, and that abdominal organs in rabbits and guinea pigs may be obscured by gaseous cecal dilation. Practice and patience ensure successful radiographic evaluation of these exotic pets.

REFERENCES

1. Silverman S: Diagnostic imaging of exotic pets. Vet Clin North Am Small Anim Pract 1993; 23:1287–1299.
2. Rubel GA, Isenbugel E, Wolvekamp P: Atlas of Diagnostic Radiology of Exotic Pets. Philadelphia, WB Saunders, 1991.

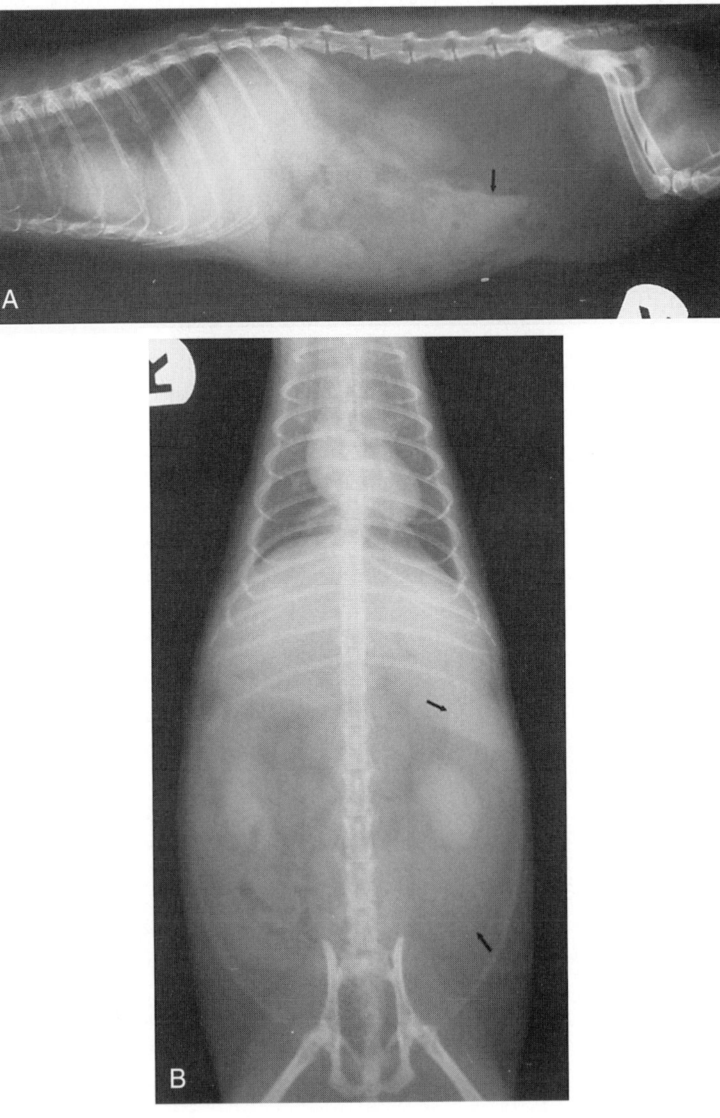

FIGURE 31–1
A and B, The normal ferret.

SIGNALMENT Four-year-old spayed female ferret.

RADIOGRAPHIC FINDINGS Splenomegaly is a common finding *(arrows)*. The large amount of intraperitoneal fat helps to improve visualization of organs such as the spleen and kidneys. Normal ferrets may have a small amount of gas in the gastrointestinal tract.

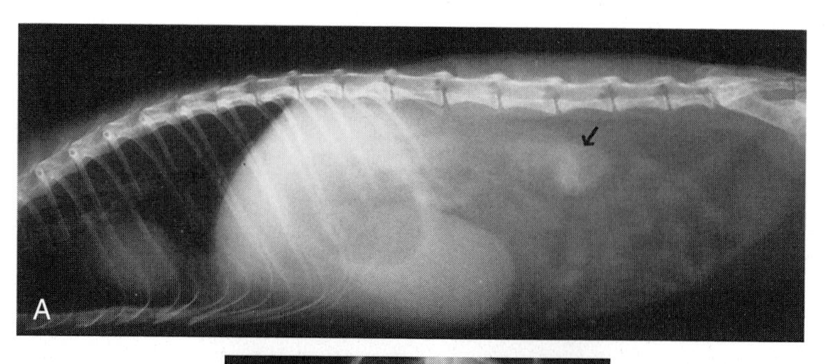

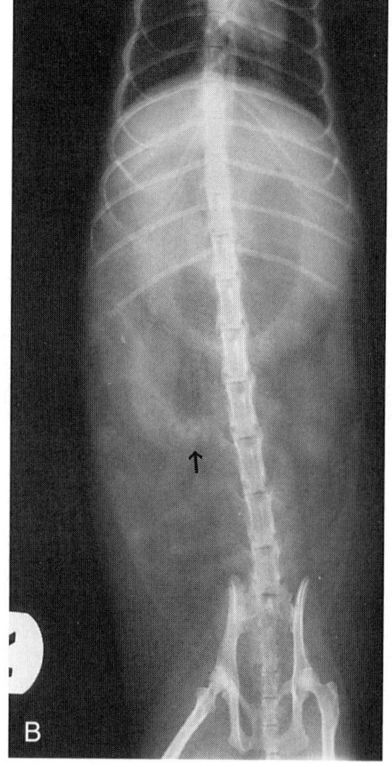

FIGURE 31–2
A and B.

SIGNALMENT	One and one half–year-old spayed female ferret.
HISTORY	Anorexia, lethargy, vomiting.
RADIOGRAPHIC FINDINGS	The stomach and proximal descending duodenum are abnormally dilated (fluid and gas). A radiopaque foreign body is present in the proximal duodenum *(arrows)*. The pulmonary blood vessels and the heart are small.
FINAL DIAGNOSIS	Duodenal foreign body (rubber). Systemic hypovolemia (dehydration).

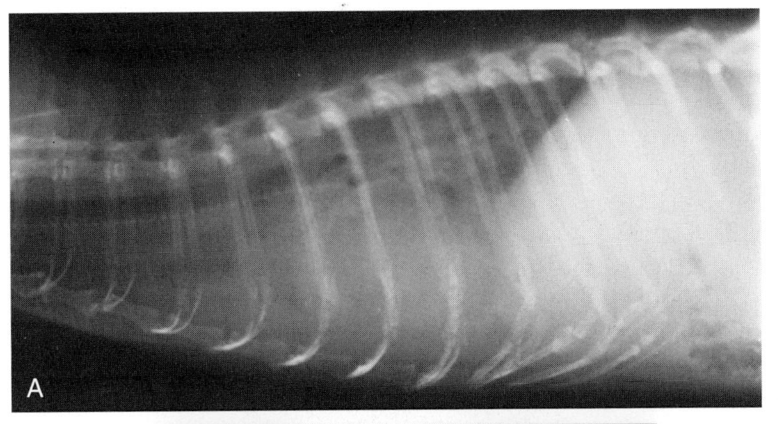

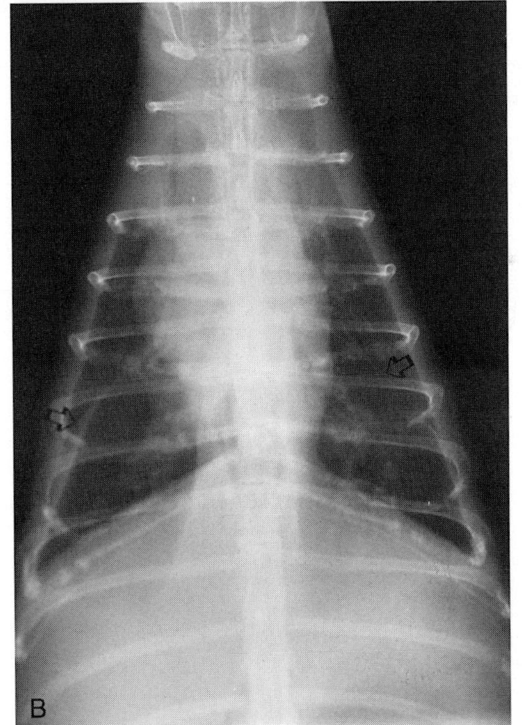

FIGURE 31–3
A and B.

SIGNALMENT Five-year-old castrated male ferret.

HISTORY Lethargy, tachypnea, respiratory distress.

RADIOGRAPHIC FINDINGS Generalized cardiomegaly is causing dorsal deviation of the trachea. Pleural effusion is present and is characterized by the appearance of pleural fissure lines *(arrows)* and a general increase in the opacity of the cranial thorax. Hepatomegaly is present.

FINAL DIAGNOSIS Dilated cardiomyopathy with mitral and tricuspid regurgitation. Hepatic congestion.

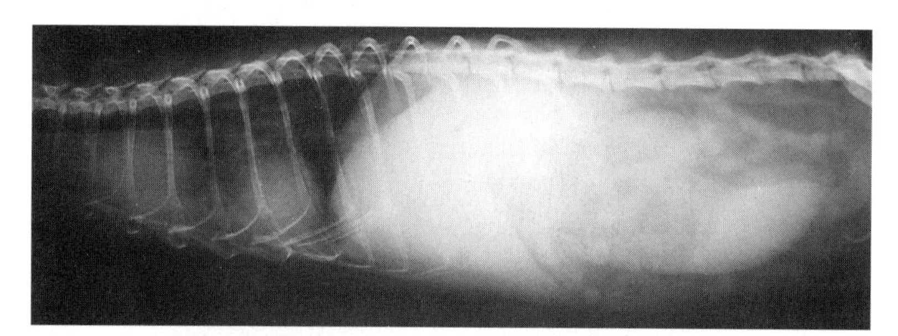

FIGURE 31–4

SIGNALMENT Seven-month-old castrated male ferret.

HISTORY Painful abdomen, diarrhea, lethargy.

RADIOGRAPHIC FINDINGS A large cranial mediastinal soft tissue mass is seen. Hepatomegaly and splenomegaly are present.

FINAL DIAGNOSIS Lymphoma.

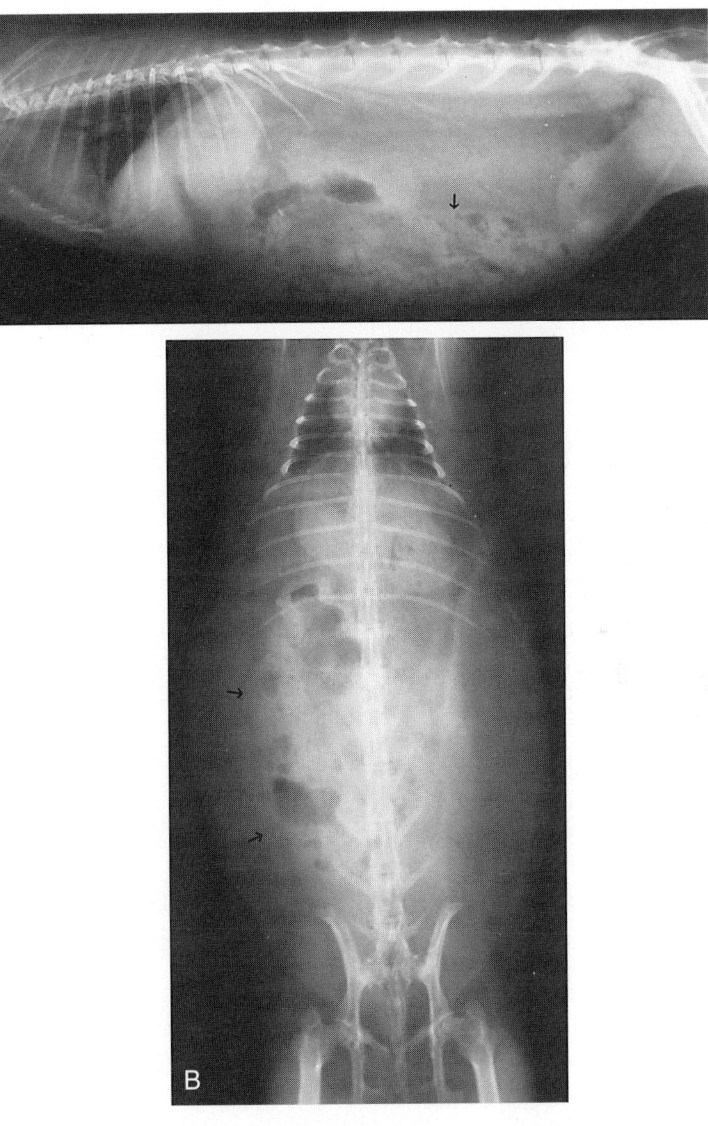

FIGURE 31–5
A and B, The normal rabbit.

SIGNALMENT Three-year-old intact female rabbit.

RADIOGRAPHIC FINDINGS Body cavity size disparity is exemplified. The cranial lung lobes are small and poorly visualized. The caudal lung lobes are well aerated. The cecum *(arrows)* is usually seen in the right hemiabdomen and contains varying amounts of gas and ingesta. A large amount of retroperitoneal fat is displacing the kidneys ventrally (lateral view).

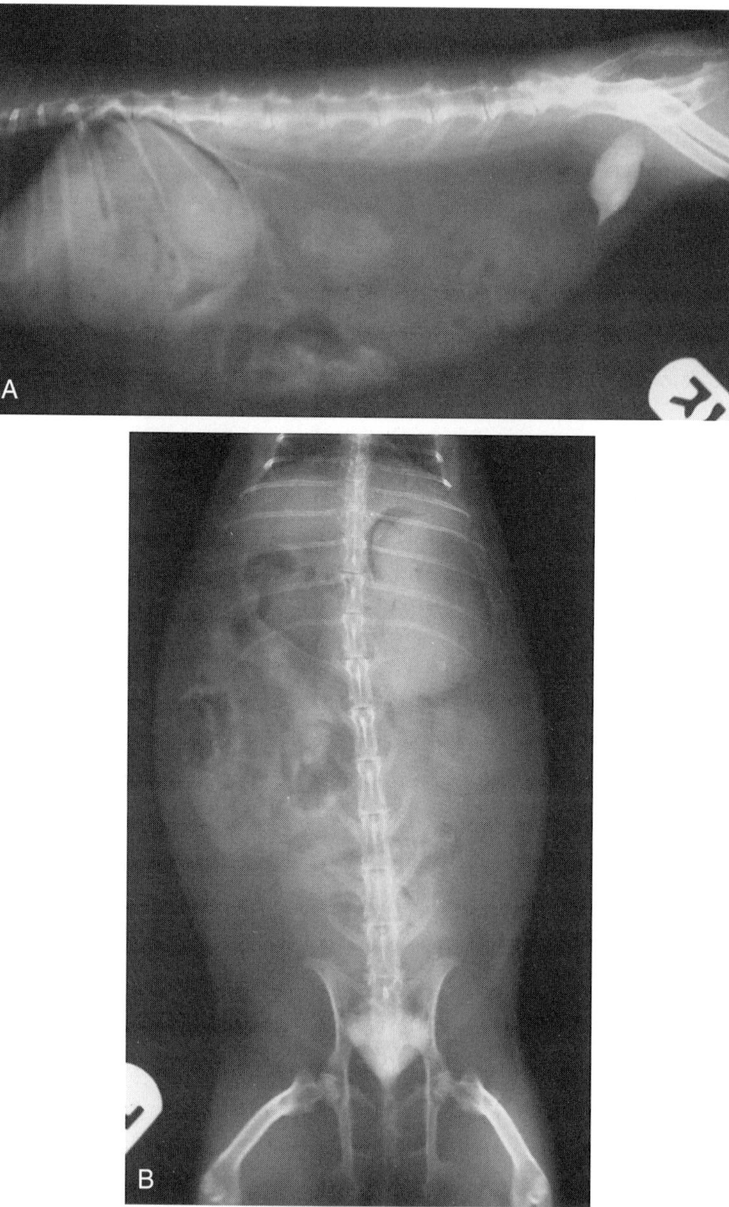

FIGURE 31–6
A and B.

SIGNALMENT Three-year-old intact female dwarf rabbit.

HISTORY Anorexia, decreased stool excretion, lethargy, dehydration.

RADIOGRAPHIC FINDINGS A large intragastric mass effect is causing gastric distention. Some gas is present around the mass. There is a mineral-opaque urinary bladder with a cranial protrusion.

FINAL DIAGNOSIS Gastric stasis (probable trichobezoar). Calciuria. Bladder diverticulum.

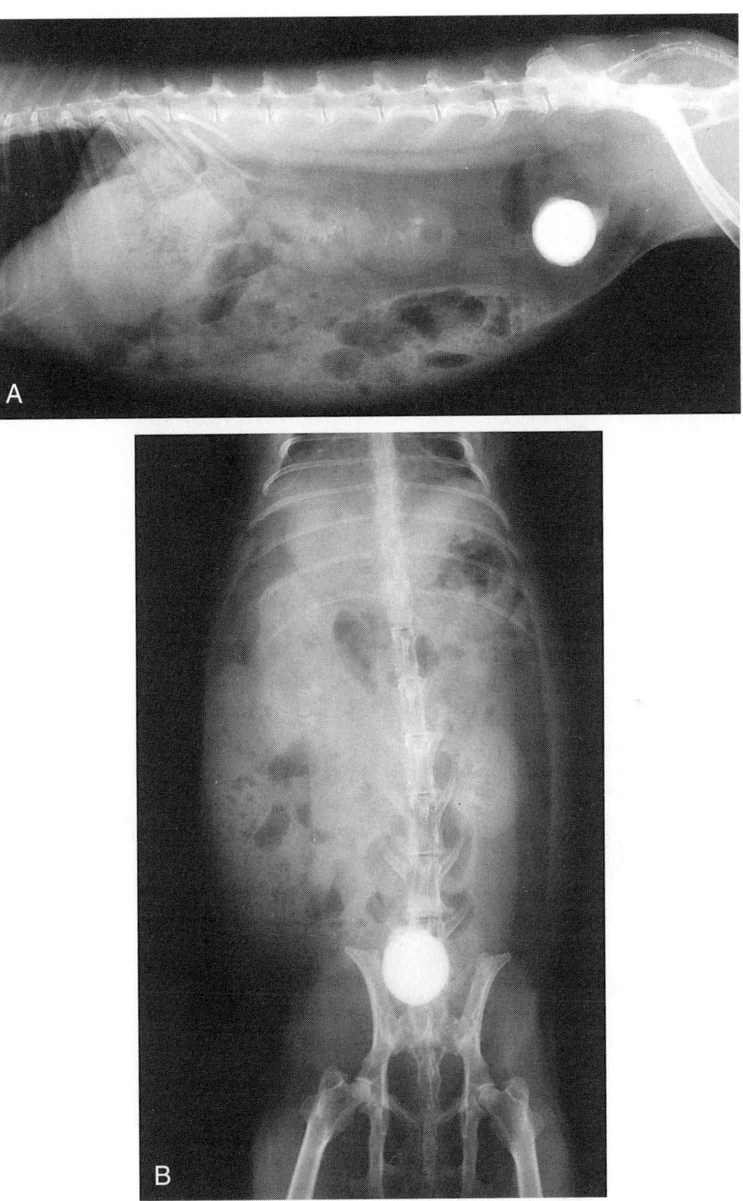

FIGURE 31–7
A and B.

SIGNALMENT Eight-year-old intact male dwarf rabbit.

HISTORY Hematuria.

RADIOGRAPHIC FINDINGS A large, round mineral opacity is seen in the caudoventral abdomen, in the same radiographic plane as the urinary bladder. Bilateral renal linear mineral striations are present.

FINAL DIAGNOSIS Calcium oxalate cystic calculus. Bilateral renal diverticular mineralization. Hypercalciuria.

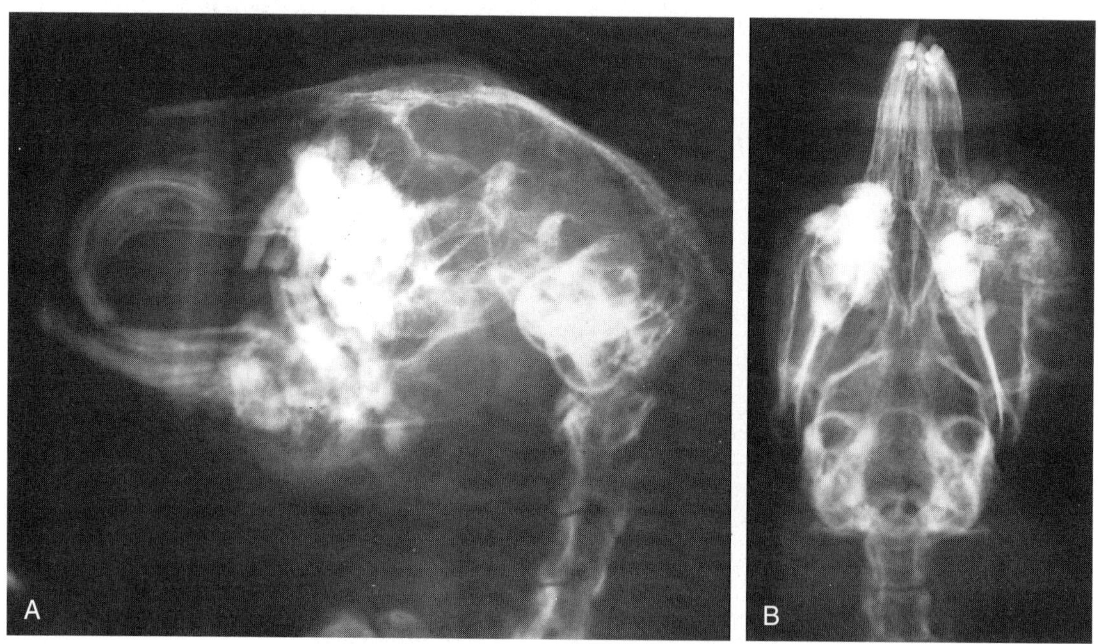

FIGURE 31–8
A and B.

SIGNALMENT	Six-year-old castrated male rabbit.
HISTORY	Mandibular mass, weight loss.
RADIOGRAPHIC FINDINGS	A diffuse soft tissue swelling is observed along the left hemimandible. There is a mixed lytic and proliferative lesion involving the left hemimandible and the bony alveoli of the left mandibular premolars and molars.
FINAL DIAGNOSIS	Chronic mandibular premolar and molar root abscessation. Secondary mandibular osteomyelitis. Molar, premolar, and incisor malocclusion.

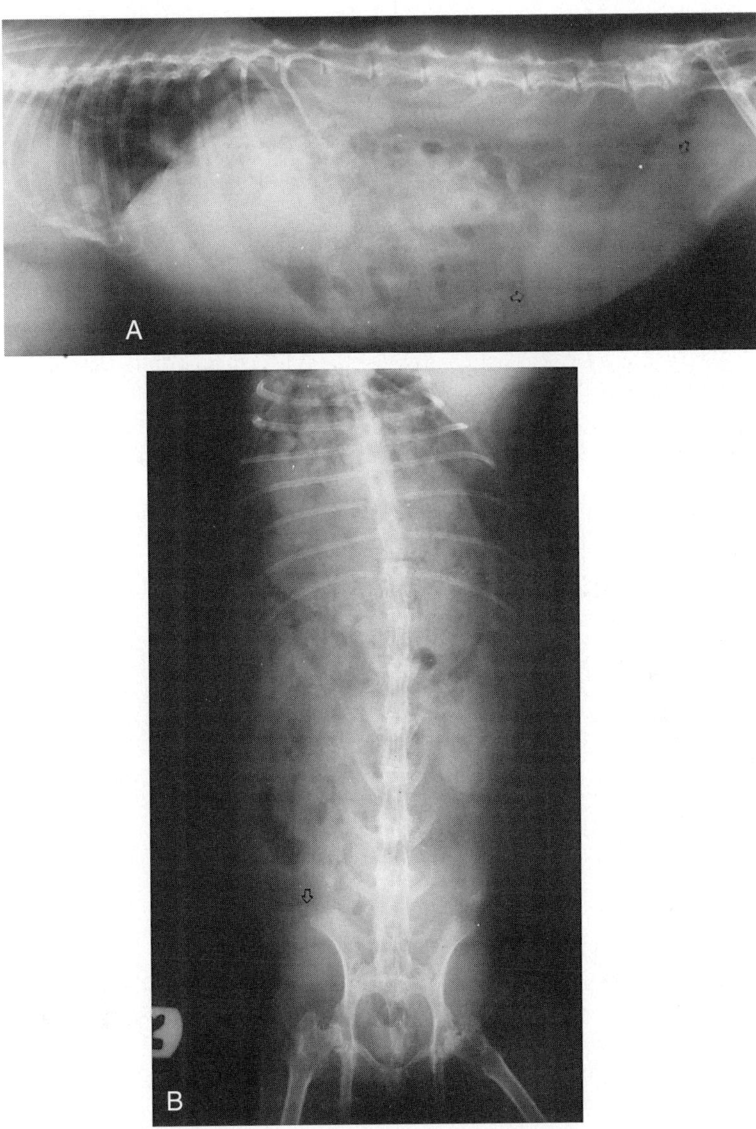

FIGURE 31–9
A and B.

SIGNALMENT Five-year-old intact female rabbit.

HISTORY Large axillary mass.

RADIOGRAPHIC FINDINGS A large soft tissue mass with mineralization is seen at the left thoracic body wall. A large, tubular soft tissue mass with mineralization is observed in the caudal abdomen *(arrows)*. Pulmonary nodules are located throughout the lung lobes.

FINAL DIAGNOSIS Uterine adenocarcinoma. Pulmonary and axillary metastasis.

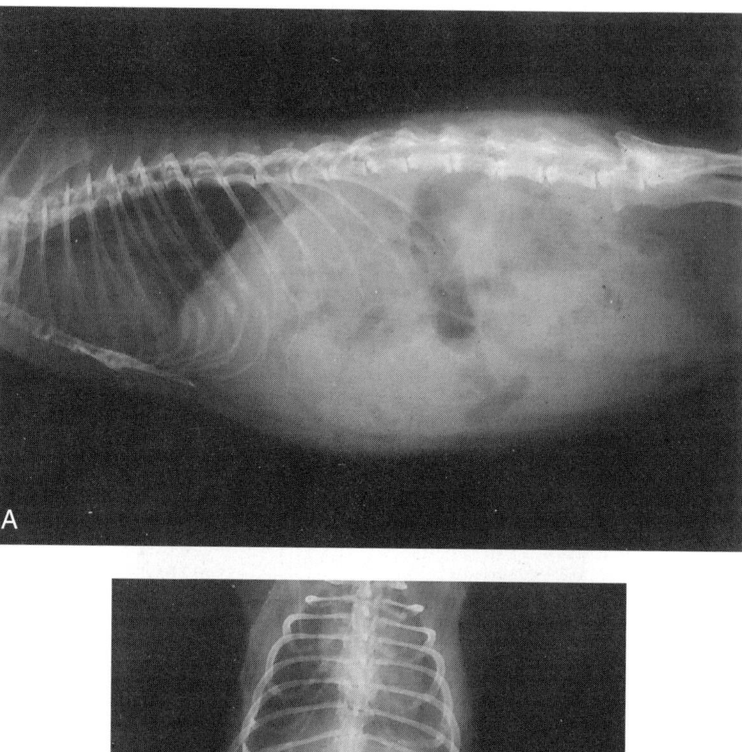

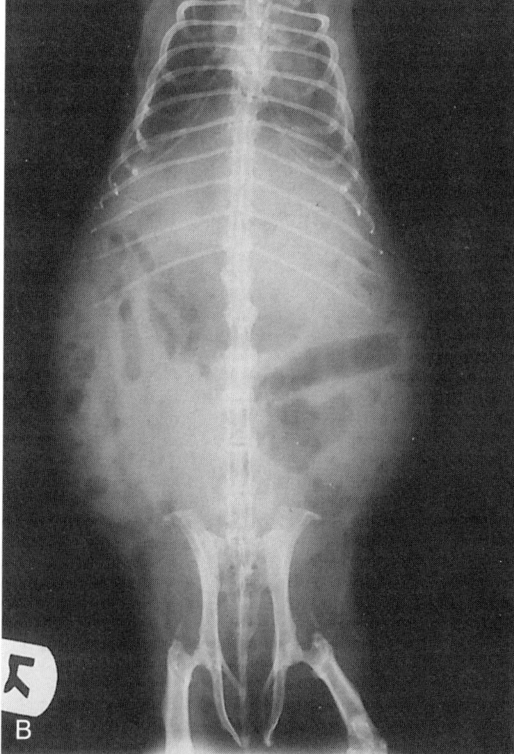

FIGURE 31–10
A and B, The normal guinea pig.

SIGNALMENT Two-year-old intact female guinea pig.

RADIOGRAPHIC FINDINGS The abdominal cavity is relatively large. The gastrointestinal tract of this herbivore contains varying amounts of ingesta and gas. Because of this, poor visualization of abdominal viscera is common. The cranial lung lobes are small and typically not well visualized; the caudal lung lobes are larger and well aerated.

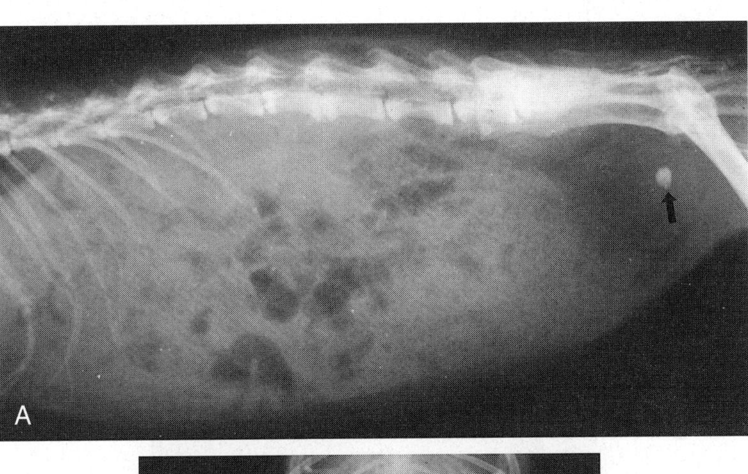

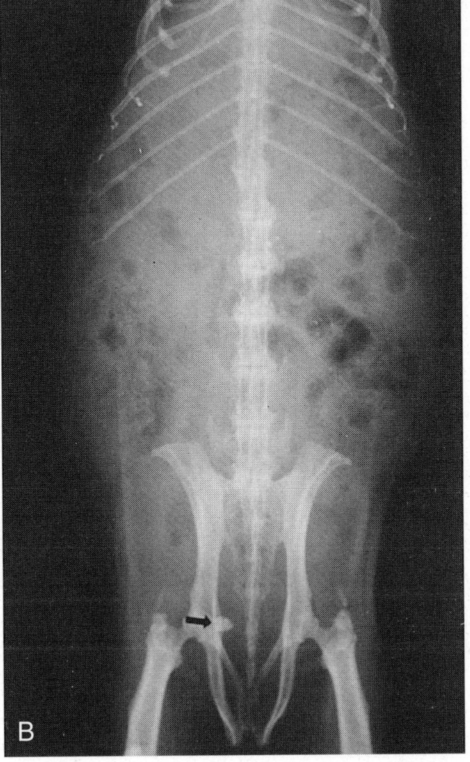

FIGURE 31–11
A and B.

SIGNALMENT Four and one half–year-old intact female guinea pig.

HISTORY Hematuria, inappetence.

RADIOGRAPHIC FINDINGS A round mineral-opaque object is present in the urinary bladder *(arrow).*

FINAL DIAGNOSIS Calcium oxalate cystic calculus.

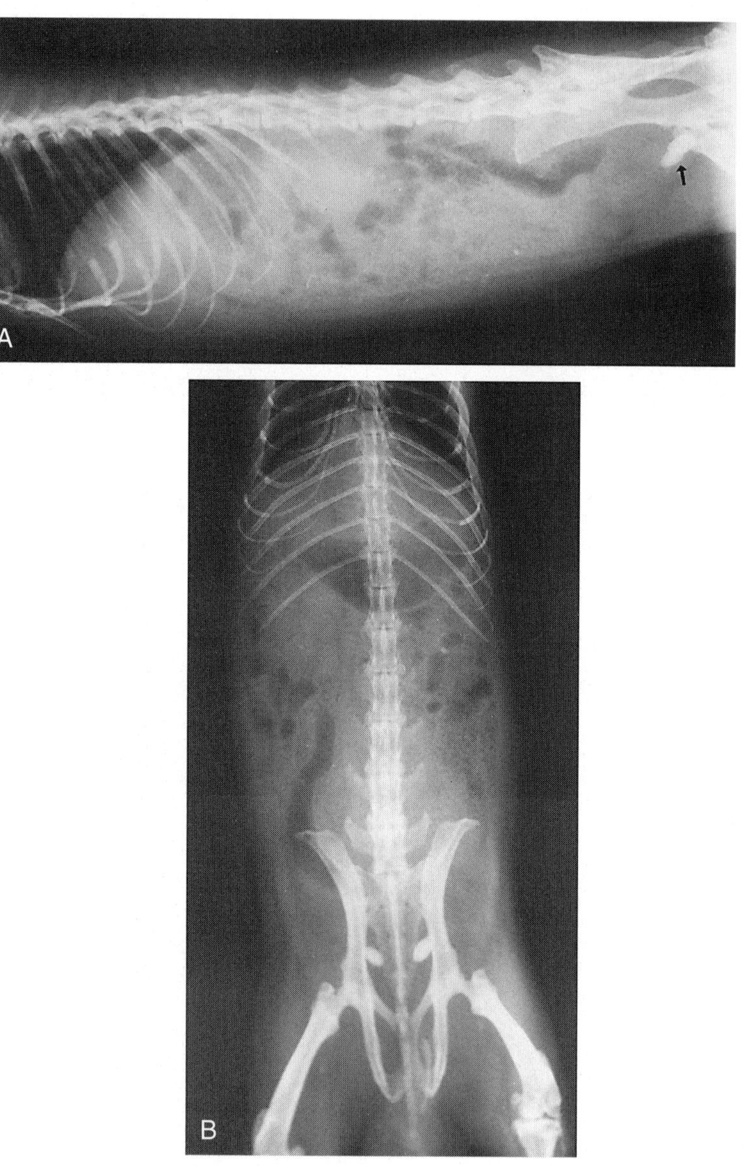

FIGURE 31–12
A and B.

SIGNALMENT Five-year-old intact male guinea pig.

HISTORY Weight loss, abdominal discomfort.

RADIOGRAPHIC FINDINGS Oval mineral opacities are present bilaterally in the caudal abdomen, adjacent to the urinary bladder *(arrow).*

FINAL DIAGNOSIS Bilateral calcium oxalate ureteral calculi.

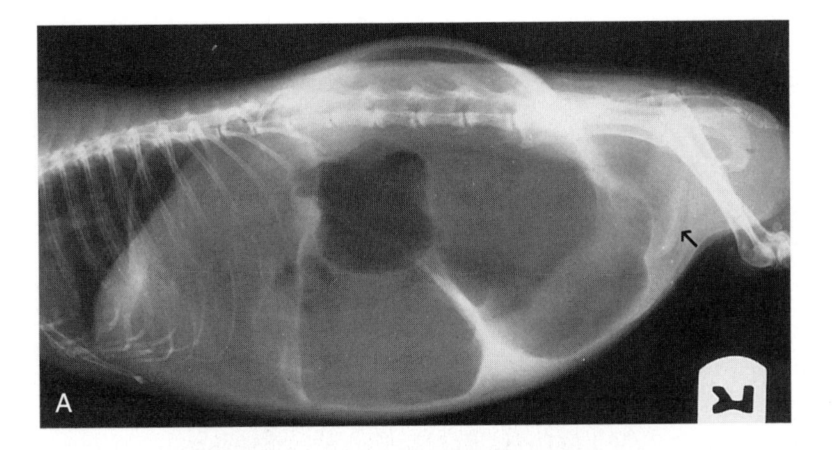

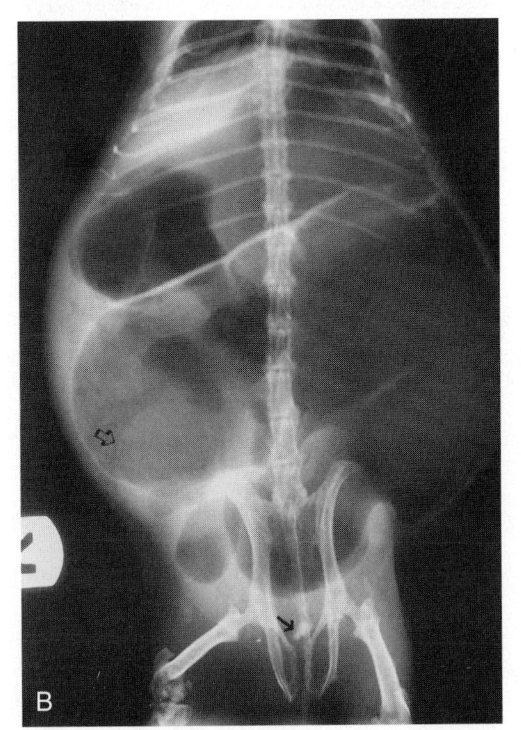

FIGURE 31–13
A and B.

SIGNALMENT Five-year-old intact female guinea pig.

HISTORY Distended abdomen, inappetence.

RADIOGRAPHIC FINDINGS The cecum and stomach are severely dilated. In the ventrodorsal view, an oval-shaped soft tissue mass can be seen in the right caudal abdomen *(open arrow)*. Mineral opacity is seen in the urinary bladder *(closed arrow)*.

FINAL DIAGNOSIS Right cystic ovary. Gastrointestinal dilation of unknown cause. Calciuria.

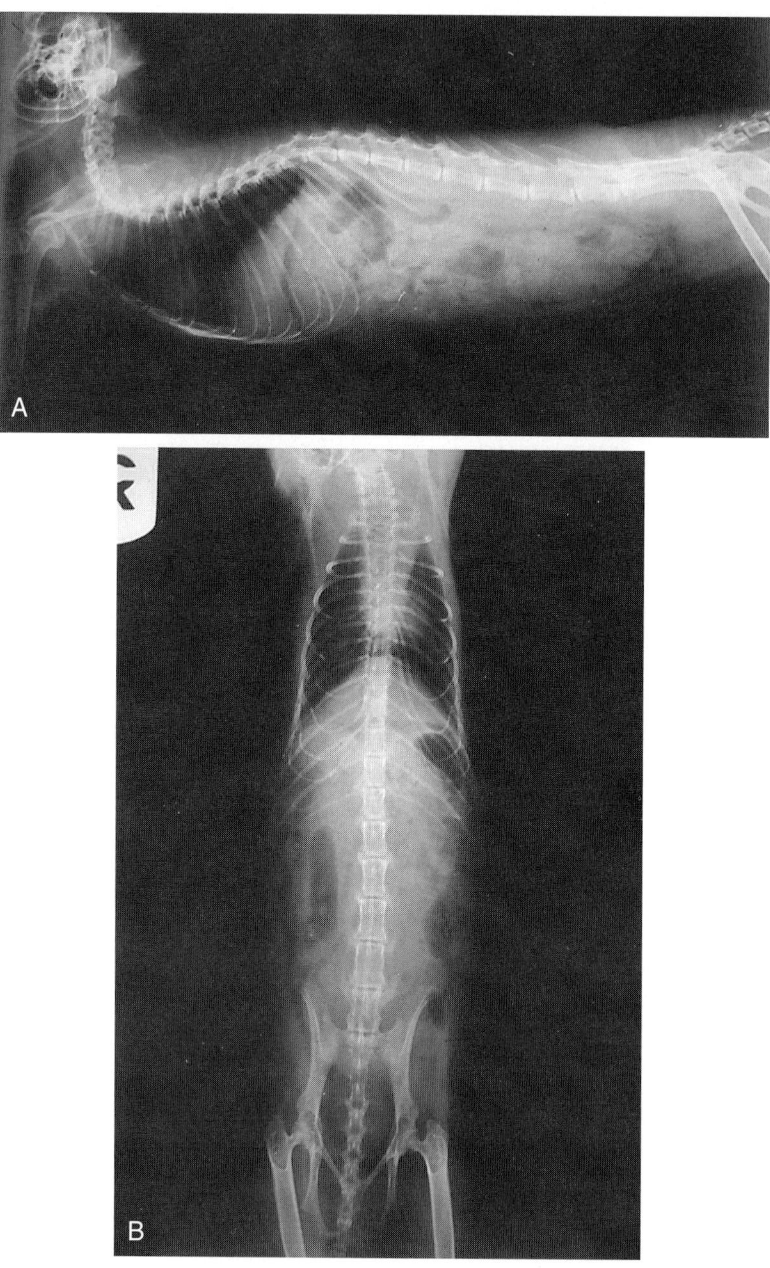

FIGURE 31–14
A and B. The normal chinchilla.

SIGNALMENT Three-year-old intact female chinchilla.

RADIOGRAPHIC FINDINGS As in other hindgut fermenters, variable amounts of gastrointestinal gas and ingesta are present in the abdomen, and serosal detail is poor. The small body size allows full survey radiography to be done. Note the large, thin-walled auditory bullae in the lateral view.

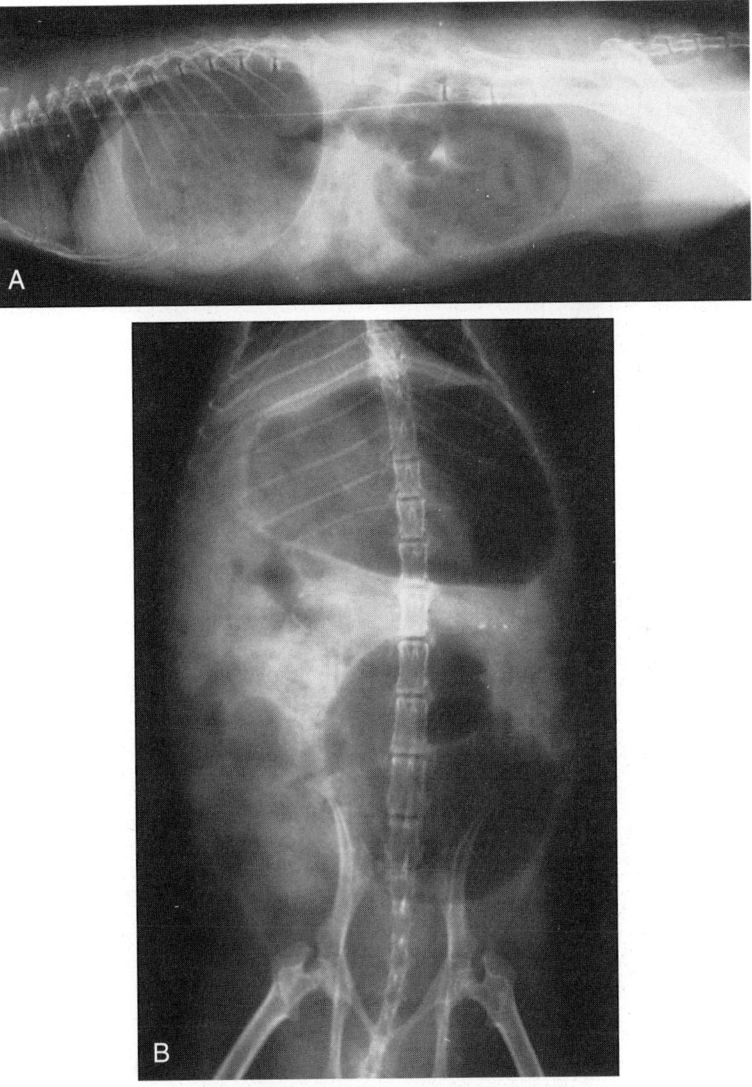

FIGURE 31–15
A and B.

SIGNALMENT Four-year-old intact male chinchilla.

HISTORY Anorexia, lethargy.

RADIOGRAPHIC FINDINGS The stomach and cecum are severely dilated. Ingesta is present in the stomach and in much of the small intestinal tract. The linear horizontal white line seen in the lateral view is an artifact.

FINAL DIAGNOSIS Segmental mechanical ileus of the cecum secondary to hairball impaction at the ileocecal junction.

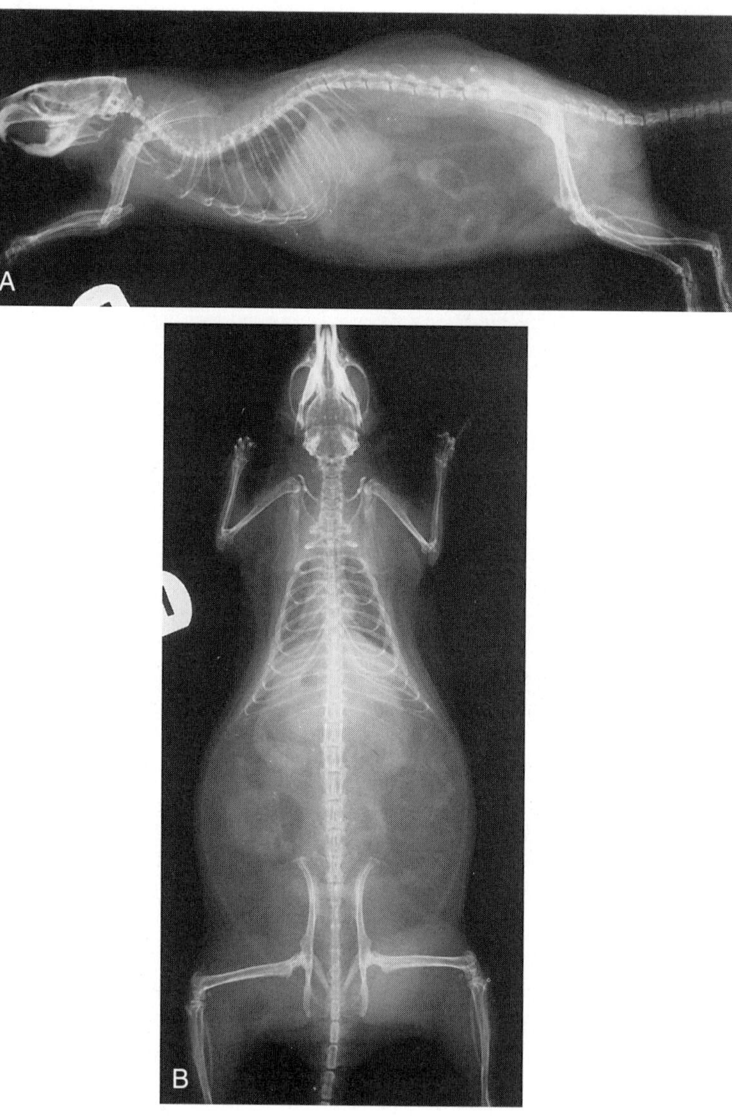

FIGURE 31–16
A and B, The normal rat.

SIGNALMENT One and one half–year-old intact female rat.

RADIOGRAPHIC FINDINGS A major disparity in body cavity size is observed. The abdomen is much larger than the thorax, making visualization of thoracic structures difficult. The heart and caudal lung lobes are seen and can be evaluated. Feces and a small amount of gas are in the large intestine. Isoflurane anesthesia was used for restraint.

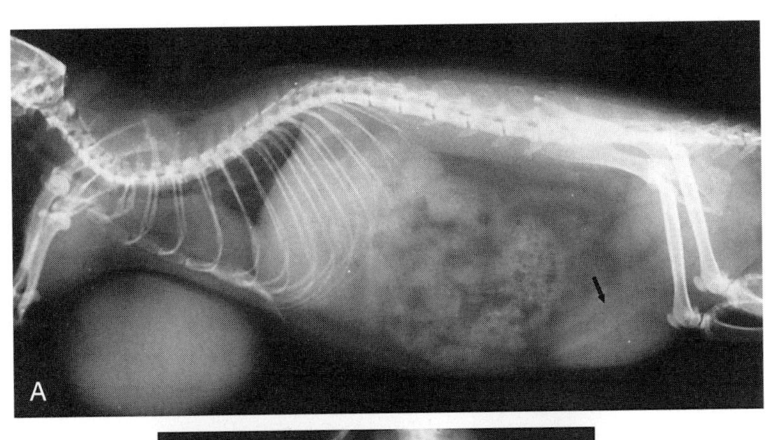

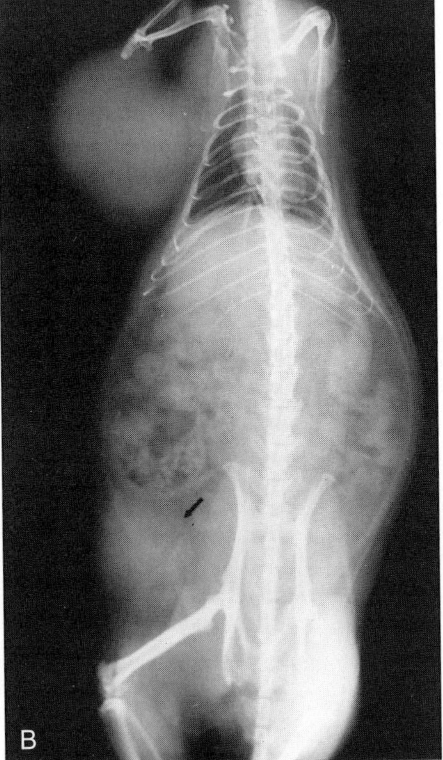

FIGURE 31–17
A and B.

SIGNALMENT One and one half–year-old female rat.

HISTORY Rapidly enlarging axillary mass.

RADIOGRAPHIC FINDINGS A large, round soft tissue mass is seen in the right axillary region. A second, similar, smaller mass is present in the right caudoventral body wall *(arrow)*.

FINAL DIAGNOSIS Mammary gland fibroadenomas.

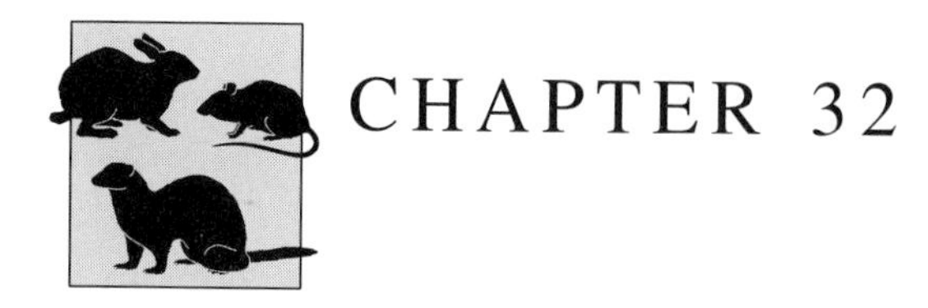

CHAPTER 32

Anesthesia, Analgesia, and Sedation for Small Mammals

Diane E. Mason, DVM

Many small mammals other than the traditional dog and cat are commonly kept as pets. Whether you commonly see these types of animals in your veterinary practice or see them only rarely, you must be prepared to provide chemical restraint or anesthesia in many instances. Fortunately, many of the same drugs and equipment used in traditional small animal practice are suitable for the treatment of ferrets, rabbits, and rodents, with some minor modifications. Therefore, the key to successfully providing chemical restraint and anesthesia for these small species is the recognition of any unique anatomic or physiologic differences among species, even though these differences often impact more on intraoperative management and monitoring than on choice of anesthetic regime. In this chapter, sedation and anesthesia are addressed individually for ferrets, rabbits, and rodents, and important species differences that influence anesthetic management are pointed out. Tables of recommended drug dosages are provided within the chapter.

Isoflurane is an integral component of most anesthetic regimens for exotic small mammals and should be available in all hospitals where these patients are seen commonly. It is a valuable anesthetic agent for use both as a "sedative" administered by face mask for short procedures and as a general anesthetic administered by face mask or endotracheal tube for surgical procedures. Induction and recovery are rapid with isoflurane, and the drug is a safer alternative to other inhalation agents, both for the patient and for hospital personnel.

GENERAL PRINCIPLES

The small size of many of these species has a large impact on the course of anesthesia for a number of reasons. Small body size is accompanied by a high specific metabolic rate (metabolic rate divided by body mass).[15] A high metabolic rate results in the rapid metabolism and elimination of drugs. As a rule, this indicates the need for increased drug dosages as well as results in a shorter duration of action than might be expected in the more typical small animal species, dogs and cats. A high metabolic rate also indicates high oxygen consumption. As a result, these species have a decreased ability to tolerate even short periods of hypoxemia or apnea. A high metabolic rate also implies the more rapid use of metabolic substrates and therefore a greater susceptibility to the development of hypoglycemia after fasting.

The small size presents difficulty in accessing the patient's airway (for intubation), veins (for IV drug or fluid administration), or muscle mass (for IM drug administration); thus, drug delivery, anesthetic monitoring, and intraoperative support likewise can be more difficult than in larger animals.

Small body size confers a large ratio of surface area to volume; thus, the likelihood of body heat loss is greater during anesthesia, when the normal thermoregulatory mechanisms are disturbed. Hypothermia results in a decrease in the requirement for anesthesia over time (predisposing to overdose); it also tends to prolong recovery. Following are recommendations for minimizing heat loss in ferrets, rabbits, and rodents:

1. Warm the immediate environment with the use of circulating water blankets or heat lamps.
2. Clip the minimum amount of hair from the body surface at and around the surgical site.
3. Use warmed surgical scrub solution for surgical site preparation.
4. Avoid alcohol rinses for surgical preparation, substituting warmed saline.
5. Cover the exposed surface of the animal with a drape (clear plastic "sticky" drapes allow visualization, facilitating respiratory monitoring).
6. Minimize the duration of surgery and anesthesia.

Following is a general summary of basic guidelines for ensuring a favorable outcome in any unfamiliar small exotic species:

1. Obtain an accurate measurement of body weight.
2. Know the appropriate preoperative fasting interval.
3. Know where to inject drugs, diluting when necessary for accurate dosing.
4. Minimize stress through proper handling or with premedication.
5. Provide oxygen even when using only injectable anesthesia.
6. Provide warming carefully and continue warming throughout recovery.
7. Be aware of the magnitude of blood and fluid losses and provide replacement fluids accordingly.

FERRETS

Drug Administration

Ferrets respond well to many routinely administered veterinary anesthetics. Often, the anesthetic routine you are accustomed to using with a cat works equally well with a ferret. Ferrets, like many carnivores, readily vomit. A preanesthetic fasting period of 8 hours is recommended for young animals; however, do not fast a ferret older than 3 years of age for longer than 4 hours unless you are certain that the ferret does not have an insulinoma (see Chapter 9) because of the possibility of precipitating a hypoglycemic episode. Ferrets also have a tendency to salivate in response to the administration of ketamine or tiletamine-zolazepam (Telazol, Fort Dodge Laboratories, Fort Dodge, IA); thus, premedication with an anticholinergic also is recommended. Perhaps the greatest challenge in anesthetizing ferrets lies in the variety of medical illnesses with which a ferret may present for treatment. Anemia, adrenal tumors, lymphoma, endocrine disorders, and cardiomyopathy are relatively common in the pet ferret population. All of these problems markedly affect anesthesia and influence the types of drugs that one might choose in the anesthetic regime. The value of a thorough physical examination and appropriate diagnostic testing cannot be overemphasized in the preanesthetic workup of a ferret. At the very least, a physical examination that includes thoracic auscultation and abdominal palpation and a laboratory workup that includes a complete blood count, blood glucose and electrolyte determination, and assess-

TABLE 32–1
SITES FOR PARENTERAL INJECTIONS IN VARIOUS SPECIES

	Injection Sites	
Species	***Intramuscular***	***Intravenous***
Ferret	Thigh muscles Epaxial muscles	Cephalic vein Lateral saphenous vein Jugular vein
Rabbit	Epaxial muscles	Cephalic vein Lateral saphenous vein
Rat	Thigh muscles	Lateral tail vein
Mouse	Thigh muscles	Lateral tail vein
Gerbil	Thigh muscles	Lateral tail vein
Hamster	Thigh muscles	Dorsal penile vein
Guinea pig	Thigh muscles	Cephalic vein Lateral saphenous vein Ear vein Dorsal penile vein
Chinchilla	Thigh muscles	Cephalic vein Lateral saphenous vein

ment of renal parameters should be conducted before anesthesia.

Ferrets have small but accessible cephalic, lateral saphenous, and jugular veins that can be used for administration of IV drugs and fluids (Table 32–1).[12] IM injections typically are given in the musculature of the thigh. Use caution when administering an IM injection in the lumbar region. The muscles at that site are shallow in depth, and the potential for puncture of a kidney exists if the ferret struggles during injection. A ferret can be intubated as easily as a small dog because its mouth opens widely for complete visualization of the larynx.

A comprehensive list of drugs and doses for sedation and injectable anesthesia can be found in Tables 32–2 and 32–3. Following is a discussion of some commonly used anesthetic agents.

Premedication, Sedation, and Chemical Restraint

ACEPROMAZINE. Try acepromazine, 0.1–0.3 mg/kg IM or SC, for mild tranquilization and before induction with inhalation anesthetics.

XYLAZINE. Xylazine produces very good sedation with analgesia for many routine procedures when it is given at 1 mg/kg IM or SC. Avoid using it in sick or debilitated ferrets, or in any ferret with suspected endocrine or cardiovascular disease.

KETAMINE. Ketamine alone can be used for chemical restraint at 10–20 mg/kg IM. Muscle relaxation is poor and salivation can be excessive, but this drug is relatively safe, even in ferrets with underlying disease.

ATROPINE OR GLYCOPYRROLATE. Give atropine (0.05 mg/kg IM or SC) or glycopyrrolate (0.01 mg/kg IM or SC) to decrease salivation in ferrets. In order to maintain a clear airway, it is useful to premedicate with an anticholinergic any ferret that is going to receive ketamine, tiletamine-zolazepam, or inhalation anesthesia by face mask.

COMBINATION. A useful premedicant combination is the following: midazolam, 0.3 mg/kg; ketamine, 5–10 mg/kg; and atropine, 0.02 mg/kg IM.*

Injectable Anesthesia

KETAMINE COMBINATIONS. A variety of tranquilizer/ketamine combinations are frequently used for minor surgical procedures in ferrets. Ketamine (10–30 mg/kg) can be combined with one of the following tranquilizers: xylazine (1–2 mg/kg), diaze-pam (1–2 mg/kg), or acepromazine (0.05–0.3 mg/kg). These combinations work best when administered IM.

TILETAMINE-ZOLAZEPAM. Tiletamine-zolazepam at 22 mg/kg IM is well suited for most minor surgical procedures. The injection volume is small, and it produces rapid immobilization. A disadvantage associated with its use is that the recovery time can be prolonged.

Inhalation Anesthesia

Inhalation anesthesia is the best approach for general anesthesia in ferrets. Ferrets' response to inhalation anesthesia is similar to that of dogs and cats and makes possible a predictable and stable anesthetic period. As with dogs and cats, premedication with one of the agents discussed earlier and followed by a chamber, face mask, or IV induction technique can precede intubation and maintenance on inhalation anesthesia. IV induction can be accomplished in a sedated ferret via an IV catheter placed in a cephalic or saphenous vein. Typically, ketamine (6–10 mg/kg) is used for IV induction.

*Whitehair K: Personal communication, 1996.

TABLE 32–2

TABLE OF DRUG DOSES FOR PREMEDICATION AND SEDATION OF SMALL EXOTIC ANIMALS

Drug	Ferret	Rabbit	Rat	Mouse	Gerbil	Hamster	Guinea Pig
Acepromazine	0.1–0.3	0.25–1.0	0.5–2.5	0.5–2.5	NR	0.5–5	0.5–1.5
Diazepam	2	1–5	3–5	3–5	3–5	3–5	1–5
Midazolam	1	1–2	1–2	1–2	1–2	1–2	1–2
Xylazine*	1	1–5	10–15	10–15	5–10	8–10	5–10
Atropine	0.05	0.8–1.0	0.05	0.05	0.05	0.05	0.05
Glycopyrrolate	0.01	0.01–0.02	0.01–0.02	0.01–0.02	0.01–0.02	0.01–0.02	0.01–0.02
Fentanyl-droperidol†	NR	0.13–0.22 mL/kg	0.13–0.33 mL/kg	2–5 mL/kg (1:10 dilution)	0.3–0.5 mL/kg	0.3–0.5 mL/kg	0.08–0.44 mL/kg‡

Values are milligrams per kilogram IM or SC, unless otherwise indicated.

Use lower end of dose range for debilitated, geriatric, or obese animals and for those that are relatively large for the species.

Abbreviation: NR = not recommended.

*If needed, the reversal agent is yohimbine (0.2 mg/kg IV).

†If necessary, use naloxone, 0.04 mg/kg IV or IM to reverse the opioid effects of fentanyl.

‡Fentanyl-droperidol can be associated with central nervous system stimulation in hamsters[2] and self-mutilation at injection site by guinea pigs.

TABLE 32-3
TABLE OF DRUG DOSES FOR INJECTABLE ANESTHESIA IN SMALL EXOTIC ANIMALS

Drug	Ferret	Rabbit	Rat	Mouse	Gerbil	Hamster	Guinea Pig	Chinchilla
Acepromazine	0.05–0.3	0.25–1.0	2.5–5.0	2.5–5.0	NR	2.5–5.0	0.5–1.0	0.5
with ketamine	10–30	25–40	50–150	50–150		50–150	20–50	20–40
Xylazine*	1–2	3–5	5	5–10	2–3	5–10	3–5	NA
with ketamine	10–30	20–40	90	50–200	50–70	50–150	20–40	
Diazepam	1–2	1–5	3–5	3–5	3–5	5	3–5	3–5
with ketamine	10–30	20–40	40–100	40–150	40–150	40–150	20–50	20–40
Tiletamine-zolazepam	22	5–25	50–80	50–80	50–80	50–80	20–40	20–40
Xylazine* with tiletamine-zolazepam	NA	NA	10 10–30	10 10–30	5 10–30	10 10–30	5 10–30	NA
Thiopental	NA	15–20 IV	20–40 IP	25–50 IP	NA	40 IP	20 IP	NA
Pentobarbital	NR	20–40 IV	30–50 IP	30–90 IP	60 IP	60–90 IP	15–30 IP	40 IP 30 IV
Propofol	NA	5–8 IV	10 IV	20–30 IV	NA	NA	NA	NA

Values are milligrams per kilogram IM, unless otherwise indicated.
Use lower end of dose range for debilitated, geriatric, or obese animals and for those that are relatively large for the species.
Abbreviations: NR = not recommended; NA = no dose available; IP = intraperitoneal; IV = intravenous.
*If needed, the reversal agent is yohimbine (0.2 mg/kg IV).

Intubate the ferret, using an endotracheal tube 2.5–3.5 mm in size. Apply 0.05 mL of 2% lidocaine to the glottis to prevent laryngospasm. The larynx can be visualized with the use of a laryngoscope, and despite the ferret's small size, intubation is not difficult. The inhalation agent of choice is isoflurane because it provides rapid induction and recovery. A nonrebreathing circuit is recommended for anesthetic delivery. In sick, depressed, or debilitated animals, it is often best to avoid injectable agents altogether; in these animals, use isoflurane as the sole agent for restraint or anesthesia.

Administer IV fluids throughout surgery for sick or older animals or during lengthy procedures. Administer 2.5–5% dextrose-containing fluids to ferrets with insulinoma or other cause of hypoglycemia.

RABBITS

Many rabbits weigh the same as or more than the normal domestic cat. However, comparatively, rabbits have a smaller thoracic cavity for this size, with a very large abdominal cavity. Thus, their respiratory reserve can be impaired when the gastrointestinal tract is full or by the effects of body positioning during anesthesia. Fast rabbits for 2–4 hours before anesthesia to reduce abdominal distention. A rabbit's skeleton is more fragile when compared with that of other species of similar size. A rabbit is therefore highly susceptible to injury from mishandling or struggling.

Drug Administration

Rabbits have developed the reputation of being difficult to anesthetize, probably owing to several factors. Rabbits are more easily stressed and are more difficult to intubate than dogs or cats. Rabbits are highly susceptible to the respiratory depressant effects of some drugs (most notably, barbiturates and narcotics), and the margin of safety of many drugs is narrow in rabbits. Many simple procedures in rabbits can be done with the use of injectable anesthetic agents, but more involved procedures require very high doses of the same drugs. When higher doses are used, the likelihood of respiratory depression is increased. Unfortunately, if rabbits become apneic, resuscitation is very difficult without an endotracheal tube. Anesthesia for more complicated procedures can be safely achieved with the use of injectable agents at lower doses. After good sedation has been attained and stress to the rabbit has been minimized, mask induction, endotracheal intubation, and maintenance of anesthesia with an inhalation agent follow. Alternatively, supplement injectable anesthesia with small doses of an inhalation agent delivered by face mask.

Rabbits have reasonably accessible injection sites, both for IM and IV injection of drugs. Administer drugs IM in the large thigh muscles, gluteal muscles, or lumbar muscles. IV access is possible through the cephalic veins and the lateral saphenous veins.[4] Avoid using the marginal ear veins for IV injections; use of these veins can result in irritation and can cause sloughing of part of the pinna. SC injection can be an effective technique for the administration of sedatives and tranquilizers and is less traumatic than IM administration for rabbits. In addition, intranasal administration of certain anesthetic agents has been demonstrated to be an effective and pain-free means of inducing chemical restraint in rabbits.[14]

A wide variety of drugs and techniques have been described for rabbits. A comprehensive list of drugs and doses can be found in Tables 32–2 and 32–3. The anesthetic protocols highlighted in the following section have proved useful and successful in many circumstances.

Premedication, Sedation, and Chemical Restraint

ACEPROMAZINE. For mild tranquilization, to decrease handling stress, and as a preanesthetic prior to inhalation anesthesia, acepromazine is a good choice. It works very well either given IM or SC, provided sufficient time is given for it to have an effect (15–30 minutes). The recommended dose range is 0.25–1.0 mg/kg IM or SC.

FENTANYL-DROPERIDOL INJECTION. Neuroleptanalgesia with fentanyl-droperidol injection (Innovar-Vet, Mallinckrodt Veterinary, Inc., Mundelein, IL) produces high-quality restraint in many species, including rabbits. Its analgesic action can be very helpful as an adjunct to the effects of inhalation agents, allowing a relatively lighter plane of anesthesia during the maintenance phase of a procedure. The recommended dose is 0.13–0.22 mL/kg IM or SC.

XYLAZINE. Alpha$_2$-agonists such as xylazine provide good sedation and analgesia in rabbits. Respiratory depression and bradycardia can be significant. This agent is recommended for use in healthy animals but not in rabbits that are significantly depressed or debilitated. The recommended dose range is 1–5 mg/kg IM or SC. In the event of an adverse reaction to xylazine, it is possible to reverse the effects of the alpha$_2$-agonist with the specific antagonist yohimbine (0.2 mg/kg IV).

ANTICHOLINERGICS. Approximately 30% of rabbits have the enzyme atropinesterase. This enzyme makes atropine ineffective unless it is given in very high doses.[10] Despite this fact, anticholinergics are often helpful as premedicants in rabbits for which intubation is planned to counteract the bradycardia produced by drugs such as opioids and xylazine or to counteract the salivation produced by drugs such as ketamine or tiletamine-zolazepam. To consistently provide an adequate effect in rabbits, administer 0.8–1.0 mg/kg of atropine by the IV (lower dose), IM, or SC (higher dose) routes. An alternative to atropine is the anticholinergic drug glycopyrrolate; administer glycopyrrolate at a dose of 0.01–0.02 mg/kg SC or IM.

COMBINATIONS. A useful premedicant combination is the following: midazolam, 0.3 mg/kg; ketamine, 5–10 mg/kg; and glycopyrrolate, 0.04 mg/kg IM. An alternative combination comprises acepromazine, 0.05 mg/kg; ketamine, 10 mg/kg; and glycopyrrolate, 0.04 mg/kg IM.*

Injectable Anesthesia

DIAZEPAM/KETAMINE. An injected diazepam/ketamine combination is rarely suitable as the sole anesthetic for major surgery, but it is good for sedation and light anesthesia or as a prelude to inhalation anesthesia. Use 1–5 mg/kg diazepam and 20–40 mg/kg ketamine IM. One disadvantage is the large volume of diazepam needed for IM injection at this dose. Alternatively, use diazepam (0.5 mg/kg) and ketamine (10–20 mg/kg) IV.

TILETAMINE-ZOLAZEPAM. This agent can be used across a continuum from light sedation to general anesthesia, depending on dose. The high end of the dose range, however, is associated with profound depression and slow recovery. Tiletamine-zolazepam at very high doses (32–64 mg/kg) has been shown to produce nephrotoxicity in rabbits.[5] Tiletamine-zolazepam is safe at lower doses. The recommended dose range for clinical use in rabbits is 5–25 mg/kg IM.

---

*Whitehair K: Personal communication, 1996.

XYLAZINE/KETAMINE. Xylazine/ketamine combination can be useful for some surgical procedures. Xylazine produces good analgesia and muscle relaxation, but a greater potential for complications exists as a result of xylazine-induced respiratory depression and hypotension. Dose xylazine at 3–5 mg/kg and ketamine at 20–40 mg/kg IM. Intranasal administration of this combination has been shown to be effective for short-term anesthesia.[14] The dose is modified to 3 mg/kg of xylazine and 10 mg/kg of ketamine for intranasal use.

PROPOFOL. Propofol is a substituted phenol anesthetic agent that is currently available as a 1% IV formulation (Diprivan, Zeneca Pharmaceuticals, Wilmington, DE) labeled for use in humans for induction or maintenance of anesthesia or sedation. It can be used in rabbits for induction of anesthesia or for maintenance of anesthesia for a short procedure, such as incisor extraction. The advantages of propofol are that it produces rapid and smooth induction, provides a short duration of anesthesia, and allows rapid recovery without excitement. However, it must be administered slowly because rapid administration can produce apnea. In New Zealand white rabbits (mean weight, 3.25 kg), slow IV administration of propofol produced rapid loss of consciousness and sufficient anesthesia for endotracheal intubation. The 95% effective dose (ED_{95}) in this study was 8.45 mg/kg.[1] No supplemental anesthesia was administered, and rabbits could be extubated from 1.5 to 4.5 minutes after induction with a return of righting reflex between 2 and 8.5 minutes after induction. Propofol gives better muscle relaxation with a shorter, smoother recovery than ketamine combinations for short procedures (e.g., dental procedures).

The following protocol has proven useful in clinical practice for short-term anesthesia in rabbits.* Administer an analgesic agent such as butorphanol approximately 30 minutes before induction, and, when the rabbit is relaxed, place an IV catheter. Administer propofol (5–8 mg/kg to effect) as a slow bolus over 5 minutes. When the rabbit is anesthetized, start an IV drip of isotonic fluids. Administer supplemental propofol as a slow IV bolus and as necessary during the procedure. The need for supplementation becomes less frequent with time. Diprivan is packaged without preservatives as a single-use parenteral product and must be handled with strict aseptic technique.

*Kaufman G: Personal communication, 1996.

Inhalation Anesthesia

Inhalation anesthesia is the preferred technique for many procedures in rabbits because the plane of anesthesia can be rapidly controlled, and this increases patient safety. During the course of the procedure, the animals receive an increased inspired oxygen concentration that improves patient oxygenation. Also, the animals often have a secured airway (if intubated), which decreases ventilatory compromise. Finally, recovery is usually quite rapid. Inhalation anesthesia is best delivered with the use of a nonrebreathing apparatus, such as a Bain circuit. Isoflurane is the agent of choice because it has a low solubility (blood:gas partition coefficient), which provides a more rapid onset (important for mask inductions) and recovery. In debilitated or depressed animals, use of isoflurane as the sole anesthetic agent is often the safest approach. If a significant operative procedure such as fracture repair or abdominal surgery is indicated, anesthesia with inhalants alone may be unsatisfactory because the deeper plane of inhalant anesthesia necessary for providing adequate analgesia and muscle relaxation begins to produce significant respiratory depression and hypotension. In this instance, the benefits of premedication with a sedative and analgesic drug are significant, allowing reduction of the concentration of inhalation agent necessary for maintaining a stable plane of anesthesia during surgery.

When using inhalation anesthesia for the anesthetic regimen in a rabbit, premedicate with one of the previously discussed agents, and then administer isoflurane by face mask until the rabbit relaxes sufficiently to allow intubation. Then, maintain the rabbit on inhalation anesthesia for the duration of the procedure. If intubation cannot be achieved without undue stress or trauma to the rabbit, induce anesthesia with one of the recommended injectable techniques and supplement this anesthesia with low doses of isoflurane given by face mask.

Endotracheal Intubation

Endotracheal intubation of a rabbit by the oral route requires some skill because the mouth does not open widely, the distal portion of the tongue is muscular, the larynx is deep within the oropharynx, and the prominent incisors obstruct the view of the larynx. In addition, rabbits have a tendency for laryngospasm.

Nasotracheal intubation is possible in rabbits, and like all technical skills, it becomes easier to perform with practice. Depending on the size of the rabbit, pass a 2.0-, 2.5-, or 3.0-mm outer diameter endotracheal tube into the larynx, starting at the nostril and advancing the tube through the ventral nasal meatus. This can often be accomplished in a sedated animal before the induction of general anesthesia, providing control of the airway from the outset. Unfortunately, the small-sized endotracheal tubes used with this technique may be predisposed to obstruction with respiratory tract secretions. In addition, trauma to the nasal cavity can result in nosebleeds; however, these are usually minor in severity.

Orotracheal intubation is possible in rabbits and is less difficult to perform in large rabbits than in small ones. Before any attempt at oral intubation, induce anesthesia either with injectable agents (preferred in most rabbits because of the longer duration of relaxation that they provide) or with inhalation agents given by face mask. Accomplish orotracheal intubation with the aid of a laryngoscope or an otoscope for direct visualization of the larynx.[8, 11, 16] It may be helpful to apply a small amount of local anesthetic to the larynx in order to diminish the likelihood of laryngospasm.[16] A small volume (0.05–0.1 mL) of 2% lidocaine is useful for this purpose. Benzocaine-containing topical anesthetic sprays are not recommended because of rabbits' susceptibility to toxic methemoglobinemia.[7] With the rabbit's head and neck extended, visually identify the glottis; then, advance an endotracheal tube of appropriate size (typically, 2.5- to 3.5-mm outer diameter) into the larynx. Using a small-diameter stylet to enter the larynx and then passing the endotracheal tube over the stylet is an effective means of achieving intubation because the view of the larynx is often obstructed once the larger diameter endotracheal tube has been advanced into the oral cavity. A small urinary catheter (5 or 6 French) makes a good stylet for this purpose.[8, 16]

A suggested technique for "blind" intubation of a rabbit involves attachment of an endotracheal tube to the tubing of a standard stethoscope, which has a small elliptic hole (4 mm × 2 mm) just proximal to the insertion point of the endotracheal tube. When the endotracheal tube has been advanced into the rabbit's mouth, listen through the stethoscope to the rabbit's inspiratory and expiratory sounds. In doing this, it is possible to place the tube precisely over the glottis. Then, on hearing the early sounds of inspiration, advance the tube into the open glottis.[6]

A variation of the blind technique can be perfected with some practice. After inducing anesthesia in the rabbit with an injectable agent (or agents) or with gas anesthesia administered by face mask, position the rabbit in sternal recumbency with its head up. While holding the head gently without opening the mouth, insert the endotracheal tube through the diastema and to the level of the glottis and rest it on the glottis. Watch the rabbit's respirations. When the rabbit begins to inspire, quickly advance the tube into the trachea. Successful placement of the endotracheal tube should elicit a cough.

An alternative method for orotracheal intubation is the passing of a catheter into the trachea percutaneously in the neck. Pass this catheter retrograde until it exits the mouth via the larynx. Then, pass an endotracheal tube through the larynx by slipping the tube over the catheter.[9] This technique may be difficult to perform in rabbits with a heavy dewlap and is the most invasive of the techniques described. Although it can be difficult to perform quickly, it can be a useful intubation technique for rabbits (and other species) in emergency situations.

RODENTS

Many rodents used as laboratory animal species, and presumably those kept as pets, can harbor respiratory pathogens that, upon stress to the animal, produce significant respiratory disease.[2, 10] Rodents may have significant pulmonary lesions, such as consolidation from pneumonia, with little overt sign of disease. When they are anesthetized, this pulmonary disease may impair ventilatory gas exchange and diminish the animals' tolerance of the respiratory depressant effects of drugs. The inability to easily intubate many of the small rodent species increases their risk of anesthesia as a result.

Pet rodents are sensitive to extremes of cold or heat because of their very small size. A rodent's primary mechanism for coping with temperature changes is behavioral—namely, they retreat to their burrows. This is obviously not an option for the sedated or anesthetized rat, mouse, or gerbil removed from its normal habitat. Thus, pay close attention to the maintenance of a thermoneutral environment during the anesthetic and postoperative period.

Small rodents are also sensitive to water or fluid loss as a result of their small blood volume, high metabolic rate, and large ratio of surface area to body weight. A high level of metabolic oxygen consumption, the inability to tolerate temperature changes, and susceptibility to fluid loss combine to make rodents potentially poor candidates for anesthesia and surgery unless special care is taken.

Rats, mice, and gerbils do not vomit, and because of their small size and high metabolic rate, preanesthetic fasting is not recommended. Fast guinea pigs and chinchillas 2–4 hours before anesthesia to reduce the volume of gastric contents. Do not withhold water. Guinea pigs have a very large cecum and colon; 65% of the gastrointestinal contents are present in these voluminous organs.[10]

Drug Administration

Injectable techniques are used in rodents, but inhalation techniques are rather easy to perform and allow better control of the depth of anesthesia. It is often difficult to achieve a surgical plane of anesthesia with the use of injectable agents alone. Injectable anesthetics can provide anything from sedation to anesthesia for minor surgical procedures, depending on the drugs and the doses used.

Administration of injectable drugs to small rodents is a little more problematic than drug administration in rabbits or ferrets (see Chapters 23 and 26). The available muscle mass is small in size, allowing only small volume injections. Rodents, especially guinea pigs, are susceptible to tissue necrosis when given certain drugs by the IM route. Presumably, the drugs are irritating to the tissues, and guinea pigs exacerbate the tissue damage by self-mutilation. Ketamine and fentanyl-droperidol (0.88 mL/kg IM) are known to produce this effect.[18] Using lower doses and dilutions of these drugs may prevent this complication.

To avoid muscle necrosis, administer injectable drugs either SC or intraperitoneally (IP). Many sedative drugs or anesthetic drug combinations can be administered SC in the suprascapular region of rodents. The uptake and onset of action of drugs given in this manner may be slower than when they are given IV or IM, so additional time is needed for achieving the desired effect. However, it is an easy technique that is less painful and stressful to the animal than an IM injection.

IP injection of anesthetic combinations has been used for years in laboratory animal species. The potential for complications exists, especially if improper technique is used. To perform the technique properly, temporarily tilt the restrained rodent in a head-down position, thus encouraging the abdominal viscera to slide forward. Using a small needle (25-gauge or smaller), direct the injection into the caudal left (rat) or the caudal right (gerbil, hamster, and mouse) quadrant of the abdomen, staying caudal and lateral to the umbilicus and always aspirating before injection to make sure that a visceral organ has not been punctured. Despite the use of proper technique, it has been reported that injection into viscera occurs in about 20% of IP injections in guinea pigs, so use the technique with caution.[10]

IV injection sites exist in many small rodents, but the vessels are small and not easily accessed in the nonsedated individual. Rats, mice, and gerbils have lateral tail (coccygeal) veins. Warm the tail by dipping it into warmed water as an aid to visualization and venipuncture. Guinea pigs have ear (auricular) veins, and male guinea pigs and hamsters have a dorsal penile vein; however, these vessels are small and can be accessed only after sedation or anesthesia. It is also possible to use the cephalic vein or medial and lateral saphenous veins in guinea pigs and chinchillas, after the hair over the site has been clipped for vessel localization.

Inhalation anesthesia can be used as the sole agent for a procedure or can be administered after sedation with an injectable drug, as in rabbits. Chamber inductions or open drop techniques are easily performed but contribute to pollution of the workplace with waste anesthetic gas. The use of a cone or face mask for administering inhalation agents from an anesthesia machine allows rapid change in depth of anesthesia. Nonrebreathing systems, such as the Bain circuit, should be used for anesthetic delivery.

Intubation is sometimes possible but difficult in rodents owing to their small size. Use 16- to 20-gauge IV catheters as endotracheal tubes in rats, placing them into the trachea on visualization of the glottis with the assistance of a small laryngoscope blade or otoscope. Because of the small size of these tubes, be constantly vigilant for signs of obstruction from respiratory secretions. The development of a squeaking or wheezing sound during inspiration often indicates that mucus is accumulating in the tube. The development of increased muscular effort with each breath may also indicate impending obstruction and warrants changing or removing the tube.

Rodents smaller than rats rarely benefit from attempts at intubation. Intubation is difficult, the pharyngeal region is easily traumatized, and the very small tubes are likely to become obstructed. In these species, it is sensible to deliver inhalation agents and oxygen by face mask. Face masks should be tight-fitting so that increased dead space can be avoided, and they often can be constructed from plastic syringe cases, with a small diaphragm made from a latex surgical glove.[2]

Although hystricomorph rodents such as guinea pigs and chinchillas have a greater body size than do rats, they also are poor candidates for intubation because of a peculiarity in their pharyngeal anatomy. It is not possible to visualize the glottis of hystricomorphs because their soft palate is continuous with the base of the tongue and only offers a small opening (the palatal ostium) through which an endotracheal tube could be passed for blind attempts at intubation.[17] In these species, administration of oxygen and inhalation anesthesia by face mask is recommended.

As mentioned earlier, fast all guinea pigs before anesthesia, whether injectable or inhalation anesthesia is used. Use atropine or glycopyrrolate in guinea pigs to prevent excessive salivation.

Little information is available regarding sedation and anesthesia in chinchillas. Isoflurane by face mask is the anesthetic of choice in most instances. However, injectable agents can also be given at the low end of doses for guinea pigs.

Premedication, Sedation, and Chemical Restraint

ACEPROMAZINE. Acepromazine is effective as a mild tranquilizer when given SC or IM to most of the rodent species. Approximately 20% of all pet and laboratory gerbils may suffer from spontaneous epileptiform seizures.[10] This seizure activity may be triggered by unfamiliar surroundings or by stress. Because of this potential for epilepsy, acepromazine is not recommended for use in gerbils. For the other rodent species, a dose range of 0.5–2.5 mg/kg is effective; the lower dose is appropriate for IM administration, and the higher dose for SC administration. Hamsters may require doses as great as 5 mg/kg SC for adequate tranquilization. The larger rodents, namely guinea pigs and chinchillas, require lower doses (0.5–1.5 mg/kg).

DIAZEPAM. Diazepam produces mild sedation in rodent species and can be used safely even in gerbils. A dose of 3–5 mg/kg IM is generally recommended. As in rabbits, a disadvantage may be the volume of drug injected at a single IM site. At the 5-mg/kg dose, 0.1 mL per 100 g of body weight would be injected IM (diazepam is formulated in 5-mg/mL concentration). Diazepam is not highly water soluble and is solubilized in a propylene glycol base that may be irritating to the muscle when given IM. An alternative is the use of midazolam (Versed, Roche Laboratories, Nutley, NJ), a benzodiazepine similar to diazepam but more water soluble and better suited for IM injection. The dose of midazolam should be slightly lower than that for diazepam.

FENTANYL-DROPERIDOL. Fentanyl-droperidol is an excellent sedative when given at lower doses. Because of its analgesic effect, increased doses can be suitable for minor surgery. Increased doses may predispose animals to significant narcotic-induced respiratory depression, so ventilation should be monitored closely until the animals are fully recovered. Fortunately, the effects of opioids can be rapidly antagonized by naloxone (0.04 mg/kg IV or IM). Fentanyl-droperidol is recommended primarily for rats and mice. Doses are reported for guinea pigs, but this drug should be used with caution in these animals: as mentioned earlier, IM administration of this drug may predispose guinea pigs to self-mutilation. The dose range for rats is 0.13–0.33 mL/kg IM for sedation and for anesthesia for minor procedures. The use of fentanyl-droperidol in mice requires a 1:10 dilution of the drug in physiologic saline solution. The diluted drug solution is given at 0.002–0.005 mL per gram of body weight for IM sedation in mice. Guinea pigs require a dose of fentanyl-droperidol from 0.08–0.44 mL/kg IM.

ANTICHOLINERGICS. Anticholinergics are useful as anesthetic premedication in rodents for two reasons. First, several rodent species (rats and guinea pigs, in particular) are prone to excessive salivation following administration of sialogogic drugs, such as ketamine, or from inhalation of pungent or irritating gas anesthetics. For animals in which intubation is not possible, drying up secretions aids in keeping a clear airway for the duration of the procedure. Second, a number of the injectable drugs recommended for use in these species (alpha$_2$-agonists and opioids) enhance vagal tone and can produce marked decreases in heart rate if they are unopposed by anticholinergic drug administration. Either atropine (0.05 mg/kg SC) or glycopyrrolate (0.01–0.02 mg/kg SC) is effective as an anticholinergic in any of these species.

COMBINATIONS. A useful premedicant combination for guinea pigs and chinchillas is the following: midazolam, 0.3 mg/kg; ketamine, 5 mg/kg (5–10 mg/kg for guinea pigs); and atropine, 0.04 mg/kg IM. An alternative combination comprises acepromazine, 0.05 mg/kg (0.1 mg/kg for guinea pigs); ketamine, 10 mg/kg; and atropine, 0.04 mg/kg IM.*

Injectable Anesthesia

XYLAZINE/KETAMINE. This familiar combination is widely used across species, but in small rodents it tends to have a short duration of action (30 minutes), the individual variability in response can be significant, and its use frequently must be supplemented with inhalation anesthesia for surgery. Rats respond well to xylazine at 5 mg/kg and ketamine at 90 mg/kg, given either IM or IP. Mice and hamsters need a similar xylazine dose (5–10 mg/kg), but the recommendation for ketamine is 50–200 mg/kg IM or IP for mice and 50–150 mg/kg IM for hamsters, depending on the level of anesthesia desired. In gerbils, reduce the xylazine dose to 2–3 mg/kg and the ketamine dose to 50–70 mg/kg IM or IP. Guinea pigs are the most sensitive to the effects of this combination; do not exceed 5 mg/kg xylazine and 20–40 mg/kg ketamine given IM.

ACEPROMAZINE/KETAMINE. Acepromazine can be used with ketamine in most rodent species and produces adequate restraint for some minor surgical procedures. Acepromazine does not add the analgesic effect that xylazine does in combination with ketamine, but it is much less of a respiratory depressant. IM or IP injection of acepromazine at 2.5–5 mg/kg, combined with 50–150 mg/kg ketamine IM or IP, is suitable for rats, mice, and hamsters. Acepromazine at 0.5 mg/kg IM combined with 20–50 mg/kg ketamine IM is suited for guinea pigs and chinchillas. As a general rule, the smaller the species, the greater the dose needed for adequate effect. This combination is not recommended for gerbils.

TILETAMINE-ZOLAZEPAM. This combination of the dissociative agent tiletamine and the benzodiazepine zolazepam can be used in rodents for minor surgical procedures. When used alone, doses in the range of 50–80 mg/kg IM or IP are needed for adequate restraint of small rodents; 20–40 mg/kg IM is needed in guinea pigs and chinchillas. Recoveries can be prolonged. If acepromazine or xylazine (see premedication doses presented earlier in this chapter) is used in combination with a lower dose of tiletamine-zolazepam (10–30 mg/kg), a better effect can be achieved, and a speedier recovery results.

*Kaufman G: Personal communication, 1996.

Inhalation Anesthesia

Because it is difficult to achieve surgical anesthesia with injectable agents alone, any major surgical procedure suggests the need for inhalation anesthesia. Induce general anesthesia by using inhalation anesthesia alone or a balanced technique that takes advantage of the sedative and analgesic effects of an injectable combination and supplements it with inhalation agents. Isoflurane is the agent of choice for delivery with a nonrebreathing circuit by tight-fitting face mask. In addition, because small rodents are rarely intubated and waste anesthetic gas exposure to personnel is a concern, isoflurane may be preferable to agents like methoxyflurane and halothane, which present greater health risks to people with chronic exposure.

MONITORING ANESTHESIA

Monitoring anesthesia generally becomes more difficult as the size of the animal being anesthetized decreases; thus, monitoring anesthesia in many of these species is a significant challenge. This challenge is compounded if the species you are anesthetizing is one with which you are unfamiliar. Anesthetic monitoring depends primarily on observation, and observation is limited if an animal does not have a reasonable site at which pulse strength can be palpated, or if a surgical drape covers the animal entirely so that chest wall motion can no longer be used for assessing respiratory function. Following the status of these very small patients under anesthesia often requires creativity, and ancillary monitoring equipment can often prove to be very helpful. Of fundamental importance in monitoring any animal under anesthesia is an assessment of cardiovascular and respiratory function, as well as depth of anesthesia. No one parameter holds the key to how the animal is responding to its anesthetic drugs; all systems must be evaluated.

Observational techniques are generally used for assessing depth of anesthesia. The depth of anesthesia required for an animal is determined by the type of procedure being performed. An animal that needs chemical restraint for diagnostic radiography is very different from an animal that is about to undergo an abdominal exploratory surgery. Even though both animals may be receiving isoflurane anesthesia by face mask, one animal simply needs to remain still, whereas the other has to have adequate anesthesia, analgesia, and muscle relaxation if it is to tolerate an incision and manipulation of viscera. In the first animal, adequate depth is achieved shortly after the loss of a righting reflex; in the second animal, the pedal withdrawal reflex should be absent before you begin surgery.

Observational techniques that help indicate depth of anesthesia include the level of muscle relaxation, reflex activities, and physiologic responses to surgical stimulation. A good assessment of muscle relaxation can be made by monitoring jaw tone in certain small animal species such as dogs, cats, and ferrets. This is much more difficult to evaluate in rodents and rabbits. Monitoring jaw tone is precluded in any animal that is maintained on inhalation anesthesia by face mask.

Purposeful movement is an indication of light anesthetic depth, and often occurs in response to a painful stimulus. An example of purposeful movement is the righting reflex, in which the animal tries to return to a prone position when it is placed in dorsal recumbency. The righting reflex is one of the earliest reflexes lost as anesthesia proceeds. Purposeful movement such as swallowing (which is often stimulated by the presence of saliva or an endotracheal tube) and head shaking (which is sometimes seen in rabbits and guinea pigs) are typical indications of a light plane of anesthesia. The pedal withdrawal reflex is commonly used in determining level of surgical anesthesia in small exotic species. Extend the foot and pinch the toe manually or gently with a hemostat. If the limb is withdrawn in response to the toe pinch, then the animal needs more anesthesia before a painful procedure can begin. The ears of rabbits and guinea pigs can be pinched: look for head shaking in response to the painful stimulus. A tail pinch reflex can sometimes be elicited in tailed rodents that are in a light plane of anesthesia. On pinching of the tail in a manner similar to that used for the pedal withdrawal, the tail flicks if the rodent is insufficiently anesthetized.

Ocular reflexes also can indicate anesthetic depth. The palpebral response is the blinking that occurs when the edge of the eyelid is lightly touched. Interspecies variation in this response exists with anesthesia. Most animals lose the palpebral response early in surgical anesthesia; however, rabbits may maintain a palpebral response even at deeper planes of anesthesia. The intensity of the palpebral response is also influenced by the particular anesthetic agent used. Palpebral response is lost early with most inhalation agents; however, it is well maintained with the use of ketamine. Various physiologic responses to stimuli are also used for assessing depth of anesthesia. Changes (usually an increase) in heart rate, blood pressure, and respiratory rate can be seen in response to surgical stimulation when no purposeful movement has been observed.

Monitoring the cardiovascular system of small species is often difficult because of limited access to a palpable pulse. In addition, heart rates are usually quite high in many of these species, and this makes them difficult to measure. For these reasons, ancillary monitoring devices can be extremely helpful for evaluating cardiovascular status in animals under anesthesia. An electrocardiograph (ECG) monitor works quite well even on very small animals. Although the standard "alligator clip" ECG leads that are used in dogs and cats can be oversized for rodents, small-gauge wire sutures can be easily placed in the skin of the animal. Attaching the ECG leads directly to the wire sutures produces an acceptable ECG trace, and significant increases or decreases in heart rate are usually evident on observation of the R–R interval on the monitoring screen. Remember that an ECG monitor indicates the status of cardiac electrical activity only; therefore, a normal ECG trace does not always mean that cardiac output is adequate.

Another useful monitor for assessing cardiovascular function is the Doppler ultrasound blood pressure monitor (Parks Medical Electronics, Aloha, OR). Doppler monitors can be used in virtually all species. As a blood pressure monitor, the Doppler monitor's accuracy is impaired by small patient size, extremes of heart rate (less than 40 or greater than 200 beats per minute), significant hypotension, and hypothermia (due to peripheral vasoconstriction). All of these factors apply to the various small exotic species, making accurate blood pressure measurement virtually impossible. However, a major advantage of the Doppler monitor is that in addition to its use as a blood pressure monitor it transmits the pulse sound through a speaker device. This audible signal can be used to measure heart rate and indicates whether functional cardiac activity is adequate to generate a peripheral pulse. The Doppler probe can be placed over any site where a peripheral pulse can be palpated. The auricular artery in rabbits works quite well, as does the femoral artery in ferrets. In the smallest species, in which it is difficult to palpate a peripheral pulse, the Doppler probe can be placed on the chest wall overlying the cardiac apex as if it were a stethoscope. In addition, changes in the intensity of the audible signal, although subjective, tend to correlate with changes in cardiac output. If the audible Doppler signal becomes diminished, quickly evaluate anesthetic depth to make sure that the animal is not overly anesthetized.

Because of the sensitivity of these small species to even brief periods of hypoxemia or apnea and owing to the tendency for small airways to become obstructed with secretions, monitoring the respiratory system is extremely important during sedation and anesthesia. Monitor chest wall motion, movement of the rebreathing bag, or condensation and clearing in the mask or endotracheal tube lumen to evaluate respiratory rate. The work of breathing, a subjective assessment of the muscular effort required to move air, can be a helpful indicator of impending airway obstruction, significant hypoxemia, or hypercarbia. Evaluate respiratory sounds either by listening closely at the head of the animal or with thoracic auscultation; if squeaking, wheezing, or silence develops during respiratory movements, airway obstruction is imminent.

A pulse oximeter is an instrument that makes use of a light source and photodetector to measure the light absorbance of tissues and thus indicates the level at which hemoglobin in the arterial blood is saturated with oxygen (SaO_2). Changes in hemoglobin saturation can be continuously monitored with a pulse oximeter. When the SaO_2 value falls below 90%, the animal is becoming hypoxemic; take steps to improve oxygenation, such as administering 100% oxygen and providing endotracheal intubation and assistance with ventilation. In addition to reporting the SaO_2, the pulse oximeter often gives a value for heart rate. If the reported heart rate differs significantly from the actual heart rate obtained on palpation of a pulse or on auscultation, then question the accuracy of the reported SaO_2. Several conditions produce erroneously low oximeter values. The pulse oximeter is highly dependent on good peripheral perfusion; thus, hypotension and hypothermia impair its accuracy. Motion artifacts (e.g., patient movement or shivering) and bright external light sources (e.g., fluorescent lights, surgery lights, heat lamps) interfere with the probe's ability to detect a signal. Pulse oximeter probes work best when they are placed on nonpigmented, hairless tissues such as the tongue, ears, feet, or tail. A variety of probes have been designed for veterinary species, including a probe that can be inserted rectally like a thermometer, which may be useful in very small animals (Sensor Devices Inc., Waukesha, WI).

TABLE 32–4

TABLE OF ANALGESIC DRUG DOSAGES FOR SMALL EXOTIC ANIMALS

Drug	Ferret	Rabbit	Rat	Mouse	Gerbil	Hamster	Guinea Pig*
Butorphanol	0.1–0.5 q4h	0.1–0.5 q4h	2 q2–4h	1–5 q2–4h	1–5 q2–4h	1–5 q2–4h	2 q2–4h
Buprenorphine	0.01–0.03 q8–12h	0.01–0.05 q8–12h	0.05–0.1 q8–12h	0.05–0.1 q8–12h	0.05–0.1 q8–12h	0.05–0.1 q8–12h	0.05 q8–12h
Pentazocine	5–10 q4h	5–10 q2–4h	10 q2–4h	10 q2–4h	10 q2–4h	10 q2–4h	10 q2–4h
Nalbuphine	0.5–1.5 q3h	1–2 q4h	1–4 q3h	4–8 q3h	4–8 q3h	4–8 q3h	1–4 q3h
Oxymorphone	0.05–0.2 q6–12h	0.05–0.2 q8–12h	0.2–0.5 q6–12h	0.2–0.5 q6–12h	0.2–0.5 q6–12h	0.2–0.5 q6–12h	0.2–0.5 q6–12h
Meperidine	5–10 q2–3h	5–10 q2–3h	20 q2–3h	20 q2–3h	20 q2–3h	20 q2–3h	20 q2–3h
Morphine	0.5–5.0 q2–6h	2–5 q2–4h	2–5 q2–4h	2–5 q2–4h	2–5 q2–4h	2–5 q2–4h	2–5 q4h
Flunixin†	0.5–2.0 q12–24h	1–2 q12–24h	2.5 q12–24h	2.5 q12–24h	2.5 q12–24h	2.5 q12–24h	2.5 q12–24h

Values are milligrams per kilogram given SC or IM.

*Analgesic doses have not been studied in chinchillas; however, guinea pig doses can probably be used.

†Flunixin should be given IM.

ANALGESIA

Because many of the species discussed in this chapter are extensively used in laboratory animal research, and because of the concern for the humane care of these animals, several sources describe the use of analgesics in these species.[3, 11, 13] In pet practice as in research, the outcomes of procedures can be markedly affected by the level of stress in a particular animal, and there is ample evidence indicating that pain is a very important contributor to level of stress. For this reason, do not hesitate to provide analgesia for surgery or after trauma in these small species, just as you would in dogs and cats in the same situations.

The current opinion of most anesthesiologists is that pre-emptive analgesia—namely, analgesia that is administered before the onset of pain—is most effective. Administer an analgesic as part of the preoperative protocol or before recovery from anesthesia if you anticipate postoperative pain. The choice of analgesic may vary with the species, drug availability, and the route and frequency of administration. Buprenorphine is a good choice in most species, both because of its apparent effectiveness and the fact that it can often be given only twice daily. A list of analgesic drugs and suggested dosages for ferrets, rabbits, and rodents can be found in Table 32–4.

Use of analgesics is particularly important in rabbits, which become lethargic, anorectic, and less responsive when they experience pain. Moreover, their recovery from surgery is faster if they are given analgesics for 1–2 days postoperatively.

REFERENCES

1. Aeschbacher G, Webb AI: Propofol in rabbits: I. determination of an induction dose. Lab Anim Sci 1993; 43:324–327.
2. Anderson NL: Basic husbandry and medicine of pocket pets. *In* Birchard SJ, Sherding RG, eds.: Saunder's Manual of Small Animal Practice. Philadelphia, WB Saunders, 1994, pp 1363–1389.
3. Bertens APMG, Booij LHDJ, Flecknell PA, et al: Anaesthesia, analgesia, and euthanasia. *In* von Zutphen LFM, Baumans V, Beynen AC, eds.: Principles of Laboratory Animal Science. Amsterdam, Elsevier, 1993, pp 267–298
4. Bivin WS, Timmons EH: Basic biomethodology. *In* Weisbroth SH, Flatt RE, Kraus AL, eds.: The Biology of the Laboratory Rabbit. New York, Academic Press, 1974, pp 73–90.
5. Brammer DW, Doerning BJ, Chrisp CE: Anesthetic and nephrotoxic effects of Telazol in New Zealand white rabbits. Lab Anim Sci 1991; 41:432–435.
6. Conlon KC, Corbally MT, Bading JR, et al: Atraumatic endotracheal intubation in small rabbits. Lab Anim Sci 1990; 40:221–222.
7. Davis JA, Greenfield RE, Brewer TG: Benzocaine-induced methemoglobinemia attributed to topical application of the anesthetic in several laboratory animal species. Am J Vet Res 1993; 54:1322–1326.
8. Gilroy BA: Endotracheal intubation of rabbits and rodents. J Am Vet Med Assoc 1981; 179:1295.
9. Haberstroh J, Clancy D, Bonnebrink M, et al: The orotracheal intubation over a retrograde translaryngeal guide in the rabbit. Kleinterpraxis 1993; 38:179–182.
10. Harkness JE, Wagner JE: The Biology and Medicine of Rabbits and Rodents. 4th ed. Baltimore, Williams & Wilkins, 1995.
11. Heard DJ: Principles and techniques of anesthesia and analgesia for exotic practice. Vet Clin North Am Small Anim Pract 1993; 23:1301–1327.
12. Hillyer EV, Brown SA: Ferrets: Clinical techniques. *In* Birchard SJ, Sherding RG, eds.: Saunder's Manual of Small Animal Practice. Philadelphia, WB Saunders, 1994, pp 1317–1322.
13. Huerkamp MJ: Anesthesia and postoperative management of rabbits and pocket pets. *In* Bonagura JD, ed.: Kirk's Current Veterinary Therapy XII: Small Animal Practice. Philadelphia, WB Saunders, 1995, pp 1322–1327.
14. Robertson SA, Eberhart S: Efficacy of the intranasal route for administration of anaesthetic agents to adult rabbits. Lab Anim Sci 1990; 44:159–165.
15. Schmidt-Neilsen K: Metabolic rate and body size. *In* Schmidt-Neilsen K, ed.: Scaling: Why Is Animal Size So Important? Cambridge, Cambridge University Press, 1984, pp 56–74.
16. Sedgwick CJ: Anesthesia for rabbits. Vet Clin North Am [Food Anim Pract] 1986; 2:731–736.
17. Timm KI, Jahn SE, Sedgwick CJ: The palatal ostium of the guinea pig. Lab Anim Sci 1987; 37:801–802.
18. White WJ, Field KJ: Anesthesia and surgery of laboratory animals. Vet Clin North Am Small Anim Pract 1987; 17:989–1017.

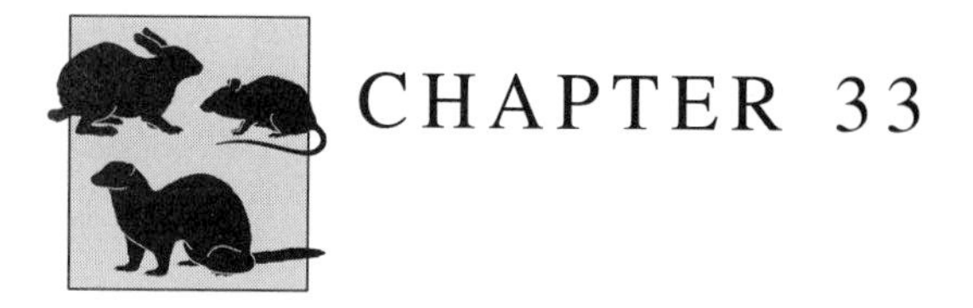

CHAPTER 33

Formulary

Dale A. Smith, DVM, DVSc, and Petra M. Burgmann, DVM

The dosages given in this chapter are derived from the published literature; however, many are empirical or are based on clinical experience. A guarantee of either safety or effectiveness under all situations is impossible. For the species discussed in this book, too few pharmacokinetic or controlled efficacy trials describing drug doses or frequency of administration have been done. As new work appears in the literature, the inappropriateness of many of the current species-to-species generalizations may become apparent, and hopefully we will be able to discard inaccurate recommendations that have become entrenched in the literature. Few drugs are specifically designed or licensed for use in rodents, rabbits, and ferrets. Owners should be made aware that the medications used are "extralabel." Veterinarians must base treatment decisions on the best available information and modify them as new facts become available.

Adverse and idiosyncratic drug reactions occur in all species; however, the sensitivity of rabbits and rodents to iatrogenic enteric disturbances is well recognized. The use of narrow-spectrum antibacterial agents can promote the overgrowth of gram-negative and anaerobic gram-positive bacteria, such as *Clostridium* species, resulting in diarrhea, enterotoxemia, and potentially death.[1] Other less common drug sensitivities also have been documented.[1] Undoubtably, as the range of medications in common use increases, so too will the number of reports of adverse responses.

Many of the drugs commonly used in small mammals are not available in suspension form, and the drug concentration in many tablets and pills is too great for use in these species. It is very difficult to administer pills to most of these animals, and gavage by gastric tubing is impractical for home treatment. Tablets sometimes can be crushed and mixed with sweet-tasting food items for administration in ferrets and rabbits. A better alternative for the treatment of all species is prescribing medications through a pharmacist who can compound drugs into suspensions. Have the suspension made in a concentration that allows the total volume given at each dosing to be easily administered to the animal. In the United States, licensed compounding pharmacists are accessible in many communities. Many compounding pharmacists advertise nationally and ship drugs anywhere in the country.

RATIONAL DRUG THERAPY

Effective drug therapy relies on choosing drugs that are appropriate for both the disease condition and the patient to be treated. A drug must reach its site of action at a sufficient concentration and for an adequate duration if it is to have the desired effect. Drug concentrations in plasma or tissue depend on drug dosages and rates of absorption. The ability of an animal to absorb a given drug and the rate at which it does so depend on the physiology of the individual and the species, the bioavailability of the drug, and the route of administration. The greatest variability in absorption occurs with PO administration. The duration of action and, therefore, the frequency of administration depend on this rate of absorption, as well as on the way in which the drug is distributed throughout and finally eliminated from the body. Body size, age, sex, genetic factors, species differences, and state of health can all affect these pharmacokinetic parameters. Some knowledge of the mode of action and basic pharmacokinetics of a drug is important for dealing with species in which the use of a particular medication may be poorly described, if at all.

Antimicrobial sensitivity testing, by dilution or agar disc diffusion methods, has become standard in veterinary practice. Minimum inhibitory concentrations (MIC) from microdilution systems are commonly included in reports from diagnostic laboratories. Organisms are most frequently classified as *susceptible* (i.e., inhibited in blood or tissue by the "usual dosage" of an antibiotic); *moderately susceptible* (i.e., inhibited by attainable concentrations of the drugs administered at higher than usual doses or in body compartments in which drug concentration occurs); or *resistant* (i.e., not inhibited by usually achievable systemic concentrations with usual dosage).[3] It is important to realize that in vitro testing is not always an accurate predictor of in vivo results, and that with little knowledge of the actual plasma or tissue antibiotic concentrations reached in a given species, minimum inhibitory concentration values may not be as broadly applicable as they are assumed to be.

ALLOMETRIC SCALING

In the veterinary medicine of nontraditional species, veterinarians are commonly forced to extrapolate drug dosages from one species to another. A standard dose per unit of body weight (i.e., milligrams per kilogram) does not take into account the fact that the rates of many physiologic processes are linked to bodyweight in a nonlinear manner. These processes affect the uptake or absorption of drugs, and pharmacokinetic parameters such as drug distribution, elimination, clearance, and volume of distribution. The specific metabolic rate, expressed in kilocalories per kilogram (kcal/kg) of a small species or individual, is much greater than that of a larger species or individual. *Allometric scaling* is a technique for the study of a variety of physiologic processes; in veterinary medicine, it is used for the calculation of pharmacologic values, such as doses and frequency of administration, and for the calculation of metabolic energy requirements for alimentary supplementation.[5]

Allometric scaling is based on a mathematic equation that multiplies an exponential function of lean bodyweight by a constant (*K* value). Animals are placed into five groups, according to their mean body core temperatures and basal energy requirements. Each group has a specific constant. The following calculations incorporate the *K* value of 70 (appropriate for placental mammals) and illustrate the use of allometric scaling for extrapolating drug dosages from those for a control species for which this information is known to another species for which it is not.[2, 4]

1. The *specific minimum energy cost (SMEC)* is calculated for both the animal for which the drug dosage is known (control) and the patient to be treated.

   $$\text{SMEC} = 70(\text{W}_{\text{kg}}^{-0.25})$$

2. The SMEC dose rate (dose per metabolic energy unit) for the control animal is calculated by dividing the drug's dose rate (mg/kg) for that species by its SMEC ($\text{SMEC}_{\text{control}}$).

   $$\text{SMEC dose rate (mg/kg)} = \text{Dose}_{\text{control}}\text{(mg/kg)/SMEC}_{\text{control}}$$

3. The dose for the patient is calculated by multiplying the $\text{SMEC}_{\text{patient}}$ by the SMEC dose rate.

   $$\text{Dose}_{\text{patient}}\text{(mg/kg)} = \text{SMEC}_{\text{patient}} \times \text{SMEC dose rate (mg/kg)}$$

4. Treatment frequency is allometrically scaled in a similar fashion for determining the frequency of administration within a 24-hour period, or the number of times that the dose should be administered.

   $$\text{SMEC frequency} = \text{Frequency}_{\text{control}}/\text{SMEC}_{\text{control}}$$

5. The frequency of administration for a 24-hour period for the patient is calculated by multiplying the SMEC frequency by the $\text{SMEC}_{\text{patient}}$

   $$\text{Frequency}_{\text{patient}} = \text{SMEC frequency} \times \text{SMEC}_{\text{patient}}$$

Note that allometric scaling assumes that all species metabolize and process drugs in the same way. In generalizing from a carnivore to a herbivore, for example, it is likely that differences in digestive physiology will affect drug uptake and absorption. The most valid extrapolations are likely to be obtained if the species are similar.

DRUG DOSAGES FOR FERRETS

Agent	Dosage
Antibacterial Agents	
Amikacin	8–16 mg/kg total per d*; divided q8–24h; SC, IM, IV
Amoxicillin	10–20 mg/kg q12–24h; PO, SC
Ampicillin	5–10 mg/kg q12h; SC, IM, IV
Cephalexin	15–25 mg/kg q8–12h; PO
Chloramphenicol	50 mg/kg q12h; PO (palmitate)†; SC, IM (succinate)
Ciprofloxacin	5–15 mg/kg q12h; PO
Clavulanic acid & amoxicillin	10–20 mg/kg q8–12h; PO
Cloxacillin	10 mg/kg q6h; PO, IM, IV
Enrofloxacin	5–15 mg/kg q12h; PO, SC, IM
Erythromycin	10 mg/kg q6h; PO
Gentamicin‡	4–8 mg/kg total per d*; divided q8–24h; SC, IM, IV
Lincomycin	10–15 mg/kg q8h; PO 10 mg/kg q12h; IM
Metronidazole	10–20 mg/kg q12h; PO
Neomycin	10–20 mg/kg q6–12h; PO
Netilmicin	6–8 mg/kg total per d*; divided q8–24h; SC, IM, IV
Oxytetracycline	20 mg/kg q8h; PO
Penicillin G procaine	20,000 U/kg q12h; IM 40,000 U/kg q24h; IM
Penicillin G, sodium or potassium	20,000 U/kg q4h; SC, IM, IV 40,000 U/kg q8h; PO
Sulfadimethoxine	25 mg/kg q24h; PO, SC, IM
Tetracycline	25 mg/kg q8–12h; PO
Trimethoprim-sulfa combinations	15–30 mg/kg q12h; PO, SC 30 mg/kg q24h for 2 weeks; PO (for the treatment of coccidiosis)
Tylosin	10 mg/kg q12–24h; PO
Antifungal Agents	
Amphotericin B	0.4–0.8 mg/kg once per wk; IV, to a total dose of 7–25 mg *or* follow published canine protocols
Griseofulvin	25 mg/kg q24h for 3–6 wk; PO
Ketoconazole	10–30 mg/kg q12–24h; PO
Antiparasitic Agents	
Amitraz	Apply to affected skin 3–6 times at 14-d intervals
Carbaryl	Treat once per wk for 3–6 wk (0.5% shampoo, 5% powder)
Diethylcarbamazine	5–11 mg/kg q24h; PO
Ivermectin	200–400 μg/kg twice at 14-d interval; PO, SC 200–500 μg/kg divided into two doses for massage into each ear 6 μg/kg once per month; PO (heartworm prevention)
Lime sulfur	Dilute 1:40 in water; wash patient once per wk for 6 wk
Lindane	0.03%; dip once per wk for 3 wk
Malathion (2% solution)	Dip every 10 d for 3 treatments
Metronidazole	20 mg/kg q12h for 5–10 d; PO
Milbemycin oxime	1.15–2.33 mg/kg once per mo; PO (heartworm prevention)
Piperazine	50–100 mg/kg once; repeat dose in 2 wk; PO
Praziquantel	12.5 mg (½ of 23-mg tablet) once; repeat dose in 2 wk; PO 5–10 mg/kg once; repeat dose in 2 wk; SC
Pyrantel pamoate	4.4 mg/kg once; repeat dose in 2 wk; PO
Pyrethrin products	Use topically as directed once per wk as needed
Sulfadimethoxine	50 mg/kg once; then, 25 mg/kg q24h for 9 d; PO
Other Agents	
Aminophylline	4 mg/kg q12h; PO
Aspirin	200 mg/kg q12h; PO
Atropine sulfate	0.5 mg/kg as a preanesthetic; IM 2–10 mg/kg as needed for organophosphate toxicity; SC
Bismuth subsalicylate	1 mL/kg q8h; PO

DRUG DOSAGES FOR FERRETS *(Continued)*

Agent	Dosage	Agent	Dosage
Buprenorphine	0.01–0.03 mg/kg q8–12h; SC, IM, IV as needed	Iron dextran	10 mg/kg once per wk as needed; IM
Butorphanol tartrate	0.05–0.4 mg/kg q8–12h; as needed; SC, IM	Kaolin, pectin	1–2 mL/kg q2–6h as needed; PO
Chlorpheniramine	1–2 mg/kg q8–12h; PO	Lactulose syrup	1.5–3 mg/kg q12h; PO
Cimetidine	10 mg/kg q8h; PO, SC, IM, IV	Megestrol acetate	Do *not* use, as predisposes patient to pyometra
Cisapride	0.5 mg/kg q8h; PO	Meperidine	5–20 mg/kg as needed q2–4h; SC, IM, IV
Dexamethasone sodium phosphate	4–8 mg/kg once; IM, IV for shock	Metoclopramide	0.2–1 mg/kg q6–8h; PO, SC
Diazepam	1–2 mg/kg as needed for seizure control; IM, IV	Oxymorphone	0.05–0.2 mg/kg q8–12h; SC, IM, IV
Diazoxide	5 mg/ferret q12h to start, up to 30 mg/kg q12h as required; PO; use in combination with prednisone for insulinoma	Oxytocin	0.2–3 USP units/kg once; SC, IM
Digoxin elixir	0.005–0.01 mg/kg q12–24h for maintenance; PO; monitor blood digoxin concentration if possible	Pentazocine	5–10 mg/kg q4h; IM
Diltiazem	1.5–7.5 mg/kg q12h; PO; adjust dosage as needed	Phenobarbital elixir	1–2 mg/kg q8–12h for seizure control; titrate dose for maintenance; PO
Diphenhydramine	0.5–2 mg/kg q8–12h; PO; q12h; IM	Prednisolone, prednisone	0.5–2.5 mg/kg q12–24h; for insulinoma, start at low dose q12h; increase dose as needed; PO, IM
Doxapram	5–11 mg/kg; IV	Proligestone	50 mg/kg once before onset of seasonal reproductive activity; IM
Enalapril	0.25–0.5 mg/kg q24–48h; PO; monitor for weakness and anorexia	Propranolol	0.5–2 mg/kg q12–24h; PO, SC
Flunixin meglumine	0.5–2 mg/kg q24h for no more than 3 d; PO, deep IM, IV	Prostaglandin $F_{2\alpha}$	0.5 mg as needed; IM
Furosemide	1–4 mg/kg q8–12h; PO, SC, IM, IV	Stanazolol	10 mg/kg once per wk as required; IM
GnRH	20 μg once after second wk of estrus; repeat in 2 wk if needed; IM	Sucralfate	25 mg/kg up to 125 mg per ferret q6–8h; PO
hCG	100 IU once after second wk of estrus; repeat in 2 wk if needed; IM	Sulfasalazine	10–20 mg/kg q12h; PO
Hydroxyzine hydrochloride	2 mg/kg q8h; PO	Theophylline elixir	4.25 mg/kg q8–12h; PO
Insulin, NPH	0.1–0.5 units/kg q12h initially; increase dose as needed; SC, IM; dilute in additional carrier if required	Vitamin B complex	Dose to thiamine content at 1–2 mg/kg as needed; IM

*An increase in the efficacy and a decrease in the toxicity of aminoglycosides may occur when the total dose is given once daily. However, neuromuscular blockade and acute renal failure can occur if the dose is given by IV bolus infusion. All aminoglycosides administered IV should be diluted with saline or sterile water at 4 mL/kg and delivered over 20 min.

†Chloramphenicol palmitate is no longer commercially available in the United States but is still obtainable in other countries.

‡Some veterinarians believe that ferrets are particularly susceptible to the toxic effects of gentamicin and that its use should be avoided in this species.

DRUG DOSAGES FOR RABBITS

Agent	Dosage	Agent	Dosage
Antibacterial Agents		***Antiparasitic Agents***	
Amikacin	8–16 mg/kg total dose*; divided q8–24h; SC, IM, IV	Amprolium 9.6% solution	1 mL/7 kg; PO q24h for 5 d, or 0.5 mL/500 mL drinking water for 10 d
Chloramphenicol palmitate†	50 mg/kg q12h; PO	Carbaryl 5% powder	Dust lightly once per wk
Chloramphenicol succinate	30–50 mg/kg q12h; SC, IM	Fenbendazole	20 mg/kg q24h for 5 d; PO
Chlortetracycline	50 mg/kg q12h; PO	Ivermectin	200–400 μg/kg; PO, SC; repeat in 8–10 d
Ciprofloxacin	5–15 mg/kg q12h; PO	Lime sulfur (2.5% solution)	Apply once per wk for 4–6 wk
Dimetridazole	0.2 mg/mL drinking water	Lindane (0.03% solution)	Dip once per wk for 3 wk
Doxycycline	2.5 mg/kg q12h; PO	Malathion (2% solution)	Dip every 10 d for 3 wk
Enrofloxacin	5–15 mg/kg q12h; PO, SC,§ IM	Piperazine adipate	0.5 g/kg q24h for 2 d; PO
Gentamicin	5–8 mg/kg total dose*; divided q8–24h; SC, IM, IV	Piperazine citrate	100 mg/kg q24h for 2 d; PO
Metronidazole	20 mg/kg q12h; PO for 3–5 d	Praziquantel	5–10 mg/kg; PO, SC, IM; repeat in 10 d
Neomycin	30 mg/kg q12h; PO	Pyrethrin (0.05%) shampoo	Shampoo weekly for 4–6 wk
Netilmicin	6–8 mg/kg total dose*; q8–24h; SC, IM, IV	Sulfadimethoxine	25–50 mg/kg q24h, or 50 mg/kg loading dose followed by 25 mg/kg q24h for 9 d; PO
Oxytetracycline	50 mg/kg q12h; PO; 15 mg/kg q24h; SC, IM	Sulfaquinoxaline	1 mg/mL drinking water
Penicillin G procaine	20,000–60,000 IU/kg q24h; SC, IM	Thiabendazole	50–100 mg/kg; PO for 5 d
Penicillin G benzathine and penicillin G procaine	47,000–84,000 IU/kg once per wk; SC, IM (for *Treponema cuniculi* infection)	***Other Agents***	
Sulfamethazine	1–5 mg/mL drinking water	Aspirin	100 mg/kg q4–6 h; PO
Tetracycline	50 mg/kg q8–12h; PO	Atropine	0.1–0.5 mg/kg; SC, IM
Trimethoprim-sulfadiazine	30 mg/kg q12–24h; SC	Buprenorphine	0.01–0.05 mg/kg q8–12h; SC, IM, IV
Trimethoprim-sulfamethoxazole	15–30 mg/kg q12h; PO	Butorphanol	0.1–0.5 mg/kg q2–4h; SC, IV
Tylosin	10 mg/kg q12h; PO, SC, IM	Calcium EDTA	27.5 mg/kg q6h; SC; dilute to 10 mg/mL with saline
Antifungal Agent			
Griseofulvin	25 mg/kg; PO q24h, or divided q12h for 28–40 d	Cimetidine	5–10 mg/kg q8–12h; PO, SC, IM, IV

DRUG DOSAGES FOR RABBITS *(Continued)*

Agents	Dosage	Agents	Dosage
Cisapride	0.5 mg/kg q8–24h; PO	Oxytocin	1–2 USP units per rabbit; SC, IM
Dipyrone	6–12 mg/kg q8–12h; PO, IM	Pentazocine	5–10 mg/kg q4h; IM, IV
Flunixin	0.3–2.0 mg/kg q12–24h for no more than 3 d; PO, deep IM	Prednisone	0.5–2 mg/kg; PO‡
Furosemide	2–5 mg/kg q12h; PO, SC, IM, IV	Tresaderm (dexamethasone, neomycin, thiabendazole)	Instill 3 drops in ear q12h for 7 d
Ibuprofen	7.5 mg/kg; PO as needed		
Meperidine	10–20 mg/kg q6h; SC, IM	Viokase (amylase, lipase, protease)	1 tsp Viokase plus 3 tbsp yogurt; let stand 15 min, then give 2–3 mL q12h
Metoclopramide	0.5 mg/kg q8h; SC		
Morphine	2–5 mg/kg q4h; SC, IM	Vitamin K_1	1–10 mg/kg; IM as needed
Naloxone	0.01–0.1 mg/kg; IM, IV		

*An increase in the efficacy and a decrease in the toxicity of aminoglycosides may occur when the total dose is given once daily. However, neuromuscular blockade and acute renal failure can occur if the dose is given by IV bolus infusion. All aminoglycosides administered IV should be diluted with saline or sterile water at 4 mL/kg and delivered over 20 min.

†Chloramphenicol palmitate is no longer commercially available in the United States but is still obtainable in other countries.

‡Corticosteroids should be used infrequently and with caution in rabbits; concurrent use of gastric protectants is advised.

§Repeated subcutaneous injection may cause skin sloughing.

DRUG DOSAGES FOR GUINEA PIGS AND CHINCHILLAS

Agent	Dosage	
	Guinea Pigs	Chinchillas
Antibacterial Agents		
Amikacin	10–15 mg/kg total per d*; divided q8–24h; SC, IM, IV	10–15 mg/kg total per d*; divided q8–24h; SC, IM, IV
Chloramphenicol palmitate†	50 mg/kg q12h; PO	50 mg/kg q12h; PO
Chloramphenicol succinate	30–50 mg/kg q12h; SC, IM	30–50 mg/kg q12h; SC, IM
Chlortetracycline	—	50 mg/kg q12h; PO
Ciprofloxacin	5–15 mg/kg q12h; PO	5–15 mg/kg q12h; PO
Doxycycline	2.5 mg/kg q12h; PO	2.5 mg/kg q12h; PO
Enrofloxacin	2.5–10 mg/kg q12h; PO, SC, IM‡	2.5–10 mg/kg q12h; PO, SC, IM‡
Gentamicin	5–8 mg/kg total per d*; divided q8–24h; SC, IM, IV	5–8 mg/kg total per d*; divided q8–24h; SC, IM, IV
Metronidazole	20–40 mg/kg q12h; PO	20–40 mg/kg q12h; PO
Neomycin	30 mg/kg q24h; PO	15 mg/kg q12h; PO
Netilmicin	6–8 mg/kg total per d*; divided q8–24h; SC, IM, IV	6–8 mg/kg total per d*; divided q8–24h; SC, IM, IV
Oxytetracycline	—	50 mg/kg q12h; PO
Tetracycline	10–20 mg/kg q8h; PO	50 mg/kg q8–12h; PO
Trimethoprim-sulfadiazine	30 mg/kg q12–24h; SC	30 mg/kg q12–24h; SC
Trimethoprim-sulfamethoxazole	15 mg/kg q12h; PO	15–30 mg/kg q12h; PO
Antifungal Agent		
Griseofulvin	25 mg/kg q24h for 14–28 d; PO	25 mg/kg q24h for 28–40 d; PO
Antiparasitic Agents		
Amitraz	Prepare according to package directions and apply topically for 3–6 treatments given at 14-d intervals	—
Carbaryl 5% powder	Dust lightly once per wk	Dust lightly once per wk
Dimetridazole	—	0.8 mg/mL drinking water
Fenbendazole	20 mg/kg q24h for 5 d; PO	20 mg/kg q24h for 5 d; PO
Ivermectin	300–400 μg/kg; SC; repeat in 8–10 d	200–400 μg/kg; PO, SC; repeat in 8–10 d
Lime sulfur (2.5% solution)	Apply once per wk for 4–6 wk	—
Lindane (0.03% solution)	Dip once per wk for 3 wk	—
Malathion	Dip every 10 d for 3 wk	—
Piperazine adipate	4–7 mg/mL drinking water for 3–10 d	500 mg/kg q24h for 2 d; PO
Piperazine citrate	10 mg/mL drinking water for 7 d; then off for 7 d, then on for 7 d	100 mg/kg q24h for 2 d; PO
Praziquantel	5–10 mg/kg; PO, SC, IM; repeat in 10 d	5–10 mg/kg; PO, SC, IM; repeat in 10 d
Pyrethrin 0.05% shampoo	Shampoo once per wk for 4–6 wk	Shampoo once per wk for 4–6 wk
Sulfadimethoxine (50mg/ml)	25–50 mg/kg q24h for 10–14 d; PO	25–50 mg/kg q24h for 10–14 d; PO

DRUG DOSAGES FOR GUINEA PIGS AND CHINCHILLAS *(Continued)*

Agents	Dosage	
	Guinea Pigs	*Chinchillas*
Sulfamethazine	1–5 mg/mL drinking water	1–5 mg/mL drinking water
Sulfaquinoxaline	1 mg/mL drinking water	—
Thiabendazole	100 mg/kg q24h for 5 d; PO	50–100 mg/kg q24h for 5 d; PO
Other Agents		
Aluminum (200 mg) and magnesium (200 mg) hydroxide per 5 mL	0.5–1 mL; PO as needed	1 mL; PO as needed
Aspirin	86 mg/kg q4h; PO	—
Atropine	0.1–0.2 mg/kg; SC, IM	—
Buprenorphine	0.05–0.1 mg/kg SC	
Cimetidine	5–10 mg/kg q6–12h; PO, SC, IM	5–10 mg/kg q6–12h; PO, SC, IM
Dexamethasone	0.1–0.6 mg/kg; IM§	—
Furosemide	2–5 mg/kg q12h; PO, SC	2–5 mg/kg q12h; PO, SC
Meperidine	10–20 mg/kg q6h; SC, IM	10–20 mg/kg q6h; SC, IM
Morphine	10 mg/kg q4h; SC, IM	—
Oxytocin	1 USP unit per guinea pig; SC, IM	1 USP unit per chinchilla; SC, IM
Prednisone	0.5–2 mg/kg; PO, SC§	0.5–2 mg/kg; PO, SC§
Vitamin C	10–30 mg/kg for maintenance; up to 50 mg/kg for treatment of deficiency; PO, SC, IM *or* 200–1000 mg/L drinking water	—
Vitamin K_1	1–10 mg/kg as needed; IM	—

*An increase in the efficacy and a decrease in the toxicity of aminoglycosides may occur when the total dose is given once daily. However, neuromuscular blockade and acute renal failure can occur if the dose is given by IV bolus infusion. All aminoglycosides administered IV should be diluted with saline or sterile water at 4 mL/kg and delivered over 20 min.

†Chloramphenicol palmitate is no longer commercially available in the United States but is still obtainable in other countries.

‡Repeated subcutaneous injection may cause skin sloughing.

§Corticosteroids should be used infrequently and with caution in guinea pigs and chinchillas. Concurrent use of gastric protectants is advised.

Agent	Dosage			
	Hamsters	*Gerbils*	*Rats*	*Mice*
Antibacterial Agents				
Amikacin	10–20 mg/kg total per d; divided q8–24h; SC, IM	10–20 mg/kg total per d; divided q8–24h; SC, IM (concurrent fluid therapy advised)	10–20 mg/kg total per d; divided q8–24h; SC, IM	10–20 mg/kg total per d; divided q8–24h; SC, IM
Ampicillin	—	20–100 mg/kg total dose divided q8h; PO, SC	20–100 mg/kg total dose divided dose q8h; PO, SC	20–100 mg/kg total dose divided dose q8h; PO, SC
Chloramphenicol palmitate*	50–200 mg/kg q8h; PO	50–200 mg/kg q8h; PO	50–200 mg/kg q8h; PO	50–200 mg/kg q8h; PO
Chloramphenicol succinate	30–50 mg/kg q12h; SC, IM	30–50 mg/kg q12h; SC, IM	30–50 mg/kg q12h; SC, IM	30–50 mg/kg q12h; SC, IM
Chlortetracycline	20 mg/kg q12h; SC, IM	—	6–10 mg/kg q12h; SC, IM	25 mg/kg q12h; SC, IM
Ciprofloxacin	10 mg/kg q12h; PO	10 mg/kg q12h; PO	10 mg/kg q12h; PO	10 mg/kg q12h; PO
Doxycycline	2.5 mg/kg q12h; PO	2.5 mg/kg q12h; PO	2.5 mg/kg q12h; PO	2.5 mg/kg q12h; PO
Enrofloxacin	—	—	2.5–10 mg/kg q12h; PO	2.5–10 mg/kg q12h; PO
Furazolidone	30 mg/kg q24h; PO			
Gentamicin	5–8 mg/kg total per d divided q8–24h; SC, IM	5–8 mg/kg total per d divided q8–24h; SC, IM (concurrent fluid therapy advised)	5–8 mg/kg total per d divided q8–24h; SC, IM	5–8 mg/kg total per d divided q8–24h; SC, IM
Metronidazole	7.5 mg/70–90-g hamster q8h; PO	—	10–40 mg/rat q24h; PO	2.5 mg/mL drinking water for 5 d
Neomycin	100 mg/kg q24h; PO	100 mg/kg q24h; PO	50 mg/kg q24h; PO	50 mg/kg q24h; PO
Oxytetracycline	16 mg/kg q24h; SC	10 mg/kg q8h; PO 20 mg/kg q24h; SC	10–20 mg/kg q8h; PO 6–10 mg /kg q12h; IM	10–20 mg/kg q8h; PO
Penicillin G procaine	—	—	22,000 IU q24h; IM	—
Tetracycline	10–20 mg/kg q8h; PO	10–20 mg/kg q8h; PO	10–20 mg/kg q8h; PO	10–20 mg/kg q8h; PO
Trimethoprim-sulfadiazine	30 mg/kg q12–24h; SC	30 mg/kg q12–24h; SC	30 mg/kg q12–24h; SC	30 mg/kg q12–24h; SC
Trimethoprim-sulfamethoxazole	15–30 mg/kg q12h; PO	15–30 mg/kg q12h; PO	15–30 mg/kg q12–24h; PO	15–30 mg/kg q12–24h; PO

Tylosin	2–8 mg/kg q12h; PO, SC, IM	10 mg/kg q12h; PO, SC, IM	10 mg/kg q12h; PO, SC, IM	10 mg/kg q12h; PO, SC, IM
Antifungal Agent				
Griseofulvin	25 mg/kg q24h for 14–28 d; PO	25 mg/kg q24h for 14–28 d; PO	25 mg/kg; q24h for 14–28 d; PO	25 mg/kg q24h for 14 d; PO
Antiparasitic Agents				
Amitraz	Prepare according to package directions and apply topically for 3–6 treatments given at 14-d intervals	—	—	—
Carbaryl 5% powder	Dust lightly once per wk	Dust lightly once per wk	Dust lightly once per wk	Dust lightly once per wk
Dichlorvos-impregnated resin strip (Vapona No Pest Strip)	Lay 1-in. square on cage for 24 h once per wk for 6 wk	Lay 1-in. square on cage for 24 h once per wk for 6 wk	Lay 1-in. square on cage for 24 h once per wk for 6 wk	Lay 1-in. square on cage for 24 h once per wk for 6 wk
Dimetridazole	0.5 mg/mL drinking water	0.5 mg/mL drinking water	1 mg/mL drinking water	1 mg/mL drinking water
Fenbendazole	20 mg/kg q24h for 5 d; PO	20 mg/kg q24h for 5 d; PO	20 mg/kg q24h for 5 d; PO	20 mg/kg q24h for 5 d; PO
Ivermectin	200–400 μg/kg; PO, SC; repeat in 8–10 d	200–400 μg/kg; PO, SC; repeat in 8–10 d	200–400 μg/kg; PO, SC; repeat in 8–10 d	200–400 μg/kg; PO, SC; repeat in 8–10 d
Lindane (0.03% solution)	—	—	Dip once per wk for 3 wk	Dip once per wk for 3 wk
Malathion	—	—	Dip every 10 d for 3 wk	Dip every 10 d for 3 wk
Piperazine adipate	3–5 mg/mL drinking water for 7 d, then off for 7 d; then on for 7 d	3–5 mg/mL drinking water for 7 d, then off for 7 d; then on for 7 d	4–7 mg/mL drinking water for 3–10 d	4–7 mg/mL drinking water for 3–10 d
Piperazine citrate	10 mg/mL drinking water for 7 d, then off for 7 d, then on for 7 d	4–5 mg/mL drinking water for 7 d, then off for 7 d, then on for 7 d	4–5 mg/mL drinking water for 7 d, then off for 7 d, then on for 7 d	4–5 mg/mL drinking water for 7 d, then off for 7 d, then on for 7 d
Praziquantel	5.1–11.4 mg/kg; PO, SC, IM; repeat in 10 d	5.1–11.4 mg/kg; PO, SC, IM; repeat in 10 d	5.1–11.4 mg/kg; PO, SC, IM; repeat in 10 d	25 mg/kg; PO, SC, IM; repeat in 10 d
Pyrethrin 0.05% shampoo	Shampoo once weekly for 4 wk	—	Shampoo once weekly for 4 wk	Shampoo once weekly for 4 wk
Sulfadimethoxine	25–50 mg/kg q24h for 10–14 d; PO	—	—	—
Sulfamethazine	1–5 mg/mL drinking water	1–5 mg/mL drinking water	1–5 mg/mL drinking water	1–5 mg/mL drinking water
Sulfaquinoxaline	1 mg/mL drinking water	1 mg/mL drinking water	1 mg/mL drinking water	—
Thiabendazole	100 mg/kg q24h for 5 d; PO	100 mg/kg q24h for 5 d; PO	100 mg/kg q24h for 5 d; PO	100 mg/kg q24h for 5 d; PO

Table continued on following page

Agent	Dosage			
	Hamsters	*Gerbils*	*Rats*	*Mice*
Other Agents				
Aluminum (200 mg) and magnesium (200 mg) hydroxide per 5 mL	0.1–0.3 mL; PO as needed	0.1–0.3 mL; PO as needed	0.2–0.3 mL; PO as needed	0.1–0.3 mL; PO as needed
Aspirin	240 mg/kg q24h; PO	240 mg/kg q24h; PO	100 mg/kg q4h; PO	120 mg/kg q4h; PO
Atropine	0.04 mg/kg; SC, IM	0.04 mg/kg; SC, IM	0.04 mg/kg; SC, IM	0.02 to 0.05 mg/kg; SC, IM
Buprenorphine	0.05–0.1 mg/kg q6–12h; SC	0.05–0.1 mg/kg q6–12h; SC	0.05–0.1 mg/kg q6–12h; SC	0.05–0.1 mg/kg q6–12h; SC
Butorphanol	—	—	0.5–2 mg/kg q6h; SC	1–5 mg/kg q6h; SC
Cimetidine	5–10 mg/kg q6–12h; PO, SC, IM	5–10 mg/kg q6–12h; PO, SC, IM	5–10 mg/kg q6–12h; PO, SC, IM	5–10 mg/kg q6–12h; PO, SC, IM
Codeine	—	—	60 mg/kg q4h; SC	10–20 mg/kg q6h; SC
Dexamethasone	0.1–0.6 mg/kg; IM	0.1–0.6 mg/kg; IM	0.1–0.6 mg/kg; IM	0.1–0.6 mg/kg; IM
Furosemide	2–5 mg/kg q12h; PO, SC, IM	2–5 mg/kg q12h; PO, SC, IM	2–5 mg/kg q12h; PO, SC, IM	2–5 mg/kg q12h; PO, SC, IM
Meperidine	10–20 mg/kg q6h; IM, SC, IP	10–20 mg/kg q6h; IM, SC, IP	10–20 mg/kg q6h; IM, SC, IP	10–20 mg/kg q6h; IM, SC, IP
Naloxone	—	—	0.01–0.1 mg/kg; IP, IV	—
Oxytocin	0.2–3 USP units/kg; IM, SC	0.2–3 USP units/kg; IM, SC	1 USP unit/kg; IM, SC	—
Pentazocine	—	—	10 mg/kg q4h; SC	10 mg/kg q4h; SC
Prednisone	0.5–2 mg/kg; PO	0.5–2 mg/kg; PO	0.5–2 mg/kg; PO	0.5–2 mg/kg; PO
Vitamin K_1	1–10 mg/kg IM as needed	1–10 mg/kg IM as needed	1–10 mg/kg IM as needed	1–10 mg/kg IM as needed

*Chloramphenicol palmitate is no longer commercially available in the United States but is still obtainable in other countries.

REFERENCES

1. Burgmann P, Percy DH: Antimicrobial drug use in rodents and rabbits. *In* Prescott JF, Baggott JD, eds.: Antimicrobial Therapy in Veterinary Medicine. 2nd ed. Ames, IA, Iowa State University Press, 1993, pp 524–541.
2. Hainsworth FR: Animal Physiology, Adaptations in Function. Menlo Park, CA, Addison-Wesley Publishing Company, 1981, pp 155–172.
3. Prescott JF, Baggott JD: Antimicrobial susceptibility and drug dosage prediction. *In* Prescott JF, Baggott JD, eds.: Antimicrobial Therapy in Veterinary Medicine. 2nd ed. Ames, IA, Iowa State University Press, 1993, pp 11–20.
4. Sedgewick CJ: Allometric scaling and emergency care: the importance of body size. *In* Fowler ME, ed.: Zoo and Wild Animal Medicine: Current Therapy 3. Philadelphia, WB Saunders, 1993, pp 34–37.
5. Sedgewick CJ, Martin JC: Concepts of veterinary practice in wild mammals. Vet Clin North Am Small Anim Pract 1994; 24:175–185.

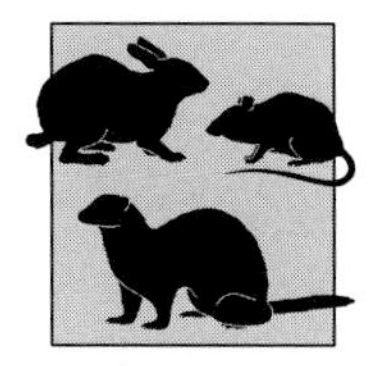

Appendices

APPENDIX 1: Differential Diagnoses for Clinical Problems in Ferrets, Rabbits, and Guinea Pigs

James K. Morrisey, DVM

DIFFERENTIAL DIAGNOSES FOR COMMON CLINICAL PROBLEMS IN FERRETS

Clinical Problem	Differential Diagnosis
Abdominal enlargement	Ascites Cardiac disease Carcinomatosis secondary to pancreatic exocrine adenocarcinoma Other intra-abdominal neoplasia Splenomegaly Intra-abdominal neoplasia, mass
Abdominal mass	*Large* Splenomegaly Urinary tract obstruction Intra-abdominal neoplasia Polycystic kidney(s) Hydronephrosis *Small* Enlargement of mesenteric lymph nodes GI foreign body Enlargement of adrenal gland Stump pyometra Intra-abdominal neoplasia
Alopecia	*Bilaterally Symmetric* Adrenocortical disease Seasonal hair loss (from tail only) Hyperestrogenism Mast cell tumor *Localized (Not Symmetric)* Dermatophytosis External parasitism Mast cell tumor
Anemia	GI bleeding (see also melena) GI foreign body Gastroenteritis, GI ulcer Lymphoma, other neoplasia Hyperestrogenism Flea infestation Lead poisoning Blood loss secondary to trauma Any chronic disease Chronic renal disease Aleutian disease
Anorexia	GI foreign body Severe metabolic disease Neoplasia Cardiac disease Dental disease
Chronic wasting disease	GI foreign body Lymphoma Other neoplasia Gastroenteritis Proliferative bowel disease GI parasitism Eosinophilic enteritis *Helicobacter mustelae* gastritis, ulcers Megaesophagus Dental disease Aleutian disease Mycotic disease
Diarrhea	GI foreign body, trichobezoar Dietary indiscretion Gastroenteritis

Table continued on following page

DIFFERENTIAL DIAGNOSES FOR COMMON CLINICAL PROBLEMS IN FERRETS *Continued*

Clinical Problem	Differential Diagnosis
Diarrhea *(Continued)*	Green slime disease GI parasites (coccidia, *Giardia* infestation) Proliferative bowel disease Eosinophilic gastroenteritis *Helicobacter mustelae* gastritis, ulcers GI neoplasia, lymphoma Aleutian disease Other gastroenteritis Salmonellosis Mycobacteriosis Viral
Dyspnea	See Respiratory disease/distress
Dysuria	Prostatic enlargement Cysts or abscesses associated with adrenocortical disease Neoplasia Urolithiasis Cystitis
Facial swelling	Salivary mucocele Dental disease Neoplasia Allergic reaction (vaccine-induced)
Gastric distention	Gastric foreign body Pyloric adenocarcinoma Overeating (bloat)
Hypersalivation	Hypoglycemia (insulinoma) GI foreign body Gastroenteritis Dental disease, gingivitis Other oral disease (neoplasia, oral foreign body) Anesthesia-related reaction
Melena	GI foreign body *Helicobacter mustelae* gastritis, ulcer GI neoplasia, lymphoma Iatrogenic disease (NSAID-induced) Toxin ingestion Aleutian disease Bleeding GI polyps Ulcers secondary to azotemia
Neurologic signs (disorientation, ataxia, inappropriate behavior)	Hypoglycemia secondary to insulinoma Trauma Toxin exposure CNS infection CNS neoplasia Canine distemper Proliferative bowel disease Rabies
Pawing at the mouth	Hypoglycemia (insulinoma) GI foreign body Gastroenteritis Anesthesia-related reaction
Pleural effusion	See Respiratory disease/distress
Pruritus	Adrenocortical disease External parasitism Mast cell tumor Dermatophytosis Dermatitis (bacterial, allergic)
Polyuria/ polydipsia	Renal disease Adrenocortical disease Hyperglycemia
Rear leg weakness/ posterior paresis	Any metabolic cause of weakness Insulinoma Lymphoma Anemia Other Cardiac disease Primary neurologic problem Trauma CNS neoplasia CNS bleeding Spinal disease (trauma, neoplasia, intervertebral disc disease) Toxicity Aleutian disease Canine distemper
Rectal prolapse	Proliferative bowel disease Coccidiosis Colitis Rectal neoplasia
Respiratory disease/ distress	Pleural effusion Cardiac disease Lymphoma, other neoplasia Infection Heartworm disease Pulmonary edema Cardiac disease Heartworm disease Electrical cord bite Intrathoracic mass Anterior mediastinal mass (lymphoma) Pneumonia Inhalation secondary to megaesophagus Bacterial Viral (canine distemper, influenza) Fungal Pneumothorax Tracheal disease Diaphragmatic hernia

DIFFERENTIAL DIAGNOSES FOR COMMON CLINICAL PROBLEMS IN FERRETS *Continued*

Clinical Problem	Differential Diagnosis
Seizures	Hypoglycemia (insulinoma) Toxin ingestion CNS infection, inflammation, trauma, or neoplasia Severe metabolic disturbance Hepatic or renal failure
Skin mass	Mast cell tumor Sebaceous epithelioma (basal cell tumor) Squamous cell carcinoma Adenocarcinoma, other neoplasm

Splenomegaly	Any disease
	Incidental finding in "normal" ferret
	Lymphoma
	Primary splenic disease
	  Hemangioma
	  Other neoplasia
	  Splenitis

Tachypnea	See Respiratory disease/distress
Upper respiratory signs	Influenza Bacterial infection Canine distemper

Urinary obstruction	Prostatic enlargement
	  Cysts or abscesses associated with adrenocortical disease
	  Neoplasia
	Urolithiasis
	Bladder neoplasia

Vomiting/ regurgitation	GI foreign body Gastroenteritis *Helicobacter mustelae* gastritis, ulcers Megaesophagus Severe metabolic disease
Vulvar swelling	Adrenocortical disease Remnant ovary in spayed female Normal estrus in intact female Hyperestrogenism

Abbreviations: GI = gastrointestinal; NSAID = nonsteroidal anti-inflammatory drug; CNS = central nervous system.

DIFFERENTIAL DIAGNOSES FOR COMMON CLINICAL PROBLEMS IN RABBITS

Clinical Problem	Differential Diagnosis
Abdominal mass	Gastric distention (trichobezoar) Lipoma/intra-abdominal fat Pregnancy Endometrial hyperplasia Neoplasia (uterine adenocarcinoma) Urinary calculi/obstruction Pyometra Metritis Cecal impaction Hydrometra
Abortion/ fetal resorption	Infection Stress Genetic predisposition Trauma Iatrogenic disease Dietary imbalance (vitamins A, E; protein) Listeriosis
Alopecia	Barbering Dermatophytosis Ectoparasitism Injection reaction Bacterial dermatitis
Anemia	Renal disease Lead toxicosis Uterine adenocarcinoma Endometrial hyperplasia Chronic metabolic disease
Anorexia	Malocclusion Trichobezoar Enterotoxemia/enteritis Pasteurellosis Renal disease Lead toxicity Uterine hyperplasia/adenocarcinoma Pregnancy toxemia Parasitism (especially coccidiosis) Septic mastitis Urolithiasis Orchitis Viral hemorrhagic disease
Ascites	Hepatic coccidiosis Abdominal neoplasia Hepatitis Cardiac disease Coronavirus infection (young rabbits)
Dermatitis, generalized	Parasitism (primarily with *Cheyletiella* species) Bacterial *(Staphylococcus aureus)* Dermatophytosis Viral infection (herpes)
Dermatitis, localized	Ptyalism secondary to malocclusion (chin) Self-trauma Dewlap dermatitis Injection reaction *Psoroptes cuniculi* infestation, face, feet Venereal spirochetosis, face, genitalia See Urine scald
Diarrhea	Low fiber/high concentrate diet Gastric stasis/trichobezoar Enteritis/enterotoxemia Coccidiosis (young rabbits) Cecal impaction Colibacillosis (neonates) Tyzzer's disease *(Bacillus piliformis)* Salmonellosis Coronavirus (young rabbits) Rotavirus Rabbit viral hemorrhagic disease (rare)
Dyspnea	See Respiratory disease/distress
Facial swelling	Abscess (mandibular or tooth root) Retrobulbar abscess Oral foreign body Acute cellulitis Myxomatosis
Hematuria	Red pigments in urine (nonpathogenic and not true hematuria) Endometrial hyperplasia Uterine adenocarcinoma Urolithiasis Cystitis Endometrial venous aneurysm Pyelonephritis Renal infarcts Bladder polyps Disseminated intravascular coagulation
Hypercalcemia	High dietary calcium and/or vitamin D Neoplasia (uncommon)
Incontinence	Hypercalciuria Urolithiasis Vertebral fracture/luxation Encephalitozoonosis Estrogen responsive (spayed rabbits)
Infertility	Stress Systemic disease Endometrial hyperplasia Metritis Uterine adenocarcinoma Malnutrition (especially vitamins A, D, and E) Inappropriate age (too old/young)

DIFFERENTIAL DIAGNOSES FOR COMMON CLINICAL PROBLEMS IN RABBITS *Continued*

Clinical Problem	Differential Diagnosis
Lameness	Pododermatitis Soft tissue trauma Fractures Joint/leg abscess Osteomyelitis Elbow luxation Intervertebral disc extrusion
Lethargy/ depression	Metabolic disease Infectious disease Toxicosis (lead)
Mammary gland enlargement	Cystic mastitis associated with: Uterine adenocarcinoma Endometrial hyperplasia Septic mastitis Mammary gland tumor Abscess Toxoplasmosis (uncommon)
Neurologic signs	Encephalitozoonosis Pasteurellosis Heat stroke Lead toxicity Trauma Cerebral nematodiasis Nutritional deficiencies (vitamins A, E; magnesium) Pregnancy toxemia Toxoplasmosis (uncommon) Hereditary disorders (uncommon) Sarcocystosis (rare) Rabies (rare)
Posterior paresis/ paralysis	Spinal fracture Spinal luxation Spinal abscess Spondylosis Intervertebral disc disease
Pyrexia	Pasteurellosis, other bacterial disease Heat stroke Mastitis (septic) Orchitis Acute cellulitis *(Pasteurella multocida, S. aureus)* Myxomatosis Viral hemorrhagic disease
Renomegaly	Renal calculi Renal cysts Neoplasia Hydronephrosis
Respiratory disease/ distress	Bacterial pneumonia (pasteurellosis, other) Pulmonary abscess Thoracic mass (thymoma) Cardiac disease Pregnancy toxemia Allergic disease; anaphylaxis Chlamydiosis
Seizures	Encephalitozoonosis Heat stroke Pregnancy toxemia Bacterial meningitis *(P. multocida)* Hypoxia (secondary to respiratory disease) Azotemia Epilepsy (rare)
Subcutaneous swelling	Bacterial abscess Lipoma Infestation with *Cuterebra* species larvae Neoplasia Myxomatosis Shope fibroma (endemic areas)
Torticollis/ataxia	Pasteurellosis Encephalitozoonosis *Baylisascaris procyonis* migration Otitis media or interna (other causes) Listeriosis
Upper respiratory tract disease	Bacterial disease *(P. multocida, S. aureus)* Allergic disease Mycoplasmosis Myxomatosis *Bordetella bronchiseptica* infection (rare)
Urine scald	Hypercalciuria Urolithiasis Posterior paresis Obesity Renal failure Polyuria/polydipsia
Vaginal discharge	Endometrial hyperplasia Uterine adenocarcinoma Pyometra Dystocia Uterine torsion (rare)
Weight loss	Dental disease Gastric stasis (trichobezoar) Pasteurellosis Renal failure Chronic enterotoxemia/enteritis Parasitism (coccidiosis, cryptosporidiosis) Pulmonary disease Urolithiasis Uterine adenocarcinoma Lead toxicosis Orchitis Tyzzer's disease *(Clostridium piliforme)*

DIFFERENTIAL DIAGNOSES FOR COMMON CLINICAL PROBLEMS IN GUINEA PIGS*

Clinical Problem	Differential Diagnosis*	Clinical Problem	Differential Diagnosis*
Abdominal distention	Gas associated with gastroenteritis Ovarian cyst	Diarrhea	Improper diet Dysbiosis associated with antibiotic therapy Gastroenteritis (all causes)
Abdominal mass	Intra-abdominal fat Ovarian cyst Urinary tract obstruction Pregnancy Ovarian tumor or other neoplasia	Dyspnea	See Respiratory disease/distress
		Dysuria	Urolithiasis
		Hematuria	Urolithiasis Cystitis
Alopecia	*Bilaterally Symmetric* Ovarian cyst Associated with pregnancy and lactation *Localized, Nonsymmetric* Sarcoptic mange *(Trixacarus caviae)* Barbering Dermatophytosis Lice Abrasion Bacterial dermatitis	Lethargy, weakness	Scurvy Any infectious or metabolic disease, toxicosis Anorexia
		Pruritus	Sarcoptic mange *(T. caviae)* Lice
		Ptyalism	Malocclusion
		Respiratory disease/ distress	Bacterial pneumonia Pulmonary neoplasm
Anemia	Chronic disease Scurvy Neoplasia (especially cavian leukemia)	Tachypnea	See Respiratory disease/distress Pregnancy toxemia
Anogenital swelling	Fecal impaction	Subcutaneous mass	Trichofolliculoma, trichoepithelioma Abscess, cervical lymphadenitis Sebaceous adenoma Other neoplasm
Anorexia†	Oral disease (especially dental malocclusion) Change in diet or environment Dysbiosis associated with antibiotic therapy Enteritis Scurvy Any infectious or metabolic disease Toxicosis (lead poisoning) Pregnancy toxemia Pyometra	Upper respiratory disease	Bacterial rhinitis Scurvy Cervical lymphadenitis Environmental irritant
		Vaginal discharge	Pyometra
		Weakness/ collapse	Septicemia Toxicosis Enterotoxemia Any severe metabolic disease

*Note: Some of the differential diagnoses may also be applicable to chinchillas.
†Forcefeeding is an integral part of the treatment of anorexia in guinea pigs (in addition to specific treatment of the cause of anorexia).

APPENDIX 2: Conversions to Système International (SI) Units

Katherine E. Quesenberry, DVM

CLINICAL CHEMISTRY

Component	Conventional Unit	Conversion Factor	SI Unit Symbol	Significant Digits*
Alanine aminotransferase (ALT)	Units/L	1	U/L	XX
Albumin	g/dL	10	g/L	XX
Alkaline phosphatase	Units/L	1	U/L	XXX
Amylase	Units/L	1	U/L	XXX
	Somogyi units/dL	1.850	U/L	XXO
Aspartate aminotransferase (AST)	Units/L	1	U/L	XX
Bile acids (total)	mg/L	2.547	μmol/L	X.X
Bilirubin	mg/dL	17.1	μmol/L	XX
Calcium	mg/dL	0.2495	mmol/L	X.XX
Calcium, ionized	mEq/L	0.5	mmol/L	X.XX
Carbon dioxide content (bicarbonate + CO_2)	mEq/L	1	mmol/L	XX
Chloride	mEq/L	1	mmol/L	XXX
Cholesterol	mg/dL	0.02586	mmol/L	X.XX
Cortisol	μg/dL	27.59	nmol/L	XXO
Creatine kinase (CK)	Units/L	1	U/L	XXX
Creatinine	mg/dL	88.40	μmol/L	XXO
Electrophoresis,	%	0.01	1	X.XX
protein	g/dL	10	g/L	XX
Fibrinogen	mg/dL	0.01	g/L	X.X
Gamma-glutamyltransferase (GGT)	Units/L	1	U/L	XX
Globulins	mg/dL	0.01	g/L	XX.XX
Glucose	mg/dL	0.05551	mmol/L	XX.X
Insulin	μU/ml	7.175	pmol/L	XXX
	μg/L	172.2	pmol/L	XXX
Iron	μg/dL	0.0179	μmol/L	XX
Lactate dehydrogenase	Units/L	1	U/L	XXX
Lipase	Units/L	1	U/L	XXO
Magnesium	mg/dL	0.4114	mmol/L	X.XX
	mEq/L	0.5	mmol/L	X.XX
Phosphate	mg/dL	0.3229	mmol/L	X.XX
Potassium	mEq/L	1	mmol/L	X.X
	mg/dL	0.2558	mmol/L	X.X
Protein (total)	g/dL	10	g/L	XX
Sodium	mEq/L	1	mmol/L	XXX
Thyroxine	μg/dL	12.87	nmol/L	XXX
Triglycerides	mg/dL	0.01129	mmol/L	X.XX
Triiodothyronine	ng/dL	0.01536	nmol/L	X.X
Urate (as uric acid)	mg/dL	59.48	μmol/L	XXO
Urea nitrogen	mg/dL	0.3570	mmol/L of urea	X.X

*Significant digits refers to the number of digits used for describing reported results. XX means that results expressed to the nearest whole number are meaningful; XXO means that results are meaningful when rounded to the nearest 10. Results reported to lower numbers or decimal points are beyond the sensitivity of the test.

Adapted from the *American Medical Association Manual of Style.* 8th ed. pp 262–295. Copyright 1989, American Medical Association.

HEMATOLOGY

Component	Conventional Unit	Conversion Factor	SI Unit Symbol	Significant Digits*
Hemoglobin	g/dL	10	g/L	XXX
Mean corpuscular hemoglobin concentration	g/dL	10	g/L	XXO
Mean corpuscular hemoglobin	pg	1	pg	XX
Mean corpuscular volume	cu μm	1	fL	XXX
Red blood cell count	10^6/cu mm or $10^6/\mu$L	1	10^{12}/L	X.X
Reticulocyte count	/cu mm or /μL	0.001	10^9/L	XX
Thrombocyte count	10^3/cu mm or $10^3/\mu$L	1	10^9/L	XXX
White blood cell count	/cu mm or /μL	0.001	10^9/L	XX.X

*Significant digits refers to the number of digits used for describing reported results. XX means that results expressed to the nearest whole number are meaningful; XXO means that results are meaningful when rounded to the nearest 10. Results reported to lower numbers or decimal points are beyond the sensitivity of the test.

Adapted from *American Medical Association Manual of Style.* 8th ed. pp 262–295. Copyright 1989, American Medical Association.

APPENDIX 3

Elizabeth V. Hillyer, DVM

RECOMMENDED VACCINES FOR SMALL MAMMALS KEPT AS PETS

Species	Recommended Vaccines	Comments
Ferrets	Canine distemper	Use modified live monovalent preparation (see Chapter 2)
	Rabies*	Use killed preparation (see Chapter 2)
Rabbits	None recommended	
Guinea pigs	None recommended	
Chinchillas	None recommended	
Rats, Mice, Hamsters, Gerbils	None recommended	

*Rabies was recently diagnosed in a ferret in New York state. Three weeks before the onset of clinical signs, the ferret had been at large for several days; it was not vaccinated against rabies at the time of presumed exposure. The isolated virus was a raccoon rabies variant. (Data from New York State Veterinary News, February 1996.)

INDEX

Note: Page numbers in italic type refer to figures; those followed by t indicate tables.